Basic ICD-10-CM/PCS Coding

Coding

2013 Edition

Lou Ann Schraffenberger, MBA, RHIA, CCS, CCS-P, FAHIMA

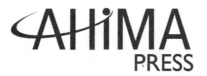

AHIMA PRESS

ISBN: 978-1-58426-368-5

AHIMA Product No.: AC200512

AHIMA Staff:
Jessica Block, MA, Assistant Editor
Angie Comfort, RHIT, CCS, Reviewer
Karen Kostick, RHIT, CCS, CCS-P, Reviewer
Jason O. Malley, Director, Creative Content Development
Theresa Rihanek, MHA, RHIA, CCS, Reviewer
Ashley R. Sullivan, Production Development Editor

For more information, including updates, about AHIMA Press publications, visit http://www.ahima.org/publications/updates.aspx.

American Health Information Management Association
233 North Michigan Avenue, 21st Floor
Chicago, Illinois 60601-5809

ahima.org

Contents

Online Resources

Available at http://www.ahimapress.org/Schraffenberger3685/.

About the Author

Lou Ann Schraffenberger, MBA, RHIA, CCS, CCS-P, FAHIMA, is employed by Advocate Health Care as the manager of clinical data in their Center for Health Information Services. Advocate Health Care is an integrated healthcare delivery system of ten hospitals and other healthcare entities, based in Oak Brook, Illinois. Her position is dedicated to systemwide health information management (HIM) and clinical data projects, and clinical coding continuing education. Prior to her current position, Lou Ann served as director of hospital health record departments, director of the Professional Practice Division of the American Health Information Management Association (AHIMA), and a faculty member at the University of Illinois at Chicago. An experienced seminar leader, Lou Ann continues to serve as part-time faculty in the health information technology and coding certificate program at Moraine Valley Community College. She has also contributed her knowledge and skills as a consultant for clinical coding projects with hospitals, ambulatory care facilities, physicians, and medical group practices. Lou Ann has been active in national, state, and local HIM associations. She has served as chair of the Society for Clinical Coding (2000). She is a current member of the AHIMA Commission on Certification of Health Informatics and Information Management. In 1997, Lou Ann was awarded the first AHIMA Volunteer Award. Lou Ann received the Legacy Award from the AHIMA Foundation in 2008 in recognition of her significant contribution to the HIM knowledge base through her authorship of coding textbooks and manuals published by AHIMA.

Acknowledgments

This book on basic ICD-10-CM/PCS coding is built on the foundation of the *Basic ICD-9-CM Coding* textbook that has been written by Lou Ann Schraffenberger since 1999. The first *Basic ICD-9-CM Coding* textbook was originally published in 1993 under the authorship of Toula Nicholas, RHIT, CCS, and Linda Ertl Bank, RHIA, CCS. Earlier ICD-9-CM instructional material authored by the late Rita M. Finnegan, MA, RHIA, was the basis for the original book. Therese M. Jorwic, RHIA, CCS, FAHIMA, updated several chapters in the 2012 Basic ICD-9-CM textbook that was also used in this edition. Chapter 2 on ICD-10-PCS procedure coding was expanded using her original work on the chapter in the previous edition. Overall, her consultation and authorship is acknowledged and appreciated. For an in-depth review of ICD-10-PCS principles and application of procedure coding rules, the reader is encouraged to examine *ICD-10-PCS: An Applied Approach* written by Lynn Kuehn and Therese Jorwic and published by AHIMA (AC201111). This is a comprehensive text for learning and mastering the new procedure coding system, ICD-10-PCS. Coding practice exercises, case study coding, and a self-test are provided to reinforce the information in the text.

Preface

The coding process requires a range of skills that combine knowledge and practice. *Basic ICD 10-CM/PCS Coding* was designed to be a comprehensive text for students. It introduces the basic principles and conventions of ICD-10-CM/PCS coding and illustrates the application of coding principles with examples and exercises based on actual case documentation. The book was written during the time when the implementation date for ICD-10-CM/PCS was uncertain, with the original implementation date of October 1, 2013 under review for possible delayed implementation to 2014.

Organization of the Book

The chapters of *Basic ICD-10-CM/PCS Coding* are organized to cover each section of ICD-10-CM. The coding self-test, appendices, and index at the back of the book make information readily accessible and provide additional resources for students.

Information Updates

This book must be used with the 2013 edition of ICD-10-CM and ICD-10-PCS code sets. The data files for the 2013 version of ICD-10-CM and ICD-10-PCS can be found at http://www.cdc.gov/nchs/icd/icd10cm.htm and http://www.cms.gov/Medicare/Coding/ICD10/index.html.

Every effort has been made to include the most current coding information in this textbook. Because coding is so dynamic, there are continuous changes. In order to keep you informed about some of them, the following information is provided to you.

Official Coding Guidelines

The full 2013 ICD-10-CM Official Guidelines for Coding and Reporting are included as Appendix E. Additional information and updates to current coding guidelines can be found on the following website: http://www.cdc.gov/nchs/icd/icd10cm.htm.

Coding guidelines are usually updated every year. The reader should check this website prior to October 1 for the updated set of guidelines that would be effective on or around October 1, 2013.

The CG icon throughout the text displays coding guidelines that directly relate to the area of ICD-10-CM/PCS being discussed in the chapter, including the coding guideline number.

Additional Practice

In addition to the student review exercises throughout and at the end of each chapter, a new student workbook, also by Lou Ann Schraffenberger, is available. *Basic ICD-10-CM/PCS Coding Exercises,* fourth edition, contains ICD-10-CM coding exercises related to each chapter of *Basic ICD-10-CM/PCS. Basic ICD-10-CM/PCS Coding Exercises* provides the student with the next level of coding practice—that is, coding from case studies or scenarios instead of one-line diagnostic or procedural statements. The *Basic ICD-10-CM/PCS Coding Exercises* can be used as a student workbook in conjunction with this textbook for the "lab" portion of a coding course or as a text for a coding practicum or lab course, or can be used for independent study for skill building.

AHIMA's publication *Clinical Coding Workout* is an excellent follow-up resource after the coder completes *Basic ICD-10-CM/PCS Coding.* Containing beginning, intermediate, and advanced exercises, it is also a perfect teaching tool for coders wanting to sharpen their ability to make critical coding decisions. The book is made up entirely of case studies that help students and coders alike understand what they need to know when it comes to correct coding practices and procedures. The case studies in the book require users to make the kinds of decisions that coding professionals must make every day on the job.

Readers who are interested in gaining more hands-on practice coding in ICD-10-CM and ICD-10-PCS should refer to the AHIMA Bookstore at www.ahimastore.org for all the available ICD-10-CM/PCS publications available.

Instructor Materials and Answer Key

AHIMA provides supplementary materials for educators who use this book in their classes. Materials include lesson plans, PowerPoint slides, and other useful instructional tips, reminders, and resources. Please visit http://www.ahima.org/publications/educators.aspx for further instruction. If you have any questions regarding the instructor materials, please contact AHIMA Customer Relations at (800) 335-5535 or submit a customer support request at https://secure.ahima.org/contact/contact.aspx.

Chapter 1

Introduction to ICD-10-CM

Objectives

At the conclusion of this chapter, you should be able to:

1. Identify the characteristics of the ICD-10-CM classification system

2. Describe the format of the Tabular List of Diseases and Injuries

3. Identify and define the chapters and subchapters or blocks used in ICD-10-CM

4. Describe the format of the Alphabetic Index to Diseases

5. Identify and define the main terms, subterms, carryover lines, nonessential modifiers, and eponyms used in ICD-10-CM

6. Explain how to accommodate the fact that all terms located in the Alphabetic Index are not included in the Tabular List

7. Identify and define the cross-reference terms and instructional notes used in ICD-10-CM

8. Describe the rules for multiple coding

9. Explain how connecting words are used in the Alphabetic Index

10. Define the symbols, punctuations, and abbreviations used in ICD-10-CM

11. List the basic steps in ICD-10-CM coding

12. Assign diagnosis codes using the Alphabetic Index and Tabular List

Key Terms

- Alphabetic Index
- Centers for Medicare and Medicaid Services (CMS)
- Classification
- Classification system
- "Code also" note
- Coding

- Colon
- Connecting words
- Cooperating Parties for the ICD-10-CM
- Default code
- Diagnosis
- Etiology
- Excludes note
- *Federal Register*
- Health Insurance Portability and Accountability Act of 1996 (HIPAA)
- ICD-10-CM Coordination and Maintenance (C&M) Committee
- Includes note
- International Classification of Diseases, Ninth Revision, Clinical Modification (ICD-9-CM)
- International Classification of Diseases, Tenth Revision
- International Classification of Diseases, Tenth Revision, Clinical Modification (ICD-10-CM)
- International Classification of Diseases, Tenth Revision, Procedure Coding System (ICD-10-PCS)
- Main terms
- Manifestation
- Medicare Prescription Drug, Improvement, and Modernization Act (MMA)
- National Center for Health Statistics (NCHS)
- Not elsewhere classified (NEC)
- Not otherwise specified (NOS)
- Nonessential modifiers
- Official Addendum to ICD-10-CM
- Parentheses
- Procedure
- "See" note
- "See also" note
- Sequela
- Slanted brackets
- Square brackets
- Tabular List
- World Health Organization (WHO)

What Is Coding?

In its simplest form, **coding** is the transformation of verbal descriptions into numbers. Coding is the process of assigning numeric or alphanumeric representations to clinical documentation. We are all very familiar with this task because we use codes every day to carry out simple business and personal transactions. For example, when we use a zip code in addressing a letter, we are transforming a street address into numbers.

In the healthcare arena, specific codes describe diagnoses and procedures. A **diagnosis** is a word or phrase used by a physician to identify a disease from which an individual suffers or a condition for which the patient needs, seeks, or receives medical care. A surgical or therapeutic **procedure** is any single, separate, systematic process upon or within the body that can be complete in itself. A procedure is normally performed by a physician, dentist, or other licensed practitioner. A procedure can be performed with or without instrumentation. It is performed to restore disunited or deficient parts, remove diseased or injured tissues, extract foreign matter, assist in obstetrical delivery, or aid in diagnosis. Whereas assigning a zip code is a rather simple activity, the assignment of diagnostic and procedural codes requires a detailed thought process that is supported by a thorough knowledge of medical terminology, anatomy, and pathophysiology.

How Are Codes Assigned and What System Is Used?

Hospitals and other healthcare facilities index healthcare data by referring and adhering to a classification system maintained by the National Center for Health Statistics and Centers for Medicare and Medicaid Services. A **classification system** is a grouping of similar diseases and procedures and organizing related information for easy retrieval. This type of system is used for assigning numeric or alphanumeric code numbers to represent specific diseases or procedures. Currently in the United States, that system (soon to be implemented) is the International Classification of Diseases, Tenth Revision, Clinical Modification (ICD-10-CM).

History of Coding

The notion of classification originated at the time of the ancient Greeks. The purpose of a classification was to present a clinical vocabulary, terminology, or nomenclature that lists words or phrases with their meanings to provide for the proper use of clinical words. A **classification** facilitates connecting standardized terms to a broader grouping for administrative and medical reasons. In the 17th century, English statistician John Graunt developed the London Bills of Mortality, which provided the first documentation of the proportion of children who died before reaching age six years. In 1838, William Farr, the registrar general of England, developed a system to classify deaths. In 1893, a French physician, Jacques Bertillon, introduced the Bertillon Classification of Causes of Death at the International Statistical Institute in Chicago.

In 1898, the American Public Health Association (APHA) recommended that the registrars of Canada, Mexico, and the United States adopt the Bertillon Classification. In addition, APHA recommended revising the system every 10 years to remain current with medical practice. As a result, the first international conference to revise the International Classification of Causes of Death convened in 1900; subsequent revisions occurred every 10 years. At that time, the classification system was contained in one book, which included an Alphabetic Index as well as a Tabular List. The book was quite small compared with current coding texts.

The revisions that followed contained minor changes; however, the sixth revision of the classification system brought drastic changes, as well as an expansion into two volumes. The sixth revision included morbidity and mortality conditions, and its title was changed to *Manual of International Statistical Classification of Diseases, Injuries and Causes of Death (ICD)*. Prior to the sixth revision, responsibility for ICD revisions fell to the Mixed Commission, a group composed of representatives from the International Statistical Institute and the Health Organization of the League of Nations. In 1948, the **World Health Organization (WHO)**, with headquarters in Geneva, Switzerland, assumed responsibility for preparing and publishing the revisions to ICD every 10 years. WHO sponsored the seventh and eighth revisions in 1957 and 1968. Today, WHO is the United Nations specialized agency responsible for ensuring the attainment of the highest possible levels of health for all people. WHO is responsible for a number of international classifications, including the International Classification of Diseases and Related Health Problems (ICD) and the International Classification of Functioning, Disability, and Health (ICF).

The entire history of coding emphasizes the determination of many people to provide an international classification system for compiling and presenting statistical data. ICD is now the most widely used statistical classification system in the world. Although some countries found ICD sufficient for hospital indexing purposes, many others believed that it did not provide adequate detail for diagnostic indexing. In addition, the original revisions of ICD did not provide for classification of operative and diagnostic procedures. As a result, interested persons in the United States began to develop their own adaptation of ICD for use in this country.

In 1959, the US Public Health Service published *The International Classification of Diseases, Adapted for Indexing of Hospital Records and Operation Classification (ICDA)*. Completed in 1962, a revision of this adaptation—considered to be the seventh revision of ICD—expanded a number of areas to more completely meet the indexing needs of hospitals. The US Public Health Service later published the *Eighth Revision, International Classification of Diseases, Adapted for Use in the United States*. Commonly referred to as ICDA-8, this classification system fulfilled its purpose to code diagnostic and operative procedural data for official morbidity and mortality statistics in the United States.

In 1978, WHO published the ninth revision of ICD (ICD-9). The US Public Health Service modified ICD-9 to meet the needs of American hospitals and called it International Classification of Diseases, Ninth Revision, Clinical Modification (ICD-9-CM). The ninth revision expanded the book to three volumes and introduced a fifth-digit subclassification. ICD-9-CM was the coding and classification system used in the United States to report diagnoses in all healthcare settings and inpatient procedures and services for morbidity and mortality reporting starting in 1979. The ICD-9-CM system is slated to be discontinued in the United States on September 30, 2014.

Background on ICD-10-CM and ICD-10-PCS

WHO published the tenth revision of ICD in 1990, and a number of countries subsequently adopted the system in either the original or an adapted form. The international version of the ICD-10 system has been used in the United States since January 1, 1999 for death certificate coding. This allows for collection of international mortality data.

A US clinical modification of the ICD-10 system was initiated in 1994 by the **National Center for Health Statistics (NCHS)**. NCHS is the federal agency responsible for collecting and disseminating information on health services utilization and the health status of the population in the United States. NCHS is responsible for developing the clinical modifications for the United States to the International Classification of Diseases for the reporting of diseases. NCHS is also responsible for the development and the use of the International Classification of Diseases, Tenth Revision (ICD-10) in the United States. The result, International Classification of Diseases, Tenth Revision, Clinical Modification (ICD-10-CM), was released in 1998 and updated several times since the initial version. ICD-10-CM will be used for the reporting of diseases and conditions of patients treated in all settings in the United States healthcare system effective October 1, 2014.

The ICD-10-CM system is more specific and contains significantly more codes than exist in ICD-9-CM. It has the same hierarchical structure as ICD-9-CM, but the codes are alphanumeric with all letters except U used. The codes can extend to up to seven characters.

The 2013 version of ICD-10-CM is available on the NCHS website, at the Classifications of Diseases, Functioning, and Disability home page (http://www.cdc.gov/nchs/icd/icd10cm .htm#10update). Although this release of ICD-10-CM is now available for public viewing, the codes in ICD-10-CM are not currently (2012) valid for any purpose or use pending the official implementation of ICD-10-CM and ICD-10-PCS in the United States. This version has been created by the NCHS, under authorization by WHO.

On January 16, 2009, the Department of Health and Human Services (HHS) published a final rule adopting ICD-10-CM (and ICD-10-PCS) to replace ICD-9-CM in HIPAA transactions, with an effective implementation date of October 1, 2013. The October 1, 2013 implementation date for ICD-10-CM/PCS was established in the original Final Rule of the HIPAA Administrative Simplification: Modifications to the Medical Data Code Set Standards to adopt ICD-10-CM and ICD-10-PCS, which was published in the *Federal Register* on January 16, 2009 (http://www.access.gpo.gov/su_docs/fedreg/a090116c.html). The *Federal Register* is the daily publication of the federal government printed by the US Government Printing Office that announces all changes in regulations and federally mandated standards, including rules concerning prospective payment systems and code sets.

The **Health Insurance Portability and Accountability Act of 1996 (HIPAA)** was federal legislation enacted to provide continuing health coverage, control fraud and abuse in healthcare, reduce healthcare costs, and guarantee the security and privacy of health information. HIPAA limits exclusions for preexisting medical conditions, prohibits discrimination against employees and dependents based on health status, guarantees availability of health insurance to small employers, and guarantees renewability of insurance to all employees regardless of size. The law is also known as Public Law 104-191 and the Kassebaum-Kennedy Law.

On April 17, 2012, the Secretary of HHS issued a proposed rule to change the compliance date for the ICD-10-CM and ICD-10-PCS code sets from October 1, 2013 to October 1, 2014. The comment period for the proposed rule closed in June 2012. The Final Rule published in the *Federal Register* on September 5, 2012 set the implementation date of October 1, 2014.

The Final Rule adopts modifications to two of the code set standards adopted in the Transactions and Code Sets Final Rule published in the *Federal Register* pursuant to certain provisions of the Administrative Simplification subtitle of HIPAA. Specifically, this Final Rule modifies the standard medical data code sets for coding diagnoses and inpatient hospital procedures by concurrently adopting the ICD-10-CM for diagnosis coding, including the *Official ICD-10-CM Guidelines for Coding and Reporting,* as maintained by the National Center for Health Statistics, and the International Classification of Diseases, Tenth Revision, Procedure Coding System (ICD-10-PCS) for inpatient hospital procedure coding, including the Official ICD-10-PCS Guidelines for Coding and Reporting, as maintained and distributed by HHS. These new codes replace ICD-9-CM, Volumes 1, 2, and 3, including the *Official Guidelines for Coding and Reporting.*

ICD-10-PCS was developed by 3M Health Information Systems under contract with **Centers for Medicare and Medicaid Services (CMS)**. CMS is a division of the Department of Health and Human Services that is responsible for developing healthcare policy in the United States, administering the Medicare program and the federal portion of the Medicaid program, and maintaining the procedure portion of the International Classification of Diseases. On October 1, 2014, ICD-10-PCS will replace ICD-9-CM, volume 3, for the reporting of hospital inpatient procedures. It is a significant improvement over ICD-9-CM, volume 3, in terms of its comprehensiveness and expandability. ICD-10-PCS is discussed in further detail in Chapter 2.

ICD-10-CM Official Guidelines for Coding and Reporting

ICD-10-CM Official Guidelines for Coding and Reporting should be used in conjunction with the official version of the ICD-10-CM as published on the NCHS website. These guidelines have been approved by the **Cooperating Parties for the ICD-10-CM** that includes representatives from the American Hospital Association (AHA), the American Health Information Management Association (AHIMA), CMS, and NCHS.

These guidelines are a set of coding rules that accompany and complement the official conventions and instructions provided within the ICD-10-CM code set. The instructions and conventions in the ICD-10-CM classification take precedence over the guidelines. The guidelines provide additional instruction for the coder and are based on the coding and sequencing instructions in the Tabular List and Alphabetic Index of ICD-10-CM.

HIPAA requires all coders adhere to these guidelines when assigning ICD-10-CM diagnosis codes. The diagnosis codes have been adopted under HIPAA for all healthcare settings.

The guidelines have been developed to identify the diagnoses and procedures that are to be reported. The importance of consistent, complete documentation in the health record cannot be overemphasized.

The conventions, general guidelines, and chapter-specific ICD-10-CM guidelines are applicable to all healthcare settings unless otherwise indicated. The guidelines for the principal and additional diagnoses are only applicable to the inpatient settings.

The *ICD-10-CM Official Guidelines for Coding and Reporting* is referenced throughout this chapter. You can find the complete document in Appendix E.

Medicare Prescription Drug, Improvement, and Modernization Act of 2003

The **Medicare Prescription Drug, Improvement, and Modernization Act (MMA)** was signed into law on December 8, 2003. Section 503 of the bill includes language that opened up the possibility for code changes two times a year, on April 1 as well as October 1. Since this legislation took effect in 2005, there have not been any April 1 code changes. However, the potential for code changes twice a year still exists if a strong and convincing case is made by the requestor that the new code is needed to describe new technologies. Otherwise, the codes will be considered for the next October 1 implementation.

Official Addendum to ICD-10-CM and ICD-10-PCS

In contrast to international ICD updates that occur less frequently, ICD-10-CM/PCS undergoes annual updates in the United States to remain current. Codes may be added, revised, or deleted. An *Official Addendum* documents the changes, which are effective April 1 and October 1 of each year. The addendum may be found at the National Center for Health Statistics' website (http://www.cdc.gov/nchs/icd/icd10cm.htm). CMS and NCHS publish the addenda with the approval of the WHO. NCHS is responsible for maintaining the diagnosis classification; CMS is responsible for maintaining the procedure classification. AHIMA and AHA give advice and assistance, as do HIM practitioners, physicians, and other users of ICD-10-CM/PCS.

Coordination and Maintenance Committee

The **ICD-10-CM Coordination and Maintenance (C&M) Committee** is chaired by a representative from the NCHS and a representative from CMS. The committee is responsible for maintaining the United States' clinical modification version of the ICD-10-CM/PCS code sets. The Coordination and Maintenance Committee holds two open meetings each year that serve as a public forum for discussing (but not making decisions about) proposed revisions to ICD-10-CM/PCS. Information about the ICD-10-CM/PCS Coordination and Maintenance Committee, including meeting minutes, can be found at http://www. cdc.gov/nchs/icd/icd9cm_maintenance.htm and at http://www.cms.gov/Medicare/Coding/ ICD9ProviderDiagnosticCodes/meetings.html.

A point to remember: To ensure accurate coding, all ICD-10-CM/PCS code books must be updated yearly with the revisions published. In addition, all coding software (encoders) must be updated. As a general rule, new ICD-10-CM/PCS codes will be effective October 1 of each year.

Characteristics of ICD-10-CM

The ICD-10-CM system will be used for all diagnosis coding beginning on October 1, 2014. The system is more extensive and specific than ICD-9-CM, but much of the hierarchical structure and conventions are similar. ICD-10-CM is divided into the Alphabetic Index, which is an alphabetic listing of terms and codes, and the Tabular List, which is a numerical list of the codes divided by chapters.

Conventions for ICD-10-CM

To assign ICD-10-CM codes accurately, a thorough understanding of the ICD-10-CM conventions is necessary. These coding conventions address the structure and format of the coding system, including how to use the Alphabetic Index and the Tabular List, as well as the rules and instructions that the coder must follow.

Alphabetic Index

The **Alphabetic Index** is divided into two parts—the Index to Diseases and Injury and the Index to External Causes of Injury. Within the Index of Diseases and Injury there is a Neoplasm Table and a Table of Drugs and Chemicals.

The Alphabetic Index in ICD-10-CM is formatted with main terms set in boldface are listed in alphabetical order. **Main terms** are entries printed in boldface type and flush with the left margin of each column in the Alphabetic Index. Main terms represent diseases, conditions, nouns, and adjectives. This is the first place the coder uses to locate the ICD-10-CM code for the patient's disease or condition. Indented beneath the main term, any applicable subterm or essential modifier is shown in their own alphabetic list. The indented subterm is always read in combination with the main term. The dash (-) at the end of an Index entry indicates that additional characters are required.

Nonessential Modifiers

A term or a series of terms that appear in parentheses following a main term or subterm are known as **nonessential modifiers**. The presence or absence of these parenthetical terms in the diagnosis statement has no effect on the selection of the codes listed for that main term or subterm.

"See" and "See Also" Instructions

The Alphabetic Index in ICD-10-CM includes both "see" and "see also" instructions following a main term to indicate that another term should be referenced.

The **"see" note** is a cross-reference term in the Alphabetic Index to Diseases and Injuries that provides direction to the coder to look elsewhere in the Index before assigning a code. The "see" cross-reference points to an alternative term. This is a mandatory instruction that must be followed to ensure accurate ICD-10-CM code assignment.

The **"see also" note** in the Alphabetic Index to Disease and Injuries provides direction to the coder to look elsewhere in the Index. It requires the review of another term in the Index if all the needed information cannot be found under the first main term. However, it is not necessary to follow the *see also* note when the original main term provides the necessary code.

> **EXAMPLE:**   **Aberrant (congenital)**—see also Malposition, congenital
> -adrenal gland Q89.1
> -artery (peripheral) Q27.8
> ---basilar NEC Q28.1
> ---cerebral Q28.3

"Code Also" Note

The **"code also" note** appears in ICD-10-CM, meaning that two codes may be required to fully describe a condition, but this note does not provide sequencing direction.

The ICD-10-CM Alphabetic Index includes manifestation of disease codes by including the manifestation code as the second code, shown in brackets, directly after the underlying or etiology code, which should always be reported first.

> **EXAMPLES:**   **Dementia**
> -with
> ---Parkinson's disease G20 *[F02.80]*
>
> **Retinitis**
> -renal N18.9 *[H32]*
> -syphilitic
> --congenital (early) A50.01 *[H32]*

Default Code

ICD-10-CM refers to the code listed next to a main term in the Alphabetic Index as a **default code.** The default code represents the condition that is most commonly associated with the main term, or is the unspecified code for the condition. If a condition is documented in the medical record without any additional information, such as whether it is acute or chronic, the default code should be assigned.

Exercise 1.1

Using the Alphabetic Index, underline the main term and assign codes to the following:

1. Breast mass

2. Primary hydronephrosis

3. Deviated nasal septum

4. Inguinal adenopathy

5. Arteriosclerotic heart disease

6. Tension headache

7. Suppurative pancreatitis

8. Neonatal tooth eruption

9. Infectious endocarditis

10. Mitral endocarditis with active aortic disease

Exercise 1.2

Using the Alphabetic Index, underline the term that is the nonessential modifier in each of the following diagnostic statements and then assign a code to each condition:

1. Congenital distortion of chest wall

2. Acute diverticulitis of large intestine

3. Bleeding external hemorrhoids

4. Functional cardiac murmur

5. Chronic maxillary sinusitis

Exercise 1.3

Review each diagnostic statement. Underline the appropriate main term to use in the Alphabetic Index. Locate the main term in the Alphabetic Index and follow all cross-reference instructions. Confirm the code in the Tabular List and enter it on the line provided.

1. Acute endomyometritis

   _____

2. Metrorrhexis, nontraumatic

   _____

3. Osteoarthrosis, shoulder

   _____

4. Cervical intervertebral disc prolapse

   _____

5. Stenosis of endocervical os

   _____

Tabular List

The ICD-10-CM **Tabular List** is a numerical listing of all the codes. The Tabular List is divided into 21 chapters. For some chapters, the body or organ system is the axis of the classification. Other chapters, such as Chapter 1, Certain infectious and parasitic diseases, group together conditions by etiology or nature of the disease process.

The 21 chapters of the ICD-10-CM classification system are as follows:

1. Certain infectious and parasitic diseases (A00–B99)

2. Neoplasms (C00–D49)

3. Diseases of the blood and blood-forming organs and certain disorders involving the immune mechanism (D50–D89)

4. Endocrine, nutritional and metabolic disorders (E00–E89)

5. Mental, behavioral and neurodevelopmental disorders (F01–F99)

6. Diseases of the nervous system (G00–G99)

7. Diseases of the eye and adnexa (H00–H59)

8. Diseases of the ear and mastoid process (H60–H95)

9. Diseases of the circulatory system (I00–I99)

10. Diseases of the respiratory system (J00–J99)

11. Diseases of the digestive system (K00–K95)

12. Diseases of the skin and subcutaneous tissue (L00–L99)

13. Diseases of the musculoskeletal system and connective tissue (M00–M99)

14. Diseases of the genitourinary system (N00–N99)

15. Pregnancy, childbirth and the puerperium (O00–O9A)

16. Certain conditions originating in the perinatal period (P00–P96)

17. Congenital malformations, deformations and chromosomal abnormalities (Q00–Q99)

18. Symptoms, signs and abnormal clinical and laboratory findings, not elsewhere classified (R00–R99)

19. Injury, poisoning and certain other consequences of external causes (S00–T88)

20. External causes of morbidity (V00–Y99)

21. Factors influencing health status and contact with health services (Z00–Z99)

Each chapter in the Tabular List of ICD-10-CM begins with a summary of the blocks to provide an overview of the categories within the chapter.

Code Format and Structure

The ICD-10-CM Coding Guidelines state the ICD-10-CM contains chapters, categories, subcategories, and codes. Chapters are further subdivided into subchapters (blocks) and subcategories that contain three character categories and form the foundation of the code.

Categories, Subcategories, and Codes

The characters for categories, subcategories, and codes may contain either letters or numbers. All categories are three characters. A three-character category that has no further subdivision is equivalent to a code.

Most three-character categories are further subdivided into four- or five-character subcategories. Codes can be three, four, five, six, or seven characters. Each level of subdivision after a category is a subcategory. Five- and six-character codes provide greater specificity or additional information about the condition being coded.

The final level of subdivision of a category is a code. Certain categories have an additional seventh character. The seventh character must always be the final character of the code. When the code contains fewer than seven characters, the placeholder X must be used to fill the empty character(s).

The fourth character 8, when placed after a decimal point (.8), is used to indicate some "other" specified category. The fourth character 9, when placed after a decimal point (.9), is usually reserved for an unspecified condition. In ICD-10-CM, the "other specified" and "unspecified" conditions each have their own code and are not combined into one code.

First Character

The first character of an ICD-10-CM code is always an alphabetic letter. All the letters of the alphabet are utilized with the exception of the letter U. The letter U has been reserved by WHO for the provisional assignment of new diseases of uncertain etiology (U00–U49) and for bacterial agents resistant to antibiotics (U80–U89.) ICD-10-CM codes may consist of up to seven characters and are formatted as shown in figure 1.1.

Figure 1.1. **ICD-10-CM code format**

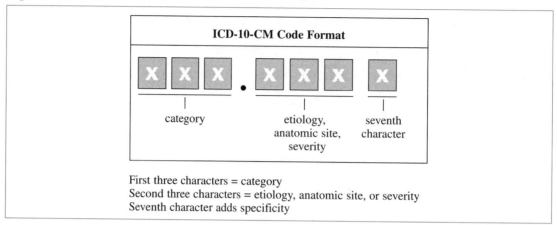

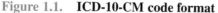

Placeholder Character

ICD-10-CM utilizes a placeholder character, which is always the letter X, and it has two uses:

1. The X provides for future expansion without disturbing the overall code structure.

   EXAMPLE: T42.3X1A, Poisoning by barbiturates, accidental, initial encounter

2. It is also used when a code has less than six characters and a seventh character extension is required. The X is assigned for all characters less than six in order to meet the requirement of coding to the highest level of specificity.

   EXAMPLE: T58.11XA, Toxic effect of carbon monoxide from utility gas, accidental, initial encounter

Seventh Character

Certain ICD-10-CM categories have applicable seventh characters. The applicable seventh character is required for all codes within the category, or as the notes in the Tabular List instruct. The seventh character must always be the seventh character in the data field. If a code that requires a seventh character does not contain six characters, a placeholder X must be used to fill in the empty characters.

   EXAMPLES: O40.1XXA, Polyhydramnios, first trimester, fetus 1
   S02.65XA, Fracture of angle of mandible

To summarize the code format and structure of ICD-10-CM, the following facts are presented:

- ICD-10-CM codes consist of three to seven characters

- The first character of an ICD-10-CM code is always an alphabetic character

- All letters are used except U in the ICD-10-CM codes

- The second character of the ICD-10-CM code is always numeric

- Characters 3 through 7 of ICD-10-CM can be alphabetic or numeric

- A decimal is placed after the first three characters of an ICD-10-CM code

- Alpha characters used in the ICD-10-CM codes are not case-sensitive

- Only complete ICD-10-CM codes are used for reporting purposes, not categories or subcategories

- When a seventh character is required but there is less than six characters, the X must be used as a placeholder for the ICD-10-CM code to be valid

Abbreviations

Two abbreviations are used in ICD-10-CM:

NEC: Not Elsewhere Classifiable

An abbreviation of **not elsewhere classifiable (NEC)** is used in ICD-10-CM. This abbreviation appears in the Alphabetic Index. When NEC appears in the Alphabetic Index, it will direct the coder to the Tabular List showing an "other specified" codes description. The NEC entry appears when a specific code is not available. The NEC code usually directs the coder to an "other specified" code in the Tabular List that includes the number 8 after the decimal point.

> **EXAMPLES:**   K65.8, Other peritonitis
> N30.80, Other cystitis without hematuria

NOS: Not Otherwise Specified

The abbreviation of **not otherwise specified (NOS)** is the equivalent of unspecified. The abbreviation "NOS" appears in the Alphabetic Index and the Tabular List. The unspecified or NOS codes are available for use when the documentation of the condition identified by the provider in the health record does not provide enough information to assign a more specific code.

> **EXAMPLES:**   I50.9, Heart failure, unspecified
> L02.93, Carbuncle, unspecified

Punctuation

The punctuation used in ICD-10-CM is brackets, parentheses, and colons.

Brackets [ ]

Square brackets [ ] are a punctuation mark used in the Tabular List to enclose synonyms, abbreviations, alternative wording, or explanatory phrases. The terms within the brackets are presented for informational purposes. The words within the square brackets are not required to be part of the diagnostic statement to use the code. **Slanted brackets** *[ ]* are used in the Alphabetic Index to identify manifestation codes. Manifestation codes represent the secondary condition that is present in addition to the underlying or primary disease that caused the secondary condition. Two codes are required when the patient has both the underlying disease and the secondary condition. The use of the slanted bracket in the Alphabetic Index provides sequencing direction. The code that appears in the slanted bracket is listed in the second position or follows the disease code listed directly after the diagnosis term in the Index. The diagnosis in the slanted brackets is not entered into a computer or data entry system in the italicized font. The italicized font is used to emphasize the presence of the second code that is required.

EXAMPLES: Tabular List:

B20, Human immunodeficiency virus [HIV] disease

The HIV that appears in the brackets is an abbreviation for human immunodeficiency virus.

Alphabetic Index:

Amyloid heart (disease) E85.4 *[143]*

For amyloid heart disease, two codes are required in the following order or sequence:

E85.4 Organ-limited amyloidosis
143 Cardiomyopathy in diseases classified elsewhere

Parentheses ( )

Parentheses are a punctuation mark that encloses supplementary words or explanatory information that may or may not be present in the statement of a diagnosis. The words within the parentheses do not affect the code assigned to the condition. Terms in parentheses are considered nonessential modifiers and appear in both the Alphabetic Index and the Tabular List.

EXAMPLES: Alphabetic Index:

Amputee (bilateral) (old) Z89.9

The diagnosis statement could be amputee, bilateral amputee, old amputee or old bilateral amputee and the code would be the same for all: Z89.9.

Tabular List:

C83.5 Lymphoblastic (diffuse) lymphoma

The diagnosis statement could be lymphoblastic lymphoma or lymphoblastic diffuse lymphoma and the code would be the same for both: C83.5.

Colon :

The **colon** is a punctuation term that is used in the Tabular List after an incomplete term that needs one or more additional terms in order to be assigned to a particular code.

In the official ICD-10-CM electronic version, the colon is used with "includes" and "excludes" notes, in which the words that precede the colon are not considered complete terms and must be appended by one of the modifiers indented under the statement before the condition can be assigned the correct code. Other publishers of the printed version of the ICD-10-CM codes have not used the colon punctuation with the "includes" and "excludes" notes.

EXAMPLE: F02 Dementia in other diseases classified elsewhere
Code first the underlying physiological condition, such as:
Alzheimer's (G30.-)
cerebral lipidosis (E75.4)
Creutzfeldt-Jakob disease (A81.0-)

Exercise 1.4

Using the Tabular List and Alphabetic Index, assign codes to the following:

1. Sepsis

   _____

2. Bacteroides infection

   _____

3. Pericarditis with effusion

   _____

4. Fifth Disease

   _____

5. Dementia with Lewy bodies

   _____

Instructional Notes

Instructional notes are included in the Tabular List to clarify information and provide additional directions for the coder. The following paragraphs describe the various types of instructional notes.

Inclusion Terms

Inclusion terms are lists of medical diagnoses under some codes in the Tabular List. These are conditions for which that code is to be used. The terms may be synonyms of the code title or the terms are a list of various conditions assigned to "other specified" codes. The inclusion terms are not an exhaustive list of terms. Additional terms found only in the Alphabetic Index may also be assigned to a code.

> **EXAMPLE:**   I51.7 Cardiomegaly
> Cardiac dilatation
> Cardiac hypertrophy
> Ventricular dilatation

Includes Notes

Another type of inclusion term is the **includes note** used in the ICD-10-CM Tabular List. Includes notes appear immediately under a three-character code title to further define, or give examples of, the content of the category.

> **EXAMPLE:**   J44 Other chronic obstructive pulmonary disease Includes:
> asthma with chronic obstructive pulmonary disease
> chronic asthmatic (obstructive) bronchitis

chronic bronchitis with airways obstruction
chronic bronchitis with emphysema
chronic emphysematous bronchitis
chronic obstructive asthma
chronic obstructive bronchitis
chronic obstructive tracheobronchitis

Excludes Notes

ICD-10-CM has two types of excludes notes. Each type of note has a different definition for use. However, they are similar in intent. The **excludes note** indicates that codes excluded from each other are independent of each other. In ICD-10-CM, there are two types of excludes notes designated either as Excludes1 or Excludes2 in their title. Either or both may appear under a category, subcategory, or code.

The Excludes1 Note

The Excludes1 note indicates that the conditions listed after it cannot ever be used at the same time as the code above the Excludes1 note. The conditions listed in the code and in the Excludes1 note are mutually exclusive. A patient cannot have both conditions at the same time. The coder must determine, based on the documentation in the health record, which condition the patient actually has in order to assign the correct code.

EXAMPLE: E06 Thyroiditis
Excludes1:   postpartum thyroiditis (O90.5)

In this example, a patient who is in the postpartum period and has thyroiditis would have the diagnosis code O90.5 assigned. Other patients who have thyroiditis and are not in the post-partum period would have the disease coded as E06. This is an either/or situation. Both codes could not be used on the same patient during the same episode of care.

The Excludes2 Note

The Excludes2 note means that two codes are applied when both conditions are present. The conditions that appear as an Excludes2 note are not part of the code that is listed above it. A patient may have both conditions at the same time. One code does not include both conditions. When both conditions are present, two codes are applied. A coder can think of it as "2" codes are required when there is documentation for a condition present in the Excludes"2" note.

EXAMPLE: G47 Sleep disorders
Excludes2:   nightmares (F51.5)
nonorganic sleep disorders (F51.-)
sleep terrors (F51.4)

In this example, a patient can have sleep disorders and nightmares at the same time. The Excludes2 note means that code G47 for sleep disorders does not include the condition of nightmares. When the patient has both a sleep disorder and nightmares, two codes must be used: a code from the category G47 and the code F51.4.

Exercise 1.5

Answer the following questions:

1. Which site is excluded from category C24?

   _____

2. According to the inclusion terms under subcategory O24.4, what conditions are included in this code?

   _____

3. According to the Excludes1 note under code R63.0, what condition is assigned to F50.0-?

   _____

4. According to the inclusion terms under category R55, what condition is included in this category?

   _____

5. According to the Excludes2 note with category K57, what condition is assigned code K38.2?

   _____

Etiology and Manifestation Convention

Some diseases produce another disease or a condition the patient would not have without the underlying disease. In ICD-10-CM, there is a coding convention that requires two codes for situations when one disease produces another condition. The first disease is considered the **etiology** and the second condition that it produces is called the **manifestation**. The etiology or the first disease must be coded first. The manifestation(s) are listed as additional codes.

"Code First" and "Use Additional Code" Notes

The coding convention used in ICD-10-CM that directs the coder as to which condition is coded first is known as a "code first" note. The "code first" note appears in the Tabular List under the manifestation code. The title of the manifestation code usually includes the phrase "in diseases classified elsewhere" in the title. It is important to remember that the "in diseases classified elsewhere" or "in other specified diseases classified elsewhere" codes are never first-listed or principal diagnosis codes nor can these codes be listed as a single code. These manifestation codes also appear in *italicized fonts*. These instructions make sure the proper sequencing of codes is followed, that is, the etiology condition is coded first, followed by the manifestation code.

There are also diseases that require two codes to completely describe the condition because all the facts of the disease are not expressed in one code. When such a condition exists, the coding convention in ICD-10-CM will remind the coder to "use additional code" to fully describe the condition. This also indicates the sequencing required with the code identified as the "use additional code" listed as an additional code.

The etiology and manifestation conventions appear in both the Alphabetic Index and the Tabular List. In the Alphabetic Index, both conditions may be listed on one line with the etiology code listed first and the manifestation code appearing in slanted brackets after it. The code in the brackets is never listed first or used as a single code. The manifestation code must be listed second. In the Tabular List, there are notes the coder must read at the category or at the code level, that is, "code first" a certain condition or "use additional code" as an additional code to the code it appears with.

An example of the etiology or manifestation convention is dementia in Alzheimer's disease. The main term is disease, subterm is Alzheimer's, with an indent term for early onset.

> **EXAMPLE:** Early onset Alzheimer's disease with dementia without behavioral disturbance
> G30.0   Alzheimer's disease with early onset
> F02.80   Dementia in other diseases classified elsewhere, without behavioral disturbance

In the above example, Alzheimer's disease with early onset is coded to G30.0. Under category G30, there is a directive to "use additional code to identify" dementia without behavioral disturbance (F02.80). If the patient had early onset Alzheimer's disease with dementia without behavioral disturbance, two codes would be required: G30.0 with F02.80. Under category F02, Dementia in other diseases classified elsewhere, there is a "code first the underlying physiological condition, such as" note directing the coder to first assign a code for the type of Alzheimer's disease present with a code from category G30.

Multiple Coding for a Single Condition

Multiple codes may be required to code a disease that includes multiple disease processes or factors. As noted in the prior section, ICD-10-CM uses such conventions as "use additional code" in the Tabular List to identify a condition that is not part of the code it appears with. Another example when a "use additional code" note appears is with an infectious disease code that does not identify the specific bacterial or viral organism that caused it, but that organism can be identified with another code.

Other requirements for multiple coding of a single condition or a condition that includes multiple parts can be identified in ICD-10-CM with such notes as "code first," code, if applicable, a causal condition first, and "code also."

"Code First"

"Code first" notes appear under certain codes that are not specifically manifestation codes. But certain conditions may be due to an underlying cause. When there is a "code first" note and an underlying condition present, the underlying condition should be sequenced first. In the following example, a patient with malignant ascites suffers from the ascites because the patient also has a malignant condition that should be coded first as it is the underlying cause of the ascites.

> **EXAMPLE:** R18.0   Malignant ascites
> Code first malignancy, such as:
> malignant neoplasm of ovary (C56.-)
> secondary malignant neoplasm of retroperitoneum and peritoneum (C78.6)

"Code, If Applicable, a Causal Condition First"

"Code, if applicable, a causal condition first" note indicates that this code may be assigned as a first-listed or principal diagnosis when the causal condition is unknown or not applicable. If a causal condition is known, then the code for that condition should be sequenced as the principal or first-listed diagnosis. In the following example, if a patient has urinary retention and the cause of the urinary retention, such as an enlarged prostate, is known, the code for the enlarge prostate is coded first followed by a second code for the urinary retention.

> **EXAMPLE:** R33.8   Other retention of urine
> Code first, if applicable, any causal condition, such as:
> Enlarged prostate (N40.1)

"Code Also"

A "code also" note indicates that two codes may be required to fully describe a condition. This code does not provide sequencing direction, that is, either code may be listed first depending on the circumstances of the medical visit or admission. In the following example, a patient may be seen for the purpose of receiving renal dialysis. The fact that the patient has end stage renal disease that requires the patient to have renal dialysis is an important fact that is reported with an additional code.

> **EXAMPLE:** Z49 Encounter for care involving renal dialysis
> Code also associated end stage renal disease (N18.6)

Cross-References and Other Terms Used in ICD-10-CM

Cross-references are used as directions for the coder to look elsewhere in the Alphabetic Index before assigning a code. Other terms are used to explain the relationships between the diagnoses and conditions included in both the Alphabetic Index and the Tabular List. To assign diagnosis codes accurately, a thorough understanding of the ICD-10-CM cross-references and other terms is essential.

And

The term "and" is interpreted to mean "and" or "or" when it appears in a code title. The term "and" means the patient may have one or the other of the statements included in the code title. In the following example, code Z51.1 is used if the patient's encounter is for the purpose of receiving antineoplastic chemotherapy or for the purpose of receiving antineoplastic immunotherapy. If the patient is receiving both chemotherapy and immunotherapy, the code is also appropriate to use.

> **EXAMPLE:** Z51.1 Encounter for antineoplastic chemotherapy and
> immunotherapy

With

The term "with" may be used by the physician to acknowledge two conditions exist but the physician may also use other phrases such as "associated with" or "due to" and the ICD-10-CM phrase of "with" also applies in the Alphabetic Index or in the Tabular List in an instructional note.

In the Alphabetic Index, the term "with" will appear immediately following the main term. The term "with" does not appear necessarily with other subterms starting with the letter "W."

In the Tabular List, the term "with" appearing in a code title means that two conditions (condition A with condition B) must be present in the patient to use that particular code.

> **EXAMPLES:** Tabular List:
> B15.0 Hepatitis A with hepatic coma

In this example, code B15.0 presents the fact that the patient has two conditions: hepatitis A and hepatic coma. Here "with" means both conditions exist at the same time.

> Alphabetic Index:
> Bronchiolitis
> with
>   bronchospasm or obstruction J21.9
>   influenza, flu, grippe - see Influenza, with, respiratory manifestations NEC
>   chemical (chronic) J68.4
>   acute J68.0
>   chronic (fibrosing)(obliterative) J44.9
>   due to
>   external agent - see Bronchitis, acute, due to

In this example, the condition of bronchiolitis with bronchospasm is found in the Alphabetic Index under the main term "bronchiolitis." The "with" connecting term, to identify that bronchospasm also exists, appears immediately under the main term and before the other terms that appear in alphabetic order such as chemical, chronic, or due to.

"See" and "See Also"

In ICD-10-CM, the "see" direction is used to instruct the coder to reference another term in the Alphabetic Index that provides more complete information about the condition to be coded. The "see" note also appears with an anatomical site main term to direct the coder to locate the disease present at that anatomic site in the Alphabetic Index. For example, if the main term of "leg" is located in the Alphabetic Index, the same line includes the phrase "see condition."

> **EXAMPLE:** Alphabetic Index:
> Angina
> with
> atherosclerotic heart disease - see Arteriosclerosis, coronary (artery)

The cross-reference note "see also" in the Alphabetic Index follows a main term if the coder should reference another term in the Index for additional information. The instruction is intended to help the coder find the most information available in the Alphabetic Index when the coder may not identify all the options that could be used. However, it is not necessary to follow the "see also" note when the original main term provides all the necessary information to assign a complete code.

> **EXAMPLE:** Alphabetic Index:
> Bruise (skin surface intact) (see also Contusion)

In this example, no codes are available under the main term of bruise that occurs on the skin. The more appropriate medical term of contusion should be referenced to identify the many anatomic sites on which a bruise may be found.

Connecting Words

Connecting words or connecting terms are subterms in the Alphabetic Index that appear after a main term to indicate a relationship between the main term and an associated condition or etiology.

Associated with
Complicated by
Due to
During
Following
In
Secondary to
With
With mention of
Without

The connecting words "with" and "without" appear in both the Alphabetic Index and in the Tabular List in code titles. "With and "without" connecting terms are sequenced before all other subterms in the Alphabetic Index but may also appear with the other subterms in alphabetic order.

Exercise 1.6

Using the Tabular List and Alphabetic Index, assign codes to the following:

1. Bleeding esophageal varices in liver cirrhosis

2. Urinary tract infection due to Escherichia coli

3. Acute duodenal ulcer with hemorrhage

4. Anemia due to prematurity

5. Patient examined following motor vehicle accident (No symptoms or complaints)

General Coding Guidelines

There are basic concepts and rules that a coder must understand in order to assign ICD-10-CM codes accurately and completely. These general coding guidelines describe how to locate a code in ICD-10-CM and how to apply all the necessary codes to fully describe a patient's condition and reason for health services.

Locating a Code in the ICD-10-CM

The coder must use both the Alphabetic Index and Tabular List when locating and assigning a code. The first step in coding is to locate the main term and applicable subterms in the Alphabetic Index. Then the code found in the Alphabetic Index is verified in the Tabular List. The coder must read and be guided by the instructional notations that appear in both the Alphabetic Index and the Tabular List.

The Alphabetic Index does not always provide the complete code. Every code listed in the Alphabetic Index must be reviewed in the Tabular List. Selection of the complete code, including laterality and any applicable seventh character can only be done in the Tabular List. If additional characters are required, a dash (-) at the end of the Alphabetic Index entry is present. The coder then uses the Tabular List to identify what additional characters are necessary to complete the code to fully describe the patient's condition. Even if it appears that a complete code is included in the Alphabetic Index, it is mandatory for the coder to review the code in the Tabular List for all the instructional notes that may require additional coding.

Level of Detail in Coding

Diagnosis codes are to be used and reported with the highest number of characters available. Codes with three characters are included in ICD-10-CM as the heading of a category of codes. A category may be further subdivided by the use of fourth, fifth, or sixth characters to provide greater detail. A seventh character may be applicable for certain codes. A three-character code is to be used only if it is not further subdivided, that is, there are no applicable fourth, fifth, sixth, or seventh characters to be used. A code is invalid if it is not coded to the full number of characters required for that code.

Signs and Symptoms

Codes that describe symptoms and physical signs are perfectly acceptable for reporting when the sign or symptom is what the physician knows for certain about the patient. There are occasions when no definitive diagnosis can be made, even after investigation or study of the patient's presenting signs and symptoms. Signs and symptoms may be transient and disappear before the physician can identify their cause. A patient may come to a physician for treatment of a sign or symptom but fail to return for further investigation and it is not determined what caused the problem. Patients with certain signs and symptoms may be referred to another physician or treatment center for investigation before the physician can identify the cause of the symptom or sign. In all of these situations and the other scenarios described at the start of Chapter 18, Symptoms, signs and abnormal clinical findings, not elsewhere classified (R00–R99), the assignment of a sign or symptom code is appropriate.

Most but not all signs and symptoms appear in Chapter 18. Signs and symptoms applicable to certain body systems appear in the body system chapter of ICD-10-CM, for example, ear pain is assigned a code from ICD-10-CM Chapter 8, Diseases of the ear and mastoid process.

Conditions That Are an Integral Part of a Disease Process

Signs and symptoms that are associated routinely with a disease process should not be assigned as additional codes, unless other instructions exist. Once the reason for the signs and symptoms are known and these complaints routinely occur with that particular disease process, the signs and symptoms are not coded. For example, abdominal pain is a common symptom of acute appendicitis and is not coded when the reason for abdominal pain is attributed to the appendicitis. The coder's knowledge of disease processes is essential to coding, especially to avoid coding the unnecessary sign and symptoms codes.

Conditions That Are Not an Integral Part of a Disease Process

Additional signs and symptoms that may not be associated routinely with a disease process should be coded when present. Again, the coder's knowledge of disease pathology is essential to coding. The coder needs to know when the physician describes accompanying signs and symptoms with a disease whether to code these conditions or not. For example, if a patient with a skull fracture is in a coma, the coma is assigned an additional code. Not every patient with a skull fracture will be in a coma.

Acute and Chronic Conditions

If a patient has both the acute form and the chronic form of one disease, the coder must identify in the Alphabetic Index if there are separate entries at the same indentation level. If there are two separate lines in the Alphabetic Index for acute and chronic forms, then both codes are assigned. The acute or subacute code is sequenced first, followed by the chronic code for the disease. For example, the doctor may describe the patient's condition as acute and chronic pancreatitis. The Alphabetic Index has the following entries:

Pancreatitis
Acute K85.9
  alcoholic induced K85.2
  biliary K85.1
  drug induced K85.3
  gallstone K85.1
  idiopathic K85.0
  specified NEC K85.8
Chronic (infectious) K86.1
  alcohol induced K86.1
  recurrent K86.1
  relapsing K86.1

The code for acute pancreatitis, K85.9, is listed first with an additional code for chronic pancreatitis, K86.1, as both conditions are listed in the Alphabetic Index at the same indentation level.

Combination Codes

A combination code is a single code used to classify two diagnoses. A combination code may also represent a diagnosis with an associated secondary process or manifestation. Finally, a combination code can be a diagnosis with an associated complication.

Combination codes are identified by referring to subterm entries in the Alphabetic Index that identify conditions that are associated with or due to each other. Combination codes are also identified by reading all the includes and excludes notes in the Tabular List. Combination codes are only assigned when the one code fully identifies the condition.

Multiple coding should not occur when the classification provides a combination code that clearly identifies all of the elements documented in the diagnosis. An additional code should be used as a secondary code only when the combination code lacks necessary specificity in describing the manifestation or complication. There may be a third condition that exists with two other conditions that requires an additional code. For example, a patient may have acute bronchitis with bronchiectasis and tobacco use. Two codes are required: J47.0, a combination code for bronchiectasis with acute bronchitis, and Z72.0, the code for tobacco use.

Sequela or Late Effects

A condition that is produced by another illness or an injury and remains after the acute phase of the illness or injury is referred to as a **sequela**. There is no time period as to when a sequela must appear or be present. The condition can be identified at the same time as the original disease, such as dysphagia that occurs with a cerebral infarction. Other conditions may occur a period of time after the acute phase of the illness is over, for example, the scar that remains after a burn heals.

Two codes are required for coding sequela conditions. The first reported code is the condition that exists at present or the sequela. The second code is the original conditions identified as the cause of the present condition. However, the code for the acute phase of an illness that led to the sequela is never used with a code for the late effect.

There are exceptions to the above guideline:

1. The code for the sequela is followed by a manifestation code identified in the Tabular List and title.

2. The sequela code has been expanded at the fourth, fifth, or sixth character levels to include the manifestations.

The main term "sequela" must be referenced in the Alphabetic Index to identify if a combination code for the sequela and the underlying cause exists. In the Tabular List, an instructional note may appear under these category codes to "code first condition resulting from (sequela of)" that particular category. In the Alphabetic Index, following the main term "sequela," is the direction term "see also condition" to remind the coder that other entries in the Alphabetic Index are also applicable to coding of these conditions.

Below is a step-by-step example of how to accurately code a sequela and the underlying condition:

A doctor documents the following condition: scar of the skin on the face due to previous third-degree burn of face. The coder must recognize the condition present today is the scar and the cause of the scar was the previous third-degree burn on the face.

First the coder accesses the term "scar" in the Alphabetic Index as follows:

Alphabetic Index:

Scar, scarring (see also Cicatrix) L90.5

Cicatrix, skin L90.5

Then the coder must confirm the code in the Tabular List as L90.5. There are no further instructions in the Tabular List. The code does not include any anatomic locations so all scars are coded here. However, the coder must know to identify the cause of the scar having been stated as due to a previous burn on the face.

The coder must translate that fact to the word "sequela" to identify the burn and use the Alphabetic Index again as follows:

Alphabetic Index:

Sequela, burn and corrosion—code to injury with seventh character S

Burn, face—see Burn, head

Burn, head, third degree, T20.30

Again, the coder must access the Tabular List to review the entry of code T20.20 to determine if more characters are required to complete the coding assignment.

T20.30 requires a seventh character of S for sequela; therefore, a placeholder character of X is needed in the sixth position, that is, T20.30XS.

After following these steps, the coder concludes that the coding of scar of the skin of the face due to previous third-degree burn of the face is coded as L90.5 and T20.30XS

Impending or Threatened Condition

According to the *ICD-10-CM Draft Official Guidelines for Coding and Reporting*, Guideline I.B.12, impending or threatened conditions are coded as follows:

If a condition described at the time of discharge as "impending" or "threatened," it should be coded as follows:

1. If the condition did occur, code as a confirmed diagnosis

2. If the condition did not occur, reference the Alphabetic Index to determine if the condition has a subentry term for "impending" or "threatened" and also reference main term entries for "Impending" and for "Threatened"

   a. If the subterms are listed, assign the given code
   b. If the subterms are not listed, code the existing underlying condition(s) and not the condition described as impending or threatened.

Reporting Same Diagnosis Code More Than Once

According to the *ICD-10-CM Draft Official Guidelines for Coding and Reporting*, Guideline I.B.13, "each unique ICD-10-CM diagnosis codes may be reported only once for an encounter. This applies to bilateral conditions when there are no distinct codes identifying laterality or two different conditions classified to the same ICD-10-CM diagnosis code."

Laterality

Some ICD-10-CM diagnosis codes include laterality or whether the condition exists on the right or left side of the body. For bilateral sites, the final character of the code indicates laterality. An unspecified side code is available for use if the side of the body is not identified in the medical record. If no bilateral code is provided and the condition is bilateral, the coder must assign separate codes for both the left and right side.

Documentation for BMI and Pressure Ulcer Stages

In the *ICD-10-CM Draft Official Guidelines for Coding and Reporting*, Guideline I.B.14 describes how to code according to the documentation of the body mass index and the pressure ulcer stages.

> For the body mass index (BMI) and pressure ulcer stage codes, the code assignment may be made based on the medical record documentation from clinicians who are not the patient's provider (such as a physician or other qualified healthcare practitioner legally accountable for establishing the patient's diagnosis.) This information is typically documented by other clinicians involved in the care of the patient, for example, a dietitian documents the BMI and nurses often document the pressure ulcer stages. However, the associated diagnosis (such as overweight, obesity or pressure ulcer) must be documented by the patient's provider. If there is conflicting medical record documentation, either from the same clinician or different clinicians, the patient's attending provider should be queried for clarification.

> The BMI codes should only be reported as secondary diagnoses. As with all other secondary diagnosis codes, the BMI codes should only be assigned when they meet the definition of a reportable additional diagnosis.

Syndromes

Guideline I.B.15 in the *ICD-10-CM Draft Official Guidelines for Coding and Reporting* describes the coding of named syndromes.

> The coder should follow the Alphabetic Index guidance when coding named syndromes. In the absence of Alphabetic Index guidance, the coder should assign codes for each of the documented individual manifestations or conditions identified as the syndrome when the multiple conditions exist at the same time.

Documentation of Complications of Care

In Guideline I.B.16 of the *ICD-10-CM Draft Official Guidelines for Coding and Reporting*, the coder is given direction on how and when to assign complication codes.

> Code assignment is based on the provider's documentation of the relationship between the condition and the care or procedure. The guideline extends to any complication of care, regardless of the chapter the code is located in. It is important to note that not all conditions that occur during or following medical care or surgery are classified as complications. There must be a cause-and-effect relationship between the care and the condition, and an indication in the documentation that it

is a complication. The physician should be queried or asked for clarification if the complication is not clearly documented.

Basic Steps in ICD-10-CM Coding

The basic steps described in this chapter should be followed when assigning a code in ICD-10-CM. To code each disease or condition completely and accurately, the coder should:

1. Identify all main terms included in the diagnostic statement

2. Locate each main term in the Alphabetic Index

3. Refer to any subterms indented under the main term. The subterms form individual line entries and describe essential differences by site, etiology, or clinical type

4. Follow the instructions (see, see also) provided in the Alphabetic Index if the needed code is not located under the first main entry consulted

5. Verify the code selected in the Tabular List

6. Read and be guided by any instructional terms in the Tabular List

7. Assign codes to their highest level of specificity, up to a total of seven characters if applicable

8. Continue coding the diagnostic statement until all the component elements are fully identified

ICD-10-CM Review Exercises: Chapter 1

Assign the correct ICD-10-CM diagnosis codes to the following exercises.

1. Acute appendicitis with perforation

   _____

2. Streptococcal pneumonia

   _____

3. Precordial chest pain

   _____

4. Acute cor pulmonale

   _____

5. Osteoarthrosis, primary of right ankle

   _____

6. Toxic nodular goiter

   _____

(Continued on next page)

ICD-10-CM Review Exercises: Chapter 1 (Continued)

7. Extra thyroid gland

8. Angiodysplasia of the colon with hemorrhage

9. Acute tracheobronchitis with bronchospasm (age 16)

10. Arteriosclerotic heart disease of native coronary artery with angina pectoris

11. Nephritis due to systemic lupus erythematosus

12. Prenatal care, normal first pregnancy, second trimester

13. Traumatic comminuted fracture of left femur involving the intertrochanteric section, initial visit

14. Prostatitis due to Trichomonas

15. Carotid artery occlusion with cerebral infarction. Essential hypertension

16. Acute hepatitis C with hepatic coma

17. Acute lymphoblastic leukemia in remission

18. Benign carcinoid tumor of the appendix

19. Enlarged prostate with urinary obstruction

20. Personal history of breast carcinoma (malignant neoplasm)

Chapter 2

Introduction to ICD-10-PCS

Learning Objectives

At the conclusion of this chapter, you should be able to:

1. Identify the design characteristics of the ICD-10 Procedure Coding System (ICD-10-PCS)

2. Describe the general design principles of the ICD-10-PCS

3. Describe the code structure of the ICD-10-PCS codes

4. Explain how the ICD-10-PCS Index is organized and used

5. Explain the general organization of the ICD-10-PCS code tables

6. Describe how a code is constructed using the Index and Tables

7. Identify the seven characters that comprise an ICD-10-PCS code

8. List the 16 sections in the Medical and Surgical and Medical and Surgical-related section of codes

9. Describe the concept of the root operation used in ICD-10-PCS

10. Specify the options to describe the approach used to perform a procedure

11. Identify the nine groups and 31 root operations

12. Define the seven different approaches used in the root operations

13. Identify how to code multiple procedures

14. Assign procedure codes using the ICD-10-PCS system

Key Terms

- Access location
- Appliances: simple, mechanical, electronic
- Approach

- Body part
- Body Part Key
- Body system
- Characters
- Completeness
- Device
- Device Aggregation Table
- Device Key
- Electronic appliances
- Expandability
- External approach
- Grafts and prostheses
- Implant
- Index
- Instrumentation
- Method of approach
- Multiaxial
- Qualifier
- Root operation
- Section
- Simple or mechanical appliances
- Standardized terminology
- Tables
- Values

ICD-10-PCS References

The Centers for Medicare and Medicaid Services (CMS) website for the 2013 ICD-10-PCS and general equivalence mappings (GEMs) has essential references for the coder who is learning ICD-10-PCS coding now and for reference in the future as their coding knowledge of ICD-10-PCS matures. The home page for ICD-10-PCS is at http://www.cms.gov/Medicare/Coding/ICD10/2013-ICD-10-PCS-GEMs.html.

The files on the website for the 2013 version of ICD-10-PCS contain the actual coding system as well as background material, references, and ICD-10-PCS guidelines. The coder should thoroughly review all the downloadable files on the site for daily use. Coders should access the CMS website to find the updated 2013 ICD-10-PCS Reference Manual.

The downloadable files on the CMS website include the following:

- 2013 Official ICD-10-PCS Coding Guidelines
- 2013 Version—What's new
- 2013 Code Tables and Index
- 2013 PCS Long and Abbreviated Titles
- 2013 Development of the ICD-10 Procedure Coding System (ICD-10-PCS)
- 2013 ICD-10-PCS Reference Manual
- 2013 Addendum

- PCS Slides for 2013

- 2013 General Equivalence Mappings (GEMS)—Procedure Codes and Guide

- 2013 Reimbursement Mappings—Procedure Codes and Guide

Especially useful to the new ICD-10-PCS coder (and the coding instructors) is the document titled "2013 Development of the ICD-10 Procedure Coding System ICD-10-PCS" written by the developers of the system. It gives the reader a thorough presentation on the design, development, and testing of the ICD-10-PCS system (Averill et al. 2013).

For the first time coders have a set of guidelines for using a procedure coding system, that is, the *ICD-10-PCS Official Guidelines for Coding and Reporting*. In the past, coding guidelines addressed only diagnosis coding. The guidelines are provided by CMS and the National Center for Health Statistics (NCHS), two federal agencies responsible for maintaining the ICD classification systems in the United States. The guidelines are to be used as a reference with the official version of ICD-10-PCS as published on the CMS website. The Cooperating Parties for ICD-10-PCS have approved the guidelines. The Cooperating Parties are representatives from the American Hospital Association (AHA), the American Health Information Management Association (AHIMA), CMS, and NCHS. The full guidelines can be found at http://www.cms .gov/Medicare/Coding/ICD10/Downloads/pcs_2013_guidelines.pdf.

The *ICD-10-PCS Official Guidelines for Coding and Reporting* is referenced throughout this chapter. A complete document is available in Appendix F.

Characteristics of the ICD-10 Procedure Coding System

In 1992, CMS began the process of replacing ICD-9-CM Volume 3 by funding a research project to design a new procedure coding system. In 1995 CMS awarded 3M Health Information Systems a three-year contract to complete the development of the new procedure coding system. The new system is the International Classification of Diseases, Tenth Revision, Procedure Coding System (ICD-10-PCS).

ICD-10-PCS is a multiaxial seven-character alphanumeric code structure. ICD-10-PCS provides a unique code for all substantially different procedures, and allows new procedures to be easily incorporated as new codes. It is exclusively designed for the United States. ICD-10-PCS was initially released in 1998 and has been updated several times since the first version. The 2013 version of ICD-10-PCS was available on the CMS website in June 2012.

ICD-10-PCS is scheduled to be implemented on October 1, 2014 for reporting inpatient procedures on electronic healthcare claims transactions, replacing Volume 3 of ICD-9-CM.

Design Considerations for ICD-10-PCS

The report *2013 Development of the ICD-10 Procedure Coding System (ICD-10-PCS)* identified four objectives that were included in the design of ICD-10-PCS: Completeness, Expandability, Multiaxial, and Standardized Terminology (Averill et al. 2013).

Completeness

The objective of **completeness** means there should be a unique code for all substantially different procedures. Different procedures performed on different body parts with differing approaches will have a unique code. To meet this objective, there are approximately 72,000 ICD-10-PCS codes.

Expandability

When new procedures are developed, the structure of ICD-10-PCS should allow a code for the new procedure to be easily identified. The concept of **expandability** means the structure of the codes allows for changes to be made easily by adding values as needed or using existing values to identify new procedures.

Multiaxial

The ICD-10-PCS consists of independent characters. **Multiaxial** is a term to describe the ability of a nomenclature to express the meaning of a concept across several axes. Each individual axis retains its meaning across broad ranges of codes as much as possible. For example, the third character is the root operation to describe the objective of the procedure. In some sections, the title of the third character changes, for example, in radiology the third character is "root type" but it still reflects the objective of the procedure.

Standardized Terminology

ICD-10-PCS includes definitions of the terminology used. ICD-10-PCS does not use multiple meanings for the same term. The **standardized terminology** in ICD-10-PCS means each term has a specific meaning or definition. The coding system tries to be as specific as possible with only limited options for "not elsewhere classified" (NEC) procedures. There are NEC options to allow for updates to the system as needed between updates. If the coder finds there is a new device being used during the year and there is not a device value for that particular procedure, the coder can use the value of "other device" until a possible update for that device is added when the coding system is updated on an annual basis.

General Design Principles

Four design principles were incorporated in the development of ICD-10-PCS according to the report *2013 Development of the ICD-10 Procedure Coding System (ICD-10-PCS)*.

There is no diagnosis included in the ICD-10-PCS procedure code description. The reason the procedure is being performed is not important for coding of the procedures. The ICD-10-CM diagnosis code identifies the diagnosis being treated. The ICD-10-PCS code identifies what procedure is being performed according to the objective of the procedure, the approach, device used, and so forth.

A second principle was to limit the "not otherwise specified" (NOS) codes available in ICD-10-PCS. The coder needs facts about the procedure in order to code it. The operative report prepared by the physician is essential; in fact, it is hard to imagine how a procedure would be coded without an operative report. The coder needs, at a minimum, the objective of the procedures, the body system and body part involved, and the approach used to perform the procedure.

Similarly, there is generally no need for an NEC code in ICD-10-PCS. NEC values in the PCS Tables are identified as the "other" specified typed. For example, in the Medical and

Surgical section there is a value for "other" for the device character. In the Imaging section, there is a value for "other" for the type of contrast used that is not high osmolar or low osmolar contrast material. In the Physician Rehabilitation section, there is a value for "other equipment" to identify when something different than the specified type of equipment is used. Otherwise, the values specifically identify the significant components of the procedure in the ICD-10-PCS codes.

Finally, the design of the system allows for all procedures to be coded with ICD-10-PCS. Each variation of a procedure can be identified with the specific values available for the body part involved, the approach used, any devices left in place, and such. Some of the combination of values that create a code may not be performed frequently or even at all at this time, yet a procedure code is available if needed.

A summary of the characteristics of the ICD-10-PCS structure is found in table 2.1.

Table 2.1. Characteristics of ICD-10-PCS codes

ICD-10-PCS	
Overall objectives	Completeness Expandability Multi-axial Standardized terminology
Design considerations	No diagnostic information included Limited NOS and NEC codes Specificity included
Codes are alphanumeric	Seven characters using digits 0–9 and letters A–H, J–N, P–Z
Consistent number of characters	All codes are seven characters long

Code Structure

The ICD-10-PCS code is constructed by the coder using the Alphabetic Index and the Code Tables. A complete seven-character code made by found in the Alphabetic Index but this should not be the expectation of the ICD-10-PCS coder. The process of constructing codes in ICD-10-PCS is intended to be logical and consistent and uses individual letters and numbers called **values** to occupy the seven digits or letters of the codes. The seven digits or letters of a code are called **characters**.

Each character has one of 34 possible values. A value can be a number from 0–9 or a letter from A–H, J–N, and P–Z. The alphabetic letters O and I are not used so they are not confused with the numbers zero (0) and one (1). An example of a complete code is 0DB68ZX for esophagogastroduodenoscopy with gastric diagnostic biopsy.

Each code is constructed by choosing a specific value for each of the seven characters. Based on the details of the procedure documented, values are assigned for each character specifying the section, the body system, root operation, body part, approach, device, and qualifier.

Because the definition of each character is a function of its physical position in the code, the same value placed in a different position means something different. For example, a drainage procedure performed in the central nervous system could have the value of 0 (zero) used in several characters:

First character 0   = Medical and Surgical

Second character 0 = Central Nervous System

Fourth character 0 = Brain

Fifth character 0   = Open approach

Sixth character 0   = Drainage device

All codes in ICD-10-PCS are seven characters long. Each character in the seven-character code represents a particular aspect of the procedure. For example, in the main section of ICD-10-PCS, Medical and Surgical, the characters are used as follows:

Character 1 = Section of ICD-10-PCS

Character 2 = Body System

Character 3 = Root Operation

Character 4 = Body Part

Character 5 = Approach

Character 6 = Device

Character 7 = Qualifier

An ICD-10-PCS code is best understood as being the result of a process rather than an isolated fixed process of accessing the Alphabetic Index to locate a code. The process consists of assigning values from among the value choices for that part of the system according to the design of the system.

More information about the specifics of the seven characters of the ICD-10-PCS code is discussed later in this chapter.

The ICD-10-PCS Format: Index and Tables

The ICD-10-PCS coding system is composed of two parts: the Index and the Tables.

The **Index** provides an alphabetic listing of procedure titles. Codes can be found in the Index based on the general type of procedure, for example, excision or resection. In addition, the Index contains entries for more commonly used procedure titles, such as cholecystectomy or percutaneous endoscopic gastrostomy (PEG).

When the term is located in the Index, the Index specifies the first three or four values of the code, for example, 0DT, or directs the coder to see another term. Each **Table** also identifies the first three values of the code. Based on the first three values of the code, the corresponding Table can be located. The Table is then used to obtain the complete code by specifying the last four values.

Each Table is composed of rows that specify the valid combinations of code values. In ICD-10-PCS, the upper portion of each Table specifies the values for the first three characters of the codes in that Table. In the Medical and Surgical section, the first three characters are the section, the body system, and the root operation.

In table 2.2, the values 0DT specify that Section = Medical and Surgical (0); Body System = Gastrointestinal System (D); and Root Operation = Resection (T).

Table 2.2. 0DT: Medical and Surgical, Gastrointestinal System, Resection

Section: 0 Medical and Surgical
Body System: D Gastrointestinal System
Root Operation: T Resection—Cutting out or off, without replacement, all of a body part

Body Part Character 4	Approach Character 5	Device Character 6	Qualifier Character 7
1 Esophagus, Upper 2 Esophagus, Middle 3 Esophagus, Lower 4 Esophagogastric Junction 5 Esophagus 6 Stomach 7 Stomach, Pylorus 8 Small Intestine 9 Duodenum A Jejunum B Ileum C Ileocecal Valve E Large Intestine F Large Intestine, Right G Large Intestine, Left H Cecum J Appendix K Ascending Colon L Transverse Colon M Descending Colon N Sigmoid Colon P Rectum Q Anus	0 Open 4 Percutaneous Endoscopic 7 Via Natural or Artificial Opening 8 Via Natural or Artificial Opening Endoscopic	Z No Device	Z No Qualifier
R Anal Sphincter S Greater Omentum T Lesser Omentum	0 Open 4 Percutaneous Endoscopic	Z No Device	Z No Qualifier

Source: CMS 2013

In Table 0DT, for the root operation, Resection, the root operation definition is provided. The lower portion of the Table specifies all the valid combinations of the remaining characters four through seven. The four columns in the table specify the last four characters. In the Medical and Surgical section the columns are labeled "Body Part," "Approach," "Device," and "Qualifier" respectively. Each row in the table specifies the valid combination of values for characters four through seven. The Tables contain only the combinations of values that result in a valid procedure code. Also, the coder must stay on one row of a Table to select a valid procedure code.

The following is an example of how to use the ICD-10-PCS Index and Tables. The procedure to be coded is an open appendectomy.

The coder accesses the Index using the term "appendectomy" and finds two entries under Appendectomy—see Excision, Appendix 0DBJ and see Resection, Appendix 0DTJ. The coder must know the definition of "excision" and "resection" for this example. Because an appendectomy is the cutting out or off the entire appendix, the entry for "resection" should be used. Using the first three values, the coder locates Table 0DT in the ICD-10-PCS code book. There are four columns to be considered with values that are appropriate with 0DT. The Index has given the code the fourth character J for appendix. The coder needs to select the fifth, sixth, and seventh characters to complete the code. The coder must stay on the same

35

row where the fourth character J for appendix is located. The choice for approach for an open appendectomy is 0 for open. There are no choices for the device and the qualifier so the sixth and seventh characters are Z and Z. By collecting the seven characters together, the coder uses 0DTJ0ZZ for coding an open appendectomy. The code for a laparoscopic appendectomy has one character different for the approach. The laparoscopic appendectomy would be coded 0DTJ4ZZ, as shown in table 2.3

Table 2.3.   **Laparoscopic appendectomy 0DTJ4ZZ**

Character	Code	Explanation
Section	0	Medical and Surgical
Body System	D	Gastrointestinal
Root Operation	T	Resection
Body Part	J	Appendix
Approach	4	Percutaneous Endoscopic
Device	Z	No Device
Qualifier	Z	No Qualifier

INDEX: Appendectomy, see Resection, Appendix 0DTJ

The ICD-10-PCS Code

All codes in ICD-10-PCS have seven characters. Each character represents an aspect of or a fact about the procedure. For example, in the first section of ICD-10-PCS, Medical and Surgical, the characters represent the following:

1	2	3	4	5	6	7
Section	Body System	Root Operation	Body Part	Approach	Device	Qualifier

Each of the characters has a defined meaning:

Character 1: Section—The first character of a code determines the broad procedure category, or **section**, where the code is located. To assign an ICD-10-PCS code, the section is identified as where the procedure is included in ICD-10-PCS structure. For example, a lung biopsy is a medical and surgical procedure, a CAT scan of the lung is an imaging procedure, and mechanical ventilation of the lungs is a procedure in the extracorporeal assistance and performance section. The 16 sections of ICD-10-PCS are shown in table 2.4. The first section of ICD-10-PCS, Medical and Surgical, includes the vast majority of codes. Codes in the Medical and Surgical section all begin with the 0 (zero) character. Other sections will be covered in the next portion of this discussion.

Character 2: Body System—The second character defines the body system, which is the general physiological system or anatomical region involved. Examples of the 31 body systems in the Medical and Surgical section include the Central Nervous System, Upper Arteries, Respiratory System, Tendons, Muscles, and Upper Joints. Note that in some of the sections of ICD-10-PCS, the second character may have an alternate meaning. For example, in the

Table 2.4. Section (Character 1) of ICD-10-PCS

0	Medical and Surgical	8	Other Procedures
1	Obstetrics	9	Chiropractic
2	Placement	B	Imaging
3	Administration	C	Nuclear Medicine
4	Measurement and Monitoring	D	Radiation Oncology
5	Extracorporeal Assistance and Performance	F	Physical Rehabilitation and Diagnostic Audiology
6	Extracorporeal Therapies	G	Mental Health
7	Osteopathic	H	Substance Abuse Treatment

Physical Rehabilitation and Diagnostic Audiology section (F), the second character indicates whether this is Rehabilitation or Diagnostic Audiology.

Character 3: Root Operation—The third character defines the root operation, or the objective of the procedure being performed. Examples of root operations are Excision, Bypass, Division, and Fragmentation. In some sections, the root operation is known as the root type. For example, in the Imaging section (B), the third character indicates the root type, not the root operation. Each of the root operations is defined in ICD-10-PCS. In addition to the discussion of root operations that is presented in this chapter, the coder should reference Appendix A: Root Operations Definitions and Appendix B: Comparison of Medical and Surgical Root Operations in the ICD-10-PCS code book.

Character 4: Body Part—The fourth character generally defines the **body part** or specific anatomical site where the procedure was performed. The second character, which represents the body system, provides only a general indication of the procedure site while this character, indicates the precise body part. Examples of body parts are Duodenum, Uterus, Liver, and Common Bile Duct. Body part values can vary in some sections of ICD-10-PCS. In the Physical Rehabilitation and Diagnostic Audiology section, for example, the fourth character represents the body system or region rather than the body part. For example, Neurological System-Whole Body and Integumentary System-Head and Neck are body system/regions in the Physical Rehabilitation section.

Character 5: Approach—The fifth character defines the **approach**, or the surgical technique used to reach the operative site. Seven different approach values are used in the Medical and Surgical section of ICD-10-PCS: Open, Percutaneous, Percutaneous Endoscopic, Via Natural or Artificial Opening, Via Natural or Artificial Opening Endoscopic, Via Natural or Artificial Opening with Percutaneous Endoscopic Assistance, and External. The meaning of the fifth character can vary in sections other than the Medical and Surgical section. For example, in the Imaging section (B), the fifth character indicates the contrast used in the imaging procedure.

Character 6: Device—The sixth character defines the device and depending on the procedure performed. There may or may not be a device left in place at the end of the procedure. Device values fall into four basic categories:

1. Grafts and Prostheses
2. Implants
3. Simple or Mechanical Appliances
4. Electronic Appliances

Again, not all sections in ICD-10-PCS include device as the sixth character. For example, in the Radiation Oncology section (D), the sixth character represents the isotope used, if applicable.

Character 7: Qualifier—The seventh character defines a qualifier for a particular code. A **qualifier** specifies an additional attribute of the procedure, if applicable. In each of the sections the qualifier has a unique meaning and even a unique meaning within different root operations in a section. For example, in the Medical and Surgical section for the root operation of Transplantation, the qualifier identifies if the organ transplanted into the body is allogeneic, syngeneic, or zooplastic in type. For the bypass procedures in the Medical and Surgical section, the qualifier with the bypass root operations identifies where in the body the bypass procedure ended. This qualifier rule does not apply to surgery on the heart and great vessels. For example, a femoral-popliteal vascular bypass procedure has the qualifier of L for the popliteal artery because the bypass is created from the femoral vessel to the popliteal vessel where it ends.

If a given character does not have a value assigned, the Z value is used. This is particularly frequent for the sixth and seventh characters, which generally represent the device and the qualifier.

In summary, the first through fifth characters are always assigned a specific value, but the device (sixth character) and the qualifier (seventh character) are not applicable to all procedures. The value Z is used for the sixth and seventh characters to indicate that a specific device or qualifier does not apply to the procedure.

Overall Organization of ICD-10-PCS

ICD-10-PCS is composed of 16 sections, represented by the numbers 0 through 9 and the letters B through D and F through H. The broad procedure categories contained in these sections range from surgical procedures to substance abuse treatment. The 16 sections are contained in three main areas: the Medical and Surgical section, the Medical and Surgical-related sections, and the Ancillary sections.

The first section, Medical and Surgical, begins with the section value of 0 and contains the majority of procedures typically reported in an inpatient setting. Sections with values 1 through 9 of ICD-10-PCS comprise the Medical and Surgical-related sections. These Medical and Surgical and Medical and Surgical-related sections include the following:

Section Value	Description
0	Medical and Surgical
1	Obstetrics
2	Placement
3	Administration
4	Measurement and Monitoring
5	Extracorporeal Assistance and Performance
6	Extracorporeal Therapies
7	Osteopathic
8	Other Procedures
9	Chiropractic

Codes in sections 1 through 9 are structured for the most part like their counterparts in the Medical and Surgical section, with a few exceptions. For example, in sections 5 and 6, the fifth character is defined as the duration instead of approach. The meaning of the sixth character is also often different in the Medical and Surgical-related section:

- In section 3 defines the sixth character represents the substance.

- In sections 4 and 5 define the sixth character represents the function.

- In sections 7 through 9 the sixth character represents the method.

Sections B through D and F through H comprise the Ancillary sections of ICD-10-PCS, which can be described as follows:

Section Value	Description
B	Imaging
C	Nuclear Medicine
D	Radiation Oncology
F	Physical Rehabilitation and Diagnostic Audiology
G	Mental Health
H	Substance Abuse Treatment

The definitions of some characters in the Ancillary sections also differ from those seen in the previous sections. For example, in the Imaging section, the third character is defined as the root type, and the fifth and sixth characters define contrast and contrast or qualifier, respectively.

The Medical and Surgical Section (0)

Since the Medical and Surgical section is the largest in ICD-10-PCS, discussion of the meanings of the second through seventh characters will concentrate on the Medical and Surgical section.

Body Systems

The second character in the Medical and Surgical section represents the general **body system**. The way in which ICD-10-PCS defines a body system, however, is a bit different than the usual meaning of the term. A review of the following list shows how some customary body systems are given multiple body-system values. For example, note the circulatory system does not have a single value.

Values	ICD-10-PCS Body Systems
0	Central Nervous System
1	Peripheral Nervous System
2	Heart and Great Vessels
3	Upper Arteries
4	Lower Arteries

(Continued)

Values	ICD-10-PCS Body Systems (Continued)
5	Upper Veins
6	Lower Veins
7	Lymphatic and Hemic System
8	Eye
9	Ear, Nose, Sinus
B	Respiratory System
C	Mouth and Throat
D	Gastrointestinal System
F	Hepatobiliary System and Pancreas
G	Endocrine System
H	Skin and Breast
J	Subcutaneous Tissue and Fascia
K	Muscles
L	Tendons
M	Bursae and Ligaments
N	Head and Facial Bones
P	Upper Bones
Q	Lower Bones
R	Upper Joints
S	Lower Joints
T	Urinary System
U	Female Reproductive System
V	Male Reproductive System
W	Anatomic Region, General
X	Anatomical Region, Upper Extremities
Y	Anatomic Regions, Lower Extremities

Root Operations

The third character in the Medical and Surgical section is the **root operation**. There are a total of 31 root operations in the Medical and Surgical section, each representing the specific objective of the procedure. These 31 root operations are divided into nine groups that share similar attributes. Appendix B of the ICD-10-PCS code book describes the nine groups of procedures.

The nine groups are as follows:

1. Procedures that take out some or all of a body part

2. Procedures that take out solids, fluids, or gases from a body part

3. Procedures involving cutting or separation only

4. Procedures that put in or put back or move some or all of a body part

5. Procedures that alter the diameter or route of a tubular body part

6. Procedures that always involve a device

7. Procedures involving examination only

8. Procedures that define other repairs

9. Procedures that define other objectives

Objective of the Procedure

In ICD-10-PCS, each component of a procedure is defined separated. The third, fourth, and fifth characters together are used to describe the objective of the procedure. The third character is the root operation, introduced just above, which technically defines the objective of the procedure, that is, to excise, to resect, or to replace for example. The fourth character identifies the body part upon which the procedure was performed. The fifth character describes the approach and further contributes to describing the procedure's objective.

The procedure coded in ICD-10-PCS is the procedure that was actually performed. If the procedure performed was not what was intended when the procedure started, that does not matter. The intended procedure may not always be completed. When the intended or anticipated procedure is changed or discontinued, the root operation is coded based on the actual procedure that was performed.

Multiple Procedures

If multiple procedures are performed that are defined by distinct objectives during a single operative episode, then multiple procedure codes are used. For example, obtaining a vein graft used for coronary artery bypass surgery is coded as a separate procedure from the bypass itself.

Multiple procedures are coded according to the following rules:

- The same root operation is performed on different body parts that have distinct body part values in ICD-10-PCS. For example, a biopsy or diagnostic excision is performed on the duodenum and rectum.

- The same root operation is repeated on different body sites that are included in the same body part value. For example, a biopsy is performed on the scalene muscle and the platysma muscle, which are both included in the neck muscle body part.

- Distinctive procedures with multiple root operations are performed on the same body part. For example, biopsy of the pancreas and partial pancreatectomy is performed.

- The intended procedure cannot be accomplished and is converted to a different approach. For example, a laparoscopic nephrectomy is attempted but must be converted to an open nephrectomy. The laparoscopic portion of the procedure is coded as an inspection and the open procedure is coded as an open resection for the nephrectomy.

Redo of Procedures

If the procedure performed is a complete or partial redo of a previous procedure, the root operation used to code the procedure is the root operation that identifies what was the actual procedure performed. The terminology used by a physician of "redo" is not necessarily always a "revision" procedure according to the definition of the root operation of 'revision." For example, a complete redo of a knee replacement procedure, which requires putting in a new prosthesis, is coded to the root operation Replacement instead of Revision. The physician is likely to describe this procedure as a "revision arthroplasty" but the coder must use the definitions of the root operations to identify the objective of a Revision as actually a replacement procedure.

The correction of complications arising from the original procedure other than device complications as defined in the root operation Revision are also coded to the procedure performed. For example, a procedure to add mesh to the abdominal wall to repair a postoperative ventral hernia is coded to Supplement rather than Revision.

Body Part

The meaning of the fourth character in the Medical and Surgical section is body part. The value chosen for this character represents the specific part of the body system (character 2) on which the surgery was performed. Body parts may specify laterality. Some examples of body parts and their body systems in ICD-10-PCS are listed in the following:

Body System	Body Part Examples
Central Nervous System	Brain, Cerebral Hemisphere, Basal Ganglia, Olfactory Nerve, Optic Nerve, and such
Heart and Great Vessels	Coronary Artery, Atrium, Ventricle, Aortic Valve, Pulmonary Artery, and such
Gastrointestinal	Esophagus, Stomach, Small Intestine, Large Intestine, Cecum, Appendix, Rectum
Endocrine System	Pituitary Gland, Pineal Body, Adrenal Gland, Thyroid Gland, Parathyroid Gland

ICD-10-PCS does not provide a specific value for every body part. In those instances the body part value selected would be either the whole body part value (for example, alveolar process is part of the mandible), or in the instance of nerves and vessels, the body part value is coded to the closest proximal branch.

Approach

ICD-10-PCS defines approach as the technique used to reach the site of the procedure (CMS 2013). It is important to know the differences between the different approaches in order to correctly assign the fifth character value in the Medical and Surgical section. The approach is composed of three components: the access location, method, and type of instrumentation.

Access Location

For procedures performed on internal organs, the **access location** specifies the external site through which the internal organ is reached. There are two types of access location: skin or mucous membrane and external orifices. Except for the External approach, every other approach value includes one of these two access locations. The skin or mucous membrane can be incised or punctured to reach the procedure site. All open and percutaneous approach values use skin or mucous membrane as the access location. The site of a procedure can also be reached through an external opening. External openings can be natural (for example, mouth) or artificial (for example, nephrostomy stoma).

Method

The method specifies how the external access location is entered for procedures performed on an internal body part. An open **method of approach** means there was cutting through the skin or mucous membrane and other body layers to expose the site of the procedure. An instrumental approach method specifies the entry of instrumentation through the access location to the internal procedure site. Instrumentation can be introduced by puncture or minor incision or through an external opening. The puncture or minor incision should not be interpreted as an Open approach. An approach can define multiple methods. For example, the approach through a natural or artificial orifice with percutaneous endoscopic assistance uses both the orifice and the percutaneous endoscopic approach to reach the procedure site.

Type of Instrumentation

Specialized equipment or **instrumentation** is used to perform a procedure on an internal body part. The instrumentation is used in all internal approaches other than the basic Open approach.

Instrumentation may or may not be used to visualize the procedure site. For example, the bronchoscope is the instrument used to perform a bronchoscopy that permits the internal site of the procedure to be visualized. Instrumentation used to perform a needle biopsy of the pancreas does not visualize the site. The term "endoscopic" as used in approach values refers to instrumentation that permits a procedure site to be visualized.

External Approaches

The **external approach** is used when procedures are performed directly on the skin or mucous membrane. External procedures may be performed indirectly by the application of external force. Examples of procedures using external approaches are skin lesion excision, closed reduction of a fracture, and tonsillectomy (because the tonsils can be reached through the mouth). There are seven different approaches, as shown in table 2.5.

Table 2.5. **Definitions of seven approaches**

Approach	Definition	Examples
Open	Cutting through the skin or mucous membrane and any other body layers necessary to expose the site of the procedure	Open cholecystectomy, open appendectomy
Percutaneous	Entry, by puncture or minor incision, of instrumentation through the skin or mucous membrane and/or any other body layers necessary to reach the site of the procedure	Needle biopsy of breast
Percutaneous Endoscopic	Entry, by puncture or minor incision, of instrumentation through the skin or mucous membrane or any other body layers necessary to reach and visualize the site of the procedure	Laparoscopic cholecystectomy, laparoscopic appendectomy
Via Natural or Artificial Opening	Entry of instrumentation through a natural or artificial external opening to reach the site of the procedure	Insertion of Foley urinary catheter, endotracheal intubation
Via Natural or Artificial Opening Endoscopic	Entry of instrumentation through a natural or artificial external opening to reach and visualize the site of the procedure	Colonoscopy, cystoscopy, esophagogastroduodenoscopy
Via Natural or Artificial Opening Endoscopic with Percutaneous Endoscopic Assistance	Entry of instrumentation through a natural or artificial external opening to reach and visualize the site of the procedure, and entry, by puncture or minor incision, of instrumentation through the skin or mucous membrane and any other body layers necessary to aid in the performance of the procedure	Laparoscopic assisted vaginal hysterectomy
External	Procedures performed directly on the skin or mucous membrane and procedures performed indirectly by the application of external force through the skin or mucous membrane	Closed reduction of fracture of radius and ulna, extraction of upper or lower teeth

Source: Averill et al. 2013

Device and Qualifier

In the Medical and Surgical section, the sixth character specifies devices that remain after the procedure is completed. The seventh character, qualifier, is used with certain procedures to define an additional attribute of the procedure.

A **device** can be one of the following four objects left in the patient's body at the conclusion of the procedure:

- **Grafts and prostheses** are biological or synthetic material that takes the place of all or a portion of a body part. Examples of grafts and prostheses are artificial skin substitute, autologous venous tissue and metal, or ceramic joint prosthesis.

- **Implants** are therapeutic material that is not absorbed, eliminated, or incorporated into a body part. The therapeutic implants can be retained permanently in the body or removed when no longer needed. Examples of implants are internal fixation devices, an intramedullary nail, or a tissue expander implanted under the skin or muscle.

- **Simple or mechanical appliances** are biological or synthetic material that assists or prevents a physiological function. Examples of implants are a tracheostomy airway device, a monoplanar external fixation device, or an intraluminal device such as a vascular graft.

- **Electronic appliances** are those that assist, monitor, or take the place of or prevent a physiological function. Examples of appliances are a cardiac pacemaker generator, cochlear implant hearing device, or neurostimulator.

The ICD-10-PCS coding system book includes a Device Key in Appendix D of the code book. The **Device Key** includes brand names and generic names of devices to help the coder determine the PCS device description by referencing the name of the device used during a procedure. For example, if the physician uses a colonic Z-Stent during a procedure, the coder could find that device name in the Device Key and determine it is coded as an Intraluminal device. The value for Intraluminal device is D in the PCS code tables.

The **Device Aggregation Table** is also found in Appendix D of the ICD-10-PCS code book to assist the coder in correctly reporting the device used during a procedure. This table crosswalks particular device character value definitions for specific root operations in a specific body part to the more general device character value to be used when the root operation covers a wide range of body parts and the device character represents an entire family of devices. For example, if the physician inserted a cardiac resynchronization pacemaker pulse generator, the coder could use the Device Aggregation Table to determine that Cardiac Rhythm Related device would be the proper general device terminology for the code assignment.

Root Operations and Devices

Devices can be removed from the body but some devices cannot be removed without being replaced with another nonbiological appliance or another substitute for the body part.

The following root operations *may or may not* have specific devices as part of the procedure:

> Alteration
> Bypass
> Creation
> Dilation
> Drainage
> Fusion
> Occlusion

Reposition
Restriction

The following root operations *must* have specific devices coded with these procedures:

Change
Insertion
Removal
Replacement
Revision

The approach includes the fact that instrumentation is used to visualize the procedure site. This information is not specified in the device value.

The Insertion root operation is used when the procedure's objective is to put in a device. If there is another objective for a procedure but it includes the use of a device, then the root operation defining the underlying objective of a procedure is used instead. For example, the objective of an angioplasty of a vessel is "dilation" and is coded with the root operation of dilation. However, a stent may be used as part of the procedure and is reported as part of the dilation as the device character. The device used is identified by the device character. For example, if the procedure is to replace the shoulder joint, the root operation is Replacement and the prosthetic device is specified in the device character. The device is being "inserted" to "replace" the joint so the objective of the procedure is "replacement."

Materials incidental to a procedure such as clips, ligatures, and sutures are not what is meant by a device and are not specified in the device character.

Because new devices can be developed at any time, the value Other Device is provided as an option for use until a specific device value may be added to the system. With this option, a procedure that involves a new device can be coded as soon as the device is available instead of waiting until the coding system is updated in the future.

The following lists illustrate examples of the sixth character available in the urinary system.

Device—Character 6	
0	Drainage Device
2	Monitoring Device
3	Infusion Device
7	Autologous Tissue Substitute
C	Extraluminal Device
D	Intraluminal Device
J	Synthetic Substitute
K	Nonautologous Tissue Substitute
L	Artificial Sphincter
M	Stimulator Lead
Y	Other Device
Z	No Device

Qualifier

The seventh character is the qualifier, which can add more information to describe the procedure. Individual procedures have unique values for the qualifier in the seventh character position. The qualifiers may have a narrow application to a specific root operation, body system, or body part. For example, the qualifier can be used to identify the destination site in a bypass procedure. Other qualifiers identify the type of transplant performed such as allogeneic, syngeneic, and zooplastic. A common qualifier is X for Diagnostic, which is used, for example, to identify when a biopsy procedure is performed.

The following list illustrates examples of the seventh character available in the Heart and Great Vessels body system.

Qualifier—Character 7	
3	Coronary Artery
4	Coronary Vein
5	Coronary Circulation
7	Atrium, Left
8	Internal Mammary, Right
9	Internal Mammary, Left
B	Subclavian
C	Thoracic Artery
D	Carotid
F	Abdominal Artery
P	Pulmonary Trunk
Q	Pulmonary Artery, Right
R	Pulmonary Artery, Left
W	Aorta

ICD-10-PCS Appendices

The OptumInsight printed versions of the ICD-10-PCS coding system include several appendices available for the coder's use to completely and accurately assign a procedure code.

Appendix A contains the root operation definitions. For each section in the ICD-10-PCS system, an alphabetic list is presented with the root operation, value code, definition, explanation, and examples of procedures that would be coded with the particular root operation. Not only are the root operations for the Medical and Surgical section included, but all root operation definitions for other sections, such as Obstetrics, Placement, Administration, and so forth.

Appendix B is a comparison of medical and surgical root operations organized into nine groups that describe related procedures. For example, one group involves procedures that involve taking out some or all of a body part, that is, excision, resection, extraction, destruction, and detachment. For each of the root operations, the action, target of the procedure, clarification of the intent of the procedure, and examples of procedure titles that may be coded with each root operation are listed.

Appendix C is the **Body Part Key**. This handy reference is a long listing of anatomical terms with the corresponding PCS description that is used for the body part values in the ICD-10-PCS codes. The same entries contained in the Body Part Key are integrated in the Alphabetic Index of ICD-10-PCS for the coder to use. This appendix supplements the coder's knowledge of anatomy by confirming specific anatomic locations with the specific PCS description used for the body part values. For example, both the Alphabetic Index and Appendix C will remind the coder that the anatomic site of the anterior cruciate ligament (ACL) is identified as knee bursa and ligament in the ICD-10-PCM codes. This appendix is likely to be used frequently by the new coder and the experienced practitioner.

Appendix D is the Device Key and Aggregation Table that helps the coder translate a specific trade name or generic name of a device to the equivalent PCS description used for the device character value. Examples of the trade names for devices include BAK/C Interbody Cervical Fusion System, GORE DUALMESH, and Rheos System Lead. Generic names such as cystostomy tube, hip joint liner, and pump reservoir are also included. It is expected Appendix D will be a useful tool for coders to identify the correct PCS description for a device.

Appendix E contains the type and type qualifier definitions for procedures coded in Sections B through H. The largest number of type qualifiers and the definitions of each are from the Physical Rehabilitation and Diagnostic Audiology section of the ICD-10-PCS codes.

Appendix F is a one-page summary of the components of the medical and surgical approach definitions. Each of the seven approaches is described with its definition, access location, method of access, type of instrumentation used, and an example.

Appendix G is a lengthy list of the character meanings for section and body system. For example, the first page identifies all the applicable root operations, body parts, approaches, devices, and qualifiers within the Medical and Surgical section that could be used for procedures performed on the central nervous system. Appendix G is not intended to be use for coding purposes. Instead it is a reference for coders to get an overview of the applicable values for particular body system procedures.

Appendix H contains the answers to the coding exercises included in the code set for coding practice.

Assigning an ICD-10-PCS Code

An ICD-10-PCS code is constructed by assigning values for each of the characters. The procedural term is referenced in the Index. The main terms listed in the Index can be either the root operation phrase, such as resection, with the subterm gallbladder, or a common procedure term, such as cholecystectomy. The Alphabetic Index of ICD-10-PCS usually provides the first three characters with the final seven characters identified by accessing the code tables that appear following the Index. The Alphabetic Index occasionally provides the complete seven-character code, which must still be confirmed by accessing the applicable code table.

As an example, to code a laparoscopic total cholecystectomy, the coder could access the Resection root operation in the Index and find:

Resection   Gallbladder, 0FT4

Alternatively, the coder could access the common procedure term "Cholecystectomy" in the Index and find:

Cholecystectomy
    See Excision, Gallbladder 0FB4
    See Resection, Gallbladder 0FT4

It is important to note that in order to choose the appropriate cross-reference, the coder must know the definitions of the root operations Excision and Resection. Excision is defined as cutting out or off, without replacement, a portion of a body part. Resection is defined as cutting out or off, without replacement, all of a body part. A cholecystectomy would be a resection of the gallbladder, as the entire gallbladder is removed during a cholecystectomy.

The next step in the process is to access the 0FT code table. The remaining four characters are assigned based on this table. The values for each of the characters must be from the same row.

For example, using table 2.6, the code for a cholecystectomy performed through a laparoscopic approach would be 0FT44ZZ. Each of the seven characters of the procedure code describes the procedure of a laparoscopic total cholecystectomy:

0 = Medical and Surgical section
F = Hepatobiliary system and pancreas body system
T = Resection root operation
4 = Gallbladder body part
4 = Percutaneous endoscopic approach
Z = No device
Z = No qualifier

Table 2.6.   Tabular List—Table for 0FT, first three characters for a surgical procedure (resection) in the hepatobiliary system and pancreas

Section: 0 Medical and Surgical
Body System: F Hepatobiliary System and Pancreas
Root Operation: T Resection—Cutting out or off, without replacement, all of a body part

Body Part Character 4	Approach Character 5	Device Character 6	Qualifier Character 7
0　Liver 1　Liver, Right Lobe 2　Liver, Left Lobe 4　Gallbladder G　Pancreas	0　Open 4　Percutaneous Endoscopic	Z　No Device	Z　No Qualifier
5　Hepatic Duct, Right 6　Hepatic Duct, Left 8　Cystic Duct 9　Common Bile Duct C　Ampulla of Vater D　Pancreatic Duct F　Pancreatic Duct, Accessory	0　Open 4　Percutaneous Endoscopic 7　Via Natural or Artificial Opening 8　Via Natural or Artificial Opening Endoscopic	Z　No Device	Z　No Qualifier

Source: CMS 2013

ICD-10-PCS Review Exercises: Chapter 2

Assign the appropriate ICD-10-PCS codes to the following statements.

1. Esophagogastroduodenoscopy (EGD)

   _____

2. Left partial mastectomy, open

   _____

3. Open left femoral-popliteal artery bypass using cadaver vein graft

   _____

4. Laparoscopy with lysis of adhesions of bilateral ovaries and bilateral fallopian tubes

   _____

5. Posterior spinal fusion of the posterior column at L2-L4 with Bak cage interbody fusion device, open

   _____

6. Cystoscopy with retrieval of right ureteral stent

   _____

7. Reattachment of severed right hand

   _____

8. Diagnostic percutaneous paracentesis for ascites

   _____

9. Transmetatarsal amputation of foot at right big toe

   _____

10. Transplant of left kidney from a living non-related donor

    _____

11. Open repair of laceration of large intestine

    _____

12. Open reduction fracture of right tibia

    _____

13. Mitral valve replacement using porcine tissue, open

    _____

14. Percutaneous transluminal coronary angioplasty right coronary artery

    _____

(Continued on next page)

ICD-10-PCS Review Exercises: Chapter 2 (Continued)

15. Endoscopic fulguration of sigmoid colon polyp

16. Thrombectomy, by incision, arteriovenous dialysis graft, right upper arm, cephalic vein

17. Revision of left knee replacement with readjustment of prosthesis, open

18. Hysteroscopy with diagnostic D&C

19. Extracorporeal shockwave lithotripsy (EWSL) of right ureter

20. Esophagogastroduodenoscopy with esophagomyotomy of esophagogastric junction

21. Skin flap transfer, open wound, right lower leg

22. Thoracotomy with banding of left pulmonary artery with extraluminal device

23. Percutaneous embolization of right uterine artery using coils

24. Construction of a vagina in a male patient using tissue bank donor graft as part of a sex change operation

25. Bilateral breast augmentation with silicone implants, open, cosmetic

26. Percutaneous insertion of spinal neurostimulator lead, lumbar spinal cord

27. Open anterior colporrhaphy with polypropylene mesh reinforcement

28. Tracheostomy tube exchange (remove and replace with new tube)

29. Intraoperative whole brain mapping by craniotomy

30. Laparotomy for control of postoperative bleeding in peritoneal cavity

Chapter 3

Introduction to the Uniform Hospital Discharge Data Set and Official ICD-10-CM Coding Guidelines

Learning Objectives

At the conclusion of this chapter, you should be able to:

1. Describe the purpose of the Uniform Hospital Discharge Data Set and identify its data elements

2. Identify the number of ICD-10-CM/PCS diagnosis and procedure codes that can appear on the Uniform Bill-04

3. Explain the purpose of the "present on admission" indicator with diagnosis codes

4. Understand the *ICD-10-CM Official Guidelines for Coding and Reporting* for selecting the principal diagnosis for inpatient care and reporting of additional diagnoses

5. Understand the *ICD-10-CM Official Guidelines for Coding and Reporting* for coding of diagnoses for outpatient services

Key Terms

- Comorbidity
- Complication
- Diagnosis
- Disposition of patient
- Expected payer
- Hospital identification
- National Uniform Billing Committee (NUBC)
- Other diagnosis
- Personal identification
- Physician identification
- Present on admission (POA)
- Principal diagnosis
- Principal procedure
- Significant procedure
- Uniform Hospital Discharge Data Set (UHDDS)

Uniform Hospital Discharge Data Set

There are many uses for the data that are created by coding activity, including compiling statistical data. In order for these data to be useful, everyone gathering the data must collect the same data the same way. The **Uniform Hospital Discharge Data Set (UHDDS)** was promulgated by the US Department of Health, Education, and Welfare in 1974 as a minimum, common core of data on individual acute care short-term hospital discharges in Medicare and Medicaid programs. It sought to improve the uniformity and comparability of hospital discharge data.

In 1985, the data set was revised to improve the original version in light of timely needs and developments. These data elements and their definitions can be found in the July 31, 1985, *Federal Register* (50 FR 31038, Vol. 50, No. 147, pp. 31038–40). Since that time, the application of the UHDDS definitions has been expanded to include all nonoutpatient settings (acute care, short-term care, long-term care, and psychiatric hospitals; home health agencies; rehabilitation facilities; nursing homes; and so forth).

Part of the current UHDDS includes the following specific items pertaining to patients and their episodes of care:

- **Personal identification:** The unique number assigned to each patient that distinguishes the patient and his or her health record from all others

- **Date of birth**

- **Sex**

- **Race**

- **Ethnicity (Hispanic–Non-Hispanic)**

- **Residence:** The zip code or code for foreign residence

- **Hospital identification:** The unique number assigned to each institution

- **Admission and discharge dates**

- **Physician identification:** The unique number assigned to each physician within the hospital (the attending physician and the operating physician [if applicable] are both to be identified)

- **Disposition of patient:** The destination of the patient upon leaving the hospital— discharged to home, left against medical advice, discharged to another short-term hospital, discharged to a long-term care institution, died, or other

- **Expected payer:** The single major source expected by the patient to pay for this bill (for example, Blue Cross/Blue Shield, Medicare, Medicaid, workers' compensation)

In keeping with UHDDS standards, medical data items for the following diagnoses and procedures also are reported:

- **Diagnoses:** All diagnoses affecting the current hospital stay must be reported as part of the UHDDS.

- **Principal diagnosis:** The principal diagnosis is designated and defined as the condition established after study to be chiefly responsible for occasioning the admission of the patient to the hospital for care.

- **Other diagnoses:** These are designated and defined as all conditions that coexist at the time of admission, that develop subsequently, or that affect the treatment received or the length of stay (LOS). Diagnoses are to be excluded that relate to an earlier episode that has no bearing on the current hospital stay. Within the Medicare Acute Care Inpatient Prospective Payment System (IPPS), other diagnoses may qualify as a major complication or comorbidity (MCC), or other complication or comorbidity (CC). The terms complication and comorbidity are not part of the UHDDS definition set but were developed as part of the diagnosis-related group (DRG) system. The presence of the complication or comorbidity may influence the MS-DRG assignment and produce a higher-valued DRG with a higher payment for the hospital.

- **Complication:** This is defined as an *additional* diagnosis that describes a condition arising after the beginning of hospital observation and treatment and then modifying the course of the patient's illness or the medical care required.

- **Comorbidity:** This is defined as a *preexisting* condition that, because of its presence with a specific principal diagnosis, will likely cause an increase in the patient's length of stay in the hospital.

- **Procedures and dates:** All significant procedures are to be reported. For significant procedures, both the identity (by unique number within the hospital) of the person performing the procedure and the date of the procedure must be reported.

- **Significant procedure:** A procedure is identified as significant when it

  ○ Is surgical in nature

  ○ Carries a procedural risk

  ○ Carries an anesthetic risk

  ○ Requires specialized training

- **Principal procedure:** This type of procedure is performed for definitive treatment rather than for diagnostic or exploratory purposes, or when it is necessary to take care of a complication. If two procedures appear to be principal, the one most related to the principal diagnosis should be selected as the principal procedure.

Uniform Bill-04

In 1975, the **National Uniform Billing Committee (NUBC)** was established with the goal of developing an acceptable, uniform bill that would consolidate the numerous billing forms hospitals were required to use. In 1982, Uniform Bill-82 (UB-82), also known as the CMS-1450 form, was implemented for use in billing services to Medicare fiscal intermediaries and other third-party payers. In 1988, the NUBC began preparations for a revised uniform bill. The resulting Uniform Bill-92 (UB-92) was implemented in October 1993 and provided for the collection of additional statistical data, including clinical information.

The NUBC approved the UB-04 as the replacement for the UB-92 at its February 2005 meeting. As of May 23, 2007, all institutional paper claims were submitted with the UB-04. The UB-04 provides alignment with the electronic HIPAA 837 transaction standard or the electronic billing format. In addition, the electronic 837 transaction standard and UB-04 accommodate the national provider identifiers, the health plan identifiers, and migration to the ICD-10-CM and ICD-10-PCS coding systems when they are implemented. There is an increased emphasis on clinical codes.

Look at the sample UB-04 claim form in figure 3.1. The UB-04 contains fields for 18 diagnosis codes. The 18 diagnosis codes are placed on form locator 67 and 67A through 67Q. There is space for one admitting diagnosis for a patient who is admitted as an inpatient (form locator 69), as well as three "patient reason" diagnosis codes (form locator 70a through 70c) to describe the patient's reason for visit at the time of outpatient registration. Additional space is allowed for reporting external cause of injury codes or E codes (form locator 72a through 72c). There is room to report three E codes on the UB-04 paper and electronic claim forms. In addition, there is a "diagnosis indicator" field to identify whether a particular final inpatient diagnosis was present at the time of admission with a yes/no (Y/N) indicator. There is space for six ICD-10-PCS procedure codes on the UB-04 (form locator 74 and 74a through 74e). These details are summarized next.

Inpatient claims:

Admitting diagnosis:	1 ICD-10-CM diagnosis code
Final diagnosis:	18 ICD-10-CM diagnosis codes
External cause of injury:	3 ICD-10-CM diagnosis codes
Total:	**22 ICD-10-CM diagnosis codes**
Procedure:	6 ICD-10-PCS procedure codes

Outpatient claims:

Reason for visit:	3 ICD-10-CM diagnosis codes
Final diagnosis:	18 ICD-10-CM diagnosis codes
External cause of injury:	3 ICD-10-CM diagnosis codes
Total:	**24 ICD-10-CM diagnosis codes**

Effective January 1, 2011, CMS expanded the number of diagnosis and procedure codes that could be processed on institutional claims through the implementation of version 5010/837I of the electronic claims transaction standards. The move to using more than the first nine diagnosis codes and the first six procedure codes for payment purposes was long awaited. This expansion will allow for 24 additional diagnosis codes, including the associated present on admission indicator, and 24 secondary procedure codes. With this expansion, CMS will process a total of 25 diagnosis codes (one principal diagnosis and 24 additional diagnoses) and a total of 25 procedure codes for its institutional electronic claims processing (CMS 2010b).

The UB-04 data elements also include the **present on admission (POA)** indicator. The purpose of the POA indicator is to differentiate between conditions present at admission and conditions that develop during an inpatient admission. The POA indicator applies to diagnosis codes for claims involving inpatient admissions to acute care hospitals or other facilities, as required by law or regulation for public health reporting. The Cooperating Parties for ICD-10-CM (AHIMA, the American Hospital Association, CMS, and NCHS) have developed comprehensive POA reporting guidelines that are included as a separate section of the *ICD-10-CM Official Guidelines for Coding and Reporting*.

Figure 3.1. **UB-04 (CMS 1450) claim form**

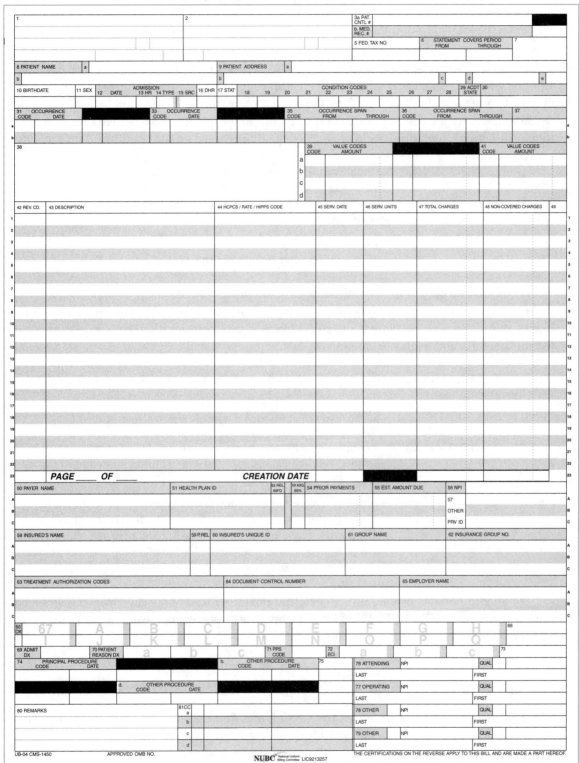

Selection of Principal Diagnosis

As the UHDDS definition states, a principal diagnosis is the condition "established after study to be chiefly responsible for occasioning the admission of the patient to the hospital for care" (NCHS 1985). Selecting the principal diagnosis depends on the circumstances of the admission, or why the patient was admitted. The admitting diagnosis has to be worked up through diagnostic tests and studies. Therefore, the words "after study" serve as an integral part of this definition. During the course of hospitalization, the admitting diagnosis, which may be a symptom or ill-defined condition, could change substantially based on the results of "further study."

> **EXAMPLE:** Patient was admitted through the emergency department with an admitting diagnosis of seizure disorder. During hospitalization, diagnostic tests and studies revealed carcinoma of the brain, which explained the seizures.
>
> The principal diagnosis was the carcinoma of the brain, which was the condition determined after study.

At times, however, it may be difficult to distinguish between the *principal* diagnosis and the *most significant* diagnosis. The most significant diagnosis is defined as the condition having the most impact on the patient's health, LOS, resource consumption, and the like. However, the most significant diagnosis may or may not be the principal diagnosis.

> **EXAMPLE:** Patient was admitted with a fractured hip due to an accident. The fracture was reduced and the patient discharged home.
>
> In this case, the principal diagnosis was fracture of the hip.

> **EXAMPLE:** Patient was admitted with a fractured hip due to an accident. While hospitalized, the patient suffered a myocardial infarction.
>
> In this case, the principal diagnosis was still the fracture of the hip, with the myocardial infarction coded as an additional diagnosis. Although the myocardial infarction may be the most significant diagnosis in terms of the patient's health and resource consumption, it was not the reason, after study, for the admission; therefore, it was not the principal diagnosis.

Another important consideration in determining principal diagnosis is the fact that the coding conventions in ICD-10-CM, volumes 1 and 2, take precedence over the Official Coding Guidelines. (See Section I.A. Conventions for the ICD-10-CM.)

ICD-10-CM Official Guidelines for Coding and Reporting

The *ICD-10-CM Official Guidelines for Coding and Reporting* is available from the Centers for Disease Control and Prevention at http://www.cdc.gov/nchs/icd/icd10cm.htm. All coding students are strongly encouraged to read the guidelines and become familiar with the rules in order to put them into practice. The application of the guidelines in everyday practice helps to ensure data accuracy in both coding and reporting for all healthcare encounters. Reporting is the process of communicating the patient's diagnoses and procedures in codes to third-party payers for reimbursement purposes and to other internal or facility databases and other external required databases for financial, quality measurement, public data, and other purposes.

The *ICD-10-CM Official Guidelines for Coding and Reporting* is referenced throughout this chapter. You can find the complete document in Appendix E.

Selecting Principal Diagnosis for Inpatient Care

The following information on selecting the principal diagnosis and additional diagnoses should be reviewed carefully to ensure appropriate coding and reporting of hospital claims.

The circumstances of inpatient admission always govern selection of the principal diagnosis in keeping with the UHDDS definition of the term as "that condition established after study to be chiefly responsible for occasioning the admission of the patient to the hospital for care."

In determining the principal diagnosis, the coding directives in ICD-10-CM, the Tabular List, and Alphabetic Index take precedence over all other guidelines.

The importance of consistent, complete documentation in the medical record cannot be overemphasized. Without such documentation the application of all coding guidelines is a difficult, if not impossible, task.

Section II of the *ICD-10-CM Official Guidelines for Coding and Reporting* address the selection of the principal diagnosis:

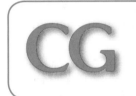 **Guideline II.A. Codes for symptoms, signs, and ill-defined conditions:** Codes for symptoms, signs, and ill-defined conditions from chapter 18 are not to be used as the principal diagnosis when a related definitive diagnosis has been established.

EXAMPLE: Patient was admitted to the hospital with chest pain to rule out myocardial infarction. After study, myocardial infarction was ruled out; the cause of the chest pain was undetermined.

Code R07.9, Chest pain, unspecified, was assigned. Although the code for chest pain (R07.9) is located in Chapter 18, a definitive diagnosis could not be made, so chest pain was coded as the principal diagnosis.

EXAMPLE: Patient was admitted to the hospital with dysphagia secondary to malignant neoplasm of the esophagus. A PEG tube was inserted.

Code C15.9, Malignant neoplasm of the esophagus, unspecified, was selected as the principal diagnosis, with code R13.10 as an additional diagnosis to describe the dysphagia. Because the dysphagia was related to the malignancy and code R13.10 is from Chapter 18, the principal diagnosis was the definitive diagnosis rather than the symptom.

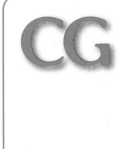 **Guideline II.B. Two or more interrelated conditions, each potentially meeting the definition for principal diagnosis:** When there are two or more interrelated conditions (such as diseases in the same ICD-10-CM chapter, or manifestations characteristically associated with a certain disease) potentially meeting the definition of principal diagnosis, either condition may be sequenced first, unless the circumstances of the admission, the therapy provided, the Tabular List, or the Alphabetic Index indicates otherwise.

EXAMPLE: Patient was admitted for initial treatment for a closed fracture of the right femur lower end and fracture of the right tibia upper end.

The following diagnosis codes were assigned: S72.401A, Fracture of femur, right, lower end, closed; S82.101A, Fracture of tibia, right, upper end, closed. Both fractures potentially met the definition of principal diagnosis; therefore, either code could be sequenced first.

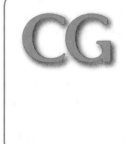 **Guideline II.C. Two or more diagnoses that equally meet the definition for principal diagnosis:** In the unusual instance when two or more diagnoses equally meet the criteria for principal diagnosis, as determined by the circumstances of admission, diagnostic workup, and/or the therapy provided, and the Alphabetic Index, Tabular List, or another coding guideline does not provide sequencing direction in such cases, any one of the diagnoses may be sequenced first.

EXAMPLE: Patient was admitted for elective surgery. A lesion on the left breast was excised and revealed fibroadenosis of breast. In addition, a right recurrent inguinal hernia was repaired.

The following diagnosis codes were assigned: N60.22, Fibroadenosis of left breast and K40.91, Unilateral inguinal hernia, without mention of obstruction or gangrene, recurrent. Both the fibroadenosis of left breast and the right recurrent inguinal hernia met the criteria for principal diagnosis. Therefore, either condition could be selected as the principal diagnosis.

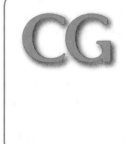 **Guideline II.D. Two or more comparative or contrasting conditions:** In those rare instances when two or more contrasting or comparative diagnoses are documented as "either/or" (or similar terminology), they are coded as if confirmed and sequenced according to the circumstances of the admission. If no further determination can be made as to which diagnosis is principal, either diagnosis may be sequenced first.

EXAMPLE: Diverticulosis of large intestine versus angiodysplasia of colon

Codes K57.30, Diverticulosis of large intestine without perforation or abscess without bleeding and K55.20, Angiodysplasia of colon without hemorrhage are assigned.

Either unconfirmed diagnosis, diverticulosis or angiodysplasia of colon, may be sequenced as the principal diagnosis.

Note: Guidelines II.A through II.D reveal that designation of the principal diagnosis is not always an exact and easy task. At times, more than one condition may have occasioned the admission. In such cases, the actual circumstances of the case dictate designation of the principal diagnosis.

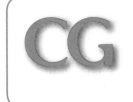

Guideline II.E. A symptom(s) followed by contrasting or comparative diagnoses: When a symptom(s) is (are) followed by contrasting or comparative diagnoses, the symptom code is sequenced first. All the contrasting or comparative diagnoses should be coded as additional diagnoses.

EXAMPLE: Patient was admitted with symptoms of periodic diarrhea and constipation during the previous 3 weeks. Following workup, physician documented the following diagnostic statement: diarrhea and constipation due to either irritable bowel syndrome or diverticulitis of large intestine.

The following codes were assigned: R19.7, Diarrhea; K59.00, Constipation; K58.0, Irritable bowel syndrome; and K57.32, Diverticulitis of large intestine (without mention of hemorrhage).

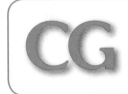

Guideline II.F. Original treatment plan not carried out: Sequence as the principal diagnosis the condition which after study occasioned the admission to the hospital, even though treatment may not have been carried out due to unforeseen circumstances.

EXAMPLE: Patient with ulcerated internal hemorrhoids was admitted for hemorrhoidectomy. Prior to the beginning of surgery, the patient developed bradycardia and the surgery was canceled.

The following codes were assigned: K64.8, Ulcerated internal hemorrhoids; R00.1, Bradycardia; and Z53.09, Procedure not carried out because of contraindication. The code for ulcerated internal hemorrhoids (R64.8) was listed as the principal diagnosis because it was the reason for admission. An additional code for bradycardia (R00.1) was reported, as well as code Z53.09, Procedure not carried out because of contraindication, to indicate that the procedure was not carried out due to the complication of bradycardia.

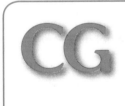

Guideline II.G. Complications of surgery and other medical care: When the admission is for treatment of a complication resulting from surgery or other medical care, the complication code is sequenced as the principal diagnosis. If the complication is classified to T80-T88 series, and the code lacks the necessary specificity in describing the complication, an additional code for the specific complication should be assigned.

EXAMPLE: Patient was being treated for an atelectasis due to recent cardiovascular surgery. The diagnosis codes would include J95.89, Other postprocedural complications and disorders of respiratory system, not elsewhere classified, and J98.11, Atelectasis

CG **Guideline II.H. Uncertain diagnosis:** If the diagnosis documented at the time of discharge is qualified as "probable," "suspected," "likely," "questionable," "possible," or "still to be ruled out," or other similar terms indicating uncertainty, code the condition as if it existed or was established. The bases for these guidelines are the diagnostic workup, arrangements for further workup or observation, and initial therapeutic approach that correspond most closely with the established diagnosis. Note: This guideline is applicable only to inpatient admissions to short-term, acute care, long-term care, and psychiatric hospitals.

Guideline II.I. Admission from observation unit:

1. Admission Following Medical Observation.

    When a patient is admitted to an observation unit for a medical condition, which either worsens or does not improve, and is subsequently admitted as an inpatient of the same hospital for this same medical condition, the principal diagnosis would be the medical condition that led to the hospital admission.

2. Admission Following Postoperative Observation.

    When a patient is admitted to an observation unit to monitor a condition (or complication) that develops following outpatient surgery, and then is subsequently admitted as an inpatient of the same hospital, hospitals should apply the UHDDS definition of principal diagnosis as "that condition established after study to be chiefly responsible for occasioning the admission of the patient to the hospital for care."

Guideline II.J. Admission from outpatient surgery: When a patient receives surgery in the hospital's outpatient surgery department and is subsequently admitted for continuing inpatient care at the same hospital, the following guidelines should be followed in selecting the principal diagnosis for the inpatient admission:

- When the reason for the inpatient admission is a complication, assign the complication as the principal diagnosis.

- When the reason for the inpatient admission is another condition unrelated to the surgery, assign the unrelated condition as the principal diagnosis.

Reporting of Additional Diagnoses

Deciding what else to code can be a challenge for coders. Doctors write many facts about the patient in terms of diagnoses and conditions that are present in the patient. However, not everything a doctor includes in a record is something to be coded. The *ICD-10-CM Official Guidelines for Coding and Reporting* help the coder decide what else to code in addition to the principal diagnosis.

In the definition of "other diagnoses," conditions that require clinical evaluation are to be coded. Clinical evaluation usually means the physician has taken the condition into consideration when examining the patient. An evaluation can mean the physician is considering testing of the condition or closely observing the condition to decide if new treatment is necessary or if the current treatment is sufficient. Frequently when a condition is being evaluated there also will be treatment or diagnostic procedures performed for it as well.

The sequencing of the additional diagnoses is not mandated by a particular coding guideline. Generally, the diagnoses that were more significant in terms of what received the most attention during the patient's hospital stay are listed first in the list of all additional diagnoses. This is a style that many coders follow but again, not a specific coding guideline.

Section III of the *ICD-10-CM Official Guidelines for Coding and Reporting* address the general rules for reporting other or additional diagnoses.

For reporting purposes, the definition for "other diagnoses" is interpreted as additional conditions that affect patient care in terms of requiring

- clinical evaluation;
- therapeutic treatment;
- diagnostic procedures;
- extended length of hospital stay; or
- increased nursing care or monitoring.

The UHDDS item #11-B defines other diagnoses as "all conditions that coexist at the time of admission, that develop subsequently, or that affect the treatment received or the length of stay. Diagnoses that relate to an earlier episode that have no bearing on the current hospital stay are to be excluded." UHDDS definitions apply to inpatients in acute care, short-term, long-term care, and psychiatric hospital settings. The UHDDS definitions are used by acute care short-term hospitals to report inpatient data in a standardized manner. These data elements and their definitions can be found in the July 31, 1985 *Federal Register* (Vol. 50, No. 147), pp. 31038–31040.

Since that time the application of the UHDDS definitions have been expanded to include all nonoutpatient settings (acute care, short-term, long-term care, and psychiatric hospitals; home health agencies; rehab facilities; nursing homes, and such).

The following guidelines are to be applied in designating "other diagnoses" when neither the Alphabetic Index nor the Tabular List in ICD-10-CM provide directions. The listing of the diagnoses in the patient record is the responsibility of the attending provider.

CG **Guideline III.A. Previous conditions:** If the provider has included a diagnosis in the final diagnostic statement, such as the discharge summary or the face sheet, it should ordinarily be coded. Some providers include in the diagnostic statement resolved conditions or diagnoses and status post procedures from a previous admission that have no bearing on the current stay. Such conditions are not to be reported and are coded only if required by hospital policy.

However, history codes (categories Z80–Z87) may be used as secondary codes if the historical condition or family history has an impact on current care or influences treatment.

EXAMPLE: The face sheet states the following diagnoses: acute diverticulitis, congestive heart failure, status post cholecystectomy, status post hysterectomy.

All are coded except the status post cholecystectomy and hysterectomy. The heart failure and the diverticulitis affect the current hospitalization and thus are coded.

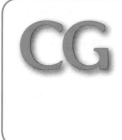

Guideline III.B. Abnormal findings: Abnormal findings (laboratory, x-ray, pathologic, and other diagnostic results) are not coded and reported unless the provider indicates their clinical significance. If the findings are outside the normal range and the attending provider has ordered other tests to evaluate the condition or prescribed treatment, it is appropriate to ask the provider whether the abnormal finding should be added.

EXAMPLE: In the inpatient setting, coders should not assign codes for conditions described in a pathology report alone without the provider's input. The provider or physician should be asked for clarification of the pathological findings if the provider has not documented the same condition in the health record.

Note: This differs from the coding practices in the outpatient setting for coding encounters for diagnostic tests that have been interpreted by a provider.

Guideline III.C. Uncertain diagnosis: If the diagnosis documented at the time of discharge is qualified as "probable," "suspected," "likely," "questionable," "possible," or "still to be ruled out," or other similar terms indicating uncertainty, code the condition as if it existed or was established. The bases for these guidelines are the diagnostic workup, arrangements for further workup or observation, and initial therapeutic approach that correspond most closely with the established diagnosis.

Note: This guideline is applicable only to inpatient admissions to short-term, acute, long-term care, and psychiatric hospitals.

Section IV: Diagnostic Coding and Reporting Guidelines for Outpatient Services

The coding of healthcare services in an outpatient setting is different from the coding of patient's diagnoses provided in an inpatient setting. Outpatient encounters are often short visits and there is not a lot of time to study the patient's condition in depth. For the outpatient visit, the goal of coding is to code what is known for certain about the patient's diagnosis, problem, or condition at that point in time and what was the focus of the healthcare attention at that time.

The coding guidelines listed below direct the coder on how to code patient visits in a hospital outpatient setting, physician's office, or other ambulatory care center.

Section IV of the *ICD-10-CM Official Guidelines for Coding and Reporting* address the general rules for diagnostic coding and reporting guidelines for outpatient services:

CG These coding guidelines for outpatient diagnoses have been approved for use by hospitals/providers in coding and reporting hospital-based outpatient services and provider-based office visits.

Information about the use of certain abbreviations, punctuation, symbols, and other conventions used in the ICD-10-CM Tabular List (code numbers and titles), can be found in Section IA of these guidelines, under "Conventions Used in the Tabular List." Information about the correct sequence to use in finding a code is also described in Section I.

The terms encounter and visit are often used interchangeably in describing outpatient service contacts and, therefore, appear together in these guidelines without distinguishing one from the other.

Though the conventions and general guidelines apply to all settings, coding guidelines for outpatient and provider reporting of diagnoses will vary in a number of instances from those for inpatient diagnoses, recognizing that:

The Uniform Hospital Discharge Data Set (UHDDS) definition of principal diagnosis applies only to inpatients in acute, short-term, long-term care and psychiatric hospitals.

Coding guidelines for inconclusive diagnoses (probable, suspected, rule out, etc.) were developed for inpatient reporting and do not apply to outpatients.

A. **Selection of first-listed condition**

In the outpatient setting, the term first-listed diagnosis is used in lieu of principal diagnosis.

In determining the first-listed diagnosis the coding conventions of ICD-10-CM, as well as the general and disease specific guidelines take precedence over the outpatient guidelines.

Diagnoses often are not established at the time of the initial encounter/visit. It may take two or more visits before the diagnosis is confirmed.

The most critical rule involves beginning the search for the correct code assignment through the Alphabetic Index. Never begin searching initially in the Tabular List as this will lead to coding errors.

(Continued)

(Continued)

1. **Outpatient Surgery**

   When a patient presents for outpatient surgery (same day surgery), code the reason for the surgery as the first-listed diagnosis (reason for the encounter), even if the surgery is not performed due to a contraindication.

2. **Observation Stay**

   When a patient is admitted for observation for a medical condition, assign a code for the medical condition as the first-listed diagnosis.

   When a patient presents for outpatient surgery and develops complications requiring admission to observation, code the reason for the surgery as the first reported diagnosis (reason for the encounter), followed by codes for the complications as secondary diagnoses.

B. **Codes from A00.0 through T88.9, Z00–Z99**

   The appropriate code(s) from A00.0 through T88.9, Z00–Z99 must be used to identify diagnoses, symptoms, conditions, problems, complaints, or other reason(s) for the encounter/visit.

C. **Accurate reporting of ICD-10-CM diagnosis codes**

   For accurate reporting of ICD-10-CM diagnosis codes, the documentation should describe the patient's condition, using terminology which includes specific diagnoses as well as symptoms, problems, or reasons for the encounter. There are ICD-10-CM codes to describe all of these.

D. **Codes that describe symptoms and signs**

   Codes that describe symptoms and signs, as opposed to diagnoses, are acceptable for reporting purposes when a diagnosis has not been established (confirmed) by the provider. Chapter 18 of ICD-10-CM, Symptoms, Signs, and Abnormal Clinical and Laboratory Findings Not Elsewhere Classified (codes R00–R99) contain many, but not all codes for symptoms.

E. **Encounters for circumstances other than a disease or injury**

   ICD-10-CM provides codes to deal with encounters for circumstances other than a disease or injury. The Factors Influencing Health Status and Contact with Health Services codes (Z00–Z99) are provided to deal with occasions when circumstances other than a disease or injury are recorded as diagnosis or problems.

See Section I.C.21. Factors influencing health status and contact with health services.

F. **Level of Detail in Coding**

1. **ICD-10-CM codes with *3, 4, 5, 6 or 7 characters***

    ICD-10-CM is composed of codes with 3, 4, 5, 6 or 7 characters. Codes with three characters are included in ICD-10-CM as the heading of a category of codes that may be further subdivided by the use of fourth, fifth, sixth or seventh characters to provide greater specificity.

2. **Use of full number of *characters* required for a code**

    A three-character code is to be used only if it is not further subdivided. A code is invalid if it has not been coded to the full number of characters required for that code, including the 7th character, if applicable.

G. **ICD-10-CM code for the diagnosis, condition, problem, or other reason for encounter/visit**

List first the ICD-10-CM code for the diagnosis, condition, problem, or other reason for encounter/visit shown in the medical record to be chiefly responsible for the services provided. List additional codes that describe any coexisting conditions. In some cases the first-listed diagnosis may be a symptom when a diagnosis has not been established (confirmed) by the physician.

H. **Uncertain diagnosis**

Do not code diagnoses documented as "probable," "suspected," "questionable," "rule out," or "working diagnosis" or other similar terms indicating uncertainty. Rather, code the condition(s) to the highest degree of certainty for that encounter/visit, such as symptoms, signs, abnormal test results, or other reason for the visit.

Please note: This differs from the coding practices used by short-term, acute care, long-term care and psychiatric hospitals.

I. **Chronic diseases**

Chronic diseases treated on an ongoing basis may be coded and reported as many times as the patient receives treatment and care for the condition(s).

(Continued)

(Continued)

J. **Code all documented conditions that coexist**

Code all documented conditions that coexist at the time of the encounter/visit, and require or affect patient care treatment or management. Do not code conditions that were previously treated and no longer exist. However, history codes (categories Z80–Z87) may be used as secondary codes if the historical condition or family history has an impact on current care or influences treatment.

K. **Patients receiving diagnostic services only**

For patients receiving diagnostic services only during an encounter/visit, sequence first the diagnosis, condition, problem, or other reason for encounter/visit shown in the medical record to be chiefly responsible for the outpatient services provided during the encounter/visit. Codes for other diagnoses (e.g., chronic conditions) may be sequenced as additional diagnoses.

For encounters for routine laboratory/radiology testing in the absence of any signs, symptoms, or associated diagnosis, assign Z01.89, Encounter for other specified special examinations. If routine testing is performed during the same encounter as a test to evaluate a sign, symptom, or diagnosis, it is appropriate to assign both the Z code and the code describing the reason for the non-routine test.

For outpatient encounters for diagnostic tests that have been interpreted by a physician, and the final report is available at the time of coding, code any confirmed or definitive diagnosis(es) documented in the interpretation. Do not code related signs and symptoms as additional diagnoses.

Please note: This differs from the coding practice in the hospital inpatient setting regarding abnormal findings on test results.

L. **Patients receiving therapeutic services only**

For patients receiving therapeutic services only during an encounter/visit, sequence first the diagnosis, condition, problem, or other reason for encounter/visit shown in the medical record to be chiefly responsible for the outpatient services provided during the encounter/visit. Codes for other diagnoses (e.g., chronic conditions) may be sequenced as additional diagnoses.

The only exception to this rule is that when the primary reason for the admission/encounter is chemotherapy or radiation therapy, the appropriate Z code for the service is listed first, and the diagnosis or problem for which the service is being performed listed second.

M. **Patients receiving preoperative evaluations only**

For patients receiving preoperative evaluations only, sequence first a code from subcategory Z01.81, Encounter for pre-procedural examinations, to describe the pre-op consultations. Assign a code for the condition to describe the reason for the surgery as an additional diagnosis. Code also any findings related to the pre-op evaluation.

N. **Ambulatory surgery**

For ambulatory surgery, code the diagnosis for which the surgery was performed. If the postoperative diagnosis is known to be different from the preoperative diagnosis at the time the diagnosis is confirmed, select the postoperative diagnosis for coding, since it is the most definitive.

O. **Routine outpatient prenatal visits**

See Guidelines for Coding and Reporting Section I.C.15. Routine outpatient prenatal visits.

P. **Encounters for general medical examinations with abnormal findings**

The subcategories for encounters for general medical examinations, Z00.0-, provide codes for with and without abnormal findings. Should a general medical examination result in an abnormal finding, the code for general medical examination with abnormal finding should be assigned as the first-listed diagnosis. A secondary code for the abnormal finding should also be coded.

Q. **Encounters for routine health screenings**

See Guidelines for Coding and Reporting Section I.C.21. Factors influencing health status and contact with health services, Screening

Note: The most recent complete version of the *ICD-10-CM Official Guidelines for Coding and Reporting* can be found at http://www.cdc.gov/nchs/icd/icd10cm.htm and are also included in Appendix E.

Review Exercises: Chapter 3

Assign the correct ICD-10-CM diagnosis codes to the following exercises.

1. What is the purpose of the Uniform Hospital Discharge Data Set and what healthcare organizations collect UHDDS?

2. What is the UHDDS definition of principal diagnosis?

3. What is the UHDDS definition of other diagnoses?

4. What is the difference between a "complication" and a "comorbidity"?

5. What is the maximum number of diagnosis codes that can appear on a UB-04 claim form for a hospital inpatient?

6. What is the maximum number of procedure codes that can appear on a UB-04 claim form for a hospital inpatient?

For exercises 7–16: Apply the *ICD-10-CM Official Guidelines for Coding and Reporting* of the Principal Diagnosis for Inpatient Care (Guidelines II A–J) to identify the principal diagnosis in the following scenarios.

7. Patient was admitted to the hospital after having a seizure at work. The admitting diagnosis was to rule out epilepsy. After testing was performed, the cause of the seizure was not determined, as the physician stated the patient did not have epilepsy.

8. Patient was admitted to the hospital with acute pyelonephritis and acute cystitis. Both infections were evaluated and treated with intravenous antibiotic therapy. The patient was discharged home to continue taking oral medications.

9. Patient was admitted to the hospital with acute exacerbation of chronic obstructive pulmonary disease and acute low back pain. Both conditions were evaluated and the patient received medical treatment. The patient was discharged home to continue to receive physical therapy for the back pain and pulmonary rehabilitation therapy for his chronic lung disease.

10. The patient was admitted to the hospital with a multitude of gastrointestinal symptoms. After diagnostic tests were performed the physician was unable to determine exactly what was causing the patient's symptoms. The physician's final diagnosis was "acute pancreatitis versus acute cholangitis."

Review Exercises: Chapter 3 (Continued)

11. The patient was admitted to the hospital with left lower quadrant abdominal pain. After study, the physician concluded the patient's abdominal pain could have been due to either of two conditions. Her final diagnosis was abdominal pain due to either a ruptured ovarian cyst or acute salpingitis.

_____

12. The patient was admitted to the hospital for a total right knee replacement for osteoarthritis of the knee. During the patient's preoperative preparation, the patient began having chest pain. The patient's knee surgery was cancelled, and the patient had extensive testing to determine the source of the chest pain, which was determined to be due to hypertensive heart disease.

_____

13. The patient was readmitted to the hospital for a postoperative wound infection. The patient had been discharged from the hospital five days ago, after having colon surgery for ruptured diverticulitis. During this hospital stay, the patient was treated for the wound infection and monitored for the remaining diverticulitis in his colon.

_____

14. The patient was admitted to the hospital with fever, cough, and shortness of breath. After study, the physician could not identify the exact cause of these symptoms but felt the most likely cause was pneumonia. The physician's final diagnosis was "possible viral pneumonia now resolving."

_____

15. The patient comes to the Emergency Department complaining of an asthma attack. The patient is placed into the observation unit to monitor his response to the asthma treatment. During the observation time the patient is determined to have status asthmaticus and is admitted for treatment of this condition. After a three-day hospital stay, the patient's asthma is better controlled, and he is discharged.

_____

16. The patient was registered as an outpatient for a left-sided cataract extraction, which was performed successfully. While the patient was preparing to leave the hospital after surgery, the patient felt faint, and it was determined the patient's blood pressure was much lower than earlier in the day. The patient was admitted to the hospital to monitor the low blood pressure. The next day, the patient felt well again and was discharged. The physician described the patient's condition as "orthostatic hypotension."

_____

For exercises 17–20: Apply the ICD-10-CM Official Guidelines for Coding and Reporting for Reporting Additional Diagnoses (Guideline Section III) to identify the other diagnosis/diagnoses in the following scenarios.

17. The physician's discharge summary includes the final diagnoses of (1) acute cholecystitis, with additional diagnosis of (2) cholelithiasis, (3) type II diabetes, (4) history of pneumonia last year, and (5) status post bunionectomy three months ago.

_____

(Continued on next page)

Review Exercises: Chapter 3 (Continued)

18. The physician's discharge summary includes the final diagnoses of (1) coronary artery disease, (2) hypertension, and (3) benign prostatic hypertrophy. The coder notes in the patient's laboratory reports that the patient has an elevated cholesterol level and an elevated PSA positive finding.

19. The physician's discharge summary includes the final diagnoses of (1) acute hemorrhagic gastritis, (2) acute duodenitis, and (3) possible acute pancreatitis.

20. The patient was admitted to the hospital with acute abdominal pain that was determined to be due to acute appendicitis, and the surgeon performed an open appendectomy on the patient. During the recovery period, the patient experienced two episodes of urinary retention that required the placement of a temporary urinary catheter. Would the second diagnosis of urinary retention be reported with a "yes" or a "no" as present on admission?

Chapter 4

Certain Infectious and Parasitic Diseases (A00–B99)

Learning Objectives

At the conclusion of this chapter, you should be able to:

1. Describe the organization of the conditions and codes included in Chapter 1 of ICD-10-CM, Certain infectious and parasitic diseases (A00–B99)

2. Review and apply the chapter specific coding guidelines for Chapter 1 of ICD-10-CM

3. Explain how and when the sequelae of infectious and parasitic disease codes are applied

4. Explain the circumstances in which codes from ICD-10-CM categories B95–B97 are used

5. Understand the coding guidelines for human immunodeficiency infection (HIV) disease reporting

6. Explain how methicillin resistant Staphylococcus aureus (MRSA) conditions are coded

7. Assign diagnosis codes for infectious and parasitic diseases

8. Assign procedure codes related to treatment of infectious and parasitic diseases

Key Terms

- Acquired immune deficiency syndrome (AIDS)
- Combination codes
- Human immunodeficiency virus [HIV]
- Methicillin resistant Staphylococcus aureus (MRSA)
- Methicillin susceptible Staphylococcus aureus (MSSA)
- Residual condition
- Sepsis
- Septic shock
- Severe sepsis

Overview of ICD-10-CM Chapter 1, Certain Infectious and Parasitic Diseases

Chapter 1 of ICD-10-CM includes categories A00–B99 arranged in the following blocks:

A00–A09	Intestinal infectious diseases
A15–A19	Tuberculosis
A20–A28	Certain zoonotic bacterial diseases
A30–A49	Other bacterial diseases
A50–A64	Infections with a predominantly sexual mode of transmission
A65–A69	Other spirochetal diseases
A70–A74	Other diseases caused by Chlamydia
A75–A79	Rickettsioses
A80–A89	Viral and prion infections of the central nervous system
A90–A99	Arthropod-borne viral fevers and viral hemorrhagic fevers
B00–B09	Viral infections characterized by skin and mucous membrane lesions
B10	Other human herpes viruses
B15–B19	Viral hepatitis
B20	Human immunodeficiency virus [HIV] disease
B25–B34	Other viral diseases
B35–B49	Mycoses
B50–B64	Protozoal diseases
B65–B83	Helminthiases
B85–B89	Pediculosis, acariasis and other infestations
B90–B94	Sequelae of infectious and parasitic diseases
B95–B97	Bacterial and viral infectious agents
B99	Other infectious diseases

In Chapter 1 a separate subchapter, or block, has been created and appropriate conditions grouped together for infections with a predominantly sexual mode of transmission (A50–A64). Two additional examples of separate blocks being created with the appropriate conditions grouped together are viral hepatitis (B15–B19) and other viral diseases (B25–B34).

The term sepsis is used throughout Chapter 1. The medical term septicemia may be found in medical records; physicians use septicemia as an equivalent term for sepsis. Category A41, Other sepsis, includes a "code first" note, and Excludes1 and Excludes2 notes to indicate how particular types of sepsis are coded as well.

Many of the codes in Chapter 1 reflect manifestations of the disease with the use of fourth or fifth characters allowing the infectious disease and manifestation to be captured in one **combination** code.

EXAMPLES: **A02.2 Localized salmonella infections**
A02.20, Localized salmonella infection, unspecified
A02.21, Salmonella meningitis
A02.22, Salmonella pneumonia
A02.23, Salmonella arthritis
A02.24, Salmonella osteomyelitis
A02.25, Salmonella pyelonephritis
A02.29, Salmonella with other localized infection

Coding Guidelines and Instructional Notes for ICD-10-CM Chapter 1

The NCHS has published chapter-specific guidelines for Chapter 1 in the *ICD-10-CM Official Guidelines for Coding and Reporting*. The coding student should review all of the coding guidelines for Chapter 1 of ICD-10-CM, which appear in an ICD-10-CM code book or at the website http://www.cdc.gov/nchs/icd/icd10cm.htm, or in Appendix E.

CG

Guideline I.C.1.a. Human Immunodeficiency Virus [HIV] Infections

1. Code only confirmed cases

   Code only confirmed cases of HIV infection/illness. This is an exception to the hospital inpatient guideline Section II, H. In this context, "confirmation" does not require documentation of positive serology or culture for HIV; the provider's diagnostic statement that the patient is HIV positive, or has an HIV-related illness is sufficient.

2. Selection and sequencing of HIV codes

   a. Patient admitted for HIV-related condition
      If a patient is admitted for an HIV-related condition, the principal diagnosis should be B20, Human immunodeficiency virus [HIV] disease followed by additional diagnosis codes for all reported HIV-related conditions.

   b. Patient with HIV disease admitted for unrelated condition
      If a patient with HIV disease is admitted for an unrelated condition (such as a traumatic injury), the code for the unrelated condition (e.g., the nature of injury code) should be the principal diagnosis. Other diagnoses would be B20 followed by additional diagnosis codes for all reported HIV-related conditions.

   c. Whether the patient is newly diagnosed
      Whether the patient is newly diagnosed or has had previous admissions/encounters for HIV conditions is irrelevant to the sequencing decision.

   (Continued)

(Continued)

d. Asymptomatic human immunodeficiency virus
    Z21, Asymptomatic human immunodeficiency virus [HIV] infection status, is to be applied when the patient without any documentation of symptoms is listed as being "HIV positive," "known HIV," "HIV test positive," or similar terminology. Do not use this code if the term "AIDS" is used or if the patient is treated for any HIV-related illness or is described as having any condition(s) resulting from his/her HIV positive status; use B20 in these cases.

e. Patients with inconclusive HIV serology
    Patients with inconclusive HIV serology, but no definitive diagnosis or manifestations of the illness, may be assigned code R75, Inconclusive laboratory evidence of human immunodeficiency virus [HIV].

f. Previously diagnosed HIV-related illness
    Patients with any known prior diagnosis of an HIV-related illness should be coded to B20. Once a patient has developed an HIV-related illness, the patient should always be assigned code B20 on every subsequent admission/encounter. Patients previously diagnosed with any HIV illness (B20) should never be assigned to R75 or Z21, Asymptomatic human immunodeficiency virus [HIV] infection status.

g. HIV Infection in Pregnancy, Childbirth and the Puerperium
    During pregnancy, childbirth or the puerperium, a patient admitted (or presenting for a health care encounter) because of an HIV-related illness should receive a principal diagnosis code of O98.7-, Human immunodeficiency [HIV] disease complicating pregnancy, childbirth and the puerperium, followed by B20 and the code(s) for the HIV-related illness(es). Codes from Chapter 15 always take sequencing priority. Patients with asymptomatic HIV infection status admitted (or presenting for a health care encounter) during pregnancy, childbirth, or the puerperium should receive codes of O98.7- and Z21.

h. Encounters for testing for HIV
    If a patient is being seen to determine his/her HIV status, use code Z11.4, Encounter for screening for human immunodeficiency virus [HIV]. Use additional codes for any associated high risk behavior. If a patient with signs or symptoms is being seen for HIV testing, code the signs and symptoms. An additional

counseling code Z71.7, Human immunodeficiency virus [HIV] counseling, may be used if counseling is provided during the encounter for the test.

When a patient returns to be informed of his/her HIV test results and the test result is negative, use code Z71.7, Human immunodeficiency virus [HIV] counseling. If the results are positive, see previous guidelines and assign codes as appropriate.

Guideline I.C.1.b. Infectious Agents as the Cause of Diseases Classified to Other Chapters

Certain infections are classified in chapters other than Chapter 1 and no organism is identified as part of the infection code. In these instances, it is necessary to use an additional code from Chapter 1 to identify the organism. A code from category B95, Streptococcus, Staphylococcus, and Enterococcus as the cause of diseases classified to other chapters, B96, Other bacterial agents as the cause of diseases classified to other chapters, or B97, Viral agents as the cause of diseases classified to other chapters, is to be used as an additional code to identify the organism. An instructional note will be found at the infection code advising that an additional organism code is required.

Guideline I.C.1.c. Infections Resistant to Antibiotics

Many bacterial infections are resistant to current antibiotics. It is necessary to identify all infections documented as antibiotic resistant. Assign a code from category Z16, Resistance to antimicrobial drugs, following the infection code only if the infection code does not identify drug resistance.

Guideline I.C.1.d. Sepsis, Severe Sepsis, and Septic Shock

1. Coding of sepsis and severe sepsis

   a. Sepsis
      For a diagnosis of sepsis, assign the appropriate code for the underlying systemic infection. If the type of infection or causal organism is not further specified, assign code A41.9, Sepsis, unspecified organism.

   A code from subcategory R65.2, Severe sepsis, should not be assigned unless severe sepsis or an associated acute organ dysfunction is documented.

   i. Negative or inconclusive blood cultures and sepsis
      Negative or inconclusive blood cultures do not preclude a diagnosis of sepsis in patients with clinical evidence of the condition, however, the provider should be queried.

(Continued)

(Continued)

    ii. Urosepsis

The term urosepsis is a nonspecific term. It is not to be considered synonymous with sepsis. It has no default code in the Alphabetic Index. Should a provider use this term, he/she must be queried for clarification.

    iii. Sepsis with organ dysfunction

If a patient has sepsis and associated acute organ dysfunction or multiple organ dysfunction (MOD), follow the instructions for coding severe sepsis.

    iv. Acute organ dysfunction that is not clearly associated with the sepsis

If a patient has sepsis and an acute organ dysfunction, but the medical record documentation indicates that the acute organ dysfunction is related to a medical condition other than the sepsis, do not assign a code from subcategory R65.2, Severe sepsis. An acute organ dysfunction must be associated with the sepsis in order to assign the severe sepsis code. If the documentation is not clear as to whether an acute organ dysfunction is related to the sepsis or another medical condition, query the provider.

  b. Severe sepsis

The coding of severe sepsis requires a minimum of 2 codes: first a code for the underlying systemic infection, followed by a code from subcategory R65.2, Severe sepsis. If the causal organism is not documented, assign code A41.9, Sepsis, unspecified organism, for the infection. Additional code(s) for the associated acute organ dysfunction are also required. Due to the complex nature of severe sepsis, some cases may require querying the provider prior to assignment of the codes.

2. Septic shock

  a. Septic shock generally refers to circulatory failure associated with severe sepsis, and therefore, it represents a type of acute organ dysfunction. For cases of septic shock, the code for the systemic infection should be sequenced first, followed by code R65.21, Severe sepsis with septic shock or code T81.12, Postprocedural septic shock. Any additional codes for the other acute organ dysfunctions should also be assigned. As noted in the sequencing instructions in the Tabular List, the code for septic shock cannot be assigned as a principal diagnosis.

3. Sequencing of severe sepsis

   If severe sepsis is present on admission, and meets the definition of principal diagnosis, the underlying systemic infection should be assigned as principal diagnosis followed by the appropriate code from subcategory R65.2 as required by the sequencing rules in the Tabular List. A code from subcategory R65.2 can never be assigned as a principal diagnosis.

   When severe sepsis develops during an encounter (it was not present on admission) the underlying systemic infection and the appropriate code from subcategory R65.2 should be assigned as secondary diagnoses.

   Severe sepsis may be present on admission but the diagnosis may not be confirmed until sometime after admission. If the documentation is not clear whether severe sepsis was present on admission, the provider should be queried.

4. Sepsis and severe sepsis with a localized infection

   If the reason for admission is both sepsis or severe sepsis and a localized infection, such as pneumonia or cellulitis, a code(s) for the underlying systemic infection should be assigned first and the code for the localized infection should be assigned as a secondary diagnosis. If the patient has severe sepsis, a code from subcategory R65.2 should also be assigned as a secondary diagnosis. If the patient is admitted with a localized infection, such as pneumonia, and sepsis/severe sepsis doesn't develop until after admission, the localized infection should be assigned first, followed by the appropriate sepsis/severe sepsis codes.

5. Sepsis due to a postprocedural infection

   a. Documentation of causal relationship
      As with all postprocedural complications, code assignment is based on the provider's documentation of the relationship between the infection and the procedure.

   b. Sepsis due to a postprocedural infection
      For such cases, the postprocedural infection code, such as, T80.2, Infections following infusion, transfusion, and therapeutic injection, T81.4, Infection following a procedure, T88.0, Infection following immunization, or O86.0, Infection of obstetric surgical wound, should be coded first, followed by the code for the specific infection. If the patient has severe sepsis the appropriate code from subcategory R65.2 should also be assigned with the additional code(s) for any acute organ dysfunction.

(Continued)

(*Continued*)

  c. Postprocedural infection and postprocedural septic shock

  In cases where a postprocedural infection has occurred and has resulted in severe sepsis and postprocedural septic shock, the code for the precipitating complication such as code T81.4, Infection following a procedure, or O86.0, Infection of obstetrical surgical wound should be coded first followed by code R65.21, Severe sepsis with septic shock and a code for the systemic infection.

6. Sepsis and severe sepsis associated with a noninfectious process

In some cases a noninfectious process (condition), such as trauma, may lead to an infection which can result in sepsis or severe sepsis. If sepsis or severe sepsis is documented as associated with a noninfectious condition, such as a burn or serious injury, and this condition meets the definition for principal diagnosis, the code for the noninfectious condition should be sequenced first, followed by the code for the resulting infection. If severe sepsis is present a code from subcategory R65.2 should also be assigned with any associated organ dysfunction(s) codes. It is not necessary to assign a code from subcategory R65.1, Systemic inflammatory response syndrome (SIRS) of non-infectious origin, for these cases.

If the infection meets the definition of principal diagnosis it should be sequenced before the non-infectious condition. When both the associated non-infectious condition and the infection meet the definition of principal diagnosis either may be assigned as principal diagnosis.

Only one code from category R65, Symptoms and signs specifically associated with systemic inflammation and infection, should be assigned. Therefore, when a non-infectious condition leads to an infection resulting in severe sepsis, assign the appropriate code from subcategory R65.2, Severe sepsis. Do not additionally assign a code from subcategory R65.1, Systemic inflammatory response syndrome (SIRS) of non-infectious origin.

See Section I.C.18. SIRS due to non-infectious process

Guidelines I.C.1.e. Methicillin Resistant *Staphylococcus aureus* (MRSA) Conditions

1. Selection and sequencing of MRSA codes

  a. Combination codes for MRSA infection
  When a patient is diagnosed with an infection that is due to methicillin resistant *Staphylococcus aureus* (MRSA), and that infection has a combination code that includes the causal organism (e.g., sepsis,

pneumonia) assign the appropriate combination code for the condition (e.g., code A41.02, Sepsis due to Methicillin resistant Staphylococcus aureus or code J15.212, Pneumonia due to Methicillin resistant Staphylococcus aureus). Do not assign code B95.62, Methicillin resistant Staphylococcus aureus infection as the cause of diseases classified elsewhere, as an additional code because the combination code includes the type of infection and the MRSA organism. Do not assign a code from subcategory Z16.11, Resistance to penicillins, as an additional diagnosis.

b. Other codes for MRSA infection

When there is documentation of a current infection (e.g., wound infection, stitch abscess, urinary tract infection) due to MRSA, and that infection does not have a combination code that includes the causal organism, assign the appropriate code to identify the condition along with code B95.62, Methicillin resistant Staphylococcus aureus infection as the cause of diseases classified elsewhere for the MRSA infection. Do not assign a code from subcategory Z16.11, Resistance to penicillins.

c. Methicillin susceptible Staphylococcus aureus (MSSA) and MRSA colonization

The condition or state of being colonized or carrying MSSA or MRSA is called colonization or carriage, while an individual person is described as being colonized or being a carrier. Colonization means that MSSA or MSRA is present on or in the body without necessarily causing illness. A positive MRSA colonization test might be documented by the provider as "MRSA screen positive" or "MRSA nasal swab positive."

Assign code Z22.322, Carrier or suspected carrier of Methicillin resistant Staphylococcus aureus, for patients documented as having MRSA colonization. Assign code Z22.321, Carrier or suspected carrier of Methicillin susceptible Staphylococcus aureus, for patient documented as having MSSA colonization. Colonization is not necessarily indicative of a disease process or as the cause of a specific condition the patient may have unless documented as such by the provider.

d. MRSA colonization and infection

If a patient is documented as having both MRSA colonization and infection during a hospital admission, code Z22.322, Carrier or suspected carrier of Methicillin resistant Staphylococcus aureus, and a code for the MRSA infection may both be assigned.

Coding Certain Infectious and Parasitic Diseases in ICD-10-CM Chapter 1

The following notes are available at the beginning of ICD-10-CM Chapter 1 in the Tabular List of Diseases and Injuries:

Includes: diseases generally recognized as communicable or transmissible

Use additional code to identify resistance to antimicrobial drugs (Z16.–).

Excludes1: Certain localized infections—see body system-related chapters Infections and parasitic diseases complicating pregnancy, childbirth and the puerperium (O98–) Influenza and other acute respiratory infections (J00–J22)

Excludes2: Carrier or suspected carrier of infectious disease (Z22.-) Infectious and parasitic diseases specific to the perinatal period (P35–P39)

In coding certain infectious and parasitic diseases, the entire health record must be reviewed to identify the following:

- Body site: for example, eye, intestine, or blood
- Specific organism responsible: for example, bacteria, virus, or fungus
- Etiology of disease: for example, parasite or food poisoning
- Severity of the disease: for example, acute or chronic

Combination Codes and Multiple Coding

Chapter 1 of ICD-10-CM includes **combination codes** to identify both the condition and the causative organism.

> **EXAMPLE:** B30.1 Conjunctivitis due to adenovirus
> B37.0 Candidal stomatitis
> A06.1 Chronic intestinal amebiasis

Mandatory multiple coding is required to describe etiology and manifestation when infectious and parasitic diseases produce a manifestation within another body system. The Alphabetic Index identifies when the etiology and manifestation convention or mandatory multiple coding is required by listing two codes after the main term with the second code listed in brackets. The first code identifies the underlying infectious or parasitic condition. The second code identifies the manifestation that occurs as a result of it.

> **EXAMPLE:** Histoplasmosis with pneumonia B39.2 *[J17]*
> The underlying cause and first listed code is B39.2. The second code describes the pneumonia caused by the histoplasmosis, J17.

Sepsis, Severe Sepsis, and Septic Shock

When coding sepsis, it is important to review the coding guidelines and the notes at the category level of ICD-10-CM.

Sepsis is a serious medical condition caused by the body's immune response to an infection. The body's immune system releases chemicals into the blood to fight the infection and triggers widespread inflammation. This inflammation causes blood clots and other complications in the vascular system. This impairs blood flow and damages the body organs by depriving the structures of oxygen and nutrients. Sepsis does not occur without another reason, especially in the lungs, abdomen, urinary tract, or skin. Surgical and invasive medical procedures can cause sepsis by introducing bacteria into the bloodstream. The pathologic organisms in the blood or tissue may include bacteria, viruses, fungi, or other organisms that produce a systemic disease.

Sepsis due to Streptococcus group A and B, and *Streptococcus pneumoniae* are classified to category A40, Streptococcal sepsis. Because streptococcal sepsis may occur after a procedure, immunization, or infusion as well as during labor or following an abortion or ectopic or molar pregnancy, a "code first" note exists to remind the coder that other codes should be assigned first to reflect those conditions.

Sepsis caused by other organisms than Streptococcus is classified to Category A41, Other sepsis. This category contains numerous codes to identify sepsis caused by a particular organism, such as Staphylococcus aureus, Hemophilus influenzae, anaerobes, other gram-negative organisms, and such. An unspecified type of sepsis is coded A41.9, Sepsis, unspecified, in cases where a specific underlying systemic infection is not further specified.

To code sepsis, the coder must review the physician's documentation to determine if the causative organism is known. By accessing the Alphabetic Index under the main term, sepsis, the coder can find the type of organism documented and its corresponding code in the list of subterms. If only the term "sepsis" is documented, code A41.9, Sepsis, unspecified is the appropriate code.

Severe sepsis is an infection with associated acute organ dysfunction. It may also be referred to as systemic inflammatory response syndrome due to an infectious process with acute organ dysfunction.

In severe sepsis, one or more of the body's organs fail. In the extreme situation, the patient suffers from very low blood pressure and heart failure. This situation advances to **septic shock**, which is potentially deadly. It causes circulatory failure and the failure of organs such as lungs, kidneys, and the liver.

Two codes at a minimum are required for the coding of severe sepsis. The first code is for the underlying infection, which may be categories A40 or A41 or codes for obstetric, puerperal, or postprocedural sepsis. A second code is from subcategory R65.2–, Severe sepsis. If septic shock is present, additional codes are required to identify the specific acute organ dysfunction, such as acute kidney failure (N17.–) or acute respiratory failure (J96.0–). The Tabular List reminds the coder that code R65.20 or R65.21 for severe sepsis without or with septic shock cannot be used as the principal, first listed, or the only code. A "code first underlying infection" note appears to direct the coder to code first the particular infection that produced the severe sepsis.

When severe sepsis is present on admission, and meets the definition of principal diagnosis, the underlying systemic infection is assigned as the principal diagnosis followed by the appropriate code from subcategory R65.2– as required by the sequencing rules in the Tabular List.

If the patient is admitted to the hospital for treatment of the sepsis and severe sepsis develops that was not present on admission, the underlying systemic infection is coded first and the appropriate code from subcategory R65.2– should be assigned as secondary diagnoses with the present on admission indicator of "no" reported.

It is possible that a patient has an infection in a particular body system that advances to a systemic infection. If this patient is admitted to the hospital for treatment of a body system or localized infection, such as pneumonia, as well as sepsis or severe sepsis, the code for the systemic infection is sequenced first. The sepsis would be the first reported or principal diagnosis. Another code would be assigned for the localized infection, such as the pneumonia. If the patient has severe sepsis, an additional code from category R65.2– would be assigned depending on whether the patient had septic shock or not.

In a different situation, a patient can be admitted to the hospital for treatment of pneumonia or another localized infection and the condition worsens while the patient is in the hospital to the extent of having sepsis or severe sepsis. In this situation, the localized infection would be coded and reported as the first code, followed by the appropriate sepsis or severe sepsis codes.

Human Immunodeficiency Virus (HIV) Disease

HIV is the medical abbreviation for **human immunodeficiency virus**. It is the virus that can lead to acquired immune deficiency syndrome (AIDS). There are two types of HIV: HIV-1 and HIV-2. In the United States, unless otherwise noted, the term "HIV" primarily refers to HIV-1. The virus damages a person's body by destroying specific blood cells called CD4+ T cells, which are essential in helping the body fight diseases.

Within a few weeks of being infected with HIV, people may develop flu-like symptoms that last for a week or two, but others have no symptoms at all. People living with HIV may appear and feel healthy for several years. However, even if they feel healthy, HIV is still affecting their bodies. Many people with HIV, including those who feel healthy, can benefit greatly from current medications used to treat HIV infection. These medications can limit or slow down the destruction of the immune system, improve the health of people living with HIV, and may reduce their ability to transmit HIV. Untreated early HIV infection is also associated with many diseases including cardiovascular disease, kidney disease, liver disease, and cancer.

Acquired immune deficiency syndrome (AIDS) is the late stage of HIV infection, when a person's immune system is severely damaged and has difficulty fighting diseases and certain cancers. Before the development of antiviral medications, people with HIV could progress to AIDS in a short period of time. Today, people can live much longer with HIV before they develop AIDS. This is because of antiviral medications that a person can tolerate over an indefinite period of time. Another treatment is to prevent opportunistic infections that can prove fatal in a person with the HIV infection.

The HIV classification includes the following categories and codes:

B20, Human immunodeficiency virus [HIV] disease. Patients with HIV-related illness should be coded to B20. Category B20 includes acquired immune deficiency syndrome [AIDS], AIDS-related complex [ARC], and HIV infection, symptomatic. This code is located under the Alphabetic Index entries of AIDS and Disease, human immunodeficiency virus [HIV], Human, immunodeficiency virus [HIV] disease.

Z21, Asymptomatic human immunodeficiency virus [HIV] infection status. Patients with physician documented asymptomatic HIV infection who have never had an HIV-related illness should be coded to Z21. This code is located under the Alphabetic Index entries of HIV, positive, seropositive or Human, immunodeficiency virus [HIV], asymptomatic.

R75, Inconclusive laboratory evidence of human immunodeficiency virus [HIV]. This code should be used for patients, including infants with nonconclusive HIV-test finding.

This code is located under the Alphabetic Index entry of Human, immunodeficiency virus, laboratory evidence.

Coding guidelines direct that only confirmed cases of HIV infection or illness be coded. The instruction to code only confirmed cases of HIV infection or HIV-related illness represents an exception to the general ICD-10-CM inpatient coding guidelines that state that diagnoses identified as suspected, possible, or other terms that reflect uncertainty as to whether or not the condition exists should be coded as if they had been established. In this context a confirmation does not mean a positive serology or culture for HIV is in the record. The physician's statement of the patient's diagnosis of AIDS or HIV-related illness is sufficient.

However, if the diagnosis of AIDS or HIV-related illness is suspected, likely, possible, probable, questionable, or another term that reflects uncertainty, it should not be coded with code B20. Instead, the physician should be asked to clarify what is known for certain about the patient, which may be symptoms of the disease or an inconclusive test result.

Patients who are diagnosed and treated for an HIV-related illness should be assigned a minimum of two codes in the following order:

1. Code B20 to identify the HIV-disease

2. Additional codes to identify all manifestations of HIV infection as directed by the "use additional code" note that appears under code B20

    EXAMPLE: Disseminated candidiasis secondary to AIDS
                           B20 Human immunodeficiency virus [HIV] disease
                           B37.7 Candidal sepsis

    EXAMPLE: Acute lymphadenitis with HIV infection
                           B20 Human immunodeficiency virus [HIV] disease
                           L04.9 Acute lymphadenitis, unspecified

During pregnancy, childbirth, or puerperium, a patient admitted because of HIV-related illness or asymptomatic HIV positive status should receive a principal diagnosis of human immunodeficiency virus [HIV] complicating pregnancy, childbirth, and the puerperium (O98.7–). An additional code is assigned to identify the type of HIV disease. See Guideline 1.C.15.a.3 that states whenever delivery occurs during current admit and there is a childbirth option, assign the in childbirth code. This is an exception to the sequencing rule discussed above.

    EXAMPLE: Pregnancy, delivered, 38 weeks, single liveborn infant in a patient with AIDS
                           O98.713 Delivery of a single liveborn male infant in a mother with AIDS, 38 weeks
                           O98.72 Human immunodeficiency virus (HIV) complicating childbirth
                           Z3A.38 Weeks of gestation pregnancy, 38 weeks
                           Z37.0 Single live birth

When a patient with HIV disease is admitted for an unrelated condition (such as a traumatic injury or a disease that was not caused by the HIV disease, such as an inguinal hernia), the code for the unrelated condition (that is, the nature of injury code) should be the principal diagnosis. Other diagnoses would be B20 followed by additional diagnosis codes for all reported HIV-related conditions.

> **EXAMPLE:** Patient with AIDS admitted with traumatic comminuted fracture femur shaft, right leg, initial encounter
> S72.351A Displaced comminuted fracture of shaft of right femur
> B20 Human immunodeficiency virus [HIV] disease

Code Z21, Asymptomatic human immunodeficiency virus [HIV] infection status, is used when the patient has the HIV virus in the blood but does not have any documented symptoms of the infection. The patient may be reported as being HIV positive or known HIV positive. Code Z21 is not used if the terms AIDS or HIV-related illness are used to describe the patient. Code Z21 is not used if the patient is being treated for any HIV-related illness or is described as having any condition resulting from his HIV positive status. Instead code B20 is used for symptomatic patients. Once a patient has conditions related to the HIV infection, even if the condition is resolved, the patient's HIV-related illness is coded as B20.

If a woman is pregnant and has HIV positive status but has no HIV-related illness, code O98.71- is used as the first-listed or principal diagnosis followed with an additional code for the HIV positive status, that is, Z21. The codes from the pregnancy chapter take sequencing priority over any other ICD-10-CM body system chapter.

Code R75, Inconclusive laboratory evidence of human immunodeficiency virus [HIV], is reported for patients who have health care services because of their inconclusive HIV serology. This code means the patient's HIV status has not been determined and he or she is likely to have additional testing in the future. This code is usually used on a short-term basis until the additional testing is completed.

A point to remember: A patient with any known prior diagnosis of an HIV-related illness should be assigned code B20. After a patient has developed an HIV-related illness, the patient should always be assigned code B20 on every subsequent visit or admission.

Testing for HIV

Patients requesting testing for HIV should be assigned code Z11.4, Encounter for screening for human immunodeficiency virus [HIV]. In addition, code Z72.5–, High risk sexual behavior, may be assigned to identify patients who are in a known high-risk group. The code for screening is used for patients who have no signs or symptoms of HIV disease. Code Z71.7, Human immunodeficiency virus [HIV] counseling, may also be assigned if these services are provided during the screening encounter.

If the results of the test are positive and the patient is asymptomatic, code Z21, Asymptomatic human immunodeficiency virus [HIV] infection status, should be assigned. If the results are positive and the patient is symptomatic with an HIV-related illness, such as Kaposi's sarcoma, the coder should assign code B20, human immunodeficiency virus [HIV] disease.

Sequelae of Infectious and Parasitic Diseases (B90–B94)

There is an important note in the Sequelae of Infectious and Parasitic Diseases (B90–B94) section that must be reviewed to understand how the codes are intended to be used. Certain infectious and parasitic diseases leave long-lasting effects after the infection is cured, which may be called a **residual condition**. The codes in categories B90–B94 are to be used to identify the original infection that produced the problem or condition the patient has as a result of it. The categories

B90–B94 are not used if the original condition is still present or if the condition is identified as a chronic infection. These categories represent the sequela of the disease. If the patient has a current chronic infection, the coder must assign codes for an active infectious disease. There is a "code first" note above the category codes B90–B94 that instructs the coder that the condition resulting from the original infectious and parasitic condition, the condition the patient has today, is coded first.

EXAMPLE: A 60-year-old female patient has a shortened right leg that is of unequal length compared to her left leg. The deformity of her right lower extremity is a result of the fact that she had acute poliomyelitis when she was 3 years old.

The residual condition is the deformity of her right tibia that is an unequal length compared to the left tibia. The deformity is the result or sequela of the past polio that she had as a child. The codes, in the correct sequence, to be assigned are

M21.761, Unequal limb length (acquired), right tibia

B91, Sequelae of poliomyelitis

Bacterial and Viral Infectious Agents (B95–B97)

ICD-10-CM contains a series of codes to identify the infective agents causing diseases. The note that appears in the Tabular List under this block heading states "These categories are provided for use as supplementary or additional codes to identify the infectious agent(s) in diseases classified elsewhere."

The infective agents are as follows:

- B95.0–B95.8, Streptococcus, Staphylococcus and Enterococcus, as the cause of diseases classified elsewhere; for example, Methicillin resistant Staphylococcus aureus (MRSA) with code B95.62

- B96.0–B96.89, Other bacterial agents, as the cause of diseases classified elsewhere; for example, Escherichia coli (E. coli) with code B96.20

- B97.0–B97.89, Viral agents, as the cause of diseases classified elsewhere; for example, respiratory syncytial virus with code B97.4

The following are examples of how to locate these conditions in the Alphabetic Index:

- Infection, infected, infective; bacterial as cause of disease classified elsewhere; Streptococcus group A—B95.0

- Streptococcus, streptococcal; group A, as cause of disease classified elsewhere—B95.0

The codes from B95–B97 will most likely be used with another code that identifies the site of an infection but does not include the causative organism. For example, to code "urinary tract infection due to E. coli" would require two codes:

N39.0 Urinary tract infection, site not specified

B96.20 Unspecified Escherichia coli [E. coli] as the cause of diseases classified elsewhere

Infection with Drug Resistant Microorganisms

ICD-10-CM allows for the coding of bacterial infections that are resistant to current antibiotics. This specificity is necessary to identify all infections documented as antibiotic resistant. The ICD-10-CM code Z16, Infection with drug resistant microorganisms, is assigned following the infection code for such cases.

Methicillin Resistant Staphylococcus aureus (MRSA) Conditions

Coding of conditions due to **methicillin resistant Staphylococcus aureus (MRSA)** bacteria are coded in one of two ways: with a combination code that identifies the infection is due to MRSA or with the use of an additional code to identify the MRSA as the causative organism with a code for the site of the infection. MRSA is called a "staph" germ that is not cured with the typical antibiotic that usually cures staphylococcus infections. When the typical antibiotic does not cure the infection, the organism is considered "resistant" to the antibiotic. The MRSA organism is resistant to methicillin or penicillins.

Examples of combination codes that identify the site of the infection and the MRSA causative organism are

A41.02, Sepsis due to Methicillin resistant Staphylococcus Aureus
J15.212, Pneumonia due to Methicillin resistant Staphylococcus aureus

An example of a condition that require two codes to identify the site of the infection and the MRSA causative organism is an infectious endocarditis due to MRSA:

I33.0, Acute and subacute infective endocarditis
B95.62, Methicillin resistant Staphylococcus aureus infection as cause of diseases classified elsewhere

To locate the additional code to identify MRSA or other bacteria that causes a disease, the coder must access the main term "infection" in the Alphabetic Index as follows:

Infection, infected, infective
bacterial
as cause of disease classified elsewhere
Staphylococcus
aureus
methicillin resistant (MRSA) B95.62

Another entry that may be used in the Alphabetic Index is

Infection, infected, infective
Staphylococcal, unspecified site
as cause of disease classified elsewhere
aureus
methicillin resistant (MRSA) B95.62

However, if the coder did not follow the subterm "as cause of disease classified elsewhere," the coder would have accessed code A49.02, Methicillin resistant Staphylococcus aureus, unspecified site. This code would not be used with another code that identifies the site of the infection. The A49.02 code is used when the site of the infection is not identified by the physician and there is no other information in the record, nor is there the opportunity to ask the physician a question to clarify the patient's condition.

Additional codes are available to capture Staphylococcus aureus that is susceptible to methicillin. These codes, A49.01 and B95.61, **Methicillin susceptible Staphylococcus aureus**, identify that the organism can be treated with methcillin antibiotics.

ICD-10-PCS Coding for Infectious and Parasitic Diseases

ICD-10-PCS codes are found in the Index based on the general type of procedure. Based on the first three values of the code found in the Index, the corresponding table is located. The upper portion of each table contains a description of the first three characters of the procedure code listed in the Index, that is, the name of the section, the body system, and the root operation performed. The lower portion of the tables specified all the valid combinations of character 4 through character 7. The four columns of the Table represent the last 4 characters of the code. The four columns are labeled body part, approach, device, and qualifier in the Medical and Surgical section. The coder constructs the code selecting characters 4 through 7 based on the facts of the procedure documented in the operative or procedure report written by the physician.

Infectious and parasitic diseases are not usually treated with surgical procedures. However, these conditions are usually treated with medication therapy. Devices such as catheters, venous access devices, and ports must be inserted into the patient for these long-term intravenous infusions.

There are six root operations that always involve a device: Insertion, Replacement, Supplement, Change, Removal, and Revision. The most commonly used root operations to code the insertion of an infusion device would be Insertion and Removal.

The root operation of Insertion is putting in a nonbiological device. The device would monitor, assist, perform, or prevent a physiologic function. The objective of these procedures is to put the device into the body. Inserting a vascular access device would be coded to the root operation of Insertion.

The main term to be used in the ICD-10-PCS for the insertion of a device would be "insertion of device in" followed by an alphabetic listing of anatomic sites where a device could be inserted. For an infusion device, the likely insertion site would be vein or vena cava. More precisely, coding of a vascular or venous access device would require the identification of the vein where the device was inserted, for example, brachial, cephalic, or subclavian in addition to the side of the body where the insertion occurred. Another site for device insertion would be vena cava, usually superior vena cava.

Table 05H would be accessed for insertion of a device in an upper vein such as subclavian, brachial, basilic, or cephalic. The approach would be Open, Percutaneous, or Percutaneous Endoscopic although Percutaneous is the typical approach. The device character gives the option of identifying the device as an Infusion device or an Intraluminal device. There are no options for a qualifier character other than Z for no qualifier. For example, the code for a percutaneous insertion of a venous access device for infusion into the right cephalic vein would be 05HD33Z. If an infusion device pump, vascular access device reservoir, or vascular access device is connected to an infusion catheter, the insertion of the device is coded separately. The ICD-10-PCS Index entry to code the insertion of the port or reservoir into subcutaneous tissue, for example, into the chest wall, would be "insertion of device in, subcutaneous tissue and fascia, chest" with the first four characters given as 0JH6. Table 0JH contains four columns for the body part, approach, device, and qualifier. The body part identifies the subcutaneous tissue and fascia's anatomic location. There are two options for the approach: Open and Percutaneous. There are numerous entries for the type of device inserted, specifically V for infusion device, pump, W for vascular access device reservoir, and X for vascular access device. For example, the insertion of an infusion pump inserted by incision (open) in the subcutaneous tissue and fascia of the abdomen would be coded 0JH80VZ in addition to the code of the device put into the vein or vena cava.

When a device is no longer needed, the root operation Removal would be the ICD-10-PCS code applied. A removal procedure takes out or takes off a device from a body part. The Index entry that should be used is "removal of device from" subcutaneous tissue or fascia (0JP), vein, lower (06PY), or vein, upper (05PY). Table 0JP, removal of device from subcutaneous tissue and fascia, includes characters 4 though 7 for the body part location, the approach, and the device (there is no qualifier option). The device option includes infusion pump, reservoir, and vascular access device. Table entries for 05P and 06P, removal of device from an upper or lower vein, are similar to those in Table 0JP, however the only device option is value 3 for Infusion device.

A patient may acquire sepsis from a disease in the digestive system, especially if there is a rupture or perforation of the intestine that allows organisms to escape and contaminate the internal cavity. Repairing the intestine likely will involve taking out some or all of a body part. The root operation Excision would be used for cutting out or off without replacement a part of the intestine as identified by the body part values in the Table. The root operation Resection would be used for cutting out or off without replacement all of a body part, as identified by one of the values of the body parts for the gastrointestinal system. For example, excision by laparotomy of a portion of the ascending colon would be 0DBK0ZZ; in comparison if the entire ascending colon was removed by laparotomy the procedure would be coded as a resection with 0DTK0ZZ. The Index entries would be "excision, colon, ascending" and "resection, colon, ascending."

Intestinal procedures may include a bypass procedure to completely treat the condition. The root operation Bypass is the altering of the route of passage of the contents of a tubular body party. A bypass can be considered a "rerouting" procedure, that is, redirecting the contents of a tubular body part, such as an intestine to travel through a different path. The bypass can send contents in a downstream route or to a similar body part or route. A bypass can also send contents to an abnormal route and different body parts such as to an external location other than a natural orifice. For noncoronary artery bypass, the body part values (character 4) indicate where the bypass originates or starts and the qualifier content indicates where the bypass goes to or ends (character 7). The Index entry is "bypass" with the subterm for the anatomic location when the bypass originates. For example, a bypass of the ascending colon as a colostomy would be coded as 0D1K0Z4. The Index entry in this example would be "bypass, ascending colon" as this is where the bypass originated. The documentation of this procedure would likely describe the open procedure as directing the contents of the ascending colon to come out of the body through the skin as a stoma. For this example, Table 0D1 would include the fourth character K for ascending colon, fifth character 0 for open, sixth character device Z for no device used, and seventh character 4 for cutaneous, which is the skin level of a colostomy.

ICD-10-CM and ICD-10-PCS Review Exercises: Chapter 4

Assign the correct ICD-10-CM diagnosis codes and ICD-10-PCS procedure codes to the following diagnoses.

1. Urinary tract infection due to Proteus mirabilis

2. *Clostridium difficile* (c. diff) colitis. This organism was resistant to multiple drugs, antibiotics

3. Acute bacterial food poisoning due to Salmonella

4. Chlamydial salpingitis

5. Kaposi's sarcoma of multiple sites on skin due to AIDS

6. Sepsis due to enterococcus from perforated diverticulitis of the small and large intestine

7. Severe sepsis due to Haemophilus influenzae with septic shock with acute renal failure

8. Whooping cough due to Bordetella pertussis with pneumonia

9. Acute hepatitis B with hepatic coma

10. Candidal esophagitis

11. PROCEDURE: Insertion of multilumen central venous catheter into the right subclavian vein for intravenous infusion by percutaneous approach

12. PROCEDURE: Exploratory laparotomy and small-bowel resection of 50 cm portion of the jejunum with side-to-side, functional end-to-end sewn anastomosis of the jejunum. The patient has peritonitis and a twisted nonviable small bowel.

(Continued on next page)

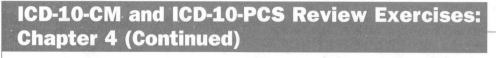

ICD-10-CM and ICD-10-PCS Review Exercises: Chapter 4 (Continued)

13.   PROCEDURE: Insertion of venous access device/port percutaneously into the subclavian vein advanced to the superior vena cava with a pocket for the port placed in the subcutaneous tissue of the chest wall for chemotherapy to treat colon carcinoma. An incision is made to create the pocket.

14.   PROCEDURE: Low anterior sigmoid colon (30 cm) open resection with end-to-end anastomosis of sigmoid to sigmoid colon

15.   PROCEDURE: Removal of implanted infusion port from patient's chest by incision following completion of infusion therapy (the port is in the subcutaneous tissue of the chest)

Chapter 5

Neoplasms (C00–D49)

Learning Objectives

At the conclusion of this chapter, you should be able to:

1. Describe the organization of the conditions and codes included in Chapter 2 of ICD-10-CM, Neoplasms

2. Review and apply the chapter specific guidelines for Chapter 2

3. Define the seven specific types of neoplasm behavior

4. Describe the organization of the Neoplasm Table

5. Explain the purpose of morphology codes

6. Understand the guidelines for using ICD-10-CM for Z codes to describe patients with neoplasms

7. Describe how to use the Alphabetic Index and Tabular List to locate a neoplasm code

8. Identify the purpose of the dash (-) in the ICD-10-CM Neoplasm Table

9. Explain how ICD-10-CM accommodates the coding of contagious sites

10. Describe how to code a primary malignant neoplasm according to its site

11. Describe how to code a secondary malignant neoplasm according to its site

12. Assign ICD-10-CM codes for neoplasms

13. Assign ICD-10-PCS codes for procedures related to treating neoplasms

Key Terms

- Benign
- Carcinoma in situ
- Histology
- Laterality

- Malignant
- Malignant primary
- Malignant secondary
- Metastasis
- Morphology
- Neoplasm
- Overlapping lesion
- Primary site
- Secondary site
- Topography
- Uncertain behavior
- Unspecified behavior

Overview of ICD-10-CM Chapter 2, Neoplasms (C00–D49)

Chapter 2 includes categories C00–D49 arranged in the following blocks:

C00–C75	Malignant neoplasms stated or presumed to be primary (of specific sites) and certain specified histologies, except neuroendocrine, and of lymphoid, hematopoietic and related tissues
C00–C14	Malignant neoplasms of lip, oral cavity, and pharynx
C15–C26	Malignant neoplasms of digestive organs
C30–C39	Malignant neoplasms of respiratory and intrathoracic organs
C40–C41	Malignant neoplasms of bone and articular cartilage
C43–C44	Malignant neoplasms of skin
C45–C49	Malignant neoplasms of mesothelial and soft tissue
C50	Malignant neoplasms of breast
C51–C58	Malignant neoplasms of female genital organs
C60–C63	Malignant neoplasms of male genital organs
C64–C68	Malignant neoplasms of urinary tract
C69–C72	Malignant neoplasms of eye, brain, and other parts of central nervous system
C73–C75	Malignant neoplasms of thyroid and other endocrine glands
C7A	Malignant neuroendocrine tumors
C7B	Secondary neuroendocrine tumors

C76–C80	Malignant neoplasms of ill-defined, other secondary and unspecified sites
C81–C96	Malignant neoplasm of lymphoid, hematopoietic and related tissue
D00–D09	In situ neoplasms
D10–D36	Benign neoplasms except benign neuroendocrine tumors
D3A	Benign neuroendocrine tumors
D37–D48	Neoplasms of uncertain behavior, polycythemia vera and myelodysplastic Syndrome
D49	Neoplasms of unspecified behavior

To properly code a neoplasm it is necessary to determine from the health record if the neoplasm is benign, in-situ, malignant, or of uncertain histologic behavior. If malignant, any secondary (metastatic) sites should be determined. Neoplasms of uncertain behavior are defined as tumors whose histologic cell type cannot determine whether the tumor is malignant or benign. Neoplasms of unspecified behavior include terms such as growth NOS (not otherwise specified), neoplasm NOS, new growth NOS, or tumor NOS. The term "mass," unless otherwise stated, is not to be regarded as a neoplastic growth.

Chapter 2 classifies neoplasms primarily by site or by topography. Included in the site codes are broad groupings for behavior (malignant, in situ, benign, and such). The Neoplasm Table should be used to identify the correct topography code. For malignant melanoma and certain neuroendocrine tumors, the morphology (histologic type) is included in the category and codes.

Neoplasm Behavior

The term **neoplasm** refers to any new or abnormal growth of body tissue. Definitions describing the behavior of the specific neoplasms include:

- **Malignant:** Malignant neoplasms are collectively referred to as cancers. A malignant neoplasm can invade and destroy adjacent structures, as well as spread to distant sites to cause death.

  - **Malignant primary:** A primary neoplasm is the site where a neoplasm originated.

  - **Malignant secondary:** A secondary neoplasm may be described as a metastatic site. **Metastasis** is the movement or spreading of cancer cells from one organ or tissue to another (MedlinePlus 2013).

    A secondary neoplasm is the site(s) to which the neoplasm has spread via

    - Direct extension, in which the primary neoplasm infiltrates and invades adjacent structures
    - Metastasis to local lymph vessels by tumor cell infiltration
    - Invasion of local blood vessels
    - Implantation in which tumor cells shed into body cavities

○ **Carcinoma in situ:** In an in situ neoplasm, the tumor cells undergo malignant changes but are still confined to the point of origin without invasion of surrounding normal tissue. The following terms also describe in situ malignancies: noninfiltrating, intracystic, intraepithelial carcinoma, and such.

- **Benign:** In benign neoplasms, growth does not invade adjacent structures or spread to distant sites but may displace or exert pressure on adjacent structures.

- **Uncertain behavior:** Neoplasms of uncertain behavior are tumors that a pathologist cannot determine as being either benign or malignant because some features of each are present.

- **Unspecified behavior:** Neoplasms of unspecified behavior include tumors in which neither the behavior nor the histological type is specified in the diagnosis.

Coding Guidelines for ICD-10-CM Chapter 2

The NCHS has published chapter-specific guidelines for Chapter 2 in the *ICD-10-CM Official Guidelines for Coding and Reporting*. The coding student should review all of the coding guidelines for Chapter 2 of ICD-10-CM, which appear in an ICD-10-CM code book or at the website http://www.cdc.gov/nchs/icd/icd10cm.htm, or in Appendix E.

CG

Guideline I.C.2. General neoplasm guidelines: The Neoplasm Table in the Alphabetic Index should be referenced first. However, if the histological term is documented, that term should be referenced first rather than going immediately to the Neoplasm Table in order to determine which column in the Neoplasm Table is appropriate. For example, if the documentation indicates "adenoma," the coder must refer to that term in the Alphabetic Index to review the entries under this term and the instructional note to "see also neoplasm, by site, benign."

Guideline I.C.2.a. Treatment directed at the malignancy: If the treatment is directed at the malignancy, designate the malignancy as the principal diagnosis. The only exception to this guideline is if a patient admission/encounter is solely for the administration of chemotherapy, immunotherapy or radiation therapy, assign the appropriate Z51.– code as the first-listed or principal diagnosis and the diagnosis or problem for which the service is being performed as a secondary diagnosis.

Guideline I.C.2.b. Treatment of secondary site: When a patient is admitted because of a primary neoplasm with metastasis and treatment is directed toward the secondary site only, the secondary neoplasm is designated as the principal diagnosis even though the primary malignancy is still present.

Guideline I.C.2.c. Coding and sequencing of complications: Coding and sequencing of complications associated with the malignancies or with the therapy thereof are subject to the following guidelines:

1. Anemia associated with malignancy: When admission/ encounter is for management of an anemia associated with the malignancy, and the treatment is only for the anemia, the appropriate code for the malignancy is sequenced as principal or first-listed diagnosis followed by the appropriate code for the anemia, such as code D63.0, Anemia in neoplastic disease.

2. Anemia associated with chemotherapy, immunotherapy and radiation therapy: When the admission/encounter is for management of an anemia associated with an adverse effect of the administration of chemotherapy or immunotherapy and the only treatment is for the anemia, the anemia code is sequenced first followed by the appropriate codes for the neoplasm and the adverse effect (T45.1X5, Adverse effect of antineoplastic and immunosuppressive drugs). When the admission/encounter is for management of an anemia associated with an adverse effect of radiotherapy, the anemia code should be sequenced first, followed by the appropriate neoplasm and code Y84.2, Radiological procedure and radiotherapy as the cause of the abnormal reaction of the patient, or of later complication, without mention of misadventure at the time of the procedure.

3. Management of dehydration due to the malignancy: When the admission/encounter is for management of dehydration due to the malignancy and only the dehydration is being treated (intravenous hydration), the dehydration is sequenced first, followed by the code(s) for the malignancy.

4. Treatment of a complication resulting from a surgical procedure: When the admission/encounter is for treatment of a complication resulting from a surgical procedure, designate the complication as the principal or first-listed diagnosis if the treatment is directed at resolving the complication.

Guideline I.C.2.d. Primary malignancy previously excised: When a primary malignancy has been previously excised and eradicated from its sites and there is no further treatment directed to that site and there is no evidence of any existing primary malignancy, a code from category Z85, Personal history of malignant neoplasm, should be used to indicate the former site of the malignancy. Any

(Continued)

(Continued)

mention of extension, invasion, or metastasis to another site is coded as a secondary malignant neoplasm to that site. The secondary site may be the principal or first-listed with the Z85 code used as a secondary code.

Guideline I.C.2.e Admissions/Encounters involving chemotherapy, immunotherapy and radiation therapy—see the complete set of Chapter 2 official coding guidelines in Appendix E.

1. Episode of care that involves the surgical removal of a neoplasm

2. Patient admission/encounter solely for administration of chemotherapy, immunotherapy, and radiation therapy

3. Patient admitted for radiation therapy, chemotherapy, or immunotherapy and develops complications

Guideline I.C.2.f. Admission/encounter to determine extent of malignancy—see complete set of Chapter 2 official coding guidelines in Appendix E.

Guideline I.C.2.g. Symptoms, signs, and abnormal findings listed in Chapter 18 associated with neoplasm—see complete set of Chapter 2 official coding guidelines in Appendix E.

Guideline I.C.2.h. Admission/encounter for pain control/management

See Section I.C.6 for information on coding admission/encounter for pain control management in Appendix E.

Guideline I.C.2.i. Malignancy in two or more contiguous site—see complete set of Chapter 2 official coding guidelines in Appendix E.

Guideline I.C.2.j. Disseminated malignant neoplasm, unspecified—see complete set of Chapter 2 official coding guidelines in Appendix E.

Guideline I.C.2.k. Malignant neoplasm without specification of site—see complete set of Chapter 2 official coding guidelines in Appendix E.

Guidelines I.C.2.l. Sequencing of neoplasm codes: Specific guidelines exist to address the coding of an encounter for treatment of primary or secondary malignancy, malignant neoplasm in a pregnant patient, encounter for complications associated with a neoplasm; complications from surgical procedures for treatment of a neoplasm; and pathologic fracture due to a neoplasm. See complete set of Chapter 2 official coding guidelines in the Appendix E.

Guideline I.C.2.m. Current malignancy versus personal history of malignancy: When a primary malignancy has been excised but further treatment, such as an additional surgery for the malignancy, radiation therapy or chemotherapy is directed to that site, the primary malignancy code should be used until treatment is completed.

When a primary malignancy has been previously excised or eradicated from its site, there is no further treatment (of the malignancy) directed to that site, and there is no evidence of any existing primary malignancy, a code from category Z85, Personal history of malignant neoplasm, should be used to indicate the former site of the malignancy.

Coding Neoplasms in ICD-10-CM Chapter 2

The coding of neoplasms requires understanding of the organization of the ICD-10-CM Neoplasm Table as well as the Index to Diseases and Injuries and the Tabular List to completely code the malignant, benign, and other neoplasms described by physicians in patients' records.

ICD-10-CM Neoplasm Table

The ICD-10-CM Neoplasm Table is a listing of codes that follows the ICD-10-CM Index of Diseases and Injuries. The ICD-10-CM Neoplasm Table is organized into seven columns. The first or the left column lists the anatomic site for the neoplasm. The next six columns provide codes for malignant primary, malignant secondary, carcinoma (CA) in situ, benign, uncertain behavior, and unspecified behavior for each anatomic site. Malignant tumor codes start with the alphabetic character C in the range of C00–C96. Benign, in situ, and neoplasms of uncertain behavior and unspecified behavior are listed in the range of D00–D49.

Topography and Histology

ICD-10-CM classifies neoplasms by topography. **Topography** is a description of a region or a special part of the body. The ICD-10-CM Neoplasm Table does not include neoplasms by histology. **Histology** is the study of the cell structures under the microscope. Certain neoplasms are identified by the histologic name of the cell structures, for example, oat cell carcinoma of the lung. For certain neoplams such as for malignant melanoma and certain neuroendocrine tumors, the histology is included in the category and codes. The term **morphology** is also used to describe neoplasms, that is, the form and structure of the tumor in the organ (Dorland 2007).

The description of the neoplasm will usually indicate which of the six columns is appropriate for coding, for example, basal cell carcinoma of skin, benign fibroadenoma of breast, or carcinoma in situ of larynx. When the name of the neoplasm does not readily identify the behavior of the neoplasm as malignant or benign, the coder should use the remainder of the Index to identify which column to use on the Neoplasm Table to assign the code. For example, giant cell glioblastoma of the brain is included in the Index to Diseases and Injuries with the following entry: see Neoplasm, malignant, by site (brain). The next step for the coder is to reference the Neoplasm Table under the anatomic site, brain, malignant, primary to assign the code.

Laterality

A feature in ICD-10-CM is the concept of **laterality**. Codes listed in the ICD-10-CM Neoplasm Table with a dash (-) following the code have a required fifth character for laterality, that is, right or left side. The Tabular List must be reviewed for the complete code. Neoplasm codes are specific as to whether the location is the right or left organ when a tumor is present in an organ that exists bilaterally. Examples of laterality would be a malignant neoplasm of the upper-outer quadrant of the right female breast (C50.411) and a benign neoplasm of the left kidney (D30.02). Codes also exist for an unspecified side of bilateral locations.

ICD-10-CM Chapter 2 Index Instructions

If the coder can identify the behavior and site of the neoplasm, the usual first step is to access the ICD-10-CM Neoplasm Table. However, the main terms and subterms in the ICD-10-CM Index to Diseases and Injuries assists the coder in locating the morphological type of neoplasms. When a specific code or site is not listed in the Index, cross-references direct the coder to the Neoplasm Table. It is essential to validate the code identified in the Neoplasm Table in the Tabular List. The assignment of the code should not be used without this step. The following instruction of classifying neoplams should be followed:

1. If the morphology is stated, the coder must locate the morphology of the tumor in the Index to Diseases and Injuries. For example, entries exist for lipoma, melanoma, sarcoma, and such, and specific codes for these types of these neoplasms are included in the Index; the coder does not need to reference the Neoplasm Table at all.

2. If the morphology is stated, the coder must locate the morphology of the tumor in the Index to Diseases and Injuries. However, not every entry in the Index will include codes. For example, if the doctor writes "subependymal glioma of the brain" as the diagnosis, the Index entry of glioma, subependymal, brain (specified site) is referenced and a cross-reference directs the coder to the following entry: see Neoplasm, uncertain behavior, by site (brain).

3. If the morphology is stated but the physician does not include and anatomic site, the coder should locate the morphology of the tumor in the Index to Diseases and Injuries. Certain types of morphology indicate the anatomic site as the only possible site where the tumor would develop. The physician would consider writing both the morphology and the site as redundant terminology. For example, the physician documents "serous papillary carcinoma" but the site is not stated. The Index entry of carcinoma, papillary, serous or carcinoma, serous, papillary is referenced and the coder will note that an entry exists for "unspecified site" and code C56.9. C56.9 is the code for malignant neoplasm of ovary, unspecified side. The coder can trust that entry because serous papillary carcinoma will only occur in an ovary.

4. If the coder is certain about the behavior of the neoplasm, for example, carcinoma is always a malignant primary tumor, the coder should reference the ICD-10-CM Neoplasm Table as the first step. The site of the neoplasm is located and the code is selected based on the behavior of the neoplasm from the appropriate column.

ICD-10-CM Chapter 2 Tabular List Instructions

In ICD-10-CM, instructional notes are found under many of the categories for malignant neoplasms. Instructional notes unique to ICD-10-CM direct coding professionals to use an additional code to identify such conditions as alcohol abuse and dependence, history of tobacco use, tobacco dependence, and history of tobacco use, exposure to environmental tobacco smoke, and other facts.

All neoplasms are classified in this chapter, whether they are functionally active or not. An additional code from Chapter 4, Endocrine, nutritional and metabolic diseases, may be used to identify functional activity associated with any neoplasm. Functional activity, such as increased or decreased hormone production, may occur when a neoplasm is present in a glandular organ. For example, when a patient has carcinoma of the ovary, she may also experience hyperestrogenism that produces excessive or frequent menstruation.

> **EXAMPLE:** C73 Malignant neoplasm of thyroid gland
>
> Use additional code to identify any functional activity

An instructional note under category D3A, Benign neuroendocrine tumor and C7A, Malignant neuroendocrine tumors instructs the coding professional to code additional disorders.

> **EXAMPLE:** D3A Benign neuroendocrine tumors
>
> Code also any associated multiple endocrine neoplasia [MEN] syndromes (E31.2-)
>
> Use additional code to identify any associated endocrine syndrome, such as: carcinoid syndrome (E34.0)

> **EXAMPLE:** C7A Malignant neuroendocrine tumors
>
> Code also any associated multiple endocrine neoplasia [MEN] syndromes (E31.2-)
>
> Use additional code to identify any associated endocrine syndrome, such as: carcinoid syndrome (E34.0)

ICD-10-CM Coding of the Anatomical Site

ICD-10-CM provides guidelines for coding the anatomical site of a neoplasm to the highest degree of specificity. These guidelines are discussed in the following sections.

Classification of Malignant Neoplasms

Malignant neoplasms are separated into primary sites (C00–C75, C7A, C76–C80) and secondary or metastatic sites (C7B, C77–C79), with further subdivisions by anatomic sites.

Neoplasms of the lymphatic and hematopoietic system are always coded to categories C81–C96, regardless of whether the neoplasm is stated as primary or secondary. Neoplasms of the lymphatic and hematopoietic system, such as leukemias and lymphomas, are considered widespread and systemic in nature and, as such, do not metastasize. Therefore, they are not coded to category C77, Secondary and unspecified malignant neoplasms of lymph nodes, which includes codes identifying secondary or metastatic neoplasms of the lymphatic system.

Neuroendocrine tumors include both malignant (C7A) and benign tumors (D3A) that arise from endocrine or neuroendrocrine cells scattered throughout the body. Neuroendocrine tumors are classified into two types: carcinoid tumors and pancreatic endocrine tumors.

Many of these tumors are associated with the multiple endocrine neoplasia syndromes identified by ICD-10-CM subcategory codes E31.20–E31.23. There is a note under subcategory E31.2- to code first any associated malignancies and other conditions associated with the syndromes. Under category C7A, Malignant neuroendocrine tumors, there is a note to code also any associated multiple endocrine neoplasia (MEN) syndrome (E31.2-). Another note instructs the coder to use an additional code to identify any associated endocrine syndrome, such as carcinoid syndrome (E34.0).

Determination of the Primary Site

The **primary site** is defined as the origin of the tumor. Physicians usually identify the origin of the tumor in the diagnostic statement. In some cases, however, the physician cannot identify the primary site. For these situations, ICD-10-CM provides an entry in the Neoplasm Table titled "unknown site or unspecified" assigned to code C80.1 for malignant (primary) neoplasm, unspecified or C79.9 for secondary malignant neoplasm of unspecified site.

Category C76

Category C76, Malignant neoplasms of other and ill-defined sites, is available for use only when a more specific site cannot be identified. This category includes malignant neoplasms of contiguous sites, not elsewhere classified, whose point of origin cannot be determined.

> **EXAMPLE:** Carcinoma of the neck
>
> C76.0 Malignant neoplasm of head, face, and neck

Primary Malignant Neoplasms Overlapping Lesion

A tumor may develop at the junction of two parts of an organ or two organs next to each other. A primary malignant neoplasm that overlaps two or more sites may be called a contiguous neoplasm or an **overlapping lesion**. When the neoplasm is identified as located at an overlapping site it will be classified to the subcategory code .8. A number of anatomic sites include an entry for an overlapping lesion with a code for the primary malignant site as the only entry on the row in the Neoplasm Table.

For multiple neoplasms of the same site that are not contiguous, codes for each site should be assigned. For example, tumors of the upper outer quadranat and lower inner quadrant of the right breast would each be assigned a separate code.

> **EXAMPLE:** A primary malignant lesion of the jejunum and ileum
>
> Neoplasm Table, Intestine, small, overlapping lesion C17.8
>
> C17.8 Malignant neoplasm of overlapping sites of small intestine

Classification of Secondary Sites

The patient's health record is the best source of information for differentiating between a primary and a secondary site. A **secondary site** may be referred to as a metastatic site in the record documentation. The following subsection describes some of the principal terms used in diagnostic statements that refer to secondary malignant neoplasms.

"Metastatic to" and "Direct Extension to"

The terms "metastatic to" and "direct extension to" are both used in classifying secondary malignant neoplasms in ICD-10-CM. For example, cancer described as "metastatic to" a specific site is interpreted as a secondary neoplasm of that site.

> **EXAMPLE:** Metastatic carcinoma of the colon to the lung
>
> C18.9 Malignant neoplasm of colon, unspecified
>
> C78.00 Secondary malignant neoplasm of lung

The colon (C18.9) is the primary site, and the lung (C78.00) is the secondary site.

"Spread to" and "Extension to"

When expressed in terms of malignant neoplasm with "spread to" or "extension to," diagnoses should be coded as primary sites with metastases.

> **EXAMPLE:** Adenocarcinoma of the stomach with spread to the peritoneum
>
> C16.9 Malignant neoplasm of stomach, unspecified
>
> C78.6 Secondary malignant neoplasm of retroperitoneum and peritoneum

The stomach (C16.9) is the primary site, and the peritoneum (C78.6) is the secondary site.

Malignant Neoplasm of Lymphatic and Hematopoietic Tissue

Chapter 2 includes the classification of malignant conditions of lymphatic and hematopoietic tissue. These conditions include lymphomas that arise out of lymph tissue, multiple myeloma that originates in bone marrow, and leukemia that forms in the blood with proliferation of abnormal leukocytes. These conditions are systemic and not isolated to a particular location, and the concept of metastatic coding discussed previously does not apply to these neoplasms. Lymphomas are classified according to their type and the specific lymph nodes involved when the diagnosis was made. Multiple myeloma is classified as to whether it is stated to be in remission, in relapse, or not having achieved remission. Leukemias are classified according to their type, such as lymphoid, myeloid, or monocytic, and how the condition currently exists (not having achieved remission, condition is in remission, or condition is in relapse). Remission occurs when the disease lessens in severity or the symptoms decrease and treatment may be discontinued. Relapse is the return of manifestations of the disease after an interval of improvement. Relapse may be considered a recurrence of the leukemia.

Neoplasm-Related Pain

A patient with primary or secondary malignant neoplasms may seek medical care because of neoplasm-related pain. Code G89.3, neoplasm-related pain (acute)(chronic) is assigned to pain documented as being related, associated, or due to a primary or secondary malignant neoplasm.

This code may be assigned for acute or chronic pain. The code may be assigned as a principal diagnosis or a first-listed diagnosis code when the stated reason for the admission or outpatient encounter is documented as pain control or pain management. The underlying neoplasm should also be reported as an additional diagnosis. When the reason for admission or outpatient care is the management of the neoplasm, and the pain associated with the malignancy is also documented, code G89.3 can be assigned as an additional diagnosis code. It is not necessary to assign an additional code for the site of the pain.

Other Conditions Described as Malignant

The medical term "malignant" has two meanings. In one context, it means resistant to treatment; occurring in severe form and frequently fatal; tending to become worse and leading to an ingravescent (increasing in severity) course. In reference to a neoplasm, malignant means having of the property of locally invasive and destructive growth and metastasis.

Effusion is the escape of fluid from blood vessels or lymphatics into the tissues or a cavity. This fluid can accumulate abnormally in the pleural cavity, pericardium, or peritoneum. Pleural effusions due to tumors may or may not contain malignant cells. When the condition is symptomatic, thoracentesis or chest tube drainage is required. Symptomatic pericardial effusion is treated by creating a pericardial window. Fluid in the peritoneum or ascites is usually treated with repeated paracentesis of small volumes of fluid.

A code for malignant ascites exists as R18.0 with a code first malignancy, such as malignant neoplasm of ovary (C56.-) or secondary malignant neoplasm of retroperitoneum and peritoneum (C78.6). Another condition described as malignant is malignant pleural effusion (J91.0). Beneath this code is a note to code first underlying neoplasm.

ICD-10-PCS Coding for Procedures Related to Neoplasms

ICD-10-PCS codes are found in the Index based on the general type of procedure. Based on the first three values of the code found in the Index, the corresponding table is located. The upper portion of each table contains a description of the first three characters of the procedure code listed in the Index, that is, the name of the section, the body system, and the root operation performed. The lower portion of the tables specified all the valid combinations of character 4 through character 7. The four columns of the table represent the last 4 characters of the code. The four columns are labeled body part, approach, device and qualifier in the Medical and Surgical section. The coder constructs the code selecting characters 4 through 7 based on the facts of the procedure documented in the operative or procedure report written by the physician.

Neoplasms are often treated with removal of tumors via surgical procedures. There are five root operations that take out some or all of a body part with three root operations that are most likely related to removing a tumor: Excision, Resection, or Destruction.

The root operation Excision would be used for cutting out or off without replacement a part of the site identified by the body part values in the table. An excision procedure may be done for the purpose of performing a biopsy of a tumor or lesion. A biopsy is the removal and examination, usually microscopic, of tissue from the body, performed to establish a precise diagnosis. The qualifier of "X" is used to indicate the excision is a diagnostic procedure.

The root operation Resection would be used for the cutting out or off without replacement of all of a body part, as identified as one of the values of the body parts for various body systems. For example, a lumpectomy to treat carcinoma of the breast is coded with the root operation Excision. If a total mastectomy was performed, the complete removal of the breast, the root operation Resection would be used. This example can be applied to many organs that are removed in part or in total to treat a malignancy.

The root operation Destruction is defined as the physical eradication of all or a portion of a body part by the direct use of energy, force, or a destructive agent. Destruction of a tumor or lesion may be performed using heat, cold, laser, or chemicals. There is usually no tissue to submit to pathology for examination after a destruction procedure as there is no tissue remaining from the site.

Antineoplastic chemotherapy is an infusion procedure coded with a procedure from the administration section of ICD-10-PCS. The root operation Introduction is used to code chemotherapy. The main term is "introduction of subsubstance in or on." The subterm identifies where the infusion is introduced which would be a vein, either a central vein or a peripheral vein. The approach is usually percutaneous as the needle is introduced in the vein through the skin. The sixth character is the substance infused with value 0 for antineoplastic. Depending on the chemical infused, there may be an appropriate qualifier assigned as the seventh character for other antineoplastic or monoclonal antibody.

ICD-10-CM and ICD-10-PCS Review Exercises: Chapter 5

Assign the correct ICD-10-CM diagnosis codes or ICD-10-PCS procedure codes for the following exercises.

1. Small cell carcinoma of the right lower lobe of the lung with metastasis to the intrathoracic lymph nodes, brain, and right rib

2. Benign carcinoid of the cecum

3. Subacute monocytic leukemia in remission

4. Type A spindle cell melanoma of right eye ciliary body

5. Patient is seen in the pain clinic for chronic neoplasm related pain that was known to be caused by the metastatic bone carcinoma of the vertebra that has spread from carcinoma of the left main bronchus of the lung.

(Continued on next page)

ICD-10-CM and ICD-10-PCS Review Exercises: Chapter 5 (Continued)

6. The patient was diagnosed with carcinoma of the descending colon five years ago with surgical excision of the descending colon. The patient had completed chemotherapy for the primary malignancy and had no cancer treatment over the past three years. The patient's colostomy is functioning well. During a follow-up examination recently, a CT scan of the liver showed a suspicious lesion that was later biopsied and found to be a secondary malignant neoplasm that originated in the colon. The patient visited the oncologist today in Oncology Clinic to review possible treatment options.

7. The reason for the encounter is to receive chemotherapy following the recent diagnosis of carcinoma of the head of the pancreas. A partial pancreatectomy was performed two months ago and the patient has been receiving chemotherapy.

8. The reason for the encounter is to receive radiation therapy following the recent diagnosis of carcinoma of the prostate to shrink the tumor prior to planned surgery to explore the tumor site in the next month.

9. The patient was treated for carcinoma of the right kidney five years ago and was treated with chemotherapy and radiation therapy at that time. During this visit the patient is being evaluated for the metastatic carcinoma of the right lung that was diagnosed recently. He will begin receiving radiation therapy again in the near future.

10. The patient was diagnosed with an advanced malignant carcinoid tumor of the ascending colon with carcinoid syndrome. Medications are being prescribed to relieve the carcinoid syndrome symptoms.

11. PROCEDURE: Ultrasound probe-guided prostate needle biopsy via rectum. One needle core biopsy submitted for diagnostic evaluation.

12. PROCEDURE: Right breast lumpectomy with open sentinel lymph node biopsy, right axilla

13. PROCEDURE: Open resection and removal of the left lobe of the liver due to metastasis from colon carcinoma

ICD-10-CM and ICD-10-PCS Review Exercises: Chapter 5 (Continued)

14. PROCEDURE: Tube thoracostomy—chest tube insertion by incision—for drainage of malignant pleural effusion from right side of pleural cavity

    _____

15. PROCEDURE: Rigid bronchoscopy with YAG laser photoresection for the destruction of tumor in the right main bronchus

    _____

Chapter 6

Diseases of the Blood and Blood-Forming Organs and Certain Disorders Involving the Immune Mechanism (D50–D89)

Learning Objectives

At the conclusion of this chapter, you should be able to:

1. Describe the organization of the conditions and codes included in Chapter 3 of ICD-10-CM, Diseases of the blood and blood-forming organs and certain disorders involving the immune mechanism (D50–D89)

2. Identify the causes of the specific types of anemia—deficiency, hemolytic, and aplastic

3. Give specific examples of coagulation defects, and briefly describe their treatment

4. Describe primary and secondary thrombocytopenia and briefly describe their treatments

5. Identify diseases of the white blood cells and give examples of these conditions

6. Assign ICD-10-CM codes for conditions categorized in ICD-10-CM Chapter 3

7. Assign ICD-10-PCS procedure codes for procedures related to diseases of the blood and blood forming organs

Key Terms

- Acute posthemorrhagic anemia
- Anemia
- Aplastic anemia
- Aspiration
- Bandemia
- Biopsy
- Coagulation defects
- Hemolytic anemia
- Hemolytic anemia—acquired
- Hemolytic anemia—hereditary
- Heparin-induced thrombocytopenia

- Neutropenia
- Pernicious anemia
- Sickle-cell disorder
- Thalassemia
- Thrombocytopenia
- Transplantation
- Von Willebrand disease (vWD)

Overview of ICD-10-CM Chapter 3, Diseases of the Blood and Blood-Forming Organs and Certain Disorders Involving the Immune Mechanism (D50–D89)

Chapter 3 includes categories D50–D89 arranged in the following blocks:

D50–D53	Nutritional anemias
D55–D59	Hemolytic anemias
D60–D64	Aplastic and other anemias and other bone marrow failure syndromes
D65–D69	Coagulation defects, purpura and other hemorrhagic conditions
D70–D77	Other disorders of blood and blood-forming organs
D78	Intraoperative and postprocedural complication of spleen
D80–D89	Certain disorders involving the immune mechanism

Diseases and disorders are grouped into subchapters or blocks making it easy to identify the type of conditions classified to ICD-10-CM Chapter 3. In Chapter 3 there is an increased level of specificity in the codes. This is intended to better identify specific disease types. The terminology used in the chapter is consistent with current clinical terminology.

Coding Guidelines and Instructional Notes for ICD-10-CM Chapter 3

At the time of this publication, there are no ICD-10-CM official coding guidelines for Chapter 3, Diseases of the blood and blood-forming organs and certain disorders involving the immune mechanism.

Instructional Notes

In ICD-10-CM Chapter 3, there are several codes with a note that states to "Use additional code for adverse effects, if applicable, to identify drug (T36–T50 with fifth or sixth character 5)."

EXAMPLES: D52.1 Drug-induced folate deficiency anemia
Use additional code for adverse effect, if applicable, to identify drug
(T36–T50 with fifth or sixth character 5)

D59.0 Drug-induced autoimmune hemolytic anemia
Use additional code for adverse effect, if applicable, to identify drug
(T36–T50 with fifth or sixth character 5)

D61.1 Drug-induced aplastic anemia
Use additional code for adverse effect, if applicable, to identify drug
(T36–T50 with fifth or sixth character 5)

Another instructional note found in this chapter is "Code first, if applicable, toxic effects of substances chiefly nonmedicinal as to source (T51–T65)."

EXAMPLE: D61.2, Aplastic anemia due to other external agents
Code first, if applicable, toxic effects of substances chiefly nonmedicinal as to source (T51–T65)

Similarly, two instructional notes appear with a code as the type of anemia is produced by either a poisoning or an adverse effect of a drug. The following type of anemia is produced by either a poisoning or an adverse effect of a drug.

EXAMPLE: D64.2 Secondary sideroblastic anemia due to drugs and toxins
Code first poisoning due to drug or toxin, if applicable (T36–T65 with fifth or sixth character 1–4, or 6)
Use additional code for adverse effect, if applicable, to identify drug
(T36–T50 with fifth or sixth character 5)

Other instructional notes apply to the entire category of codes or an individual code to use additional codes for associated conditions.

EXAMPLES: D56.0 Alpha thalassemia
Use additional code, if applicable, for hydrops fetalis due to alpha thalassemia (P56.99)

D57 Sickle-cell disorders
Use additional code for any associated fever (R50.81)

D59.3 Hemolytic-uremic syndromes
Use additional code to identify associated:
  E. coli infection (B96.2-)
  Pneumococcal pneumonia (J13)
  Shigella dysenteriae (A03.9)

D70 Neutropenia
Use additional code for any associated:
  Fever (R50.81)
  Mucositis (J34.81, K12.3-, K92.81, N76.81)

Instructions to "Code first" or "Code also" the underlying disease are also included in Chapter 3.

> **EXAMPLES:**   D61.82 Myelophthisis
> Code also the underlying disorder, such as:
> > Malignant neoplasm of breast (C50.-)
> > Tuberculosis (A15.-)
>
> D63.0 Anemia in neoplastic disease
> Code first neoplasm (C00-D49)
>
> D63.1 Anemia in chronic kidney disease
> Code first underlying chronic kidney disease (CKD) (N18.-)

Another instruction recognizes external causes can produce a blood disorder.

> **EXAMPLE:**   D59.6 Hemoglobinuria due to hemolysis from other external causes
> Use additional code (Chapter 20) to identify external cause

Certain blood disorders and disorders involving the immune mechanism are related to underlying diseases as well as influences of drugs and toxins. In addition, a blood disorder can produce other conditions or manifestations.

> **EXAMPLES:**   D70.1 Agranulocytosis secondary to cancer chemotherapy
> Use additional code for adverse effect, if applicable, to identify drug (T45.1X5)
> Code also underlying neoplasm
>
> D89.81 Graft-versus-host disease
> Code first underlying cause, such as:
> > Complications of transplanted organs and tissue (T86.-)
> > Complications of blood transfusion (T80.89)
> Use additional codes to identify associated manifestations, such as:
> > Desquamative dermatitis (L30.8)
> > Diarrhea (R19.7)
> > Elevated bilirubin (R17)
> > Hair loss (L65.9)

At least one blood disorder in Chapter 3 of ICD-10-CM has at least three instructional codes, such as the following example.

> **EXAMPLE:**   D75.81 Myelofibrosis
> Code first the underlying disorder, such as:
> > Malignant neoplasm of breast (C50.-)
> Use additional code, if applicable, for associated therapy-related myelodysplastic syndrome (D46.-)
> Use additional code for adverse effect, if applicable, to identify drug (T45.1X5)

Coding Guidelines

There are no separate chapter specific coding guidelines for Chapter 3 of ICD-10-CM. There are coding guidelines found in ICD-10-CM for Chapter 2 which apply to conditions coded in Chapter 3. Coding guideline, I.C.2.c.1, Neoplasms for anemia associated with malignancy states: "When the admission or encounter is for management of an anemia associated with the malignancy, and the treatment is only for anemia, the appropriate code for the *malignancy* is sequenced as the principal or first listed diagnosis followed by the appropriate code for the anemia (such as code D63.0, Anemia in neoplastic disease").

There are directions provided in the guidelines for anemia associated with chemotherapy, immunotherapy, and radiation therapy. For example, when the patient is seen for management of anemia associated with an adverse effect of the administration of chemotherapy or immunotherapy and the only treatment is for the anemia, the following should be coded:

1. The type of anemia treated and sequenced first

2. The neoplasm being treated with chemo- or immunotherapy

3. The adverse effect (T45.1X5) of antineoplastic and immunosuppressive drugs

Another example is when the patient is seen for management of anemia associated with an adverse effect of radiation, the following should be coded:

1. The type of anemia treated and sequenced first

2. The neoplasm being treated with radiation therapy

3. Y84.2, Radiological procedure and radiotherapy as the cause of abnormal reaction of the patient, or of later complication, without mention of misadventure at the time of the procedure

Coding Diseases of the Blood and Blood-Forming Organs and Certain Disorders Involving the Immune Mechanism in ICD-10-CM Chapter 3

Diseases of the blood include anemias, coagulation defects, purpura, and other hemorrhagic disorders as well as a variety of other disorders of blood-forming organs.

Anemias

Anemia is defined as a decrease in the number of erythrocytes (red blood cells), the quantity of hemoglobin, or the volume of packed red cells in the blood. Laboratory data reflect a decrease in red blood cells (RBCs), hemoglobin (Hgb), or hematocrit (Hct). Anemia is manifested by pallor of skin and mucous membranes, shortness of breath, palpitations of the heart, soft systolic murmurs, lethargy, and fatigability.

Nutritional Anemias (D50–D53)

Categories D50–D53 include codes for nutritional anemias. The most common type of anemia, iron deficiency anemia (category D50), is caused by an inadequate absorption of or excessive loss of iron. Iron deficiency anemia due to (chronic) blood loss is reported with code D50.0. The underlying cause of the bleeding should be coded when documented in the health record. Without further specification, iron deficiency anemia is reported with code D50.9.

Other nutritional anemias included here are as follows:

Vitamin B12 Deficiency Anemia (D51)

Specific codes exist for vitamin B12 deficiencies due to intrinsic factor deficiency, B12 malabsorption, transcobalamin II, and other dietary vitamin B12 deficiency anemia also known as vegan anemia.

Vitamin B12 and folate are important elements to enable the body to produce RBCs. The body's building blocks for its genetic code, DNA, also uses vitamin B12 in its production. The body stores vitamin B12 in the liver from various food sources, including seafood, meat, poultry, eggs, and dairy products. When the body does not have enough vitamin B12, a vitamin B12 deficiency anemia is produced and usually treated with replacement vitamin B12 orally or by injection.

Pernicious anemia is a form of vitamin B12 deficiency because of the body's inability to absorb vitamin B12 and make sufficient number of RBCs. Other conditions can also produce pernicious anemia, for example, from problems in the small intestine that prevent absorption of vitamin B12 from food. In addition, a vitamin B12 deficiency may occur with a folate deficiency.

Folate Deficiency Anemia (D52)

Specific codes exist for dietary folate deficiency and for drug-induced folate deficiency anemia as well as an unspecified folic acid deficiency anemia. A use additional code note appears under code D52.1, Drug induced folate deficiency anemia to use additional code for adverse effect, if applicable, to identify the drug (T36–T50 with fifth or sixth character 5).

Other Nutritional Anemia (D53)

Specific codes exist for protein deficiency anemia (D53.0), megaloblastic anemia (D53.1), and simple chronic anemia, which is considered an unspecified form of nutritional anemia in ICD-10-CM (D53.9).

Hemolytic Anemias

Hemolytic anemias are blood disorders when red blood cells are destroyed in a process called hemolysis that occurs before the normal time period in which the body normally destroys them, usually about 120 days after a red blood cell is created. The bone marrow that produces red blood cells cannot keep up with the rapid destruction even though it will try to speed up RBC production. With hemolysis the body has a lower number of normal levels of RBCs (HHS 2011). **Hemolytic anemia** is a condition in which your bone marrow cannot make enough new RBCs to replace the ones that are destroyed too early. There are many types and causes of hemolytic anemia. Hemolytic anemia can be acquired or inherited but the cause may not be known.

In **acquired hemolytic anemia**, the body senses that something is wrong with the RBCs even though they are normal. For example, antibodies or proteins made by the immune system may signal to the body's immune system that the RBCs do not belong. In response, the body destroys the RBCs before their usual lifespan is up. The destruction of RBCs commonly occurs in the spleen but can also occur in the bloodstream. Causes of acquired hemolytic anemia include

- Autoimmune responses
- Physical damage to RBCs from certain conditions and factors
- Exposure to certain infectious organisms and toxins
- Reactions to certain medicines

Hereditary hemolytic anemia is related to problems with the genes that control how the RBCs are made in the body. This causes defects in the outer membranes of the RBCs, enzyme deficiencies inside RBCs, or hemoglobin disorders. The abnormal RBCs are fragile and may break down as they move through the bloodstream. If this happens, the spleen may remove the faulty RBCs from the blood. Types of hereditary hemolytic anemias include

- Glucose-6 phosphate dehydrogenase (G6PD) deficiency
- Pyruvate kinase deficiency
- Thalassemia
- Sickle cell
- Hereditary spherocytosis
- Hereditary elliptocytosis

ICD-10-CM classifies hereditary hemolytic anemias to categories or codes:

Glucose-6-Phosphate Dehydrogenase (G6PD) Deficiency (D55.0)

In this type of anemia, the RBCs are missing an enzyme called G6PD. These enzymes are proteins that drive chemical reactions in the body. The missing enzyme makes the RBCs fragile and more likely to break down. If the RBCs come in contact with certain substances in the bloodstream, they rupture and die. Many factors, including those in certain medicines, foods (like fava beans), and infections, can trigger the breakdown of the RBCs. G6PD deficiency mostly affects men of African or Mediterranean descent. Some states require G6PD deficiency screening for newborns.

Pyruvate Kinase (PK) Deficiency Anemia (D55.2)

In this type of congenital anemia, the RBCs are missing an enzyme called pyruvate kinase. This causes them to break down easily. Pyruvate kinase deficiency is more common among the Amish. It may also be called ovalocytosis.

Thalassemia (D56)

Specific forms of thalassemia such as alpha, beta, delta-beta as well as thalassemia minor and other thalassemias have individual codes. **Thalassemias** are inherited blood disorders. "Inherited" means that the disorder is passed from parents to children through genes. Thalassemias cause the body to make fewer healthy red blood cells and less hemoglobin than normal. Hemoglobin is an iron-rich protein in red blood cells. It carries oxygen to all parts of the body. Hemoglobin also carries carbon dioxide from the body to the lungs, where it is exhaled. People who have thalassemias can have mild or severe anemia. Anemia is caused by a lower than normal number of red blood cells or not enough hemoglobin in the red blood cells. Thalassemias often affect people of Southeast Asian, Indian, Chinese, Filipino, Mediterranean, or African descent. The treatment for thalassemias are blood transfusions to replace destroyed RBCs, and blood and marrow stem cell transplants (HHS 2011).

Sickle-Cell Disorders (D57)

Different forms of sickle-cell disorders are included in category D57. For example, specific codes exist for Hb-SS disease with crisis, including acute chest syndrome and splenic sequestration each in a single code. Codes for other forms of sickle-cell disorders including Hb-C, sickle-cell trait, sickle-cell thalassemia, Hb-SD, and Hb-SE disease are included in this category. In **sickle-cell disorder**, the body makes abnormal hemoglobin that causes RBCs to have a sickle, or "C," shape. These sickle cells are sticky and do not travel easily through the blood vessels. Sickle cells live only about 10 to 20 days, and the bone marrow cannot make new RBCs fast enough to replace the dying ones. In the United States, sickle-cell anemia mainly affects people of African and Hispanic descent. Some states require sickle-cell anemia screening for newborn babies. The treatments for sickle-cell anemia include folic acid supplements made from the synthetic form of folate, antibiotics to prevent infection, medicine to reduce the number of faulty RBCs in the blood, and a medicine called hydroxyurea. Hydroxyurea may help the body make more healthy hemoglobin and reduce the amount of faulty hemoglobin that leads to sickle cells.

Other Hereditary Hemolytic Anemias (D58)

Hereditary Spherocytosis (D58.0)

Hereditary spherocytosis is caused by a defect in the RBCs' outer membranes that causes them to have a spherical, or ball-like, shape. The ball-shaped RBCs have a shorter than normal lifespan. Hereditary spherocytosis is the most common cause of hemolytic anemia among people of Northern European descent.

Hereditary Elliptocytosis (D58.1)

Hereditary elliptocytosis is caused by a defect in the RBCs' outer membranes that makes them oval-shaped and less flexible than normal. The RBCs have a shorter than normal lifespan. Disorders of the RBC outer membrane, both hereditary spherocytosis and hereditary elliptocytosis, are treated with folic acid supplements, blood transfusions, and removal of the spleen (rarely).

Acquired Hemolytic Anemia

Typically, **acquired hemolytic anemias** are caused by extrinsic factors such as drugs or toxins, systemic diseases, liver or renal disease, or abnormal immune responses. Treatments for acquired hemolytic anemia include different treatments depending on the type of anemia. Examples of these treatments are:

- Corticosteroids and other medicines to suppress the immune system
- Intravenous gammaglobulin, a medication than can increase the lifespan of RBCs and possibly reduce the amount of antibodies produced
- Iron and folic acid supplements

- Eculizumab, an antibody that blocks the destruction of RBCs in this form of anemia
- Plasmapheresis or a procedure to remove antibodies from the blood
- Blood transfusion
- Removal of the spleen
- Avoidance of cold temperatures

ICD-10-CM classifies acquired hemolytic anemia to category D59, with the fourth character describing the specific type or cause of disorder; for example:

D59.0 Drug-induced autoimmune hemolytic anemia with the instructional note "use additional code for adverse effect, if applicable, to identify drug (T36–T50 with fifth or sixth character 5)."

D59.1 Other autoimmune hemolytic anemia, which may be described as cold agglutinin disease or cold or warm type hemolytic anemia

D59.3 Hemolytic-uremic syndrome with the instructional note "use additional code to identify associated E. Coli infection, pneumococcal pneumonia or shigella dysenteriae."

Aplastic and Other Anemias and Other Bone Marrow Failure Syndromes

Aplastic anemia is a condition in which the bone marrow is damaged. As a result, the stem cells are destroyed or develop abnormally. In this situation the body cannot make enough RBCs, WBCs, or platelets. This type of anemia is rare, but it can be fatal. Aplastic anemia can be acquired or inherited. Many times, the cause of the aplastic anemia or the condition that triggers it is unknown. There are known causes of acquired aplastic anemia that include:

1. High-dose radiation or chemotherapy: These cancer treatments kill cancer cells, but they also may damage other cells, such as stem cells. When stem cells are damaged, healthy RBCs, WBCs, and platelets cannot develop. Aplastic anemia may resolve after these cancer treatments are stopped.

2. Environmental toxins: Substances such as pesticides, arsenic, and benzene can damage bone marrow, causing aplastic anemia.

3. Certain medicines: Certain medications used to treat rheumatoid arthritis and some antibiotics, such as chloramphenicol (which is rarely used in the United States), can damage the bone marrow and cause aplastic anemia.

4. Viral infections: Hepatitis, Epstein-Barr virus, parvovirus B-19, human immunodeficiency virus (HIV), mononucleosis, and cytomegalovirus can damage the bone marrow and lead to aplastic anemia.

5. Autoimmune diseases: These diseases, such as lupus and rheumatoid arthritis, may cause the immune system to attack its own cells. This can damage bone marrow cells and prevent them from making healthy new blood cells.

6. Other hereditary conditions can damage your stem cells, leading to aplastic anemia. These conditions include Fanconi anemia, Shwachman-Diamond syndrome, dyskeratosis congenita, Diamond-Blackfan anemia, and a megakaryocytic

thrombocytopenia. Some women may develop mild aplastic anemia during pregnancy. This anemia tends to go away after the baby is born.

7. In some cases, aplastic anemia is associated with another blood disorder called paroxysmal nocturnal hemoglobinuria (PNH). A genetic mutation causes PNH. The disorder develops when abnormal stem cells in the bone marrow make blood cells with a faulty outer membrane (outside layer). This destroys RBCs and prevents the body from making enough WBCs and platelets (HHS 2011). Aplastic anemia may only last a short time if it is due to a short-term condition, illness, or other factor. However, aplastic anemia can be a long-term condition if its cause is unknown or if an inherited condition or long-term illness or other factor causes it.

ICD-10-CM classifies aplastic anemias to categories D60–D64, with the fourth, fifth, and sixth characters indicating the specific type, for example:

Other Aplastic Anemias and Other Bone Marrow Failure Syndromes (D61)

Within this category are codes for constitutional anemias such as Blackfan-Diamond syndrome (D61.01), Fanconi's anemia (D61.09), drug induced aplastic anemia (D61.09), and aplastic anemia due to other external agents (D61.2). The codes for pancytopenia are included in category D61. Specific codes exist for antineoplastic chemotherapy induced pancytopenia (D61.810) and other drug-induced pancytopenia.

Acute Posthemorrhagic Anemia (D62)

Acute posthemorrhagic anemia or anemia due to acute blood loss is reported with code D62. It is defined as a normocytic, normochromic anemia developing as a result of rapid loss of large quantities of RBCs during bleeding. It may occur as a result of a massive hemorrhage that may be due to spontaneous or traumatic rupture of a large blood vessel, rupture of an aneurysm, arterial erosion from a peptic ulcer or neoplastic process, or complications of surgery from excessive blood loss. Coders should not assume that anemia following a procedure, or postoperative anemia, is acute blood loss anemia. But coding postoperative anemia as a diagnosis needs more information than this phrase. Postoperative anemia must be specified as due to (acute) blood loss (D62) or due to chronic blood loss (D50.). If the doctor specifies the postoperative anemia further, it is assigned to D64.9, anemia, unspecified.

Anemia in Chronic Diseases Classified Elsewhere (D63)

These conditions develop in a patient with chronic diseases, for example:

1. Anemia in neoplastic disease (D63.0)

   This code includes an instructional note to "code first neoplasm (C00-D49)."

2. Anemia in chronic kidney disease (CKD) (D63.1)

   This condition is also known as erythropoietin resistant anemia (EPO resistant anemia). The code includes an instructional note to "code first underlying chronic kidney disease (CKD) (N18.-)."

3. Anemia in other chronic disease classified elsewhere (D63.8)

   The "code first underlying disease, such as:" instruction note is included here. Examples of the underlying diseases that may be coded here are hypothyroidism, malaria, symptomatic late syphilis, and tuberculosis.

Coagulation Defects

Coagulation defects are disorders of the platelets that result in serious bleeding due to a deficiency of one or more clotting factors. ICD-10-CM classifies coagulation defects to categories D65–D68. Coagulation defects include:

1. Disseminated intravascular coagulation [defibrination syndrome], D65

2. Hereditary factor VIII deficiency, D66

   This category includes classical hemophilia or hemophilia A.

3. Hereditary factor IX deficiency, D67

   Factor IX deficiency disorder includes Christmas disease or hemophilia B.

4. Other coagulation defects, D68

Subcategory D68.0 classifies **von Willebrand disease (vWD)**. This is a bleeding disorder that affects the blood's ability to clot. If the blood does not clot, the person will have heavy, difficult to control hemorrhage after an injury. The bleeding can damage the internal organs and can be life threatening. In vWD, there is one of two low levels of a certain protein in the blood or the protein does not function well. The protein is called von Willebrand factor, and it helps to make the blood clot. Small blood cell fragments called platelets clump together to plug the hole in the blood vessel and stop the bleeding. Von Willebrand factor acts like glue to help the platelets stick together and form a blood clot. Von Willebrand factor also carries clotting factor VIII (8), another important protein that helps the blood clot. Factor VIII is the protein that is missing or nonfunctioning in people who have hemophilia, another bleeding disorder. VWD is more common and usually milder than hemophilia. In fact, VWD is the most common inherited bleeding disorder. VWD affects both males and females, while hemophilia mainly affects males.

Purpura and Other Hemorrhagic Conditions

Category D69 includes codes that describe purpura, thrombocytopenia, and other hemorrhagic disorders. **Thrombocytopenia** is diagnosed when the platelets fall below 100,000/mm. Two types of thrombocytopenia are recognized: primary or idiopathic and secondary. Idiopathic or immune thrombocytopenic purpura (ITP) is an autoimmune disorder with development of antibodies to one's own platelets. In children, the condition often resolves without treatment. In adults, medications such as corticosteroids or thrombopoietins are given. In severe cases, the spleen may be removed to eliminate the platelet destruction by phagocytosis. Primary thrombocytopenia may also be congenital or hereditary. Primary thrombocytopenia is classified in ICD-10-CM to D69.4- subcategory depending on the type.

Secondary thrombocytopenia is a complication of another disease. The treatment of the secondary form of this condition centers on treating the underlying disease or changing medication. ICD-10-CM classifies secondary thrombocytopenia to code D69.59. Posttransfusion purpura (PTP) is coded to D69.51. This condition is characterized by a sudden and severe thrombocytopenia (a platelet count of less than 10,000), usually occurring 5 to 10 days following transfusions of whole blood, plasma, platelets, or red blood cells. PTP is a reaction associated with the presence of antibodies directed against the Human Platelet Antigen (HPA) system.

Other Disorders of Blood and Blood-Forming Organs

ICD-10-CM classifies neutropenia to category D70 with fourth character codes for the various specific forms of neutropenia. **Neutropenia** is a decrease in the number of neutrophils, a type of white blood cell. Codes in the range of D70.0–D70.9 describe congenital agranulocytosis, agranulocytosis secondary to cancer chemotherapy, other drug-induced agranulocytosis, neutropenia due to infection, and cyclic neutropenia as well as other and unspecified forms of neutropenia.

Bandemia is defined as the presence of an excess number of immature WBCs or band cells, while the total WBC count is normal. Bandemia is frequently present in patients with bacterial infections. However, bandemia may be identified when a diagnosis of infection has not been established. Pediatricians frequently use this diagnosis in children when the source of an infection is unknown. ICD-10-CM specifically identifies bandemia with code D72.825. Category D72, other disorders of white blood cells, also includes codes for eosinophilia and leukopenia.

Diseases of the spleen, a blood-forming organ, are included in category D73. Specific codes exist for hyposplenism, hypersplenism, chronic congestive splenomegaly, abscess, cyst, and infarction of spleen.

Methemoglobinemia, both congenital and acquired forms, are classified to codes within category D74.

Other and unspecified diseases of blood and blood-forming organs are included in category D75.

It includes myelofibrosis, a chronic progressive disease in which fibrous tissue replaces normal bone marrow. A progressive anemia results even though the spleen attempts to replace the lost blood production and splenomegaly can occur. Secondary polycythemia occurs as a result of tissue hypoxia and is associated with chronic obstructive pulmonary disease, congenital heart disease, and prolonged exposures to high altitudes (higher than 10,000 feet). ICD-10-CM classifies secondary polycythemia to code D75.1. Myelofibrosis can be a primary hematologic disease or a secondary process. Code D47.1, Chronic myeloproliferative disease, is the primary form of the disease. Code D75.81 is used to code the unspecified form or the secondary form of myelofibrosis.

Heparin-induced thrombocytopenia (HIT) is a life-threatening clinical event that can occur in 3 to 5 percent of all patients receiving unfractionated heparin for at least five days or in about 0.5 percent of patients receiving low molecular-weight heparin. HIT is a hypercoagulable state, not a hemorrhagic condition. The diagnosis is first suspected based on a fall in the platelet count by 50 percent or more occurring 5 to 12 days after beginning heparin therapy. Treatment involves the initiation of an alternative anticoagulant or direct thrombin inhibitor drugs. Code D75.82 is included in ICD-10-CM for HIT.

Intraoperative and Postprocedural Complications of the Spleen

Category D78, Intraoperative and postprocedural complications of the spleen, includes codes for intraoperative hemorrhage and hematoma of the spleen, accidental puncture and laceration of the spleen, and postprocedural hemorrhage and hematoma of the spleen. These combination codes identify the specific complication and whether the complication occurred during a procedure on the spleen or the complication occurred during another surgical procedure. Two codes, D78.81 and D78.89, are available to identify another specified type of complication of the spleen beyond the codes in the range of D78.01–D78.22. An additional code is used to further identify what the complication was.

ICD-10-PCS Procedure Coding

The types of procedures that are most closely related to the treatment of blood disorders are administration for transfusions, aspiration, biopsy and transplant.

Administration

Transfusion of blood and blood components is a treatment for various types of blood disorders. Transfusions are coded with ICD-10-PCS codes from the Administration section. There are seven characters to the administration codes:

Character 1: Section

Character 2: Physiological System and Anatomical Region

Character 3: Root Operation

Character 4: Body System/Region

Character 5: Approach

Character 6: Substance

Character 7: Qualifier

Administration codes represent procedures for putting in or on a therapeutic, prophylactic, protective, diagnostic, nutritional, or physiological substance. This section includes codes for transfusions, infusions, and injections as well as similar procedures such as irrigations.

Section

Character 1, which represents the section, uses the value 3.

Body System

Character 2 for the body part contains only three values: Indwelling Device, Physiological Systems and Anatomical Regions, or Circulatory System.

Root Operation

Character 3 is for the root operation. There are only three root operations in the Administration section.

Introduction: Putting in or on a therapeutic, diagnostic, nutritional, physiological, or prophylactic substance except blood or blood products

Irrigation: Putting in or on a cleansing substance

Transfusion: Putting in blood or blood products

Body/System Region

Character 4 specifies the body system/region. This character identifies the site where the substance is administered, not the site where the substance administered takes effect.

119

Sites include Skin and Mucous Membrane, Subcutaneous Tissue, and Muscle. The other sites include Eye, Respiratory Tract, Peritoneal Cavity, and Epidural Space. The body systems/regions for arteries and veins are Peripheral Artery, Central Artery, Peripheral Vein, and Central Vein.

Approach

Character 5 specifies the approach. The Percutaneous approach is for intradermal, subcutaneous, and intramuscular introductions or injections. Other approaches are Open, Via Natural or Artificial Opening, External, and Via Natural or Artificial Opening Endoscopic approaches as defined in the Medical and Surgical section.

Substance

Character 6 specifies the substance being administered or introduced. Broad categories of substances are defined, for example, Anesthetic, Contrast, Dialysate, and Blood Products.

Qualifier

Character 7 is the qualifier and is used for limited factors. A qualifier for autologous and non-autologous specifies the type of substance. Other qualifiers further specify a substance.

When accessing the Index to identify a code for a transfusion, the main term is transfusion followed by subterms for artery, products of conception, and vein for further indentations. Under artery, the coder must know if it is a central or peripheral artery. Under the type of artery, the coder must identify the substance being administered, such as antihemophilic factors, blood, bone marrow, and such. The same factors are found under the subterm vein, that is, is it a central vein or a peripheral vein where the administration is the site where the substance is to be administered. For transfusions, under both artery and vein, the type of blood products must be known: platelets, red cells, frozen red cells, white cells, or whole blood.

Aspiration, Biopsy, and Transplant

Biopsies are common procedures that are used to diagnose blood disorders and disorders of blood-forming organs. In the ICD-10-PCS Index, the entry for biopsy states "see Drainage with qualifier Diagnostic" and "see Excision with qualifier Diagnostic." A **biopsy** or another procedure may also be described as an aspiration biopsy or simply an aspiration. The Index entry for aspiration tells the coder to see Drainage. **Aspiration** or drainage is defined as taking or letting out fluids or gases from a body part.

Two common sites for biopsies for these conditions in blood and blood-forming organs are bone marrow and lymph nodes. A bone marrow aspiration is found in the Index under the main term Drainage, bone marrow with a four-character code of 079T. An aspiration is taking out fluids from the bone marrow through a needle. The coder must identify the approach for this procedure as Open, Percutaneous, or Percutaneous Endoscopic. There is no choice for the device. The seventh character for an aspiration that is a diagnostic procedure would be value X.

When the coder access the Index for a bone marrow biopsy under the main term Excision there is no entry for bone marrow. This is not a mistake. A bone marrow biopsy does not meet the definition of an Excision as there is cutting out or off of a body part. A bone marrow "biopsy" is by definition of how it is performed an Extraction, that is; the bone marrow is pulled or stripped out or off all or a portion of a body part by the use of force. Under the main term Extraction, bone marrow, the coder must know the location of the extraction, that is, iliac, sternum, or vertebral. All three entries lead to the three-character code of 07D. The fourth character is value Q for Sternum, R for Iliac, or S for Vertebral. The approach is either Open or Percutaneous, which is the typical approach. There is no value for device except for Z for no device. The qualifier is either X for diagnostic or Z for no qualifier.

A bone marrow transplant is coded as a transfusion in ICD-10-PCS as it meets the definition of the root operation of "putting in blood or blood products." **Transplantation** is defined as putting in or on all or a portion of a living body part taken from another individual or animal to physically take the place or function of all or a portion of a similar body part. A bone marrow transplant is a procedure to replace damaged or destroyed bone marrow with healthy bone marrow stem cells. Bone marrow is the soft, fatty tissue inside your bones. Stem cells are immature cells in the bone marrow that give rise to all of your blood cells. Stem cell transplants are also coded with the root operation Transfusion.

Coding of a lymph node biopsy is coded to the root operation Excision or Aspiration depending on how the specimen is removed. Usually a lymph node biopsy is performed by cutting or excision. The main term Excision is located in the ICD-10-PCS Index. The body part needs to be identified as the location of the lymphatic structure, for example, Axillary, Inguinal, Neck, and such. The three-character code given is 07B. The approach options are Open, Percutaneous, or Percutaneous Endoscopic. There is no option for device other than Z for no device. A biopsy would have the "qualifier" of X for diagnostic.

ICD-10-CM and ICD-10-PCS Review Exercises: Chapter 6

Assign the correct ICD-10-CM diagnosis codes and ICD-10-PCS procedure codes for the following exercises.

1. Iron deficiency anemia due to blood loss

2. Von Willebrand disease

3. Chronic congestive splenomegaly

4. Congenital nonspherocytic hemolytic anemia

5. Idiopathic thrombocytopenic purpura

6. Fanconi's anemia

(*Continued on next page*)

ICD-10-CM and ICD-10-PCS Review Exercises: Chapter 6 (Continued)

7. Disseminated intravascular coagulation

8. Acute blood loss anemia

9. Cooley's anemia

10. Polycythemia secondary to living in high altitude region

11. Glucose-6 phosphate dehydrogenase (G6PD) anemia

12. Heparin induced thrombocytopenia (HIT)

13. Sickle cell thalassemia with crisis

14. Anemia in end stage renal disease (ESRD)

15. Neutopenic fever

16. PROCEDURE: Transfusion via peripheral vein through percutaneous approach, blood platelets, nonautologous donor blood

17. PROCEDURE: Therapeutic plasmapheresis, single session

18. PROCEDURE: Bone marrow needle extraction biopsy, iliac

19. PROCEDURE: Laparoscopic total splenectomy

20. PROCEDURE: Lymph node open biopsy by excision, right axilla

Chapter 7

Endocrine, Nutritional and Metabolic Diseases (E00–E89)

Learning Objectives

At the conclusion of this chapter, you should be able to:

1. Describe the organization of the conditions and codes included in Chapter 4 of ICD-10-CM, Endocrine, nutritional and metabolic diseases (E00–E89)

2. Identify the eight major endocrine glands

3. Describe the different types of diabetes and how the type of diabetes impacts code selection in ICD-10-CM

4. Identify the codes included in Chapter 4 of ICD-10-CM that describe nutritional and metabolic disorders

5. Assign ICD-10-CM diagnosis codes for endocrine, nutritional and metabolic diseases

6. Assign ICD-10-PCS procedure codes for procedures related to endocrine, nutritional and metabolic diseases

Key Terms

- Cystic fibrosis
- Dehydration
- Diabetes mellitus
- Diabetes type 1
- Diabetes type 2
- Endocrine glands
- Excision
- Hypoglycemia
- Hypovolemia
- Kwashiorkor
- Malnutrition
- Marasmus
- Resection
- Stereotactic radiosurgery

Overview of ICD-10-CM Chapter 4, Endocrine, Nutritional and Metabolic Diseases

Chapter 4 includes categories E00–E89 arranged in the following blocks:

E00–E07	Disorders of thyroid gland
E08–E13	Diabetes mellitus
E15–E16	Other disorders of glucose regulation and pancreatic internal secretion
E20–E35	Disorders of other endocrine glands
E36	Intraoperative complications of endocrine system
E40–D46	Malnutrition
E50–E64	Other nutritional deficiencies
E65–E68	Overweight, obesity and other hyperalimentation
E70–E88	Metabolic disorders
E89	Postprocedural endocrine and metabolic complications and disorders not elsewhere classified

Diabetes mellitus and malnutrition have their own subchapter codes in this chapter. Additional codes can be found for other diseases of other endocrine glands and nutritional deficiencies.

All neoplasms, whether functionally active or not, are classified in Chapter 2. Appropriate codes in Chapter 4 (namely, E05.8-, E07.0, E16–E31, and E34.-) may be used as additional codes to indicate either functional activity by neoplasms and ectopic endocrine tissue or hyperfunction and hypofunction of endocrine glands associated with neoplasms and other conditions classified elsewhere.

Coding Guidelines and Instructional Notes for ICD-10-CM Chapter 4

The NCHS has published chapter-specific guidelines for Chapter 4 in the *ICD-10-CM Official Guidelines for Coding and Reporting*. The coding student should review all of the coding guidelines for Chapter 4 of ICD-10-CM, which appear in an ICD-10-CM code book or at the website http://www.cdc.gov/nchs/icd/icd10cm.htm, or in Appendix E.

Guideline I.C.4.a. Diabetes mellitus

The diabetes mellitus codes are combination codes that include the type of diabetes mellitus, the body system affected, and the complications affecting that body system. As many codes within a particular category as are necessary to describe all of the complications of the disease may be used. They should be sequenced based on the reason for a particular encounter. Assign as many codes from categories E08–E13 as needed to identify all of the associated conditions that the patient has.

1. Type of diabetes

   The age of a patient is not the sole determining factor, though most type 1 diabetics develop the condition before reaching puberty. For this reason type 1 diabetes mellitus is also referred to as juvenile diabetes.

2. Type of diabetes mellitus not documented

   If the type of diabetes mellitus is not documented in the medical record the default is E11.-, Type 2 diabetes mellitus.

3. Diabetes mellitus and the use of insulin

   If the documentation in a medical record does not indicate the type of diabetes but does indicate that the patient uses insulin, code E11, Type 2 diabetes mellitus, should be assigned. Code Z79.4, Long-term (current) use of insulin, should also be assigned to indicate that the patient uses insulin. Code Z79.4 should not be assigned if insulin is given temporarily to bring a type 2 patient's blood sugar under control during an encounter.

4. Diabetes mellitus in pregnancy and gestational diabetes

   See Section I.C.15. Diabetes mellitus in pregnancy.
   See Section I.C.15. Gestational (pregnancy induced) diabetes

5. Complications due to insulin pump malfunction

   a. Underdose of insulin due to insulin pump failure

      An underdose of insulin due to an insulin pump failure should be assigned to a code from subcategory T85.6, Mechanical complication of other specified internal and external prosthetic devices, implants and grafts, that specifies the type of pump malfunction, as the principal or first-listed code, followed by code T38.3x6-, Underdosing of insulin and oral hypoglycemic [antidiabetic] drugs. Additional codes for the type of diabetes mellitus and any associated complications due to the underdosing should also be assigned.

   b. Overdose of insulin due to insulin pump failure

      The principal or first-listed code for an encounter due to an insulin pump malfunction resulting in an overdose of insulin, should also be T85.6-, Mechanical complication of other specified internal and external prosthetic devices, implants and grafts, followed by code T38.3x1-, Poisoning by insulin and oral hypoglycemic [antidiabetic] drugs, accidental (unintentional).

(Continued)

(*Continued*)

6. Secondary diabetes mellitus

   Codes under categories E08, Diabetes mellitus due to underlying condition, and E09, Drug or chemical induced diabetes mellitus, identify complications/manifestations associated with secondary diabetes mellitus. Secondary diabetes is always caused by another condition or event (e.g., cystic fibrosis, malignant neoplasm of pancreas, pancreatectomy, adverse effect of drug, or poisoning).

   a. Secondary diabetes mellitus and the use of insulin

      For patients who routinely use insulin, code Z79.4, Long-term (current) use of insulin, should also be assigned. Code Z79.4 should not be assigned if insulin is given temporarily to bring a patient's blood sugar under control during an encounter.

   b. Assigning and sequencing secondary diabetes codes and its causes

      The sequencing of the secondary diabetes codes in relationship to codes for the cause of the diabetes is based on the Tabular List instructions for categories E08 and E09. For example, for category E08, Diabetes mellitus due to underlying condition, code first the underlying condition; for category E09, Drug or chemical induced diabetes mellitus, code first the drug or chemical (T36–T65).

      i. Secondary diabetes mellitus due to pancreatectomy

         For postpancreatectomy diabetes mellitus (lack of insulin due to the surgical removal of all or part of the pancreas), assign code E89.1, Postprocedural hypoinsulinemia. Assign a code from category E13 and a code from subcategory Z90.41-, Acquired absence of pancreas, as additional codes.

      ii. Secondary diabetes due to drugs

         Secondary diabetes may be caused by an adverse effect of correctly administered medications, poisoning or sequela of poisoning. *See section I.C.19.e for coding of adverse effects and poisoning, and section I.C.20 for external cause code reporting.*

Coding Endocrine, Nutritional and Metabolic Diseases in ICD-10-CM Chapter 4

Chapter 4 of ICD-10-CM, Endocrine, nutritional and metabolic Diseases (E00–E89) contains many frequently coded conditions such as disorders of the thyroid gland, obesity, dehydration, and diabetes mellitus. There is an Excludes1 note at the beginning of ICD-10-CM, Chapter 4 for transitory endocrine and metabolic disorders specific to the newborn (P70–P74).

Disorders of Thyroid Gland (E00-E07)

This block of codes contains the frequently coded conditions of hypothyroidism, nontoxic goiter, thyrotoxicosis or hyperthyroidism, and thyroiditis. For the conditions that are related to drugs, there are notes to "code first" poisoning due to drug or toxin and use additional code for adverse effect. For acute thyroiditis, another note reminds the coder to use additional code (B95–B97) to identify the infectious agent.

Diabetes Mellitus (E08-E13)

Diabetes mellitus is a metabolic disease in which the pancreas does not produce insulin normally. The cause of diabetes mellitus can be attributed to both hereditary and nonhereditary factors, such as obesity, surgical removal of the pancreas, or the action of certain drugs. When the pancreas fails to produce insulin, glucose (sugar) is not broken down to be used and stored by the body's cells. As a result, too much sugar accumulates in the blood, causing hyperglycemia and resulting in spill-over into the urine, causing glycosuria. Saturating the blood and urine with glucose draws water out of the body, causing dehydration and thirst. Other symptoms include excessive hunger, marked weakness, and weight loss. Treatment may consist of insulin regulation by either insulin injection or oral antidiabetic agents, along with physical activity and a healthy diet. Over time, high blood glucose can lead to serious problems in the heart, eyes, kidneys, nerves, gums, and teeth.

Diabetes type 1 is usually diagnosed in children and young adults, and was previously known as juvenile diabetes but can appear at any age. In type 1 diabetes, the body does not produce insulin. Only 5 percent of people with diabetes have this form of the disease. Symptoms of type 1 diabetes include frequent urination, unusual thirst, extreme hunger, unusual weight loss, and extreme fatigue and irritability.

The most common type of diabetes is **diabetes type 2**. The body does not produce enough insulin or the cells ignore the insulin or use insulin well. The patient who is older, obese, has a family history of diabetes, and does not exercise is at higher risk of type 2 diabetes. The symptoms of type 2 diabetes appear slowly. Symptoms include the same symptoms type 1 diabetic patients experience in addition to frequent infections, blurred vision, cuts and bruises that are slow to heal, and tingling and numbness in the hands and feet. However, some people do not notice symptoms at all.

There are five categories for diabetes mellitus in ICD-10-CM. The diabetes mellitus codes reflect manifestations and complications of the disease by using the fourth or fifth characters. ICD-10-CM classifies inadequately controlled, out of control, and poorly controlled diabetes mellitus by reporting diabetes mellitus, by type, with hyperglycemia.

The diabetes mellitus codes are combination codes that include the

- type of diabetes (type 1, type 2, due to underlying condition or due to drug or chemical),

- body system affected, and

- complications affecting that body system.

For type 1 and type 2 diabetes, the diabetes code contains the details about the type of diabetes and most of the associated complications. A few of the diabetes codes require the use of an additional code, for example to identify the stage of the chronic kidney disease caused by the diabetes. For other types of diabetes, the underlying condition is listed first, followed by the diabetes code that includes any associated complication.

Each type of diabetes has a particular category of codes:

- E08, Diabetes mellitus due to underlying condition

  ○ Code first the underlying condition, such as forms of Cushing's Syndrome (category E24.-)

- E09, Diabetes or chemical induced diabetes mellitus

  ○ Code first poisoning (T36–T65) to identify drug or toxin, if applicable (T36–T65 with fifth or sixth character 1–4 or 6)

  ○ Use additional code for adverse effect, if applicable, to identify drug (T36–T50 with fifth or sixth character 5)

  ○ Use additional code to identify any insulin use (Z79.4)

- E10, Type 1 diabetes mellitus

  ○ Includes: brittle diabetes (mellitus), diabetes (mellitus) due to autoimmune process, diabetes (mellitus) due to immune mediated pancreatic islet beta-cell destruction, idiopathic diabetes (mellitus), juvenile onset diabetes (mellitus) and ketosis-prone diabetes (mellitus)

- E11, Type 2 diabetes mellitus

  ○ Includes: diabetes (mellitus) due to insulin secretory defect, diabetes NOS, insulin resistant diabetes (mellitus)

  ○ Use additional code to identify any insulin use (Z79.4)

- E13, Other specified diabetes mellitus

  ○ Includes: diabetes mellitus due to genetic defects of beta-cell function, diabetes mellitus due to genetic defects in insulin action, postpancreatectomy diabetes mellitus, postprocedural diabetes mellitus, secondary diabetes mellitus NEC

  ○ Use additional code to identify any insulin use (Z79.4)

Other forms of diabetes are coded elsewhere in ICD-10-CM:

- Gestational diabetes (O24.4-)
- Neonatal diabetes mellitus (P70.2)

In addition to identifying the type of diabetes, the ICD-10-CM code includes one or more of the complications or manifestations that exists in a particular body system. For example,

- E08.21, Diabetes mellitus due to underlying condition with diabetic nephropathy
- E09.610, Drug or chemical induced diabetes mellitus with diabetic neuropathic arthropathy
- E10.321, Type 1 diabetes mellitus with mild nonproliferative diabetic retinopathy with macular edema

- E11.51, Type 2 diabetes mellitus with diabetic peripheral angiopathy without gangrene

- E13.620, Other specified diabetes mellitus with diabetic dermatitis

The coder may assign as many codes from categories E08–E13 as needed to identify all the associated conditions that a patient may have had treated. Except for type 1 diabetes, an additional code of Z79.4 is used to identify patients who routinely use insulin for the management of their type 2 or other forms of diabetes. Type 1 diabetes mellitus is typically treated with insulin and therefore the additional code Z79.4 would be not be used with type 1 diabetes. Other forms of diabetes may or may not use insulin as part of the treatment. When insulin is used with other types of diabetes, for example with type 2 diabetes, the additional code of Z79.4 provides more information about the patient's disease and what is required to treat it.

Other Disorders of Glucose Regulation and Pancreatic Internal Secretion (E15–E16)

Codes for nondiabetic hypoglycemic coma, other hypoglycemic conditions, and Zollinger-Ellison syndrome are included in this block of codes. Code E16.0, Drug-induced hypoglycemia without coma, has an "use additional code" note to add a code for adverse effect, if applicable, to identify a drug (T36–T50 with fifth or sixth character 5).

Codes for specified forms of hypoglycemia or the unspecified diagnosis of hypoglycemia are included in category E16, other disorders of pancreatic internal secretion. The body needs glucose, a form of sugar, to have enough energy. After a meal, the person's blood absorbs glucose. If the person eats more sugar than needed, muscles and the liver store the extra. When the blood sugar declines, a hormone causes the liver to release glucose. Usually this raises blood sugar. If it does not elevate the blood sugar level, the person has a condition called **hypoglycemia**. In some situations, the blood sugar can be dangerously low. Physical signs and symptoms of hypoglycemia include hunger, confusion, shakiness, dizziness, weakness, anxiety, and sometimes difficulty speaking.

Hypoglycemia is usually a side effect of diabetes medicine. However, a person can also have hypoglycemia without having diabetes. In order to find the cause of hypoglycemia certain laboratory tests will be performed to measure blood glucose, insulin, and other chemicals that play a part in the body's use of energy. The code for unspecified hypoglycemia in the category E16 will likely be used for the patient's reason for theses diagnostic studies.

Disorders of Other Endocrine Glands (E20–E35)

The endocrine system is made up of the endocrine glands that secrete hormones. There are eight major **endocrine glands**: pituitary, pineal, thyroid, thymus, adrenal, pancreas, testes in males, and ovaries in females. These glands are scattered throughout the body but are considered one body system because of their similar functions and mechanisms of influence as well as important interrelationships.

Codes for disorders of the parathyroid gland, pituitary gland, adrenal gland, thymus gland, as well as testicular and ovarian dysfunction are included here. Some of the commonly coded conditions in this block of codes are Cushing's syndrome, Addison's disease, polycystic ovarian syndrome, premature menopause, multiple endocrine neoplasia (MEN) syndromes, and carcinoid syndrome. For conditions related to the use of medications, notes are included to "use additional code" for adverse effect to identify the drug or drugs that are responsible for the gland's dysfunction.

Malnutrition (E40–E46)

Malnutrition is the condition that occurs when the body does not get enough nutrients. There are a number of causes of malnutrition. It may result from inadequate or unbalanced diet, problems with digestion or absorption, and certain medical conditions. Malnutrition can occur if a person does not eat enough food. Starvation is a form of malnutrition. A person may develop malnutrition if there is a lack of a single vitamin in the diet. In some cases, malnutrition is very mild and causes no symptoms. However, sometimes it can be so severe that the damage done to the body is permanent.

ICD-10-CM contains a code for **kwashiorkor,** a severe malnutrition with nutritional edema with dyspigmentation of skin and hair. This condition is most common in areas where there is famine, limited food supply, and low levels of education of how to eat a proper diet. This disease is more common in very poor countries. It often occurs during a drought or other natural disaster, or during political unrest. These conditions are responsible for a lack of food, which leads to malnutrition. Kwashiorkor is very rare in children in the United States. When kwashiorkor does occur in the United States, it is usually a sign of child abuse and severe neglect.

Marasmus is a severe deficiency of calories and protein. It tends to develop in infants and very young children. It typically results in weight loss and dehydration. Breastfeeding usually protects against marasmus.

ICD-10-CM contains a limited number of malnutrition codes in this chapter. Codes are included for severe malnutrition, moderate and mild degree protein-calorie malnutrition, and malnutrition unspecified. The documentation required to best describe the type of malnutrition would include the degree of malnutrition (first, mild, moderate, second, severe, third), or the type of protein calorie or protein energy malnutrition (mild, moderate, or severe).

Other Nutritional Deficiencies (E50–E64)

Codes in this section classify a variety of vitamin and other nutrient deficiencies. For example, the conditions included here are vitamin A, thiamine, B group, D, and K deficiencies. Other conditions include dietary deficiencies of calcium, zinc, iron, magnesium, and other specified nutrient elements. Also in this block of codes is category E64, Sequelae of malnutrition and other nutritional deficiencies. This category is used to indicate conditions in categories E43, E44, E46, E50–63 as the cause of sequelae, which are themselves classified elsewhere. These are the "late effects" of diseases classifiable to the above categories if the disease itself is no longer present. A "code first" note to code the condition resulting from (sequela) of malnutrition and other nutritional deficiencies is included here.

Overweight, Obesity, and Other Hyperalimentation (E65–E68)

With category E66, overweight and obesity, two instructional notes are included. A code first note appears here to code obesity complicating pregnancy, childbirth, and the puerperium if applicable, that is if the patient is pregnant or in the postpartum period. Another note states "use additional code to identify body mass index (BMI) if known (Z68.1-)" for all the codes in category E66. Coding guideline 1.B.14 addresses documentation for BMI and pressure ulcer stages. The BMI level can be coded based on other clinicians' documentation if the BMI meets the requirements for a reportable additional diagnosis.

Metabolic Disorders (E70–E88)

This block of codes is a mixture of common and not-so-common diseases. The commonly coded conditions here are hypercholesterolemia, hyperlipidemia, cystic fibrosis, dehydration, hyper- and hypokalemia, electrolyte imbalance, and metabolic syndrome. Less commonly occurring conditions coded here are a variety of metabolism disorders including fatty-acid, amino-acid, purine, and porphyrin metabolism.

Volume depletion may refer to depletion of total body water (dehydration) or depletion of the blood volume (hypovolemia). **Dehydration**, a lack of adequate water in the body, can be a medical emergency. This condition is classified to E86.0. Common in infants and elderly people, severe dehydration can occur with vomiting, excessive heat and sweating, diarrhea, or lack of food or fluid intake. Blood volume may be maintained despite dehydration, with fluid being pulled from other tissues. Conversely, hypovolemia may occur without dehydration when "third-spacing" of fluids occurs, for example, with significant edema or ascites. **Hypovolemia** is an abnormally low circulating blood volume and is classified to E86.1. Blood loss may be due to internal bleeding from the intestine or stomach, external bleeding from an injury, or loss of blood volume and body fluid associated with diarrhea, vomiting, dehydration, or burns. If hypovolemia is severe, hypovolemic shock can occur with symptoms such as rapid or weak pulse, feeling faint, pale skin, cool or moist skin, rapid breathing, anxiety, overall weakness, and low blood pressure. Emergency medical attention must be sought. Given that the nature of these two conditions and their respective treatments are different, coding of hypovolemia is different from dehydration.

> **EXAMPLE:** Patient admitted with severe dehydration and gastroenteritis.
> Treatment was directed toward resolving the dehydration.
> E86.0 Dehydration
> K52.9 Gastroenteritis

Cystic fibrosis is an inherited disease of the exocrine glands that affects the gastrointestinal and respiratory systems. Category codes for cystic fibrosis (CF) (category E84) describe the complications that occur with CF in the respiratory system, digestive system, and other manifestations that often occur. Cystic fibrosis is characterized by chronic obstructive pulmonary disease, pancreatic insufficiency, and abnormally high sweat electrolytes. The degree of pulmonary involvement usually determines the course of the disease. The patient's demise is often the result of respiratory failure and cor pulmonale. A "use additional code to identify any infectious organism present, such as: Pseudomonas (B96.5)" appears under code E84.0 for cystic fibrosis with pulmonary manifestations.

Postprocedural Endocrine and Metabolic Complications and Disorders, Not Elsewhere Classified (E89)

A limited number of postprocedural, postsurgical, or postirradiation complications and disorders are coded in Chapter 4 of ICD-10-CM. Such conditions include postprocedural hypothyroidism, hypoinsulinemia, hypoparathyroidism, hypopituitarism, and postprocedural ovarian failure. As in other chapters, postprocedural hemorrhage and hematoma of an endocrine system organ are included at the end of the block of codes.

ICD-10-PCS Procedure Codes for Procedures Related to Chapter 4, Endocrine, Nutritional and Metabolic Disorders

The root operations that represent the objectives of procedures for diseases of the endocrine system are Change, Destruction, Division, Drainage, Excision, Extirpation, Insertion, Inspection, Reattachment, Release, Removal, Repair, Reposition, Resection, and Revision. The more common procedures on the endocrine glands are Excision, Resection, and Destruction.

The surgical removal of all (**Resection**) or part (**Excision**) of endocrine glands are coded based on the body part involved, such as Adrenal Glands, Thyroid, and Parathyroid Glands. The body parts have individual values that include laterality when a pair of glands exists. The approach for the excision and resection procedures include Open, Percutaneous, and Percutaneous Endoscopic approaches as applicable. The qualifier value of X for diagnostic procedure is available for the root operation of Excision. The coder should review the ICD-10-PCS guideline for B3.8 and B4.1a for a complete description of coding excision and resection procedures.

Stereotactic radiosurgery using a gamma beam, particulate type, or other photon radiosurgery is available to destroy lesions on endocrine glands such as the adrenal, parathyroid, pineal body, pituitary, and thyroid glands. Stereotactic radiosurgery is classified in the radiation oncology section of ICD-10-PCS. The main term to use in the Index to locate these procedures is "stereotactic radiosurgery" with subterms of gamma beam, other photon and particulate with additional entries of the body part involved. **Stereotactic radiosurgery** is a form of radiation therapy that focuses high-powered x-rays on a small area of the body. Other types of radiation therapy can affect nearby healthy tissue; stereotactic radiosurgery better targets the abnormal area. Despite its name, radiosurgery is a treatment, not a surgical procedure.

ICD-10-CM and ICD-10-PCS Review Exercises: Chapter 7

Assign the correct ICD-10-CM diagnosis codes and ICD-10-PCS procedure codes for the following exercises.

1. Type 2 diabetic with nephropathy due to the diabetes

   _____

2. Toxic diffuse goiter with thyrotoxic storm

   _____

3. Cushing's syndrome

   _____

4. Hypokalemia

   _____

5. Cystic fibrosis with pulmonary manifestations

   _____

ICD-10-CM and ICD-10-PCS Review Exercises: Chapter 7 (Continued)

6. Uncontrolled (hyperglycemia) type 2 diabetes mellitus; mild degree malnutrition

7. Panhypopituitarism

8. Lower extremity ulcer on skin of left heel secondary to brittle diabetes mellitus, type 1, uncontrolled

9. Diabetic proliferative retinopathy in a patient with controlled type 1 diabetes

10. Overweight adult with a body mass index (BMI) of 26.5

11. Syndrome of inappropriate secretion of antidiuretic hormone (SIADH)

12. Hypoglycemia in type 1 diabetes with coma

13. Postsurgical hypothyroidism

14. Folic acid deficiency

15. Partial androgen insensitivity syndrome

16. PROCEDURE: Open total thyroidectomy

17. PROCEDURE: Partial left lobectomy, thyroid gland, open

18. PROCEDURE: Right carotid body biopsy, open, by excision

19. PROCEDURE: Laparoscopic partial left adrenalectomy

20. PROCEDURE: Stereotactic gamma beam radiosurgery, parathyroid gland tumor

Chapter 8

Mental, Behavioral and Neurodevelopmental Disorders (F01–F99)

Learning Objectives

At the conclusion of this chapter, you should be able to:

1. Describe the organization of the conditions and codes included in Chapter 5 of ICD-10-CM, Mental and behavioral disorders (F01–F99)

2. Describe the *DSM-IV-TR* and explain its purpose

3. Describe the multiple coding rules related to the coding of mental disorders

4. Review the inclusion and exclusion notes for the classification of mental disorders

5. Describe the ICD-10-CM coding guidelines for the selection of principal diagnosis for patients admitted for alcohol or drug dependence treatment

6. Assign ICD-10-CM codes for mental and behavioral disorders

7. Assign ICD-10-PCS codes for mental and behavioral disorders related procedures

Key Terms

- Alcoholism
- Bipolar disorder
- Borderline personality disorder
- Detoxification
- *The Diagnostic and Statistical Manual of Mental Disorders, Fourth Edition, Text Revision* (DSM-IV-TR)
- Drug dependence
- Eating disorder
- Generalized anxiety disorder (GAD)
- Intellectual disabilities
- Rehabilitation
- Schizophrenia

Overview of ICD-10-CM Chapter 5 Mental, Behavioral and Neurodevelopment Disorders (F01–F99)

Chapter 5 organizes mental and behavioral disorders in the following blocks:

F01–F09	Mental disorders due to known physiological conditions
F10–F19	Mental and behavioral disorders due to psychoactive substance use
F20–F29	Schizophrenia, schizotypal and delusional, and other non-mood psychotic disorders
F30–F39	Mood [affective] disorders
F40–F48	Anxiety, dissociative, stress-related, somatoform and other nonpsychotic mental disorders
F50–F59	Behavioral syndromes associated with physiological disturbances and physical factors
F60–F69	Disorders of adult personality and behavior
F70–F79	Mental retardation
F80–F89	Pervasive and specific developmental disorders
F90–F98	Behavioral and emotional disorders with onset usually occurring in childhood and adolescence
F99	Unspecified mental disorder

Chapter 5, Mental, behavioral, and neurodevelopmental disorders (F01–F99), allows for more specific coding of these conditions consistent with the language of behavioral health and substance abuse services as documented in health and client records today. For example, mental and behavioral disorders due to psychoactive substance use (F10–F19) include an extensive number of codes that link the substance involved (alcohol or specific drug) with the specific disorder caused by it. For instance, code F14.280 identifies cocaine dependence with cocaine-induced anxiety disorder. The Index to Diseases and Injuries provides access to these codes under the main term "dependence," with the substance and subterms beneath it to identify the behavioral disturbance associated with the substance.

There are unique codes for alcohol and drug use (not specified as abuse or dependence), and abuse and dependence, so careful review of the documentation is required. There are changes to the codes for drug and alcohol abuse and dependence. A history of drug or alcohol dependence is coded as "in remission" but the diagnosis of history or in remission requires the provider's clinical judgment and must be specifically documented in the patient's record. Further, there are combination codes for drug and alcohol use and associated conditions, such as withdrawal, sleep disorders, or psychosis. Under the category F10, there is a "use additional code" note for blood alcohol level (Y90.-), if applicable. Blood alcohol level can be indexed in the External Cause of Injuries Index.

Other categories in this chapter, including schizophrenia, mood disorders, anxiety, dissociative, or other nonpsychotic disorders, allow for more specific reporting of the current episode of illness. Chapter 5 also includes codes for eating disorders, sleep disorders not due to a substance or known physiological condition, impulse disorders, and gender identity disorders, as well as specific developmental disorders.

DSM-IV-TR

The codes in Chapter 5 of ICD-10-CM parallel the codes in *The Diagnostic and Statistical Manual of Mental Disorders, Fourth Edition, Text Revision* (**DSM-IV-TR**), in most cases.

DSM-IV-TR provides clear descriptions of diagnostic categories that allow clinicians and investigators to diagnose, communicate about, study, and treat people with various mental disorders. Definitions of mental disorders classified in Chapter 5 of ICD-10-CM can be found in DSM-IV-TR. Keep in mind that coders must assign diagnosis codes based on medical record documentation by a provider who is legally qualified to render a medical diagnosis. However, coders might find the definitions useful for a basic understanding of the mental disorders documented in the medical record.

DSM-IV-TR uses a multiaxial system involving an assessment on five different axes:

- Axis I (Clinical Disorders and Other Conditions That May Be a Focus of Attention) includes all psychiatric disorders except personality disorders and mental retardation.

- Axis II includes personality disorders and mental retardation.

- Axis III identifies the presence of general medical conditions.

- Axis IV is used to note clinically relevant psychosocial and environmental problems.

- Axis V is used to indicate the individual's overall psychological, social, and occupational functioning.

In addition, axes I, II, and III provide diagnostic information.

Coding Guidelines and Instructional Notes for ICD-10-CM Chapter 5

The NCHS has published chapter-specific guidelines for chapter 5 in the *ICD-10-CM Official Guidelines for Coding and Reporting*. The coding student should review all of the coding guidelines for Chapter 5 of ICD-10-CM, which appear in an ICD-10-CM code book or at the website http://www.cdc.gov/nchs/icd/icd10cm.htm, or in Appendix E.

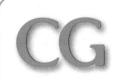

Guideline I.C.5.a. Pain disorders related to psychological factors

Assign code F45.41 for pain that is exclusively related to psychological disorders. As indicated in the Excludes 1 note under category G89, a code from category G89 should not be assigned with code F45.41.

Code F45.42, Pain disorders with related psychological factors, should be used with a code from category G89, Pain, not elsewhere classified, if there is documentation of a psychological component for a patient with acute or chronic pain.

(Continued)

(Continued)

See Section I.C.6 Pain

Guidelines I.C.5.b. Mental and behavioral disorders due to psychoactive substance use

1. In Remission

   Selection of codes for "in remission" for categories F10–F19, mental and behavioral disorders due to psychoactive substance use (categories F10–F19 with -.21) requires the provider's clinical judgment. The appropriate codes for "in remission" are assigned only on the basis of provider documentation (as defined in the Official Guidelines for Coding and Reporting).

2. Psychoactive Substance Use, Abuse, and Dependence

   When the provider documentation refers to use, abuse and dependence of the same substance (that is, alcohol, opioid, cannabis, etc.), only one code should be assigned to identify the pattern of use based on the following hierarchy:

   • If both use and abuse are documented, assign only the code for abuse

   • If both abuse and dependence are documented, assign only the code for dependence

   • If use, abuse, and dependence are all documented, assign only the code for dependence

   • If both use and dependence are documented, assign only the code for dependence.

3. Psychoactive Substance Use

   As with all other diagnoses, the codes for psychoactive substance use (F10.9-, F11.9-, F12.9-, F13.9-, F14.9-, F15.9-, F16.9-) should only be assigned based on provider documentation and when they meet the definition of a reportable diagnosis (see Section III, Reporting Additional Diagnoses). The codes are to be used only when the psychoactive substance use is associated with a mental or behavioral disorder, and such a relationship is documented by the provider.

Coding Mental, Behavioral and Neurodevelopmental Disorders in ICD-10-CM Chapter 5

The codes in this chapter include disorders of psychological development, but exclude symptoms, signs, and abnormal clinical laboratory findings (R00–R99).

Within Chapter 5 of ICD-10-CM, the behavioral health conditions are organized into related sections. Each section has specific Index entries with Includes, Excludes1, and Excludes2 notes, along with directional notes to further explain the coding of the conditions. The terminology used by the physicians must be carefully followed in the Index and Tabular List to code accurately.

The diagnosis codes must be used and reported to the highest level of specificity provided by the physician. In this chapter many of the codes have been expanded to include related conditions and manifestations. An understanding of the diseases and updated clinical terminology in the behavioral health setting is crucial to accurately code the conditions treated. Coders should make no assumptions about the meaning of physician diagnostic statements; when in doubt the physician should be asked for clarification.

Direction notes are included in the chapter to direct the coder how to use the codes appropriately. A note appears to explain what conditions are included in a section. For example, under the block of codes for mental disorders due to known physiological conditions (F01–F09), a note explains these codes include a group of mental disorders that have a common etiology in cerebral disease, brain injury, or other disorder leading to cerebral dysfunction. Other instructional notes appear to direct the coder when multiple coding is required to describe the coexistence of physical and psychological conditions.

Multiple Coding

When coding mental disorders, instructional notations to assign additional codes to fully describe the patient's condition are frequently encountered. Examples of such instructional notations follow:

- Instructional note to assign an additional code to identify any associated behavioral disorder

    EXAMPLE: F01.51 Vascular dementia with behavioral disturbance

    Use additional code, if applicable, to identify wandering in vascular dementia (Z91.83)

- Instructional note to code first the underlying physiological condition

    EXAMPLE: F07.0 Personality change due to known physiological condition

    Code first the underlying physiological condition

- Instructional note to code first the associated physical disorder

    EXAMPLE: F54 Psychological and behavioral factors associated with disorders or disease classified elsewhere

    Code first the associated physical condition, such as:

    Asthma (J45.-)

    Dermatitis (L23–L25)

    Gastric ulcer (K25.-)

    Mucous colitis (K58.-)

    Ulcerative colitis (K51.-)

    Urticaria (L50.-)

- Instructional note to use additional code to identify other conditions

> **EXAMPLE:**   F84 Pervasive developmental disorders
>
> Use additional code to identify any associated medical condition and intellectual disabilities

Inclusion and Exclusion Notes

Chapter 5 of ICD-10-CM contains many special inclusion notes, such as those in the following two examples.

> **EXAMPLE:**   F16   Hallucinogen related disorders
> Includes: ecstasy
> PCP
> phencyclidine

The preceding inclusion note says that ecstasy, PCP, and phencyclidine are included in hallucinogen related disorders, as these are hallucinogen drugs.

> **EXAMPLE:**   F44   Dissociative and conversion disorders
> Includes: conversion hysteria
> conversion reaction
> hysteria
> hysterical psychosis

The preceding inclusion note serves to advise that conditions described as conversion hysteria, conversion reaction, hysteria, and hysteria psychosis are coded to category F44.

Exclusion notes also are used frequently in Chapter 5 to warn that specified forms of a condition are classified elsewhere, such as

> **EXAMPLE:**   F10.1   Alcohol abuse
> Excludes1: Alcohol dependence (F10.2-)
> Alcohol use, unspecified (F10.9-)

The preceding Excludes1 note advises that the codes for alcohol dependence and alcohol use cannot be used with code F10.1- for alcohol abuse as these terms are mutually exclusive. Patients will have only one of these conditions: abuse, dependence, or use.

> **EXAMPLE:**   F15   Other stimulant related disorders
> Excludes2: cocaine-related disorders (F14.-)

The Excludes2 notes indicates that a code for cocaine-related disorders (F14.-) can be used with a code from other stimulant related disorders (F15.-) because a patient can have both a stimulant-related disorder and a cocaine-related disorder. An Excludes2 note indicates that both conditions can be coded when a patient is treated for both conditions.

Alcoholism and Alcohol Abuse and Use

Alcoholism (alcohol dependence) is a chronic condition in which a patient has become dependent on alcohol with increased tolerance and is unable to stop using it, even while facing strong incentives such as impairment of health, deteriorated social interactions, and interference with job performance. Such patients often experience physical signs of withdrawal during any sudden cessation of drinking.

According to DSM-IV-TR, the definition of alcohol dependence is the following:

A. A maladaptive pattern of drinking, leading to clinically significant impairment or distress, as manifested by three or more of the following occurring at any time in the same 12-month period:

- Need for markedly increased amounts of alcohol to achieve intoxication or desired effect; or markedly diminished effect with continued use of the same amount of alcohol

- The characteristic withdrawal syndrome for alcohol; or drinking (or using a closely related substance) to relieve or avoid withdrawal symptoms

- Drinking in larger amounts or over a longer period than intended

- Persistent desire or one or more unsuccessful efforts to cut down or control drinking

- Important social, occupational, or recreational activities given up or reduced because of drinking

- A great deal of time spent in activities necessary to obtain, to use, or to recover from the effects of drinking

- Continued drinking despite knowledge of having a persistent or recurrent physical or psychological problem that is likely to be caused or exacerbated by drinking

B. No duration criterion separately specified, but several dependence criteria must occur repeatedly as specified by duration qualifiers associated with criteria (that is, "persistent," "continued") (APA 2004).

Alcoholism is classified to subcategory F10.2-, Alcohol dependence. The fifth characters identify the following:

- alcohol dependence, uncomplicated (F10.20)

- alcohol dependence, in remission (F10.21)

- alcohol dependence with intoxication (F10.22-) with a sixth character to identify alcohol dependence with intoxication, uncomplicated, with delirium, or unspecified as to the type

- alcohol dependence with withdrawal (F10.23-)

- alcohol dependence with alcohol-induced mood disorder (F10.24)

- alcohol dependence with alcohol-induced psychotic disorder (F10.25-) with a sixth character to identify alcohol dependence with delusions, hallucinations, or unspecified as to the type

- alcohol dependence with alcohol-induced persisting amnestic disorder (F10.26)

- alcohol dependence with alcohol-induced persisting dementia (F10.27)

- alcohol dependence with other alcohol-induced disorders (F10.28-) with a sixth character to identify alcohol dependence with anxiety disorder, sexual dysfunction, sleep disorder and other alcohol-induced disorder

- alcohol dependence with unspecified alcohol-induced disorder (F10.29)

Other codes exist in ICD-10-CM for alcohol abuse (F10.1-) with fifth and sixth characters to classify alcohol abuse with intoxication, alcohol-induced mood disorder, alcohol-induced psychotic disorder, and other alcohol-induced disorders. When the terminology of "alcohol use" is used by a health care provider without further specification as to whether the disorder is a dependence or an abuse type, there are ICD-10-CM codes with five and six characters for alcohol use, unspecified (F10.9-).

Drug Dependence and Abuse

Drug dependence or drug addiction is a chronic mental and physical condition related to the patient's pattern of taking a drug or a combination of drugs. It is characterized by behavioral and physiological responses such as a compulsion to take the drug, to experience its psychic effects, or to avoid the discomfort of its absence. There is increased tolerance and an inability to stop the use of the drug, even with strong incentives.

According to DSM-IV-TR, the criteria or definition of substance or drug dependence is as follows:

> Substance dependence is defined as a maladaptive pattern of substance use leading to clinically significant impairment or distress, as manifested by three (or more) of the following, occurring any time in the same 12-month period:
>
> 1. Tolerance, as defined by either of the following: (a) A need for markedly increased amounts of the substance to achieve intoxication or the desired effect or (b) Markedly diminished effect with continued use of the same amount of the substance.
>
> 2. Withdrawal, as manifested by either of the following: (a) The characteristic withdrawal syndrome for the substance or (b) The same (or closely related) substance is taken to relieve or avoid withdrawal symptoms.
>
> 3. The substance is often taken in larger amounts or over a longer period than intended.
>
> 4. There is a persistent desire or unsuccessful efforts to cut down or control substance use.
>
> 5. A great deal of time is spent in activities necessary to obtain the substance, use the substance, or recover from its effects.
>
> 6. Important social, occupational, or recreational activities are given up or reduced because of substance use.
>
> The substance use is continued despite knowledge of having a persistent physical or psychological problem that is likely to have been caused or exacerbated by the substance (for example, current cocaine use despite recognition of cocaine-induced depression or continued drinking despite recognition that an ulcer was made worse by alcohol consumption) (APA 2004).

ICD-10-CM includes a series of three-character categories for drug related disorders:

F11 Opioid related disorders
F12 Cannabis related disorders

F13 Sedative, hypnotic or anxiolytic-related disorders
F14 Cocaine related disorders
F15 Other stimulant related disorders
F16 Hallucinogen related disorders
F17 Nicotine dependence
F18 Inhalant related disorders
F19 Other psychoactive substance related disorders

All of the categories have a similar outline: four-character codes for drug abuse, drug dependence, and drug use, unspecified. The codes are further divided into drug abuse, drug dependence and drug use that exist with intoxication, mood disorder, psychotic disorder, and other drug induced disorders.

Codes exist in other chapters of ICD-10-CM to describe the current or past use of nicotine or tobacco. For example, if a patient is no longer smoking or using tobacco products, a personal history of nicotine dependence, Z87.891, is present in Chapter 21, The factors influencing health status and contact with health services. If the provider simply documents tobacco use as a diagnosis for the patient, another code in Chapter 21 provides a description of the patient's status, that is, tobacco use, Z72.0. If a pregnant woman uses tobacco during her pregnancy, a code in Chapter 15, Pregnancy, childbirth and the puerperium is available to describe smoking or tobacco use complicating the pregnancy (O99.33-), with a sixth character to identify the trimester of pregnancy of the woman. An additional code appears under this code to use additional code from F17 to identify the type of tobacco used.

Other Mental, Behavioral, and Neurodevelopmental Disorders (F20-F69)

Categories F20–F29 are a block of codes that classify schizophrenia, schizotypal, delusional, and other non-mood psychotic disorders. Specific forms of schizophrenia are contained in category F20, Schizophrenia, such as paranoid, disorganized, catatonic, undifferentiated, residual, and other forms of schizophrenia. **Schizophrenia** is a chronic mental health condition that can be a severe and disabling disorder in some patients while other individuals with the condition can cope with the symptoms and lead normal lives. New medications have proven to be effective for more patients. Some individuals with schizophrenia hear voices, may not make sense when they talk, and believe other people are controlling their thoughts or intending to harm them. While some patients can be independent while taking their medications other patients have difficulty holding a job or caring for themselves so they rely on family and others for assistance with their day-to-day lives.

Mood (affective) disorders are classified with the codes in the block of codes from F30–F39. A **bipolar disorder** is also known as manic-depressive illness. Various forms of this illness are classified with category F31 to the fifth character level for the specific forms of the illness. Bipolar disorder or manic-depressive illness, psychosis, or reaction is a mental health disorder that produces unusual mood swings in a patient as well as varying levels of functioning, for example, in handling the everyday activities of daily life. The bipolar disorder usually develops when a person is in their late teen or early adult years. Patients with bipolar disorder experience intense emotional episodes that can be overly excited, which is called a manic episode. The patient can experience a sad and hopeless state that is called a depressive episode. Doctors may also describe a patient as having a mixed state, which includes symptoms of both mania and depression. A patient with bipolar disorder may be very irritable and explosive during a mood episode. People with bipolar disorder may also abuse alcohol or other substances, have difficulty maintaining positive personal relationships, and perform poorly in school or on the job. Often these problems are not recognized as a sign of this major mental illness. Bipolar disease is a long-term illness and patients need long-term treatment to maintain control of their symptoms. There are effective treatments using medications and psychotherapy for reducing the severity of a patient's symptoms and preventing a relapse.

Code F41.1 classifies **generalized anxiety disorder** (GAD). This condition is usually diagnosed in patients who are excessively worried about many things even when there is little to no reason to worry about them. The patient is very anxious about activities of daily life. They expect things will go poorly for them and this keeps them from doing normal everyday tasks. GAD may be an inherited condition. It may develop slowly, often starting during the teen years or early adult life. Symptoms get better and worse over time and are often severe during times of stress. Better treatments have been developed as researchers learn more about fear and anxiety as it is produced in the brain. The condition is first suspected in a patient who complains about headaches, stomach and muscle aches, unexplained pain, and difficulty sleeping with feeling tired all the time. It is hard to diagnosis as it develops slowly and may take time to be diagnosed while other causes are ruled out. Patients worry about everyday things, have trouble controlling their constant worries, have a hard time concentrating in school and on the job, and are not able to relax. GAD is usually treated with psychotherapy, medication, or both. Cognitive behavior therapy is often useful for the patient by teaching the patient different ways to think, behave, and react to situations that they worry about. Two types of medications that may be beneficial include antianxiety medications and antidepressants.

An **eating disorder** is an illness that causes disturbances in eating, such as consuming very small amounts of food or confusing excessive amounts of food. A person with an eating disorder usually has severe concerns about their body weight or appearance. Eating disorders frequently begin during teen and young adult years but may also start in childhood or later in life. Common eating disorders are anorexia nervosa, bulimia nervosa, and binge-eating disorder. These conditions are treatable medical and mental illnesses. Frequently the conditions coexist with other mental illnesses such as depression, anxiety disorders, and substance abuse. If a patient does not seek or receive treatment the conditions can be life threatening. Some patients who do not continue their treatment are frequently hospitalized. Patients with anorexia nervosa require hospital care because of severe metabolic disorder and nutritional deficiencies that result from the condition that make the individual very ill. ICD-10-CM classifies the various forms of eating disorders that exist. Code F50.01, Anorexia nervosa restricting type and code F50.02, anorexia nervosa binger eating/purging type are available to classify the patient. Other codes exist for bulimia nervosa (F50.2), other eating disorders (F50.3), and unspecified types of eating disorders (F50.9) in ICD-10-CM.

ICD-10-CM provides a block of codes for disorders of adult personality and behavior (F60-F69). One example of a condition classified with a code from this section is **borderline personality disorder**, code F60.3. This is a serious mental illness marked by unstable moods with difficulty in controlling behavior and maintaining positive interpersonal relationships. Most people who suffer from borderline personality disorder have problems regulating their emotions and thoughts and exhibit impulsive and reckless behavior. As a result the patients have unstable relationships with other people including multiple marriages and alienating friends. Patients with this disorder also have other mental health illnesses such as depression, anxiety, substance abuse, and eating disorders. The condition is difficult to identify and often underdiagnosed or misdiagnosed. Borderline personality disorder can be treated with different types of psychotherapy, such as cognitive behavioral therapy, dialectical behavior therapy, and schema-focused therapy. It is important for the therapy to be effective so the patient must get along with and trust their therapist, otherwise the patient often abandons the treatment.

Unfortunately there are no medications recognized as effective to treat the condition. However, some patients benefit from medications to treat their symptoms of anxiety, depression, and aggression.

Intellectual disabilities (F70–F79) is another description for mental retardation. The phrase intellectual disabilities is used to describe a person's ability to learn and function at an expected level for their age in the activities of daily life. The level of intellectual disability can vary for both children and adults with this condition. Some individuals have very minor problems while others are severely disabled by the lack of ability to function at a normal level (CDC 2012).

There is an instructional note that follows the section heading to code first any associated physical or developmental disorder. In ICD-10-CM, the associated physical or developmental disorder is listed first, followed by the appropriate code from F70–F79.

ICD-10-PCS Coding for Behavioral Health Procedures

Therapies for patients that include behavior health procedures have ICD-10-PCS procedures in the Mental Health (GZ1–GZJ) and Substance Abuse (HZ2–HZ9) sections.

Detoxification

Detoxification is the active management of withdrawal symptoms in a patient who is physically dependent on alcohol and/or drugs. Treatment includes evaluation, observation, and monitoring, as well as administration of thiamine and multivitamins for nutrition and other medications, such as methadone, clonidine, long-acting barbiturates, benzodiazepines, and carbamazepine.

Rehabilitation

Rehabilitation is a structured program that results in controlling the alcohol or drug use and in replacing alcohol or drug dependence with activities that are nonchemical in nature. Modalities may include individual counseling, group counseling, individual psychotherapy, family counseling, medication management, and pharmacotherapy for substance abuse treatment.

Mental Health Therapies

Specific mental health therapies include psychological tests, crisis intervention, medication management, individual psychotherapy, counseling, family psychotherapy, electroconvulsive therapy, biofeedback, hypnosis, narcosynthesis, group psychotherapy, and light therapy.

ICD-10-PCS Index

There are Index entries for mental health and substance abuse treatment procedures under "substance abuse treatment" and under the titles of the various procedures for both mental health and substance abuse therapy. For example, under substance abuse treatment are entries for counseling, detoxification services, medication management, pharmacotherapy, and psychotherapy. These same procedure titles are listed under separate entries in the Index as well.

Currently there are no specific coding guidelines published for coding mental health and substance abuse treatment procedures.

Two pages of tables for mental health procedures are included in the ICD-10-PCS code book. The seven characters for this section are as follows:

Character 1—Mental Health (G)
Character 2—Body system, which is always none (Z)
Character 3—Root type. The third character includes 12 types of mental health procedures, such as psychological tests, crisis intervention, individual psychotherapy, counseling, family psychotherapy, electroconvulsive therapy, biofeedback, hypnosis, narcosynthesis, group psychotherapy, and light therapy.
Character 4—The type qualifier indicates more about the root type procedure, for example, whether counseling was vocational or educational
Characters 5, 6, and 7—All three of these characters are not specified and always have the value "none" (Z).

Similarly, two pages of tables for substance abuse treatments are included in the ICD-10-PCS code book. The seven characters for this section are as follows:

Character 1—Substance Abuse Treatment (H)
Character 2—Body system, which is always none (Z)
Character 3—Root type. The third character includes seven types of substance abuse treatment, such as detoxification services, individual counseling, group counseling, family counseling, individual psychotherapy, medication management, and pharmacotherapy.
Character 4—The type qualifier depends on the root type procedure. For example, detoxification contains only the value Z for none and family counseling contains only the value 3 for other family counseling. However, the other root type procedures include specific options, such as the type of individual and group counseling modalities.
Characters 5, 6, and 7—All three of these characters are not specified and always have the value "none" (Z).

ICD-10-CM and ICD-10-PCS Review Exercises: Chapter 8

Assign the correct ICD-10-CM diagnosis codes and ICD-10-PCS procedure codes to the following exercises.

1. Marijuana (cannabis) addiction with drug related anxiety disorder

   _____

2. Chronic undifferentiated schizophrenia

   _____

3. Seasonal depression, current episode, moderate

   _____

ICD-10-CM and ICD-10-PCS Review Exercises: Chapter 8 (Continued)

4. Acute alcoholic intoxication with delirium, blood alcohol level of 200 mg/100 ml

5. Chronic posttraumatic stress disorder (PTSD)

6. Steroid drug abuse

7. Anorexia nervosa, restricting type

8. Bipolar disorder, current episode mixed, moderate

9. Anxiety depression

10. Conduct disorder, oppositional defiant type

11. Adult attention deficit hyperactivity disorder hyperactivity type

12. Arteriosclerotic dementia, due to cerebral arteriosclerosis

13. Postpartum depression

14. Childhood onset stuttering

15. Developmental expressive dysphasia; moderate intellectual disabilities

16. Münchhausen's syndrome with predominantly physical symptoms

17. Heroin addiction with withdrawal

18. Explosive personality disorder

(*Continued on next page*)

ICD-10-CM and ICD-10-PCS Review Exercises: Chapter 8 (Continued)

19. Current cigarette smoker (listed as a diagnosis by physician as part of the final diagnoses in the discharge summary)

_____

20. Cocaine abuse with hypersomnia

_____

21. PROCEDURE: Individual cognitive psychotherapy for mental health treatment

_____

22. PROCEDURE: Electroconvulsive therapy, bilateral, single seizure

_____

23. PROCEDURE: Intellectual and psychoeducational psychological test

_____

24. PROCEDURE: Cognitive-behavioral group counseling for substance abuse treatment

_____

25. PROCEDURE: Drug detoxification treatment for substance abuse

_____

Chapter 9

Diseases of the Nervous System (G00–G99)

Learning Objectives

At the conclusion of this chapter, you should be able to:

1. Describe the organization of the conditions and codes included in Chapter 6 of ICD-10-CM, Diseases of the nervous system (G00–G99)

2. Differentiate the coding of hemiplegia and hemiparesis and other paralytic conditions

3. Differentiate the coding of epilepsy, seizures, and convulsions

4. Describe different types of headaches coded with ICD-10-CM

5. Assign ICD-10-CM codes for diseases of the nervous system

6. Assign ICD-10-PCS code for procedures related to diseases of the nervous system

Key Terms

- Central pain syndrome
- Cerebral palsy
- Dementia
- Epilepsy
- Hemiparesis
- Hemiplegia
- Meningitis
- Migraine
- Mild cognitive impairment
- Neoplasm-related pain
- Release
- Repair
- Reposition
- Seizure
- Transfer

Overview of ICD-10-CM Chapter 6, Diseases of the Nervous System

Chapter 6 of ICD-10-CM includes categories G00–G99 arranged in the following blocks:

G00–G09	Inflammatory diseases of the central nervous system
G10–G14	Systemic atrophies primarily affecting the central nervous system
G20–G26	Extrapyramidal and movement disorders
G30–G32	Other degenerative diseases of the nervous system
G35–G37	Demyelinating diseases of the central nervous system
G40–G47	Episodic and paroxysmal disorders
G50–G59	Nerve, nerve root and plexus disorders
G60–G65	Polyneuropathies and other disorders of the peripheral nervous system
G70–G73	Diseases of myoneural junction and muscle
G80–G83	Cerebral palsy and other paralytic syndromes
G89–G99	Other disorders of the nervous system

Chapter 6 only contains diseases of the nervous system. A number of codes include a combination of conditions, such as persistent migraine aura with cerebral infarction, intractable (G43.61-). Additionally, a number of codes for diseases of the nervous system include facts concerning the onset of the disease. For example, G30.0, Alzheimer's disease with early onset and G30.1, Alzheimer's disease with late onset are available in ICD-10-CM. ICD-10-CM has codes for the nervous system disease that exist with and without associated symptoms. For example, there are two codes for phantom limb syndrome, differentiating whether pain is present or not (G54.6–G54.7).

Classification of sleep disorders are now included in Chapter 6 rather than signs and symptoms. Sleep apnea has its own subcategory with fifth character specificity identifying the type.

Epilepsy and recurrent seizures are classified to category G40 in ICD-10-CM. The Alphabetic Index also refers the coder to category G40 for the diagnosis of "seizure disorder." In contrast, the diagnoses of "seizure(s)" or "convulsion(s)" or "convulsive seizure" are classified to a symptom code, R56.9 in category R56, Convulsions, not elsewhere classified. Coders must follow the Alphabetic Index entries cautiously to distinguish these diagnoses when coding.

Coding Guidelines and Instructional Notes for ICD-10-CM Chapter 6

At the start of Chapter 6 in ICD-10-CM, a series of excluded conditions are listed that are applicable to all conditions classifiable to Chapter 6. Additional modifications were made to specific codes. Throughout the chapter there are instructional notes to "use additional code to identify organism," "code first underlying disease," "use additional code for adverse effect, if applicable, to identify drug," and "code also any associated condition." Multiple coding is frequently required to fully describe diseases of the nervous system.

In ICD-10-CM beneath category G89, Pain, not elsewhere classified, there is a note that states, "Code also related psychological factors associated with pain (F45.42). There is an Excludes1 note here that reminds the coders what is not coded with codes from category G89, specifically generalized pain (R52), pain disorders exclusively related to psychological factors (F45.41), or pain unspecified (R52). In addition, there is an Excludes2 note that reminds the coder what other pain codes can be assigned with a code from category G89, Pain, not elsewhere classified. The category G89 codes describe acute pain, chronic pain, and neoplasm related pain. Included in the Excludes2 codes under category G89 are codes for the site of the pain, such as abdominal or back, with other terms such as myalgia or pain from prosthetic devices, implants, and grafts.

The NCHS has published chapter-specific guidelines for Chapter 6 in the *ICD-10-CM Official Guidelines for Coding and Reporting*. The coding student should review all of the coding guidelines for Chapter 6 of ICD-10-CM, which appear in an ICD-10-CM code book or at the website http://www.cdc.gov/nchs/icd/icd10cm.htm, or in Appendix E.

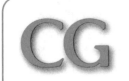

Guideline I.C.6.a. Dominant/nondominant side: Codes from category G81, hemiplegia and hemiparesis, and subcategories G83.1–G83.3, Monoplegia of lower limb, upper limb or unspecified, identify whether the dominant or non-dominant side is affected. Should the affected side be documented, but not specified as dominant or non-dominant, and the classification does not indicate a default, code selection is as follows:

- For ambidextrous patients, the default should be dominant
- If the left side is affected, the default is non-dominant
- If the right side is affected, the default is dominant

Guidelines I.C.6.b. Pain—Category G89

1. General coding information

   Codes in category G89, Pain, not elsewhere classified, may be used in conjunction with codes from other categories and chapters to provide more detail about acute or chronic pain and neoplasm-related pain, unless otherwise indicated below.

   If the pain is not specified as acute or chronic, post-thoracotomy, postprocedural, or neoplasm-related, do not assign codes from category G89.

   A code from category G89 should not be assigned if the underlying (definitive) diagnosis known, unless the reason

   (Continued)

(Continued)

for the encounter is pain control/management and not management of the underlying condition

When an admission or encounter is for a procedure aimed at treating the underlying condition (e.g., spinal fusion, kyphoplasty), a code for the underlying condition (e.g., vertebral fracture, spinal stenosis) should be assigned as the principal diagnosis. No code from category G89 should be assigned.

a. Category G89 Codes as Principal or First-Listed Diagnosis

Category G89 codes are acceptable as principal diagnosis or the first-listed code:

- When pain control or pain management is the reason for the admission/encounter (e.g., a patient with displaced intervertebral disc, nerve impingement and severe back pain presents for injection of steroid into the spinal canal). The underlying cause of the pain should be reported as an additional diagnosis, if known.

- When a patient is admitted for the insertion of a neurostimulator for pain control, assign the appropriate pain code as the principal or first-listed diagnosis. When an admission or encounter is for a procedure aimed at treating the underlying condition and a neurostimulator is inserted for pain control during the same admission/encounter, a code for the underlying condition should be assigned as the principal diagnosis and the appropriate pain code should be assigned as a secondary diagnosis

b. Use of Category G89 Codes in Conjunction with Site Specific Pain Codes

  i Assigning Category G89 and Site-Specific Pain Codes

  Codes from category G89 may be used in conjunction with codes that identify the site of pain (including codes from chapter 18) if the category G89≈code provides additional information. For example, if the code describes the site of the pain, but does not fully describe whether the pain is acute or chronic, then both codes should be assigned.

  ii Sequencing of Category G89 Codes with Site-Specific Pain Codes

  The sequencing of category G89 codes with site-specific pain codes (including chapter 18 codes), is dependent on the circumstances of the encounter/admission as follows:

- If the encounter is for pain control or pain management, assign the code from category G89 followed by the code identifying the specific site of pain (e.g., encounter for pain management for acute neck pain from trauma is assigned code G89.11, Acute pain due to trauma, followed by code M54.2, Cervicalgia, to identify the site of pain).

- If the encounter is for any other reason except pain control or pain management, and a related definitive diagnosis has not been established (confirmed) by the provider, assign the code for the specific site of pain first, followed by the appropriate code from category G89.

2. Pain due to devices, implants and grafts

   See Section I.C.19. Pain due to medical devices

3. Postoperative Pain

   The provider's documentation should be used to guide the coding of postoperative pain, as well as *Section III. Reporting Additional Diagnoses and Section IV. Diagnostic Coding and Reporting in the Outpatient Setting.*

   The default for post-thoracotomy and other postoperative pain not specified as acute or chronic is the code for the acute form.

   Routine or expected postoperative pain immediately after surgery should not be coded.

   a. Postoperative pain not associated with specific postoperative complication

   Postoperative pain not associated with a specific postoperative complication is assigned to the appropriate postoperative pain code in category G89.

   b. Postoperative pain associated with specific postoperative complication

   Postoperative pain associated with a specific postoperative complication (such as painful wire sutures) is assigned to the appropriate code(s) found in Chapter 19, Injury, poisoning, and certain other consequences of external causes. If appropriate, use additional code(s) from category G89 to identify acute or chronic pain (G89.18 or G89.28).

   (Continued)

(Continued)

4. Chronic pain

Chronic pain is classified to subcategory G89.2. There is no time frame defining when pain becomes chronic pain. The provider's documentation should be used to guide use of these codes.

5. Neoplasm Related Pain

Code G89.3 is assigned to pain documented as being related, associated or due to cancer, primary or secondary malignancy, or tumor. This code is assigned regardless of whether the pain is acute or chronic.

This code may be assigned as the principal or first-listed code when the stated reason for the admission/encounter is documented as pain control/pain management. The underlying neoplasm should be reported as an additional diagnosis.

When the reason for the admission/encounter is management of the neoplasm and the pain associated with the neoplasm is also documented, code G89.3 may be assigned as an additional diagnosis. It is not necessary to assign an additional code for the site of the pain.

See Section I.C.2 for instructions on the sequencing of neoplasms for all other stated reasons for the admission/encounter (except for pain control/pain management).

6. Chronic pain syndrome

Central pain syndrome (G89.0) and chronic pain syndrome (G89.4) are different than the term "chronic pain," and therefore codes should only be used when the provider has specifically documented this condition.

See Section I.C.5. Pain disorders related to psychological factors

Coding Diseases of the Nervous System for ICD-10-CM Chapter 6

ICD-10-CM's Chapter 6, Diseases of the nervous system (G00–G99), includes diseases of the central and peripheral nervous systems as well as epilepsy, migraine, and other headache syndromes. Laterality is included in the nerve root and plexus disorders to identify whether the mononeuropathy occurs on the right or left side. Codes from category G81, Hemiplegia and hemiparesis, and subcategories G83.1–G83.2–G83.3-, Monoplegias, identify whether the right or left dominant or nondominant side is affected.

Meningitis

Meningitis is the inflammation of the meninges, which cover the brain and the spinal cord. A variety of microorganisms or viruses can cause meningitis, which is classified in ICD-10-CM in Chapter 6, Diseases of the nervous system and Chapter 1, Certain infectious and parasitic diseases. Because of this particular classification, the instructions provided in the Alphabetic Index to Diseases must be followed to ensure accurate code assignment.

> **EXAMPLE:**   Meningitis G03.9
> abacterial G03.0
> actinomycotic A42.81
> adenoviral A87.1
> arbovirus A87.8
> aseptic (acute) G03.0
> bacterial G00.9

Organic Sleep Disorders (G47)

The category G47, Sleep disorders, includes fourth and fifth digit codes to classify various types of insomnia, hypersomnia, circadian rhythm sleep disorders, sleep apnea, narcolepsy and cataplexy, parasomnia, and sleep-related movement disorders. Several of the subclassification codes contain the direction "Code first underlying condition" and "Code also associated medical condition." Additional codes for sleep disorders not due to a substance or known physiological condition (F51) and due to substance related conditions are included in Chapter 5, Mental, behavioral and neurodevelopmental disorders.

Other Degenerative Diseases of the Nervous System (G30–G32)

Categories G30-G32 describe hereditary and degenerative diseases of the central nervous system that range in severity from mild to severe.

Alzheimer's Disease (G30)

Four digit codes are available to classify Alzheimer's disease with early onset (G30.0) and Alzheimer's disease with late onset (G30.1), as well as other and unspecified Alzheimer's disease. An important note is included to use an additional code to identify

Delirium, if applicable, (F05)
Dementia with behavioral disturbance (F02.81)
Dementia without behavioral disturbance (F02.80)

There is an Excludes1 note that reminds the coder the certain senile degeneration of brain, senile dementia, unspecified and senility, unspecified is not coded with category G30 codes for Alzheimer's disease.

A patient with **dementia** can experience a variety of symptoms that are attributed to a neurological disorder with behavioral features. The patient's relatives may first notice a loss of the patient's memory of recent events. Memory loss by itself does not establish the diagnosis of dementia. However, if a patient has other symptoms such as language difficulties and the ability to carry out normal everyday functions, the diagnosis of dementia is more likely to be made. Patients with dementia can have difficulty handling their financial responsibilities, such as writing checks, or taking care of their home, such as cooking, cleaning, washing dishes, and laundry. As the disease progresses, the patient may lose their problem solving thought processes and may have personality changes. Patients with dementia may become agitated and experience visual delusions, such as seeing objects that are not present. Another classic symptom is memory loss that progresses from mild to severe. Patients with dementia may not recognize loved ones as their disease progresses and lose their ability to express themselves or to even speak (MedlinePlus 2013).

Other Degenerative Diseases of the Nervous System, Not Elsewhere Classified (G31)

This category also has the instruction to use an additional code to identify dementia with and without behavioral disturbance.

Acute and chronic forms of cerebral degenerative disease are included in this category, such as Pick's disease, G31.01; Degeneration of nervous system due to alcohol, G31.2; and Dementia with Lewy bodies, G31.83.

Code G31.84 identifies the condition described by physicians as **mild cognitive impairment**. This disease entity is defined as impairment in memory (or any other cognitive domain) that is beyond what is normal for age, with relatively intact function in the other cognitive domains. The patient will first have a memory complaint that is corroborated by other individuals and, for this reason, seek medical evaluation. The diagnosis is used by physicians as the reason for diagnostic testing services.

Other Degenerative Disorders of the Nervous System in Diseases Classified Elsewhere (G32)

Included in this category are *italicized codes* to identify degenerative disorders that are the consequence of other diseases. "Code first underlying disease" directions remind the coder that entries such as vitamin B12 deficiency, amyloidosis, and cerebellar ataxia in neoplastic disease should be coded first when these conditions are the known causes of the degenerative disorder.

Pain, Not Elsewhere Classified (G89)

This category in ICD-10-CM has unique codes for encounters for pain management. A "use additional code" note appears at the top of this category to direct the coder to assign a code for pain associated with psychological factors, as documented by the physician. Excludes notes under this category state that generalized pain is coded to the ICD-10-CM symptoms chapter (R52), and localized pain should be coded to pain by the site identified. The excludes note also states that a pain disorder exclusively attributed to psychological factors should not be coded with category G89, but instead with code F45.41.

Code G89.0, **central pain syndrome**, describes the condition that can be caused by damage to the central nervous system by trauma or brain-related disease (for example, cardiovascular accident [CVA], multiple sclerosis, tumors, epilepsy, or Parkinson's disease.) The condition may also be described as "thalamic pain syndrome."

Other codes exist for acute pain (G89.11–G89.19) and chronic pain (G89.21–G89.29) due to trauma or surgery. There is no timeframe defining when pain becomes chronic. The physician's documentation should be used to guide the use of chronic pain codes.

Neoplasm-related pain may be described with code G89.3 for pain due to the primary or secondary malignancy or tumor. This code is assigned regardless of whether the pain is described as acute or chronic. Code G89.4 can be used as a principal diagnosis or first-listed diagnosis if the reason for the admission or outpatient visit is for pain control or pain management. The underlying neoplasm should be reported as an additional diagnosis code. The neoplasm-related pain code can be reported as an additional diagnosis when the reason for the admission or outpatient visit is management of the neoplasm, and the pain associated with the neoplasm is also documented.

Finally, a single code, G89.4, is provided for the diagnostic statement "chronic pain syndrome," often stated as the reason for ongoing pain management services. The code for chronic pain syndrome should only be used when the physician has specifically documented this condition.

Category G89 codes are acceptable as the principal or first-listed diagnosis codes. Codes from category G89 can be reported with codes that identify the site of the pain, including symptom codes from the ICD-10-CM body system or symptoms chapters, if the category G89 code provides additional information. For example, if a code from the body system or symptoms chapters identifies the site of the pain but does not describe the pain as acute or chronic, both codes should be assigned.

The sequencing of category G89 codes with site-specific pain codes depends on the circumstances of the admission or outpatient visit.

If the encounter is for pain control or pain management, the code from category G89 is sequenced first, followed by the code for the specific site of the pain or the underlying cause of the pain, if known. For example, assume a patient with known displacement of lumbar intervertebral disc is seen in the Pain Clinic for management of his chronic low back pain secondary to displacement of the lumbar intervertebral disc. For this encounter the chronic pain, G89.29, would be listed first with an additional code M51.26 for the underlying condition of the displacement of the lumbar intervertebral disc.

When an admission or encounter is for a procedure aimed at treating the underlying condition, a code for the underlying condition should be assigned as the principal or first-listed diagnosis. No code from category G89 should be assigned. For example, assume a patient with known displacement of lumbar intervertebral disc and chronic back pain due to the displaced disc is admitted for a laminectomy with excision of the herniated intervertebral disc. This patient's principal diagnosis is the displacement of the lumbar intervertebral disc, M51.26

When an admission or encounter is for any other reason except pain control or pain management, and a related definitive diagnosis has not been established or confirmed by the provider, the coder should assign the code for the specific site of pain first, followed by the appropriate code from category 338. For example, assume a patient comes to the physician's office complaining of left hip pain that has been present for several months. The physician orders x-rays to be performed and concludes the patient has chronic hip pain of unknown etiology. For this encounter the code for the left hip pain, M25.552, is listed as the first code with an additional code for the chronic pain, 338.29.

Codes for postoperative or post-thoracotomy pain are classified to the subcategories of G89.1 or G89.2 depending on whether the pain is acute or chronic. If the postoperative pain is not specified as acute or chronic, G89.18 is the default code for the acute form. Postoperative pain may be a principal or first-listed diagnosis when the reason for the admission or outpatient visit is documented as postoperative pain control or management. Postoperative pain can be reported as a secondary diagnosis code when a patient has outpatient surgery and develops an unusual amount of postoperative pain. Routine or expected postoperative pain immediately after surgery is not coded.

Cerebral Palsy and Other Paralytic Syndromes (G80–G83)

The following subsections discuss the categories of other disorders of the nervous system, including paralytic conditions and epilepsy.

Cerebral Palsy, Category G80

Cerebral palsy is a nonprogressive, brain-damaging disturbance that originates during the prenatal and perinatal period. It is characterized by persistent, qualitative motor dysfunction, paralysis, and, in severe cases, mental retardation. Fourth-digit subcategories identify the different forms of infantile cerebral palsy.

A note on how to use the codes in the categories G81 (Hemiplegia and hemiparesis), G82 (Paraplegia and quadriplegia), and G83 (Other paralytic syndromes) is provided: the categories are to be used only when the listed conditions are reported without further specification, or are stated to be old or longstanding but of unspecified cause. The category is also for use in multiple coding to identify these conditions resulting from any cause. Paralytic sequelae of cerebral infarct/stroke are in Chapter 9, Diseases of the circulatory system.

Hemiplegia and Hemiparesis, Category G81

The terms **hemiplegia** and **hemiparesis** both refer to the paralysis of one side of the body. Category G81 has fourth- and fifth-digit subcategories that differentiate between flaccid and spastic hemiplegia. Flaccid refers to the loss of muscle tone in the paralyzed parts with the absence of tendon reflexes, whereas spastic refers to the spasticity of the paralyzed parts with increased tendon reflexes. The G81 codes often are assigned when the health record provides no further information, when the cause of the hemiplegia and hemiparesis is unknown, or as an additional code when the condition results from a specified cause.

A fifth-digit subclassification is included in category G81-G83 to identify whether the dominant or nondominant side of the body is affected. This type of specificity may not be available in the health record; if the information is not available, assign the fifth digit 0. However, if the affected side is documented but not specified as the dominant or nondominant side for the patient, and the classification does not provide a default code, the code is based on the following guideline:

For ambidextrous patients, the default should be the dominant side.
If the left side is affected, the default is nondominant.
If the right side is affected, the default is dominant.

Epilepsy and Recurrent Seizures, Category G40

An instructional note appears under the category heading G40, Epilepsy and recurrent seizures; it explains that terminology that is the same as "intractable" may be documented as pharmacoresistant, pharmacologically resistant, treatment resistant, refractory, medically refractory, and poorly controlled. If the physician uses any of these terms, the coder can assign the ICD-10-CM diagnosis code for the intractable form of the disease.

The term **epilepsy** denotes any disorder characterized by recurrent seizures. A **seizure** is a transient disturbance of cerebral function caused by an abnormal paroxysmal neuronal discharge in the brain.

Physicians often document "recurrent seizure" or "seizure disorder" as well as epilepsy in a health record. Recurrent seizures or seizure disorders are classified in the same category as epilepsy because the terminology is synonymous in medicine. Localization-related epilepsy is the terminology used today for an older term, partial epilepsy.

Other terms used to describe convulsions are not classified to category G40. Such phrases as convulsion or convulsive disorder, convulsive seizures, fits, or recurrent convulsions are not accepted as equivalent to epilepsy or recurrent seizures. Instead the codes for the convulsive conditions are included in category R56 within ICD-10-CM Chapter 18 for symptoms. The term seizure and the plural term seizures are also coded to the symptom code R56.9 by following the Alphabetic Index carefully. Coders must not use the terms seizures and convulsions interchangeably. By using the physician's description of the patient's condition and following the Alphabetic Index precisely, different terminology will produce different ICD-10-CM diagnosis codes. Conditions documented as convulsions, posttraumatic seizures, seizures, and convulsive seizures are not coded to category G40, Epilepsy and recurrent seizures. Instead these conditions are coded to category R56, Convulsions, not elsewhere classified. Recurrent seizures, epileptic convulsions, and seizure disorders are assigned to category G40, Epilepsy and recurrent seizures.

Migraine, Category G43

A note with G43, Migraine provides the following terms to be considered equivalent to intractable: pharmacoresistant (pharmacologically resistant), treatment resistant, refractory (medically), and poorly controlled.

Migraine headaches are recurrent headaches that produce moderate to severe head pain for the patient. The pain may be pulsing or throbbing and may appear on only one side of the head. In addition to pain, the patient often experiences nausea and vomiting. The patient prefers to rest in a darkened, quiet room as light and sound exacerbates the patient's symptoms. Some patients experience what is called an "aura," that is a warning to the patient that they are about to have a migraine headache. The aura may be flashing lights or zigzag lines that the patient sees in their visual field. Some patients have momentary loss of vision during their aura stage. Some research has suggested that migraines may be linked to the alternating dilation and narrowing of blood vessels in the brain. Migraines may be an inherited condition and have a genetic component that affects the activity of brain cells. Some medications have helped to prevent the severity of migraine attacks while other medications relieve the symptoms that patients with migraines experience. Some patients experience migraines for most of their adult life, while other patients report fewer migraines as the person ages (MedlinePlus 2013).

The classification of migraine headaches is reported with category codes G43, Migraine. Many types of migraine headaches can be identified with specific codes in subcategories for migraine with aura, migraine without aura, hemiplegic migraine, persistent migraine aura with and without cerebral infarction, chronic migraine, and other forms of migraine. Category G43 codes include a sixth digit to identify the manifestation of the migraine in several of the individual codes. For example, migraine, not intractable with status migrainous and migraine, intractable, without status migrainous are both options for the sixth character.

An additional code to identify the cerebral infarction (codes from I63.-) is required with subcategory codes from G43.6, Persistent migraine aura with cerebral infarction. The definition of "chronic" in primary episodic headache disorders is a headache that occurs on more days than not for more than three months.

ICD-10-CM provides codes for other types of headaches. Chapter 6, Diseases of the nervous system, also includes category G44, other headache syndromes. This includes cluster headaches, tension-type headaches, posttraumatic headache, drug-induced headache, and complicated headache syndromes. Headaches without a known cause are included in Chapter 18, Signs, symptoms and ill-defined conditions.

Intraoperative and Postprocedural Complications, Category G97

Also in this chapter are the intraoperative and postprocedural complication codes. For example, cerebrospinal fluid leak from spinal puncture is coded here with G97.0. Other codes identify intraoperative hemorrhage or hematoma, accidental puncture of dura or other nervous system organ or postprocedural hemorrhage, or hematoma that occurred during a nervous system procedure or affecting a nervous system organ during another procedure.

Procedure Coding for ICD-10-PCS Chapter 6

Procedures performed on the central nervous system are included in the tables from 001–00X with the root operations Bypass, Change, Destruction, Division, Drainage, Excision, Extirpation, Extraction, Fragmentation, Insertion, Inspection, Map, Release, Removal, Repair, Reposition, Resection, Supplement, Revision, and Transfer. One frequently performed procedure in the central nervous system is the creation of a shunt to drain fluid from one site to another cavity. For example, shunting from the cerebral ventricle to a peritoneal location is coded as a Bypass in ICD-10-PCS. Guideline B3.6a includes the instruction that a bypass procedure is coded using the body part that is the origin of the shunt in the fourth character code of the code and the destination of the shunt in the seventh character (qualifier). Bypass procedures therefore are coded as "from" a body part "to" another body part.

Procedures frequently performed on the peripheral nervous system include release, repair, reposition and transfer procedures. The Index entries for **Release** include a subterm of "nerve" with the peripheral nerves as well as other nerves listed beneath it. A release is freeing a nerve from a body part from an abnormal physical constraint. The three-digit code for release of a peripheral nerve is "01N." The fourth character identifies the nerve released, such as ulnar, median, radial, and such. The approach choices are Open, Percutaneous, or Percutaneous Endoscopic. There is no device or qualifier option in this table, as neither will apply to this type of procedure. A **Repair** of a nerve is restoring the nerve to the extent position or restoring the nerve to its normal anatomic structure and function. The broad terms of neuroplasty or neurorrhaphy refer the coder to the root operations of Repair and Supplement. The suture repair of a nerve is coded as a Repair. Supplement of a nerve would involve an autologous tissue substitute to reinforce the nerve structure.

Other procedures performed on nerves may be described as a transposition. Transposition is not a root operation in ICD-10-PCS. Instead the Index refers the coder to the root operations of **Reposition** or **Transfer** for a transposition of a nerve. A Reposition of a nerve is moving it to its normal location or other suitable location all of a portion of the nerve. Under the main term Reposition in the Index, the coder will find a subterm of nerve with specific nerves listed beneath it. Table 01S for reposition of a peripheral nerve includes the identified nerve as the fourth body part character. The approach for a Reposition is Open, Percutaneous, or Percutaneous endoscopic. There is no applicable value for the sixth or seventh characters of device or qualifier.

A nerve transfer is coded to the root operation Transfer. In ICD-10-PCS, a nerve transfer is the moving, without taking it out, all of a portion of the nerve to another location to take over the function of all or a portion of the nerve. Transfer is a main term in the Index with nerve as a subterm and the specific nerves listed with the three-digit code table "01X." Again the "from" and "to" concept is used for transfers with the body part used for the nerve transferred from and the qualifier as the nerve transferred to. There are two choices for the approach used, that is, Open and Percutaneous Endoscopic, and there is no choice for a device as it does not apply.

ICD-10-CM and ICD-10-PCS Review Exercises: Chapter 9

Assign the correct ICD-10-CM diagnosis codes and ICD-10-PCS procedure codes to the following exercises.

1. A patient had been noted to have dementia and forgetfulness. He has been leaving his home and forgetting where he is or where he is going. The diagnosis of dementia due to early-onset Alzheimer's was established.

2. Juvenile myoclonic epilepsy with intractable seizures.

3. Episodic cluster headache, not described as intractable

4. Chronic Migraine without aura, not intractable with status migrainous

5. Autonomic dysreflexia due to urinary tract infections

6. Idiopathic normal pressure hydrocephalus

7. The patient, a Type 2 diabetic with neuropathy, developed weakness of the left arm and leg. The patient was brought to the emergency room where he could speak but was unable to use his left arm and leg. The patient was able to ambulate with no neurological deficits within 24 hours. Due to the complete recovery, it was determined that the patient had experienced a TIA. During this encounter the patient also was treated for an intractable classical migraine.

8. Myasthenia gravis in crisis

9. Alcoholic encephalopathy

10. Complex regional pain syndrome I, bilateral lower legs

11. Intracranial subdural abscess due to methicillin resistant *Staphylococcus aureus*

12. Carpal tunnel syndrome and tarsal tunnel syndrome, both on left side

(Continued on next page)

ICD-10-CM and ICD-10-PCS Review Exercises: Chapter 9 (Continued)

13. Spastic diplegic cerebral palsy

    _____

14. Dementia with Parkinsonism

    _____

15. Postpolio Syndrome

    _____

16. PROCEDURE: Diagnostic lumbar spinal puncture

    _____

17. PROCEDURE: Transposition/reposition radial nerve, open, right arm

    _____

18. PROCEDURE: Ulnar nerve release by fasciotomy, left arm

    _____

19. PROCEDURE: Cerebral ventricular-peritoneal shunt using synthetic shunt material for shunt creation via open technique

    _____

20. PROCEDURE: Open neurorrhaphy, left tibial nerve

    _____

Chapter 10

Diseases of the Eye and Adnexa (H00–H59)

Learning Objectives

At the conclusion of this chapter, you should be able to:

1. Describe the organization of the conditions and codes included in Chapter 7 of ICD-10-CM, Diseases of the eye and adnexa (H00–H59)

2. Identify and describe the various types of eye disorders, including retinopathy, glaucoma, and cataract

3. Describe how the glaucoma stage relates to the coding of glaucoma

4. Assign ICD-10-CM codes for diseases of the eyes and adnexa

5. Assign ICD-10-PCS codes for procedures related to diseases of the eyes and adnexa

Key Terms

- Bullous keratoplasty
- Cataract
- Chemical conjunctivitis
- Cortical cataract
- Cystoid macular edema (CME)
- Glaucoma
- Glaucoma suspect
- Infantile and juvenile cataract
- Morgagnian type cataract
- Nuclear cataracts
- Retained lens fragment
- Retinal detachment
- Retinopathy of prematurity (ROP)
- Rhegmatogenous (retinal) detachment
- Subcapsular cataract
- Traction (retinal) detachment

Overview of ICD-10-CM Chapter 7, Diseases of the Eye and Adnexa

Chapter 7 of ICD-10-CM includes categories H00–H59 arranged in the following blocks:

H00–H05	Disorders of eyelid, lacrimal system and orbit
H10–H11	Disorders of conjunctiva
H15–H22	Disorders of sclera, cornea, iris and ciliary body
H25–H28	Disorders of lens
H30–H36	Disorders of choroid and retina
H40–H42	Glaucoma
H43–H44	Disorders of vitreous body and globe
H46–H47	Disorders of optic nerve and visual pathways
H49–H52	Disorders of ocular muscles, binocular movement, accommodation and refraction
H53–H54	Visual disturbances and blindness
H55–H57	Other disorders of eye and adnexa
H59	Intraoperative and postprocedural complications and disorders of eye and adnexa, not elsewhere classified

Chapter 7 was introduced with ICD-10-CM. The structure of the codes is by site for diseases of the eye and adnexa. The terminology for some of the categories in Chapter 7 has been updated to reflect current terminology. For example, senile cataract terminology has been updated to age-related cataract. There has been an expansion of the number of characters in the codes for eye and adnexa diseases to describe right side, left side, and in some cases bilateral conditions. There is also a code for "unspecified" side to use when the health record documentation does not specify the laterality of the condition.

Coding Guidelines and Instructional Notes for ICD-10-CM Chapter 7, Diseases of the Eye and Adnexa

At the start of Chapter 7 in ICD-10-CM, a "use an external cause code" appears following the code for the eye condition, if applicable, to identify the cause of the eye condition.

A series of Exclude2 conditions are listed that are applicable to all conditions classifiable to Chapter 7. The conditions described in the Excludes2 note are diseases that can be coded in addition to the Chapter 7 codes for eye conditions.

The NCHS has published chapter-specific guidelines for Chapter 7 in the *ICD-10-CM Official Guidelines for Coding and Reporting.* The coding student should review all of the coding guidelines for Chapter 7 of ICD-10-CM, which appear in an ICD-10-CM code book or at the website http://www.cdc.gov/nchs/icd/icd10cm.htm, or in Appendix E.

CG

Guideline I.C.7.a Glaucoma

1. Assigning Glaucoma Codes

   Assign as many codes from category H40, Glaucoma, as needed to identify the type of glaucoma, the affected eye, and the glaucoma stage.

2. Bilateral glaucoma with same type and stage

   When a patient has bilateral glaucoma and both eyes are documented as being the same type and stage, and there is a code for bilateral glaucoma, report only the code for the type of glaucoma, bilateral, with the seventh character for the stage.

   When a patient has bilateral glaucoma and both eyes are documented as being the same type and stage, and the classification does not provide a code for bilateral glaucoma (i.e. subcategories H40.10, H40.11 and H40.20) report only one code for the type of glaucoma with the appropriate seventh character for the stage.

3. Bilateral glaucoma stage with different types or stages

   When a patient has bilateral glaucoma and each eye is documented as having a different type or stage, and the classification distinguishes laterality, assign the appropriate code for each eye rather than the code for bilateral glaucoma.

   When a patient has bilateral glaucoma and each eye is documented as having a different type, and the classification does not distinguish laterality (i.e. subcategories H40.10, H40.11 and H40.20), assign one code for each type of glaucoma with the appropriate seventh character for the stage.

   When a patient has bilateral glaucoma and each eye is documented as having the same type, but different stage, and the classification does not distinguish laterality (i.e. subcategories H40.10, H40.11 and H40.20), assign a code for the type of glaucoma for each eye with the seventh character for the specific glaucoma stage documented for each eye.

4. Patient admitted with glaucoma and stage evolves during the admission

(Continued)

(Continued)

> If a patient is admitted with glaucoma and the stage progresses during the admission, assign the code for highest stage documented.
>
> 5. Indeterminate stage glaucoma
>
>   Assignment of the seventh character "4" for "indeterminate stage" should be based on the clinical documentation. The seventh character "4" is used for glaucomas whose stage cannot be clinically determined. This seventh character should not be confused with the seventh character "0", unspecified, which should be assigned when there is no documentation regarding the stage of the glaucoma.

Coding Diseases of the Eye and Adnexa in ICD-10-CM Chapter 7

Chapter 7 of ICD-10-CM contains specific codes for diseases of the eye that include infections, inflammations, lesions, deformities, and visual impairments among the many afflictions that a person can experience in the eye and the supporting structures. As stated in the Excludes2 note, diseases of the eye can be coded with conditions classified in other chapters. Diseases of the eye and adnexa coexist with infectious and parasitic diseases, diabetes, eye injuries, and other conditions. Coding diseases of the eye require the coder's attention to detail including the specific forms of the disease and whether the condition occurs on the right side, left side, or is present in both eyes.

Disorders of the Eyelid, Lacrimal System and Orbit (H00–H05)

ICD-10-CM codes in the range of H00–H05 describes disorders of the eyelid, lacrimal, and orbit such as hordeolum, chalazion, entropion, ectropion, blepharochalasis, inflammations, deformities of the lacrimal system and orbit, and other conditions. The codes include specific codes for the right eye, left eye, and bilateral eyes, and a code for those conditions that do not have the laterality documented.

Disorders of Conjunctiva (H10–H11)

Disorders of the conjunctiva are classified in the rage of H10–H11. Acute and chronic conjunctivitis, blepharoconjunctivitis, pterygium, conjunctival scars, hemorrhages, cysts, and other disorders of the conjunctiva are included in this block of codes. Right eye, left eye, bilateral eyes, and unspecified sides of these conditions are classified with individual codes.

A note follows the code for acute chemical conjunctivitis (H10.21-) to direct the coder to "code first" T51–T65 to identify the chemical and intent of the toxic chemical that caused the damage to the eye. The toxic chemicals could be alcohol, organic solvents, corrosive substances, soaps, and detergents as well as pesticides and other substances. **Chemical conjunctivitis** occurs when a person develops an inflammation of the conjunctiva after a substance gets in the eye. Technically this event is an injury and that is the reason the T51–T65 code is used first. As a result of the exposure to the chemical, the patient suffers eye pain, redness, and swelling. Often this is an occupational injury with workers in the construction, manufacturing, and agriculture industry injured when working with chemicals. The treatment usually occurs in an Emergency Department or Urgent Care Center with prolonged eye washing, antibiotic eyedrops, and artificial tears prescribed.

Disorders of Sclera, Cornea, Iris and Ciliary Body (H15–H22)

The block of codes H15–H22 describes disorders of the sclera, cornea, iris, and ciliary body. Conditions classified with these codes include many inflammations of these sites such as episcleritis, keratitis, keratoconjunctivitis and iridocyclitis. Other corneal conditions such as bullous keratopathy, corneal edema, keratoconus, and other corneal deformities are also included. Diseases of the iris and ciliary body such as hyphema and cysts of the iris as well as anterior and posterior synechiae complete the block of codes. Right eye, left eye, bilateral, and unspecified laterality are included for the conditions in these codes.

Disorders of Lens (H25–H28)

Disorders of the lens (H25–H28) included commonly coded conditions of the eye. These conditions are age-related cataract, infantile and juvenile cataract, traumatic cataract, cataract secondary to ocular disorders, drug-induced cataract, and other disorders of the lens including aphakia and dislocation of the lens. Again codes exist for laterality and bilateral conditions.

Age-Related Cataract (Category H25)

A **cataract** is the opacity of the crystalline lens of the eye, or its capsule, which results in a loss of vision. ICD-10-CM identifies different types of age-related or senile cataracts. The most common senile cataract in the elderly is a **cortical cataract** (H25.0-), which creates an opacity and swelling of the entire lens in a mature cataract. The cataract is white wedgelike opacities that look like spokes around the periphery of the cortex of the lens that is part of the lens surrounding the central nucleus. Other common cataracts produce an opacity at the anterior subcapsular (anterior pole cataract, H25.03-) or the posterior subcapsular (posterior pole cataract H25.04-) pole of the lens. **Subcapsular cataracts** develop in the back of the eye and are more common in patients with diabetes or patients taking high doses of steroid medications. Other age related cataracts are **nuclear cataracts** or an opacity in the central nucleus of the eye (H25.1-) or **Morgagnian type cataracts** (H25.2-), which are a mature cataract in which the cortex has liquefied and the nucleus moves freely in the lens.

Infantile and Juvenile Cataract (H26.0-)

Infantile and juvenile cataracts are congenital cataracts that are present at birth but may not be identified until the child is older. Cataracts that require treatment include lamellar, polar, total, or nuclear types. Not all congenital cataracts are significant for the patient but require surgery when it begins to obstruct the vision. About a quarter of children with congenital cataracts inherit the condition due to a family genetic condition. The most common causes of a congenital cataract include intrauterine infections and metabolic disorders in the mother. If the mother contracts rubella, rubeola, chicken pox, cytomegalovirus, herpes simplex or herpes zoster, or Epstein-Barr virus, the fetus is at risk for developing a congenital cataract. These cataracts are coded according to the type: cortical, lamellar, zonular, nuclear, or polar.

Disorders of Choroid and Retina (H30–H36)

Codes in the range of H30–H36 are describing disorders of choroid and retina including the laterality. The more frequently coded conditions in this section are retinal detachments, retinopathy due to hypertension, vasculitis, prematurity, and macular degeneration of various types.

Retinal Detachments and Breaks (H33)

A **retinal detachment** is the separation of the inner layers of the retina from the underlying retinal pigment epithelium that is attached to the choroid. The choroid is a vascular membrane containing large branched pigment cells sandwiched between the retina and sclera. Separation of the sensory retina from the underlying epithelium occurs in different ways. A hole, tear, or break occurs with fluid from the vitreous cavity seeping in between and separate sensory and epithelium. This type is called a **rhegmatogenous detachment** or a retinal detachment with a retinal break (H33.0-). This is the most common type of detachment. Rhegma means a break. Vitreous fluid enters the break and separates the sensory retina from the epithelium resulting in the "detachment."

The second type is a **traction detachment** of the retina (H33.4-), which is caused by traction from inflammatory or vascular fibrous membranes on the surface of the retina, which attaches to the vitreous. The most common causes of tractional retinal detachment are proliferative diabetic retinopathy, sickle cell disease, advanced retinopathy of prematurity, and penetrating trauma. Vitreoretinal traction increases with age, as the vitreous gel shrinks and collapses over time, frequently causing posterior vitreous detachments in approximately two-thirds of persons older than 70 years.

Symptoms of a retinal detachment are what is described as vitreous "floaters," which is a floating spot or oval in the patient's vision. Another symptom a patient may describe is tiny black flecks appearing suddenly. Later as the condition progresses, the patients describe cobwebs in their vision. Another common symptoms described by patients are flashing lights or prisms with floaters in their vision.

Retinopathy of Prematurity (H35.1-)

Retinopathy of prematurity (ROP) is a serious vasoproliferative disorder involving the developing retina in premature infants. ROP is the disease name used to describe the acute retinal changes seen in premature infants. Mild forms usually cause little or no vision loss. Severe forms lead to vision loss due to retinal scarring and damage. Even with optimal treatment, many preterm infants will develop some level of ROP, especially the smallest and most premature infants. Rentolental fibroplasia is an older medical term used to describe the condition in which the retina is actually scarred. Codes in the range of H35.10- through H35.17- identify the specific stages of ROP as well as rentolental fibroplasia. Codes for retinopathy of prematurity identify the stage of the disorder and the right eye, left eye, or bilateral status of the disease.

Glaucoma (H40–H42)

Detailed glaucoma coding guidelines appear in the Official Coding and Reporting Guidelines. Part I.C.7a1–a5 must be reviewed prior to coding these conditions. Specific forms of glaucoma are coded with ICD-10-CM codes in the block of codes from H40 and H42. The official coding guidelines describe the requirement to assign as many codes from category H40, Glaucoma, as needed to identify the type of glaucoma, the affected eye, and the glaucoma stage. The stage of glaucoma is specified with a seventh character:

0—stage unspecified

1—mild stage

2—moderate stage

3—severe stage

4—indeterminate stage

The assignment of the seventh character 4 for "indeterminate stage" of glaucoma should be based on the clinical documentation. The seventh character 4 is used for glaucomas whose stage cannot be clinically determined. The seventh character 4 should not be confused with seventh character 0 for unspecified stage. Unspecified stage should be assigned when there is no documentation regarding the stage of the glaucoma.

Glaucoma is the result of high pressure in the eye that causes damage to the optic nerve. The space in the front of the eye is the anterior chamber. The anterior chamber is filled with fluid known as aqueous humor that is produced continually and protects the tissues of the eye. In a normal eye, the aqueous humor flows in and out of the anterior chamber maintaining a constant pressure. In a diseased eye, the fluid does not drain out of the eye as it should and pressure builds up in the anterior chamber. This pressure over time damages the optic nerve. Damage to the optic nerve impairs vision and is irreversible. If the high pressure is not treated, the damage to the optic nerve can lead to blindness. Ocular hypertension is another term that describes the high intraocular pressure in the eye that has not damaged the optic nerve at a point in time.

Category H40 is subdivided to identify the various types of glaucoma. Subcategory codes exist for glaucoma suspect (H40.0-), open-angle glaucoma (H40.1-) and primary angle-closure glaucoma (H40.2-). Other forms of glaucoma are the result of eye trauma (H40.3-), eye inflammation (H40.4-), secondary to other eye diseases (H40.5-), or due to the adverse effects of prescription drugs (H40.6-).

Glaucoma suspect (H40.0-) is a condition identified in a patient who has risk factors that may cause glaucoma in the future. When described as having glaucoma suspect the patient does not have damage to the optic nerve as the result of the increased pressure in the anterior chamber but there is an abnormal appearance of the optic nerve upon examination. The patients are monitored over time to begin treatment if glaucoma is found. Glaucoma suspect is the name of this condition and should not be considered the equivalent of a diagnosis stated as "suspected" glaucoma.

Open-angle glaucoma (H40.1-) is a chronic form of glaucoma that gets its name from the fact that the angle between the iris and the cornea remains open and looks normal upon examination of the eye. However, for an unknown reason, the draining system in the eye fails to function correctly. This causes pressure to build up in the eye slowly and gradually damages the optic nerve. The patient has no visual symptoms, no pain in the eye, and only experiences vision problems as the nerve damage progresses. Physicians may describe this form of glaucoma as simple chronic glaucoma or low-tension glaucoma and it usually affects both eyes.

Primary angle-closure glaucoma (H40.2-) is an acute form of the disease. This form occurs suddenly with significant eye pain and visual defects. The disease is called angle-closure because the angle between the iris and the cornea closes and prevents the aqueous humor from draining raising pressure in the anterior chamber. Usually this "attack" of glaucoma affects one eye. The occurrence of primary angle-closure glaucoma is a medical emergency and if left untreated will result in permanent damage to the patient's vision in less than two days. The emergency is usually treated with surgery to open the blockage and allow normal flow of aqueous humor. Physicians may describe this form of glaucoma is acute angle-closure glaucoma, acute glaucoma, or a glaucoma attack or crisis. It may also be described as narrow-angle glaucoma. A chronic and intermittent form of angle-closure glaucoma also exists when the normal flow of drainage cannot be sustained.

There are also secondary forms of glaucoma that develop as a complication of other diseases. Secondary glaucoma can be the result of eye trauma and eye inflammations such as uveitis, as well as a complication of eye surgery or a complication of advanced cataracts left untreated. Secondary forms of glaucoma are coded in ICD-10-CM as glaucoma secondary to eye trauma (H40.3-), secondary to eye inflammation (H40.4-), secondary to other eye disorders (H40.5-), and glaucoma secondary to drugs (H40.6-).

Some patients developing glaucoma as a result of corticosteroid therapy are classified to subcategory H40.6. A "use additional code" note appears beneath subcategory H40.6 to code the drug that is causing the adverse effect of glaucoma that would be in the range of T36–T50 with the fifth or sixth character 5. Subcategory H40.83- includes codes for aqueous misdirection, also known as malignant glaucoma. It is not "malignant" as in the sense of a cancerous condition. The term "malignant" is used in medicine to identify any condition that is severe and becomes progressively worse over time. Aqueous misdirection is usually a complication of eye surgery and requires additional surgical treatment. It is neither angle-closure nor open-angle glaucoma. In this form of glaucoma, the aqueous flows into the vitreous or posteriorly instead of flowing into the anterior chamber. Finally, if documentation in the health record states glaucoma only, code H40.9, Unspecified glaucoma, should be assigned.

Intraoperative and Postprocedural Complications and Disorders of Eye and Adnexa, Not Elsewhere Classified

The final category in this chapter is H59, for intraoperative and postprocedural complications and disorders of eye and adnexa, not elsewhere classified. These include disorders of the eye following cataract surgery as well as eye conditions that are complications of ophthalmic and other procedures. Codes in this section also identify if the right eye, left eye, or both eyes (bilateral) are affected by the complication.

There are three specific disorders of the eye that occur following cataract surgery: keratopathy (bullous aphakic), cataract (lens) fragments in the eye, and cystoid macular edema. Codes in the range of H59.0- to H59.09- identify these conditions. **Bullous keratopathy** (H59.01-) is a condition of the cornea with excess accumulation of fluid in the cornea. It occurs occasionally after cataract extraction from the loss of corneal endothelium as the result of surgery. The patient reports that their vision is not as clear as it was immediately after surgery. Any type of intraocular surgery, especially cataract surgery, may damage endothelial cells and hasten the decline in endothelial cell count. Various treatments exist for this condition from simple observing to see if the condition resolves after the surgery to the most intensive therapy being a corneal transplant (Aquavella 2013).

An infrequent but well-known complication of cataract surgery is some form of **retained lens fragments**, particularly posterior dislocation of lens fragments. This is coded as H59.02-, Cataract (lens) fragments in eye following cataract surgery. Depending on the severity of the case, associated side effects range from uncomfortable inflammation and elevated intraocular pressure to cystoid macular edema and retinal detachment. With timely and appropriate management, the final visual outcome for the majority of patients with retained lens material is positive. Removing the retained lens fragments is usually a straightforward task for the ophthalmologist with a pars plana vitrectomy, effective for removing retained lens fragments, lowering the intraocular pressure, and reducing inflammation.

Cystoid macular edema (CME) (H59.03-) is a complication that occurs during the first year after cataract surgery in a very small number of patients who have had a lens extraction procedure. It is a disease of the macula or the central retina. It is painless with multiple cyst-like areas of fluid that causes retinal swelling. The symptoms of the edema include blurred, decreased central vision and a painless swelling of the eye. The retinal inflammation is treated with anti-inflammatory medications that can be administered by as eye drops, by injection, or as medications taken orally. Sometime diuretics help reduce the swelling. If necessary, a vitrectomy is done to relieve the pressure of the vitreous pulling on the macular (University of Michigan 2013).

The other intraoperative and postprocedural complications include:

- Intraoperative hemorrhage and hematoma of eye and adnexa complicating a ophthalmic procedure (H59.11-)

- Intraoperative hemorrhage and hematoma of eye and adnexa complicating other procedure (H59.12-)

- Accidental puncture and laceration of eye and adnexa during an ophthalmic procedure (H59.21-)

- Accidental puncture and laceration of eye and adnexa during other procedure (H59.22-)

- Postprocedural hemorrhage and hematoma of eye and adnexa following an ophthalmic procedure (H59.31-)

- Postprocedural hemorrhage and hematoma of eye and adnexa following other procedure (H59.32-)

- Inflammation (infections) of postprocedural bleb (H59.4-)

- Chorioretinal scars after surgery for detachment (H59.81-)

ICD-10-PCS Procedure Coding

Procedures performed on the eye are included in the tables from 080–08X with the root operations Alteration, Bypass, Change, Destruction, Dilation, Drainage, Excision, Extirpation, Extraction, Fragmentation, Insertion, Inspection, Occlusion, Reattachment, Release, Removal, Repair, Replacement, Reposition, Resection, Supplement, Restriction, Revision, and Transfer. Like procedures in other body systems, in order to code eye procedures, the coder needs to know the definition of root operations and the anatomy of the eye to identify the body parts.

Using strictly the titles of operations of eye procedures is not sufficient to code in ICD-10-PCS. A term used by a physician may be the equivalent of multiple possible root operations that the coder has to analyze by reading the operative report to determine the primary objective of the procedure (what the procedure accomplished). For example, consider the following eye procedure terminology and the possible root operations that may be used based on what was performed:

Keratoplasty:
- Repair (LASIK to correct refractive error)
- Replacement (Corneal transplant)
- Supplement (Lamellar keratoplasty)

Phacoemulsification
- Replacement (if an intraocular lens (IOL) is inserted)
- Extraction (if there is no IOL inserted)

ICD-10-PCS procedures are produced by building a code using the values provided for each root operation performed on a particular body system and body part. A keratoplasty is surgery on the cornea that may also be called corneal transplant or corneal grafting. A penetrating keratoplasty is the removal of the full thickness of the cornea and replacing it with donor corneal tissue; usually this is called a corneal transplant. A lamellar keratoplasty is a partial thickness graft of the cornea. In this procedure, only the epithelium and superficial stroma of the cornea is removed and is replaced with donor tissue that supplements the remaining corneal tissue that was not removed from the eye. Based on the type of keratoplasty performed, the root operation may be Repair as the procedure is restoring, to the extent possible, a body part to its normal anatomic structure and function. A Replacement is defined as putting in or on biological or synthetic material that physically takes the place or function of all or a portion of a body part. The Supplement root operation, defined as putting in or on biological or synthetic material that physically reinforces or augments the function of a portion of a body part, is used for the lamellar keratoplasty as the donor tissue reinforces the existing cornea in the patient's eye (Dorland 2007).

For cataract surgery, the root operation may be Replacement or Extraction depending on whether the intraocular lens is placed in the eye at the same procedure. Replacement, defined as putting in or on biological or synthetic material that physically takes the place or function of all or a portion of a body part, is used when the artificial lens is placed in the eye to replace the lens that was removed with the cataract. Extraction, defined as pulling or stripping out or off all or a portion of a body part by the use of force, is the root operation when the cataract or the diseased lens in the eye is removed without replacement by an artificial lens during the same procedure.

Other examples of eye procedures and the possible root operations used to code them:

Blepharoplasty: Alteration, Repair, Replacement, Reposition, or Supplement

Dacryocystostomy or sclerotomy: Drainage

Enucleation or evisceration: Replacement or Resection

Photocoagulation: Destruction or Repair

Probing lacrimal duct: Inspection or Dilation

Removal of foreign body: Extirpation

Scleral buckling: Supplement

Strabismus: Reposition

Trabeculectomy: Drainage

Vitrectomy: Excision or Resection

ICD-10-CM and ICD-10-PCS Review Exercises: Chapter 10

Assign the correct ICD-10-CM diagnosis codes or ICD-10-PCS procedure codes to the following exercises.

1. Macular drusen, right eye

    _____

2. Irregular astigmatism, both eyes

    _____

3. Presenile cortical cataract, left eye

    _____

4. Retained metal foreign body fragments, right upper eyelid

    _____

5. Low tension glaucoma, mild stage, both eyes

    _____

6. Floppy iris syndrome, right eye, due to the patient's prescription Flomax taken as prescribed, follow-up visit

    _____

7. Single break retinal detachment, left eye

    _____

8. Acute chemical conjunctivitis, right eye

    _____

9. Bilateral retinopathy of prematurity, stage 2

    _____

10. Monocular exotropia with V pattern, left eye

    _____

11. Low vision, visual impairment category two, both eyes

    _____

(*Continued on next page*)

ICD-10-CM and ICD-10-PCS Review Exercises: Chapter 10 (Continued)

12. Bullous keratopathy, left eye, due to cataract surgery

   _____

13. Chronic iridocyclitis and cataract with neovascularization, right eye

   _____

14. Acute lacrimal canaliculitis, right eye

   _____

15. Essential hypertensive with hypertensive retinopathy

   _____

16. PROCEDURE: Removal of foreign body (glass) from left cornea

   _____

17. PROCEDURE: Transnasal endoscopy for dilation and stent placement in left lacrimal duct

   _____

18. PROCEDURE: Penetrating keratoplasty of right cornea with donor matched cornea for transplant, percutaneous approach

   _____

19. PROCEDURE: Cataract extraction by phacoemulsification, left eye, with prosthetic lens immediate insertion

   _____

20. PROCEDURE: Lamellar keratoplasty, onlay supplement type, right cornea, using autograft

   _____

Chapter 11

Diseases of the Ear and Mastoid Process (H60–H95)

Learning Objectives

At the conclusion of this chapter, you should be able to:

1. Describe the organization of the conditions and codes included in Chapter 8 of ICD-10-CM, Diseases of the ear and mastoid process (H60–H95)

2. Identify and describe the various types of ear infections, including otitis externa and otitis media

3. Identify and describe the various types of hearing loss

4. Assign ICD-10-CM codes for diseases of the ear and mastoid process

5. Assign ICD-10-PCS codes for procedures related to the ear and mastoid process

Key Terms

- Conductive hearing loss
- Deaf nonspeaking
- Dizziness
- Otitis externa
- Otitis media (OM)
- Mastoiditis
- Meniere's disease
- Otosclerosis
- Salpingitis
- Sensorineural hearing loss
- Vertigo

Overview of ICD-10-CM Chapter 8, Diseases of the Ear and Mastoid Process (H60–H95)

Chapter 8 of ICD-10-CM includes categories H60–H95 arranged in the following blocks:

H60–H62	Diseases of external ear
H65–H75	Diseases of middle ear and mastoid
H80–H83	Diseases of inner ear
H90–H94	Other disorders of ear
H95	Intraoperative and postprocedural complications and disorders of ear and mastoid process, not elsewhere classified

Chapter 8 is introduced in ICD-10-CM to classify the diseases of the ear and mastoid process. Blocks of codes have been created to identify the types of conditions that would occur in the external ear, middle ear and mastoid, and inner ear. Like many chapters, the intraoperative and postprocedural complications are grouped at the end of the chapter rather than included in different categories. The codes include greater specificity at the fourth-, fifth-, and sixth-character levels, for example, acute otitis media with and without spontaneous rupture of ear drum with specific codes for the type of perforation. Also included are codes for laterality for the right, left, bilateral, and unspecified sides of the body for the sites and more "code first underlying disease" notes.

> **EXAMPLES:** H65, Nonsuppurative otitis media
> H71, Cholesteatoma of middle ear
> H81, Disorders of vestibular function

Coding Guidelines and Instructional Notes for ICD-10-CM Chapter 8, Diseases of the Ear and Mastoid Process (H60–H95)

At the time of this publication, the NCHS has not published chapter-specific guidelines for Chapter 8 in the *ICD-10-CM Official Guidelines for Coding and Reporting*. The coding student should review all of the coding guidelines for ICD-10-CM, which appear in an ICD-10-CM code book or at the website http://www.cdc.gov/nchs/icd/icd10cm.htm, or in Appendix E.

There are instructional notes throughout Chapter 8 to direct the coder for correct and complete coding. At the start of Chapter 8 in ICD-10-CM, there is a note to use an external cause code following the code for the ear condition, if applicable, to identify the cause of the ear condition. An Excludes2 note includes a series of excluded conditions that are applicable to all conditions classifiable to Chapter 8. For example, certain conditions originating in the perinatal period of the first 28 days of life are coded to Chapter 16 of ICD-10-CM and certain infectious and parasitic diseases are coded to Chapter 1 instead of to the chapter for diseases of the ear and mastoid process.

An example of an instructional note appears at category H72, Perforation of tympanic membrane, to recognize the importance of coding first the associated otitis media with the diagnosis of perforation of the tympanic membrane. The Excludes1 note that follows explains other conditions that are not to be coded to category H72 as these excluded conditions cannot occur together.

EXAMPLE: H72, Perforation of tympanic membrane
Code first any associated otitis media (H65.-, H66.1-, H66.2-, H66.3-, H66.4-, H66.9-, H67.-)
Excludes1:
acute suppurative otitis media with rupture of the tympanic membrane (H66.01-)
traumatic rupture of ear drum (S09.2-)

There is an instructional note in categories H65, H66, and H67 to use an additional code for any associated perforated tympanic membrane (H72.-). This is a reminder to the coder that two codes are required when a patient has both otitis media and perforated tympanic membrane.

Another instructional note is found under the category for suppurative and unspecified otitis media (H66). The note instructs coding professionals to use an additional code to identify:

exposure to environmental tobacco smoke (Z77.22),

exposure to tobacco smoke in the perinatal period (P96.81),

history of tobacco use (Z87.891),

occupational exposure to environmental tobacco smoke (Z57.31),

tobacco dependence (F17.-), or

tobacco use (Z72.0).

Coding Diseases of the Ear and Mastoid Process in ICD-10-CM Chapter 8

The chapter is organized into four blocks of codes. The first block is diseases of the external ear (H60–H62). These codes include otitis externa, other disorders of the external ear such as chondritis and perichondritis, noninfective disorders of the pinna, and acquired stenosis of the external ear canal. Laterality is included with codes for right, left, bilateral, and unspecified ears.

Diseases of External Ear (H60–H62)

The external ear is the part of the ear consisting of the auricle and the auditory canal or the passage leading to the ear drum. It may also be called the outer ear. **Otitis externa** (external otitis, swimmer's ear) is an infection of the external auditory canal that may be classified as acute or chronic. Acute otitis externa is characterized by moderate to severe pain, fever, regional cellulitis, and partial hearing loss. Instead of pain, chronic otitis externa is characterized by pruritus, which leads to scaling and a thickening of the skin.

ICD-10-CM classifies otitis externa to category H60, Otitis externa. Subcategories H60.0 for abscess of external ear, H60.1 for cellulitis of external ear, and H60.2 for malignant otitis externa include codes for unspecified, right, left, and bilateral ears. Similarly, subcategory H60.3 includes fifth and sixth character codes for diffuse otitis externa, hemorrhagic otitis externa, swimmer's ear, and other infective otitis media with specific codes for unspecified, right, left, and bilateral ears.

Subcategories H62.4 and H62.8 classify otitis externa and other disorders of the external ear in diseases classified elsewhere. These codes require the reporting of the underlying disease that has caused the external ear condition. A "code first underlying disease" note appears under each subcategory, such as coding erysipelas, impetigo, or gout as the underlying disease.

Diseases of Middle Ear and Mastoid (H65–H75)

Diseases of the middle ear and mastoid (H65–H75) is a large block of codes. A note to use additional code for any associated perforated tympanic membrane is included with the otitis media codes at the H65 and H66 category level. Other notes to use additional codes for exposure to smoke from environment and personal use of tobacco products are also included with the codes for otitis media or middle ear infections.

Otitis Media

Otitis media (OM) is an inflammation of the middle ear that may be further specified as suppurative or secretory, and acute or chronic. These variations and their symptoms follow:

- Acute suppurative OM is characterized by severe, deep, throbbing pain; sneezing and coughing; mild to high fever; hearing loss; dizziness; nausea; and vomiting. Suppurative infections involve the formation of pus.

- Acute secretory or serous OM results in severe conductive hearing loss and, in some cases, a sensation of fullness in the ear with popping, crackling, or clicking sounds on swallowing or with jaw movement. Secretory infections produce a secretion or serous exudate.

- Chronic OM has its origin in the childhood years but usually persists into adulthood. Cumulative effects of chronic OM include thickening and scarring of the tympanic membrane, decreased or absent tympanic mobility, cholesteatoma, and painless purulent discharge.

Acute, chronic and unspecified types of otitis media can be coded with laterality identified for right, left, bilateral, or unspecified ears. ICD-10-CM classifies OM to categories H65, Nonsuppurative otitis media, and H66, Suppurative and unspecified otitis media. Both of these categories are subdivided to identify acute and chronic forms of OM and other specific types of OM. The following subcategory codes identify common forms of otitis media that require fifth and sixth characters to further specify the type and the laterality:

EXAMPLE:

H65.0	Acute serous otitis media
H65.2	Chronic serous otitis media
H65.3	Chronic mucoid otitis media

H65.9	Unspecified nonsuppurative otitis media
H66.0	Acute suppurative otitis media that includes fifth characters for without or with spontaneous rupture of ear drum
H66.1–H66.3	Chronic (forms) suppurative otitis media
H66.4	Suppurative otitis media, unspecified
H66.9	Otitis media, unspecified

There are instructional notes with categories H65, H66, and H67 to use an additional code for any associated perforated tympanic membrane. Another instructional note is found under the categories H65 and H66 to use an additional code to identify use of or exposure to tobacco products.

Eustachian Salpingitis and Obstruction (H68)

Acute and chronic infections of the Eustachian tube as well as obstruction of the Eustachian tube can be coded with category H68. The term "salpingitis" is included in the codes. **Salpingitis** is the inflammation of a tubular site, such as a fallopian tube in the female reproductive tract as well as the Eustachian tube in the middle ear.

Mastoiditis and Related Conditions (H70)

Category H70, Mastoiditis and related conditions, includes four-, five-, and six-character codes to identify acute mastoidits, chronic mastoidits, petrositis, and other related conditions. Laterality is included in this category to identify if the patient's right, left, or bilateral ears are involved. Codes for an unspecified ear is also included.

The definition of **mastoiditis** includes all inflammatory processes of the mastoid air cells of the temporal bone. As the mastoid bone is an extension of the middle ear cleft, many children or adults with acute otitis media (AOM) or chronic middle ear inflammatory disease will have mastoiditis. In most cases, middle ear symptoms are more obvious in the patients (that is, fever, pain, conductive hearing loss), and the disease within the mastoid is not considered a separate disease when it occurs together.

Acute mastoiditis is present with AOM. In some patients, the infection spreads and patients develop osteitis or periosteitis of the mastoid process. These patients have acute surgical mastoiditis (ASM), a complication of otitis media.

Chronic mastoiditis most commonly occurs with chronic suppurative otitis media and with cholesteatoma formation. Cholesteatomas are growths in the lining of the middle ear that invade and change the normal structure and function of surrounding soft tissue and bone. It is a destructive process accelerated in the presence of active infection.

With acute otitis media as the underlying disease, the most common organism causing surgical mastoiditis is *Streptococcus pneumoniae*, followed by *Haemophilus influenzae* and group A *Streptococcus pyogenes*. Gram-negative organisms and *Staphylococcus aureus* are the organisms that develop more frequently in patients with chronic mastoiditis.

Most of the children admitted with acute mastoiditis have no history of recurrent AOM. In those children, *Streptococcus pneumoniae* has been the leading pathogen, while *Pseudomonas aeruginosa* causes the disease in children with recurrent AOM. Persistent otorrhea that persists more than 3 weeks is the most consistent sign that a process involving the mastoid has evolved.

A patient with acute mastoiditis may have a high and unrelenting fever. Some of this symptomatology may be related to the associated acute otitis media (AOM). However, if a patient has a persistent fever, particularly when the patient is receiving adequate and appropriate antimicrobial agents, this is the indication the patient has acute surgical mastoiditis.

The patient feels pain deep in and behind the ear with mastoiditis and it is typically worse at night when the patient is laying down and trying to sleep. This persistent pain is a warning sign of mastoid disease. Hearing loss is common with all infectious processes that involve the middle ear (Devan 2011).

Perforation of Tympanic Membrane (H72)

The most common use of the codes in category H72 is to classify the condition of a "ruptured" tympanic membrane that can occur at the same time as acute and chronic middle ear infections. However, the "includes" note under category H72 states that persistent posttraumatic perforation of the ear drum and postinflammatory perforation of the ear drum are included in this category. There is a note to "code first" any associated otitis media with the codes from category H72 when the two conditions occur together. The "code first" note acknowledges that the otitis media is the cause of the perforation in many patients.

Diseases of the Inner Ear (H80–H83)

Disease of the inner ear includes such conditions as otosclerosis, disorders of vestibular function such as Meniere's disease, and different types of vertigo. Vertiginous syndromes in diseases classified elsewhere as well as other diseases of the inner ear may be coded with laterality.

Otosclerosis (H80)

Otosclerosis is the growth of spongy bone in the inner ear where it causes obstruction. It causes slowly progressive conductive hearing loss. Otosclerosis affects 10 percent of the white population and is more likely to occur in women. Frequency is thought to be decreasing because more people now are receiving the measles vaccination. Often the patient with otosclerosis has a family history of the disease. Pregnancy and estrogen therapy is suspected to increase the progression of otosclerosis. Symptom onset usually occurs by age 40 but can also occur later in life. The most common symptom is slowly progressive bilateral hearing loss. Vertigo is uncommon but tinnitus or ringing in the ears may be present. These symptoms often resolve after successful surgical treatment. On physical examination, patients with conductive hearing loss often speak softly but do not realize it because they hear their voices as louder because of the enhanced bone conduction of sound (Shohet 2011).

Meniere's Disease (H81.0-)

Meniere's disease is a disorder of the inner ear that may be documented as idiopathic endolymphatic or labyrinthine hydrops. Endolymphatic hydrops is increased pressure within the inner ear lymphatic system. Excess pressure accumulation causes symptoms of fluctuating hearing loss, occasional episodic vertigo, tinnitus, and pressure or fullness sensation in the ears. The terms of Meniere's disease, Meniere's syndrome, and endolymphatic hydrops may be used as synonymous terms. However, Meniere's disease has an unknown cause but Meniere's syndrome is due to endocrine abnormalities, trauma, electrolyte imbalance, autoimmune dysfunction, medications, parasitic infections, or hyperlipidemia. Finding the cause and treatment can be a difficult medical task. The cause may be a simple condition like dehydration or a serious disease such as a brain tumor. Medical therapy can be directed toward treatment of the actual symptoms of the acute attack or directed toward prophylactic prevention of the attacks. If Meniere's syndrome is the final diagnosis, treatment is directed as the primary disease (that is, thyroid disease). In ICD-10-CM, Meniere's disease, labyrinthine hydrops, Meniere's syndrome, or vertigo is coded to one subcategory, H81.0-, with fifth characters for right ear, left ear, bilateral ears, or unspecified ear.

Benign Paroxysmal Vertigo (H81.1-)

A common type of vertigo is benign paroxysmal positional vertigo (BPPV). The subcategory of codes V81.10–V81.13 identify laterality for right, left, bilateral, and unspecified ear. Patients describe their **vertigo** as a feeling that their surroundings seem to whirl around them. Dizziness is not the same as vertigo. **Dizziness** is a sensation of unsteadiness accompanied by a feeling of movement within the head. Many patients who present to their physician's office complaining of the vertigo sensation are diagnosed with BPPV. In addition, BPPV can occur at the same time with other inner ear diseases, for example with Meniere's disease.

Classic BPPV is usually triggered by sitting up quickly from a supine position. Patients describe the feeling of the room spinning around them. The onset is typically sudden. Patients state they are more likely to experience the condition in the morning while trying to sit up when they are getting out of bed. The symptoms resolve quickly. However, the sensation can occur again when the person moves to a sitting position when they are getting out of bed. This sensation can occur for a period of days to weeks. Some patients report the symptoms periodically resolve but later recur. The condition is more common in women than men and usually in women over the age of 60 and older. Patients report that if they get up slowly and pause while sitting on the edge of the bed before standing they do not have the same vertigo sensations. People who have BPPV may not feel dizzy, but can experience severe dizziness triggered by head movements. Many patients have few or no symptoms between the episodes of vertigo. However, some patients complain of a continual "foggy or cloudy" sensation after their vertigo starts. The cause of the vertigo may never be found. Patients who are at risk for vertigo are people who have been inactive, such as patient's recovering from surgery and illnesses and spending a lot of time lying down in bed. It is also common in patients with central nervous system diseases and ear diseases but the connection has not been established. Vertigo is also common in patients with acute alcoholism. Treatment of the condition may be vertigo-suppressant medications that relieve some of the symptoms. However, many patients simply experience a resolution of the problem on its own but continue to observe the pattern of rising slowly from bed or from a reclining position to prevent a recurrence (Li 2012).

Other Disorders of Ear (H90–H94)

The block of codes H90–H94 includes specific codes with laterality for many different types of hearing loss. Other conditions such as ostalgia, tinnitus, and disorders of acoustic or the eighth cranial nerve can be coded with laterality.

Conductive and Sensorineural Hearing Loss, Other and Unspecified Hearing Loss (H90–H91)

ICD-10-CM category codes H90 and H91 contain several subcategory codes that describe various forms of hearing loss or deafness. **Conductive hearing loss** is the decreased ability to hear sounds because of a defect of the sound-conducting apparatus of the ear. Conductive hearing loss in one ear (unilateral) is classified with codes H90.11–H90.12 when the patient has unrestricted hearing on the contralateral or opposite site. Conductive hearing loss that occurs bilaterally is classified with code H90.0. There is also the option for unspecified conductive hearing loss with code H90.2.

Sensorineural hearing loss is the decreased ability to hear sounds due to a defect in the sensory mechanisms within the ear or the nerves within the ear. Sensorineural hearing loss may be described as sensory, neural, or central hearing loss. Sensorineural hearing loss with unrestricted hearing in the opposite ear is classified with codes H90.41–H90.42. The code for bilateral conductive hearing loss is H90.3. Again there is a code H90.5 for unspecified sensorineural hearing loss.

Specific codes exist for unilateral mixed conductive and sensorineural hearing loss (H90.7-) and bilateral mixed hearing loss (H90.6), as well as code H90.8 for use when the condition is not specified as unilateral or bilateral. Another condition described as **deaf nonspeaking** or "deafmutism" is classified with code H91.3 to identify the condition when a patient has the absence of both hearing and the faculties of speech.

Intraoperative and Postprocedural Complications and Disorders of Ear and Mastoid Process, Not Elsewhere Classified (H95)

Finally, intraoperative and postprocedural complications and disorders of ear and mastoid process, not elsewhere classified are the block of codes at the end of the chapter. These codes identify conditions such as the following:

- Recurrent cholesteatoma of postmastoidectomy cavity (H95.0-)

- Other disorders of ear and mastoid process following mastoidectomy (H95.1-)

- Intraoperative hemorrhage and hematoma of ear and mastoid procedure complicating a procedure on the ear and mastoid process (H95.2-)

- Accidental puncture and laceration of ear and mastoid process during a procedure on the ear and mastoid process (H95.3-)

- Postprocedural hemorrhage and hematoma of ear and mastoid process following a procedure on the ear and mastoid process (H95.4-)

- Postprocedural stenosis of external ear canal (H95.81-)

ICD-10-PCS Procedure Coding for Chapter 8, Diseases of the Ear and Mastoid Process

Procedures performed on the ear, nose, and sinus are included in the tables from 090–09W with root operations Alteration, Bypass, Change, Destruction, Dilation, Division, Drainage, Excision, Extirpation, Extraction, Insertion, Inspection, Reattachment, Release, Removal, Repair, Replacement, Reposition, Resection, Supplement, and Revision. Like procedures in other body systems, in order to code ear, nose, and sinus procedures, the coder needs to know the definition of root operations and the anatomy to identify the body parts.

Using strictly the titles of operations of eye procedures is not sufficient to code in ICD-10-PCS. A term used by a physician may be the equivalent of multiple possible root operations that the coder has to analyze by reading the operative report to determine the primary objective of the procedure—what did the procedure accomplish? Different types of devices are inserted into the body for hearing assistance, for example, bone conduction hearing implants and cochlear devices. Numerous other surgical and diagnostic procedures are performed in the ear, nose, and sinuses. For example, consider the following ear, nose, and sinus procedure terminology and the possible root operations that may be used based on what was performed:

Rhinoplasty may be performed for a variety of objectives as described by these root operations:

- Alteration: cosmetic repair for improved appearance
- Repair: restoring, to the extent possible, the body part to its normal anatomic structure and function
- Replacement: putting in or on biological or synthetic material that physically takes the place or function of all or a portion of a body part
- Supplement: putting in or on biological or synthetic material that physically reinforces or augments the function of a portion of a body part

Ethmoidectomy, myringectomy, sinusotomy, stapedectomy, and turbinectomy procedures all involve the removal of these body parts as described by these root operations:

- Excision: cutting out or off, without replacement, a portion of a body part
- Resection: cutting out or off, without replacement, all of a body part

Otoplasty, septoplasty, and turbinoplasty are procedures that correct a condition at the body part as described by these root operations:

- Repair: restoring, to the extent possible, the body part to its normal anatomic structure and function
- Replacement: putting in or on biological or synthetic material that physically takes the place or function of all or a portion of a body part
- Reposition: moving to its normal location or other suitable location all or a portion of a body part
- Supplement: putting in or on biological or synthetic material that physically reinforces or augments the function of a portion of a body part

Otoscopy, rhinoscopy, and sinusoscopy may be performed without an accompanying surgical procedure through the scope. When the procedure is strictly an examination it is coded with the following root operation:

- Inspection: visually or manually exploring a body part

Myringotomy or turbinotomy are procedures performed to drain or destroy a lesion in the body part and are described by one of the following operations:

- Drainage: taking or letting out fluids or gases from a body part
- Destruction: physical eradication of all or a portion of a body part by the direct use of energy, force, or a destructive agent

Removal of foreign body is a common procedure performed on the ear. The root operation is

- Extirpation: taking or cutting out solid matter from a body part

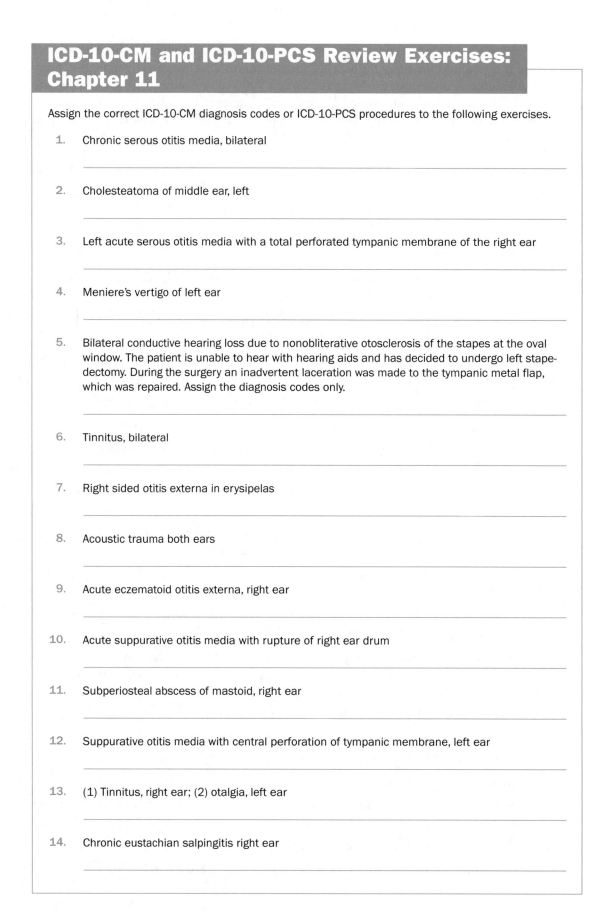

ICD-10-CM and ICD-10-PCS Review Exercises: Chapter 11

Assign the correct ICD-10-CM diagnosis codes or ICD-10-PCS procedures to the following exercises.

1. Chronic serous otitis media, bilateral

2. Cholesteatoma of middle ear, left

3. Left acute serous otitis media with a total perforated tympanic membrane of the right ear

4. Meniere's vertigo of left ear

5. Bilateral conductive hearing loss due to nonobliterative otosclerosis of the stapes at the oval window. The patient is unable to hear with hearing aids and has decided to undergo left stapedectomy. During the surgery an inadvertent laceration was made to the tympanic metal flap, which was repaired. Assign the diagnosis codes only.

6. Tinnitus, bilateral

7. Right sided otitis externa in erysipelas

8. Acoustic trauma both ears

9. Acute eczematoid otitis externa, right ear

10. Acute suppurative otitis media with rupture of right ear drum

11. Subperiosteal abscess of mastoid, right ear

12. Suppurative otitis media with central perforation of tympanic membrane, left ear

13. (1) Tinnitus, right ear; (2) otalgia, left ear

14. Chronic eustachian salpingitis right ear

ICD-10-CM and ICD-10-PCS Review Exercises: Chapter 11 (Continued)

15. Chronic postmastoidectomy cavity inflammation, left ear

16. PROCEDURE: Stapedectomy (removal of entire stapes), right ear

17. PROCEDURE: Removal of impacted foreign body (bead) left external auditory canal through ear canal

18. PROCEDURE: Endoscopic partial nasal turbinectomy

19. PROCEDURE: Bilateral myringotomy and placement of tubes behind the tympanic membrane

20. PROCEDURE: Excision of cholesteatoma, left eye

Chapter 12

Diseases of the Circulatory System (I00–I99)

Learning Objectives

At the conclusion of this chapter, you should be able to:

1. Describe the organization of the conditions and codes included in Chapter 9 of ICD-10-CM, Diseases of the circulatory system (I00–I99)

2. Apply the ICD-10-CM coding guidelines for the correct coding of circulatory diagnoses

3. Describe the circulatory system diseases of rheumatic fever, chronic rheumatic heart disease, hypertension, hypertensive disease, angina, acute myocardial infarction, chronic ischemic heart disease, heart failure, cardiac arrhythmias, cardiac arrest, cerebrovascular disease, and sequelae of cerebrovascular disease

4. Assign ICD-10-CM codes for ICD-10-CM Chapter 9, Diseases of the circulatory system

5. Assign ICD-10-PCS codes for procedures related to diseases of the circulatory system

Key Terms

- Abdominal-coronary artery bypass
- Acute myocardial infarction (AMI)
- Angina pectoris
- Aortocoronary bypass
- Arteriosclerotic heart disease
- Atherosclerotic heart disease
- Atrial fibrillation
- Atrial flutter
- Automatic implantable cardioverter-defibrillator (AICD)
- Atherosclerosis
- Benign hypertension
- Cardiac arrhythmia

- Cardiac catheterization
- Cerebral infarction
- Cerebrovascular accident (CVA)
- Cerebrovascular disease
- Congestive heart failure
- Coronary angiography
- Coronary arteriography
- Deep vein thrombosis (DVT)
- Electrode
- Heart block: First-, Second-, and Third-degree
- Heart failure
- Hypertensive chronic kidney disease
- Hypertensive heart disease
- Hypertensive heart and chronic kidney disease
- Internal mammary-coronary artery bypass
- Intravenous tissue plasminogen activator (tPA)
- Left-sided heart failure
- Malignant hypertension
- Non-ST elevation myocardial infarction (NSTEMI)
- Normal blood pressure (BP)
- Pacing lead
- Paroxysmal tachycardia
- Percutaneous transluminal coronary angioplasty (PTCA)
- Pulse generator
- Rheumatic chorea
- Rheumatic fever
- Rheumatic heart disease
- Right-sided heart failure
- Secondary hypertension
- Sick sinus syndrome (SSS)
- ST elevation myocardial infarction (STEMI)
- Supraventricular tachycardia
- Unstable angina
- Ventriculography
- Venous thrombo-embolism (VTE)
- Ventricular fibrillation
- Wolff-Parkinson-White (WPW) syndrome

Overview of ICD-10-CM Chapter 9, Diseases of the Circulatory System

Chapter 9 of ICD-10-CM includes categories I00–I99 arranged in the following blocks:

I00–I02	Acute rheumatic fever
I05–I09	Chronic rheumatic heart diseases
I10–I15	Hypertensive diseases

I20–I25	Ischemic heart disease
I26–I28	Pulmonary heart disease and diseases of pulmonary circulation
I30–I52	Other forms of heart disease
I60–I69	Cerebrovascular disease
I70–I79	Diseases of arteries, arterioles and capillaries
I80–I89	Diseases of veins, lymphatic vessels and lymph node, not elsewhere classified
I95–I99	Other and unspecified disorders of the circulatory system

The terminology used to describe several cardiovascular conditions has been revised to reflect more current medical practice. For example, acute myocardial infarction is now identified as **ST elevation myocardial infarction (STEMI)** and **non-ST myocardial infarction elevation (NSTEMI)**. Intermediate coronary syndrome is identified in ICD-10-CM as unstable angina. Acute coronary occlusion without myocardial infarction is better classified in ICD-10-CM as acute coronary thrombosis not resulting in myocardial infarction. Hypertension codes do not identify the type of hypertension such as benign or malignant.

The terminology used to describe several cardiovascular conditions has been revised to reflect more current medical practice.

EXAMPLES: I21, ST elevation (STEMI) and non-ST elevation (NSTEMI) myocardial infarction
I20.0, Unstable angina
I24.0, Acute coronary thrombosis not resulting in myocardial infarction

The type of hypertension that may be used to describe a patient's condition (benign, malignant, unspecified) is not used as an axis for the ICD-10-CM hypertension codes. There is only one code for essential hypertension (I10).

The category for late effects of cerebrovascular disease is titled "Sequelae of cerebrovascular disease." The codes in the category include the type of stroke, such as hemorrhage or infarction, and the specific sequela, such as cognitive or speech deficits, monoplegia or hemiplegia, and aphasia or dysphagia. In addition, the laterality of the affliction and whether the dominant or nondominant side is affected is included in the codes' descriptions.

Coding Guidelines and Instructional Notes for ICD-10-CM Chapter 9

At the start of Chapter 9, a series of excluded conditions are listed that are applicable to all conditions classifiable to Chapter 9. For example, the Excludes2 note includes conditions that can be coded with codes from Chapter 9. Such conditions include certain conditions originating in the perinatal period, certain infectious and parasitic diseases, and complications of pregnancy, childbirth, and the puerperium.

Under several blocks of codes including hypertensive disease (I10–I15) and ischemic heart disease (I20–I25), there are "use additional code to identify" notes to code exposure to environmental tobacco smoke, history of tobacco use, occupational exposure to environmental tobacco smoke, tobacco dependence, and tobacco use.

Other codes including cardiomyopathy in diseases classified elsewhere (I43) and paroxysmal tachycardia (I47) include "code first" notes such as underlying diseases of amyloidosis; glycogen storage disease; gout and thyrotoxicosis; or abortion, ectopic, or molar pregnancy; and obstetric surgery and procedures.

The NCHS has published chapter-specific guidelines for Chapter 9 in the *ICD-10-CM Official Guidelines for Coding and Reporting.* The coding student should review all of the coding guidelines for Chapter 9 of ICD-10-CM, which appear in an ICD-10-CM code book, at the website http://www.cdc.gov/nchs/icd/icd10cm.htm, or in Appendix E.

CG

Guideline I.C.9.a.1. Hypertensive with Heart Disease: Heart conditions classified to I50.- or I51.4–I51.9 are assigned to a code from category I11, Hypertensive heart disease, when a causal relationship is stated (due to hypertension) or implied (hypertensive). Use an additional code from category I50, Heart failure, to identify the type of heart failure in those patients with heart failure.

The same heart conditions (I50.-, I51.4-, I51.9) with hypertension, but without a stated causal relationship, are coded separately. Sequence according to the circumstances of the admission/encounter.

Guideline I.C.9.a.2. Hypertensive Chronic Kidney Disease: Assign codes from category I12, Hypertensive chronic kidney disease, when both hypertension and a condition classifiable to category N18, Chronic kidney disease (CKD), are present. Unlike hypertension with heart disease, ICD-10-CM presumes a cause-and-effect relationship and classifies chronic kidney disease with hypertension as hypertensive chronic kidney disease.

The appropriate code from category N18 should be used as a secondary code with a code from category I12 to identify the stage of chronic kidney disease.

See Section I.C.14.a. Chronic kidney disease.

If a patient has hypertensive chronic kidney disease and acute renal failure, an additional code for the acute renal failure is required.

Guideline I.C.9.a.3. Hypertensive Heart and Chronic Kidney Disease: Assign codes from combination category I13, Hypertensive heart and chronic kidney disease, when both hypertensive kidney disease and hypertensive heart disease are stated in the diagnosis. Assume a relationship between the hypertension and the chronic kidney disease, whether or not the condition is so designated. If heart failure is present, assign an additional code from category I50 to identify the type of heart failure.

The appropriate code from category N18, Chronic kidney disease, should be used as a secondary code from category I13 to identify the stage of chronic kidney disease.

See Section I.C.14.a. Chronic kidney disease.

The codes in category I13, Hypertensive heart and chronic kidney disease, are combination codes that include hypertension, heart disease and chronic kidney disease. The Includes note at I13 specifies that the condition included in I11 and I12 are included together in I13. If a patient has hypertension, heart disease and chronic kidney disease then a code from I13 should be used, not individual codes for hypertension, heart disease and chronic kidney disease, or codes from I11 or I12.

For patients with both acute renal failure and chronic kidney diseases an additional code for acute renal failure is required.

Guideline I.C.9.a.4. Hypertensive Cerebrovascular Disease: For hypertensive cerebrovascular disease, first assign the appropriate code from categories I60–I69, followed by the appropriate hypertension code.

Guideline I.C.9.a.5. Hypertensive Retinopathy: Subcategory I35.0, Background retinopathy and retinal vascular changes, should be used with a code from category I10-I15, Hypertensive disease to include the systemic hypertension. The sequencing is based on the reason for the encounter.

Guideline I.C.9.a.6. Hypertension, Secondary: Secondary hypertension is due to an underlying condition. Two codes are required: one to identify the underlying etiology and one from category I15 to identify the hypertension. Sequencing of codes is determined by the reason for admission/encounter.

Guideline I.C.9.a.7. Hypertension, Transient: Assign code R03.0, Elevated blood pressure reading without diagnosis of hypertension, unless patient has an established diagnosis of hypertension. Assign code O13.-, Gestational [pregnancy-induced] hypertension without significant proteinuria, or O14, Pre-eclampsia, for transient hypertension of pregnancy.

Guideline I.C.9.a.8. Hypertension, Controlled: This diagnosis statement usually refers to an existing state of hypertension under control by therapy. Assign the appropriate code from categories I10-I15, Hypertensive diseases.

Guideline I.C.9.a.9. Hypertension, Uncontrolled: Uncontrolled hypertension may refer to untreated hypertension or hypertension not responding to current therapeutic regimen. In either case, assign the appropriate code from categories I10-I15, Hypertensive diseases.

Guideline I.C.9.b. Atherosclerotic Coronary Artery Disease and Angina: ICD-10-CM has combination codes for atherosclerotic heart disease with angina pectoris. The subcategories for these codes are I25.11, Atherosclerotic heart disease of native coronary artery with angina pectoris and I25.7, Atherosclerosis of coronary

(Continued)

(Continued)

artery bypass graft(s) and coronary artery of transplanted heart with angina pectoris.

When using one of these combination codes it is not necessary to use an additional code for angina pectoris. A causal relationship can be assumed in a patient with both atherosclerosis and angina pectoris, unless the documentation indicates the angina is due to something other than atherosclerosis.

If a patient with coronary artery disease is admitted due to an acute myocardial infarction (AMI), the AMI should be sequenced before the coronary artery disease.

See Section I.C.9.e. Acute myocardial infarction (AMI).

Guideline I.C.9.c Intraoperative and Postprocedural Cerebrovascular Accident: Medical record documentation should clearly specify the cause-and-effect relationship between the medical intervention and the cerebrovascular accident in order to assign a code for intraoperative or postprocedural cerebrovascular accident.

Proper code assignment depends on whether it was an infarction or hemorrhage and whether it occurred intraoperatively or postoperatively. If it was a cerebral hemorrhage, code assignment depends on the type of procedure performed.

Guideline I.C.10.d.1. Category I69, Sequelae of Cerebrovascular Disease: Category I69 is used to indicate conditions classifiable to categories I60–I67 as the causes of sequela (neurologic deficits), themselves classified elsewhere. These "late effects" include neurologic deficits that persist after initial onset of conditions classifiable to categories I60–I67. The neurologic deficits caused by cerebrovascular disease may be present from the onset or may arise at any time after the onset of the condition classifiable to categories I60–I67.

Codes from category I69, Sequelae of cerebrovascular disease, that specify hemiplegia, hemiparesis and monoplegia identify whether the dominant or nondominant side is affected. Should the affected side be documented, but not specified as dominant or nondominant, and the classification system does not indicate a default, code selection is as follows:

- For ambidextrous patients, the default should be dominant.
- If the left side is affected, the default is nondominant.
- If the right side is affected, the default is dominant.

Guideline I.C.10.d.2. Codes from category I69 with codes from I60–I67: Codes from category I69 may be assigned on a health care record with codes from I60–I67, if the patient has a current cerebrovascular disease and deficits from an old cerebrovascular disease.

Guideline I.C.10.d.3. Codes from category I69, Personal history of transient ischemic attack (TIA) and cerebral infarction (Z86.73): Codes from category I69 should not be assigned if the patient does not have neurologic deficits.

See Section I.C.21.c.4. History (of) for use of personal history codes

Guideline I.C.9.e.1. Acute myocardial infarction (AMI) ST Elevation Myocardial Infarction (STEMI) and Non-ST Elevation Myocardial Infarction (NSTEMI): The ICD-10-CM codes for acute myocardial infarction (AMI) identify the site, such as anterolateral wall or true posterior wall. Subcategories I21.0–I21.2 and code I21.3 are used for ST elevation myocardial infarction (STEMI). Code I21.4, Non-ST elevation (NSTEMI) myocardial infarction, is used for non-ST elevation myocardial infarction (NSTEMI) and nontransmural MIs.

If NSTEMI evolves to STEMI, assign the STEMI code. If STEMI converts to NSTEMI due to thrombolytic therapy, it is still coded as a STEMI.

For encounters occurring while the myocardial infarction is equal to, or less than, four weeks old, including transfers to another acute setting or a postacute setting, and the patient requires continued care for the myocardial infarction, codes from category I21 may continue to be reported. For encounters after the 4 week time frame and the patient is still receiving care related to the myocardial infarction, the appropriate aftercare code should be assigned, rather than a code from category I21. For old or healed myocardial infarctions not requiring further care, code I25.2, Old myocardial infarction, may be assigned.

Guideline I.C.9.e.2. Acute myocardial infarction, unspecified: Code I21.3, ST elevation (STEMI) myocardial infarction of unspecified site, is the default for unspecified acute myocardial infarction. If only STEMI or transmural MI without the site is documented, assign code I21.3

Guideline I.C.9.e.3. AMI documented as nontransmural or subendocardial but site provided: If an AMI is documented as nontransmural or subendocardial, but the site is provided, it is still coded as subendocardial AMI.

See Section I.C.21.3 for information on coding status post administration of tPA in a different facility within the last 24 hours.

Guideline I.C.9.e.4. Subsequent acute myocardial infarction: A code from category I22, Subsequent ST elevation (STEMI) and non-ST elevation (NSTEMI) myocardial infarction is to be used

(Continued)

(Continued)

when a patient who has suffered an AMI has a new AMI within the 4 week time frame of the initial AMI. A code from category I22 must be used in conjunction with a code from category I21. The sequencing of I22 and I21 codes depends on the circumstances of the encounter.

Coding Diseases of the Circulatory System in ICD-10-CM Chapter 9

Chapter 9 contains an expanded number of specific codes that describe coronary, cerebral, and vascular diseases. "Use additional code to identify" notes appear throughout the chapter to direct the coder to identify exposure to, history of current use of, and dependence on tobacco. Codes also specify the laterality of vessels to identify the specific location of disease, for example, left middle cerebral artery.

Beneath categories I21, I22, and I23 for acute myocardial infarction are notes that state the specific category to be used to identify myocardial infarctions specified as acute or with a stated duration of four weeks (28 days) or less from onset.

The instructional notes and guidelines are very important for these three categories to indicate correct code usage. A code from category I22, Subsequent acute myocardial infarction, must be used in conjunction with a code from category I21, STEMI and NSTEMI. A code from category I23, Certain current complications following STEMI and NSTEMI must be used in conjunction with a code from category I21 or I22.

Acute Rheumatic Fever and Rheumatic Heart Disease (I00–I09)

Acute and chronic diseases of rheumatic origin are classified in categories I00 through I09. This section also covers diseases of mitral and aortic valves. Rheumatic heart disease continues to be the most common cause for mitral stenosis, and rarely do other factors cause the condition (PubMed Health 2010).

Acute Rheumatic Fever (I00–I02)

Rheumatic fever occurs after a streptococcal sore throat (Group A *Streptococcus hemolyticus*). The acute phase of the illness is marked by fever, malaise, sweating, palpitation, and polyarthritis, which varies from vague discomfort to severe pain felt chiefly in the large joints. Most patients have elevated titers of antistreptolysin antibodies and increased sedimentation rates.

The importance of rheumatic fever derives entirely from its capacity to cause severe heart damage. Salicylates markedly reduce fever, relieve joint pain, and may reduce joint swelling, if present. Because rheumatic fever often recurs, prophylaxis with penicillin is recommended and has markedly reduced the incidence of rheumatic heart disease in the general population.

ICD-10-CM codes for acute rheumatic fever include categories for rheumatic fever without heart involvement (I00), rheumatic fever with heart involvement (I01), and rheumatic chorea (I02).

Rheumatic chorea is also known as Sydenham's chorea. The condition occurs more often in children but can also occur in adults. Chorea is the result of acute rheumatic fever but may not be evident for as long as 6 months after the original streptococcal infection. It can be present with or without rheumatic fever damage to the heart. A patient with rheumatic chorea will have a variety of symptoms including muscle weakness, difficulty in gripping objects, difficulty walking, and a slurred or garbled speech pattern. Psychological symptoms may be present with the physical signs. The patient may have emotional displays that are out of proportion with the events occurring around the patient. The patient may also have attention deficits, experience anxiety when separated from parents or caregivers, and have some obsessive-compulsive tendencies. In adult women, poststreptococcal chorea may complicate pregnancy, known as chorea gravidarum (Vertrees 2012).

Chronic Rheumatic Heart Disease (I05–I09)

Instructional notes that clarify code usage are also found under specific codes. Under code I05, Rheumatic mitral valve diseases, is a note that states this category includes conditions classifiable to both I05.0 and I05.2–I05.9, whether specified as rheumatic or not.

Rheumatic heart disease develops with an initial attack of rheumatic fever in about 30 percent of cases. The cardiac involvement may affect all three layers of the heart muscle, causing pericarditis, scarring and weakening of the myocardium, and endocardial involvement of heart valves. The latter condition occurs more often in children who have had rheumatic fever and, to a lesser extent, in adults with rheumatic fever. A murmur heard over the heart is symptomatic of a valvular lesion. Rheumatic fever causes inflammation of the valves, thus damaging the valve cusps so that the opening may become permanently narrowed (stenosis). The mitral valve is involved in the great majority of such cases; the aortic valve is involved to a lesser extent; and the tricuspid and pulmonary valves are involved in a small percentage of the patients. In about 10 percent of patients, two of these valves are involved.

When stenosis affects the mitral valve, blood flow decreases from the left atrium into the left ventricle. As a result, blood is held back in the lungs, then in the right side of the heart, and, finally, in the veins of the body. Incompetence of a valve may also occur because the cusps will not retract. If the mitral valve cannot close, blood escapes from the mitral valve back into the left atrium. In the case of the aortic valve, blood escapes from the aorta into the left ventricle. In such cases, plastic and metal replacement valves that function as well as normal valves may be surgically inserted.

In coding diseases of the mitral valve and diseases affecting both the mitral and aortic valves, the Index to Diseases offers direction to codes from categories I05–I09. Remember to always trust the Index to Diseases and assign the code it indicates.

EXAMPLE: Insufficiency, insufficient.
    mitral (valve) I34.0
        with
            aortic (valve) disease I08.0
                with tricuspid (valve) disease I08.3
        obstruction or stenosis I05.2
            with aortic valve disease I08.0
        congenital Q23.3
        rheumatic I05.1
            with
                aortic valve disease I08.0
                    with tricuspid (valve) disease I08.3
        obstruction or stenosis I05.22
            with aortic valve disease I08.0
                with tricuspid valve disease I08.3

Diseases of the mitral valve, aortic valve, tricuspid valve, and pulmonary valve that are identified by the physician as nonrheumatic are classified to categories I34–I37 as directed by the Index to Diseases and the Excludes1 notes under the chronic rheumatic heart disease subcategory codes.

Hypertensive Disease (I10–I15)

The Index to Diseases uses the main terms "hypertension" and "hypertensive" to list the disease of hypertension and the other conditions caused by hypertension. ICD-10-CM has one category for "hypertension," I10, even though different forms of hypertension may be described by a physician for a particular patient. Hypertension is one of the most important treatable conditions and is a major risk factor for coronary heart disease, stroke, congestive heart failure, end-stage renal disease, and peripheral vascular disease.

Definition of Hypertension

Blood pressure (BP) readings, which is described in mm Hg, for adults aged 18 years or older is as follows:

- Normal: systolic lower than 120 mm Hg, diastolic lower than 80 mm Hg
- Prehypertension: systolic 120 to 139 mm Hg, diastolic 80 to 89 mm Hg
- Stage 1 hypertension: systolic 140 to 159 mm Hg, diastolic 90 to 99 mm Hg
- Stage 2 hypertension: systolic 160 mm Hg or greater, diastolic 100 mm Hg or greater

The definition above is based on the average of two or more readings taken at each of two or more visits after the initial measurement. **Normal blood pressure (BP)** with respect to cardiovascular risk is less than 120/80 mm Hg (Riaz 2012).

The prevalence of hypertension increases with age. About 90 to 95 percent of hypertension is primary (essential hypertension), and its cause is unknown. The remaining 5 to 10 percent is secondary to renal disease. Both essential and secondary hypertension can be either benign or malignant. Complications of hypertension include left ventricular failure, arteriosclerotic heart disease, retinal hemorrhages, cerebrovascular insufficiency, and renal failure.

Benign Hypertension (I10)

In most cases, **benign hypertension** remains fairly stable over many years and is compatible with a long life. If untreated, however, it becomes an important risk factor in coronary heart disease and cerebrovascular disease. Benign hypertension is also asymptomatic until complications develop. Effective antihypertensive drug therapy is the treatment of choice.

Malignant Hypertension (I10)

Malignant hypertension is far less common, occurring in only a small percent of patients with elevated blood pressure. It is also known as accelerating hypertension. The malignant form is frequently of abrupt onset. It often ends with renal failure or cerebral hemorrhage. Usually a person with malignant hypertension will complain of headaches and difficulties with vision. Blood pressures of 180/120 are common, and an abnormal protrusion of the optic nerve (papilledema) occurs with microscopic hemorrhages and exudates seen in the retina. The initial event appears to be some form of vascular damage to the kidneys. This may result from long-standing benign hypertension with damage of the arteriolar walls, or it may derive from arteritis of some form. The chances for long-term survival depend on early treatment before significant renal insufficiency has developed.

Hypertensive Heart Disease (I11)

Hypertensive heart disease refers to the secondary effects on the heart of prolonged sustained systemic hypertension. The heart has to work against greatly increased resistance in the form of high blood pressure. The primary effect is thickening of the left ventricle, finally resulting in heart failure. The symptoms are similar to those of heart failure from other causes. Many persons with controlled hypertension do not develop heart failure. However, when a patient has heart failure due to hypertension, additional codes are required to be used with category I11 to specify the type of heart failure that exists, such as I50.1–I50.9, if known. The separate hypertensive heart disease codes are

I11.0   Hypertensive heart disease with heart failure
     Hypertensive heart failure
     Use additional code to identify type of heart failure (I50.-)

I11.9   Hypertensive heart disease without heart failure
     Hypertensive heart disease NOS

Heart conditions such as heart failure and other forms of heart disease (I50.- or I51.4–I51.9) are assigned to a code from category I11, Hypertensive heart disease, when a causal relationship is stated (due to hypertension) or implied (hypertensive). The physician must make the connection that the hypertension caused the heart disease. The same heart conditions (I50.-, I51.4–I51.9) with hypertension, but without a stated causal relationship, are coded separately.

Hypertensive Chronic Kidney Disease (I12)

Hypertensive chronic kidney disease is any chronic kidney disease (N18,-) or contracted kidney (N26.-) that is due to hypertension. A code from category I12, Hypertensive chronic kidney disease, is assigned when both the diagnosis of hypertension and chronic kidney disease are present and documented by the physician. Unlike hypertension with heart disease, ICD-10-CM presumes a cause-and-effect relationship and classifies chronic kidney disease with hypertension as hypertensive chronic kidney disease. An additional code from category N18 should be used with a code from category I12 to identify the stage of chronic kidney disease. If a patient has hypertensive chronic kidney disease and acute renal failure, an additional code for the acute renal failure is required. Separate codes exist for hypertension with different stages of chronic kidney disease:

I12.0   Hypertensive chronic kidney disease with stage 5 chronic kidney disease or end stage renal disease
     Use additional code to identify the stage of chronic kidney disease (N18.5, N18.6)

I12.9   Hypertensive chronic kidney disease with stage 1 through stage 4 chronic kidney disease, or unspecified chronic kidney disease
Use additional code to identify the stage of chronic kidney disease (N18.1–N18.4, N18.9)

Hypertensive Heart and Chronic Kidney Disease (I13)

Hypertensive heart and chronic kidney disease is any heart disease due to hypertension (I11) with chronic kidney disease and hypertension (I12). Separate subcategory codes exist for hypertensive heart disease with chronic kidney disease, stage 1 through stage 4, and hypertensive heart disease with chronic kidney disease, stage 5 or end stage renal disease:

I13.0   Hypertensive heart and chronic kidney disease with heart failure and stage 1 through stage 4 chronic kidney disease or unspecified chronic kidney disease
Use additional code to identify type of heart failure (I50.-)
Use additional code to identify the stage of chronic kidney disease (N18.1–N18.4, N18.9)

I13.10   Hypertensive heart and chronic kidney disease without heart failure with stage 1 through stage 4 chronic kidney disease, or unspecified chronic kidney disease
Use additional code to identify the stage of chronic kidney disease (N18.1–N18.4, N18.9)

I13.11   Hypertensive heart and chronic kidney disease without heart failure with stage 5 or end stage renal disease
Use additional code to identify the stage of chronic kidney disease (N18.5, N18.6)

I13.2   Hypertensive heart and chronic kidney disease with heart failure and with stage 5 or end stage renal disease
Use additional code to identify type of heart failure (I50.-)
Use additional code to identify the stage of chronic kidney disease (N18.5, N18.6)

Secondary Hypertension (I15)

Secondary hypertension is due to another disease or underlying condition. Two codes are required: one to identify the underlying etiology and one from category I15 to identify the hypertension. Beneath category code I15 is an instructional note to "code also underlying condition." The sequencing of the two codes depends on the circumstances of the visit or admission, that is, what the primary focus of attention is. The codes in category I15 include a broad description of the underlying cause:

I15.0   Renovascular hypertension
I15.1   Hypertension secondary to other renal disorders
I15.2   Hypertension secondary to endocrine disorders
I15.8   Other secondary hypertension
I15.9   Secondary hypertension, unspecified

Secondary hypertension identified as renovascular hypertension is hypertension usually due to renal artery or renal vascular disease. This is the opposite of the conditions in category I12.0 where the chronic kidney disease is due to hypertension, not the other way around as in secondary hypertension (I15.0).

Ischemic Heart Disease (I20–I25)

Combination codes in ICD-10-CM include atherosclerotic heart disease with angina and appear in category I25, Chronic ischemic heart disease. This placement eliminates the need to use an additional code for angina pectoris or unstable angina. The I25 category codes in ICD–10-CM contain details about the location of the coronary artery disease, such as native vessel or bypass graft, and the type of angina, such as unstable, with documented spasm, as well as other forms of angina pectoris.

Angina Pectoris (I20)

There are two types of angina: unstable angina and angina pectoris.

Unstable Angina

Unstable angina, also known as crescendo and preinfarction angina, is defined as the development of prolonged episodes of anginal discomfort, usually occurring at rest and requiring hospitalization to rule out a myocardial infarction. ICD-10-CM classifies unstable angina with code I20.0. Code I20.0 is assigned when a patient is admitted to the hospital and treated for unstable angina without documentation of infarction, occlusion, or thrombosis.

Angina Pectoris

Angina pectoris refers to chest pain due to ischemia (loss of blood supply to a part) of the heart. The blood flow, with its supply of oxygen, is reduced because of atherosclerosis (hardening of arteries). Immediate causes of angina pectoris can be exertion, stress, cold weather, or digestion of a large meal. Pain is most commonly felt beneath the sternum, and a vague or a sharp pain sometimes radiates down the left arm. Blood pressure and heart rate are increased during an attack; however, angina lasts only a few minutes and is relieved by rest and/or sublingual nitroglycerin. Angina pectoris is a warning of more severe heart disease, such as myocardial infarction or congestive heart failure.

ICD-10-CM classifies angina pectoris to category I20. The fourth-digit subcategories identify specific types of angina pectoris, such as angina pectoris with documented spasm, which may also be described as Prinzmetal angina, variant angina or spasm induced angina (I20.1). The definition of Prinzmetal or variant angina is chest pain at rest secondary to myocardial ischemia. Other forms of angina pectoris are classified as I20.8 and may be described as angina equivalent or coronary slow flow syndrome. There is also a code I20.9 for angina pectoris NOS or angina NOS, which may also be described as ischemic chest pain.

ICD-10-CM has combination codes for atherosclerotic heart disease with angina pectoris. The subcategories for these codes are I25.11, Atherosclerotic heart disease of native coronary artery with angina pectoris and I25.7, Atherosclerosis of coronary artery bypass graft(s) and coronary artery of transplanted heart with angina pectoris. When using one of these combination codes it is not necessary to use an additional code for angina pectoris. A causal relationship can be assumed in a patient with both atherosclerosis and angina pectoris, unless the documentation indicates the angina is due to something other than atherosclerosis. If a patient with coronary artery disease is admitted due to an acute myocardial infarction (AMI), the AMI should be sequenced before the coronary artery disease.

Angina and Coronary Disease

Keep in mind the definition of principal diagnosis: "the condition established after study to be chiefly responsible for occasioning the admission of the patient to the hospital for care." This definition must be used when a patient suffers from angina.

> **EXAMPLE:** A patient was admitted with angina. Diagnostic cardiac catheterizations determined that the angina was due to coronary arteriosclerosis of the native vessels. The patient was discharged on antianginal medications.
> The combination code, I25.119, Atherosclerotic heart disease of native coronary with unspecified angina pectoris, is listed as the principal diagnosis. There is no requirement to add an additional code for the angina.

> **EXAMPLE:** A patient was admitted with symptomatic angina that evolved into an AMI.
> The AMI is sequenced as the principal diagnosis, I21.3, ST elevation (STEMI) of unspecified site. No additional code is assigned for angina as it is an inherent part of the condition.

> **EXAMPLE:** A patient with unstable angina was admitted to the hospital for left heart cardiac catheterization. He was found to have significant four-vessel coronary atherosclerosis. He had four-native-vessel coronary artery bypass surgery performed during the same admission.
> The combination code I25.110, Atherosclerotic heart disease of native coronary artery with unstable angina, is the principal diagnosis. The diagnosis of unstable angina, 411.1, is not assigned as an additional diagnosis because it is included in code I25.110.

Acute and Subsequent STEMI and NSTEMI and Certain Complications (I21–I23)

Acute myocardial infarction (AMI) usually occurs as a result of a sudden inadequacy of coronary flow. The first symptom of AMI is the development of deep substernal pain described as aching or pressure, often with radiation to the back or left arm. The patient may be pale, diaphoretic (sweaty), and in severe pain, however, the symptoms may vary between men and women. Peripheral or carotid cyanosis may be present, as well as arrhythmias. Treatment is designed to relieve the patient's distress, reduce cardiac work, and prevent and treat complications. Major complications include tachycardia, frequent ventricular premature beats, Mobitz II heart block, and ventricular fibrillation. Heart failure often occurs. Physicians may refer to an AMI as a STEMI or NSTEMI.

Included under category I21, STEMI and NSTEMI myocardial infarction, is the terminology of cardiac infarction, coronary (artery) embolism, coronary (artery) occlusion, coronary (artery) rupture, coronary (artery) thrombosis, and infarction of heart, myocardium or ventricle. This code is intended to represent a myocardial infarction specified as acute or with a stated duration of 4 weeks (28 days) or less from onset. Specific ICD-10-CM coding guidelines exist for the coding of current and subsequent AMIs with AMI complication codes and likely will challenge new ICD-10-CM coders as they begin to use the classification system.

The note with category I22 says that a code from category I22 must be used in conjunction with a code from category I21. The I22 code should be sequenced first, if it is the reason for encounter, or, it should be sequenced after the I21 code if the subsequent MI occurs during the encounter for the initial MI. Also watch for notes to use additional codes to identify body mass index (BMI), if known, and tobacco use or exposure. Should a patient who is in the hospital due to an AMI have a subsequent AMI while still in the hospital, code I21 would be sequenced first as the reason for admission, with code I22 sequenced as a secondary code. Should a patient have a subsequent AMI after discharge for care of an initial AMI, and the reason for admission is the subsequent AMI, the I22 code should be sequenced first followed by the I21. An I21 code must accompany an I22 code to identify the site of the initial AMI, and to indicate that the patient is still within the four-week time frame of healing from the initial AMI.

Certain current complications following STEMI and NSTEMI myocardial infarctions are reported with category I23 codes when the condition occurs within 28 days after the infarction. Code I25.2, Old myocardial infarction, is assigned when the diagnostic statement mentions the presence of a healed MI presenting no symptoms during the current episode of care.

Diagnostic Tools for AMI

The diagnosis of AMI depends on the patient's clinical history, the physical examination, interpretation of the electrocardiogram (EKG) and chest radiograph, and measurement of serum levels of cardiac enzymes, such as troponins or the MB isoenzyme of creatine kinase (CK-MB).

Diagnostic uncertainty frequently arises because of various factors. Many patients with acute AMI have atypical symptoms. Other people with typical physical symptoms do not have AMI. EKGs may also be nondiagnostic. Laboratory tests known as biochemical or serum markers of cardiac injury are commonly relied upon to diagnose or exclude an AMI.

Creatine kinase and lactate dehydrogenase have been the "gold standard" for the diagnosis of AMI for many years. However, single values of these tests have limited sensitivity and specificity. Serum markers currently in use are troponin T and I, myoglobin, and CK-MB. These markers are used instead of, or along with, the standard markers.

EKGs also prove useful in diagnosing myocardial infarctions. The initial EKG may be diagnostic in acute transmural myocardial infarction, but serial EKGs may be necessary to confirm the diagnosis for other myocardial infarction sites.

A patient diagnosed with an acute myocardial infarction or an acute ischemic stroke may be given **intravenous tissue plasminogen activator (tPA)**, which is a thrombolytic agent also known as a "clot-busting drug." Studies have shown that tPA and other clot-dissolving agents can reduce the amount of damage to the heart muscle and save lives. In order to be effective, tPA must be given within the first three hours after the onset of symptoms. The fact that a patient has received tPA is important information. A patient may be seen in Hospital A and receive tPA intravenously and then be transferred to Hospital B for further management of the acute myocardial infarction. If the patient has received tPA within the 24 hours prior to admission to the current facility then the coder at Hospital B should code Z92.82, Status post administration of tPA (rtPA) in a different facility within the last 24 hours prior to admission to the current facility. The condition requiring the tPA administration is coded first, such as acute MI or acute cerebral infarction. Hospital A does not use diagnosis code Z92.82.

Chronic Ischemic Heart Disease (I25)

ICD-10-CM classifies chronic ischemic heart disease to category I25. Chronic ischemic heart disease or **atherosclerotic** or **arteriosclerotic heart disease** refers to those cases in which ischemia has induced general myocardial atrophy and scattered areas of interstitial scarring. This heart disease results from slow, progressive narrowing of the coronary arteries. This course may be altered by episodes of sudden severe coronary insufficiency. The patient with chronic ischemic heart disease may develop angina or an AMI.

Atherosclerosis

Atherosclerosis is the formation of lesions on the inside of arterial walls from the accumulation of fat cells and platelets. Another term for atherosclerosis is arteriosclerosis. The gradual enlargement of the lesion eventually weakens the arterial wall and narrows the lumen, or channel of the blood vessel, decreasing the volume of blood flow. The large arteries—the aorta and its main branches—are primarily affected, but smaller arteries such as the coronary and cerebral arteries can also be affected. In such a case, the patient experiences chest pain, shortness of breath, and sweating. Blood pressure is high; pulse is rapid and weak. An x-ray reveals cardiomegaly and narrowing, or occlusion, of the affected vessel wall. Blood tests may show hypercholesterolemia.

Atherosclerosis is the major cause of ischemia of the heart, brain, and extremities. Its complications include stroke, congestive heart failure, angina pectoris, myocardial infarction, and kidney failure. Treatment is directed toward the specific manifestation.

Subcategories of I25, Chronic Ischemic Heart Disease

ICD-10-CM classifies atherosclerotic heart disease and coronary artery disease to category I25, Chronic ischemic heart disease. The fourth-, fifth-, and sixth-digit subcategories describe specific types of ischemic heart diseases. The ICD-10-CM subcategories under I25 describe specific types of ischemic heart disease, such as

I25.1   Atherosclerotic heart disease of native coronary artery, with and without types of angina pectoris

I25.10   Atherosclerotic heart disease of native coronary artery without angina pectoris

I25.11   Atherosclerotic heart disease of native coronary artery with angina pectoris
Sixth characters are used to identify the atherosclerotic heart disease with unstable angina, angina pectoris with documented spasm, with other forms of angina pectoris and unspecified angina pectoris.

I25.2   Old myocardial infarction

I25.3   Aneurysm of heart

I25.4   Coronary artery aneurysm and dissection

I25.5   Ischemic cardiomyopathy

I25.6   Silent myocardial ischemia

I25.7   Atherosclerosis of coronary artery bypass graft(s) and coronary artery of transplanted heart with angina pectoris, specifying the type of graft involved

       I25.70   Atherosclerosis of coronary artery bypass graft(s), unspecified, with angina pectoris

I25.71   Atherosclerosis of autologous vein coronary artery bypass graft(s), with angina pectoris

I25.72   Atherosclerosis of autologous artery coronary artery bypass graft(s), with angina pectoris

I25.73   Atherosclerosis of nonautologous biological coronary artery bypass graft(s), with angina pectoris

I25.75   Atherosclerosis of native coronary artery of transplanted heart with angina pectoris

I25.76   Atherosclerosis of bypass graft of coronary artery of transplanted heart with angina pectoris

I25.79   Atherosclerosis of other coronary artery bypass graft(s) with angina pectoris

Sixth characters represent the atherosclerosis with unstable angina, angina pectoris with documented spasm, with other forms of angina pectoris and unspecified angina pectoris.

I25.8   Other forms of chronic heart disease

I25.81   Atherosclerosis of other coronary vessels without angina pectoris
Sixth characters represent the type of coronary artery such as bypass graft(s), native coronary artery of transplanted heart, bypass graft of coronary artery of transplanted heart.

I25.82   Chronic total occlusion of coronary artery

I25.83   Coronary atherosclerosis due to lipid rich plaque

I25.84   Coronary atherosclerosis due to calcified coronary lesion

I25.89   Other forms of chronic ischemic heart disease

I25.9   Chronic ischemic heart disease, unspecified

Important "use additional code" notes appear throughout category I25, Chronic ischemic heart disease. These notes remind the coder to add a code, depending on the particular subcategory code:

Chronic total occlusion of coronary artery, I25.82
Coronary atherosclerosis due to calcified coronary lesion, I25.84
Coronary atherosclerosis due to lipid rich plaque, I25.83
Various codes for tobacco use and exposure to tobacco smoke

The instructional code of "code first coronary atherosclerosis (I25.1-, I25.7-, I25.8-)" appears under codes for chronic total occlusion of coronary artery, coronary atherosclerosis due to lipid rich plaque, and coronary atherosclerosis due to calcified coronary lesion.

Subcategory code I25.4 differentiates between aneurysms and dissections of the heart. Code I25.42 is included for dissection of the coronary artery. An arterial dissection is characterized by blood coursing within the layers of the arterial wall and is not an aneurysm.

Subcategory I25.82, Chronic total occlusion of coronary artery, is used as an additional code when a patient with coronary atherosclerosis (I25.1-, I25.7- and I25.81-) also has the complete blockage of a coronary artery. There is an increased risk of myocardial infarction or death for individuals with chronic total occlusion of a coronary artery. Chronic total occlusion of a coronary artery may be treated with angioplasty or stent placement, which is technically more difficult to perform than an angioplasty or stent placement in a patient with less than total occlusion of a coronary artery.

Subcategory I25.83, Coronary atherosclerosis due to lipid rich plaque, identifies the type of plaque within a coronary artery. This diagnostic information is important to the cardiologist in determining the most appropriate type of stent (drug-eluting or bare metal) to place in the vessel depending on the location and amount of lipid-rich plaque present. Code I25.83 is used in addition to a code for the location and type of coronary artherosclerosis (I25.1-, I25.7-, and I25.81-) that exists in the patient.

Heart Failure (I50)

Heart failure is the heart's inability to contract with enough force to properly pump blood. This condition may be caused by coronary artery disease (usually in a patient with a previous myocardial infarction), cardiomyopathy, hypertension, or heart valve disease. Sometimes the exact cause of heart failure is not found. Heart failure may develop gradually or occur acutely. Heart failure can involve the heart's left side, right side, or both sides. However, it usually affects the left side first.

Heart failure has the following three effects:

- Pressure in the lungs is increased. Fluid collects in the lung tissue, inhibiting O_2 and CO_2 exchange.

- Kidney function is hampered. Blood does not filter well, and body sodium and water retention increase, resulting in edema.

- Blood is not properly circulated throughout the body. Fluid collects in tissues, resulting in edema of the feet and legs.

Symptoms of heart failure include:

- Sudden weight gain, such as three or more pounds a day or five or more pounds a week
- Shortness of breath or difficulty breathing, especially while at rest or when lying flat in bed
- Waking up breathless at night, trouble sleeping, using more pillows
- Frequent dry, hacking cough, especially when lying down
- Increased fatigue and weakness, feeling tired all the time
- Dizziness or fainting
- Swollen feet, ankles, and legs
- Nausea with abdominal swelling, pain, and tenderness

Left-Sided Heart Failure

The heart's pumping action moves oxygen-rich blood from the lungs to the left atrium and then on to the left ventricle, which pumps it to the rest of the body. The left ventricle supplies most of the heart's pumping power, so it is larger than the other chambers and essential for normal function. In left-sided or left ventricular (LV) heart failure, the left side of the heart must work harder to pump the same amount of blood.

There are two types of **left-sided heart failure**. Drug treatments are different for the two types.

- Systolic failure: The left ventricle loses its ability to contract normally. The heart cannot pump with sufficient force to push enough blood into circulation.

- Diastolic failure: The left ventricle loses its ability to relax normally (because the muscle has become stiff). The heart cannot properly fill with blood during the resting period between each beat.

Right-Sided Heart Failure

The heart's pumping action also moves deoxygenated blood, which returns through the veins to the heart, through the right atrium, and into the right ventricle. The right ventricle then pumps the blood back out of the heart into the lungs to be replenished with oxygen.

Right-sided heart failure usually occurs as a result of left-sided failure. When the left ventricle fails, increased fluid pressure is, in effect, transferred back through the lungs, ultimately damaging the heart's right side. When the right side loses pumping power, blood backs up in the body's veins. This usually causes swelling in the legs and ankles.

Congestive Heart Failure

Congestive heart failure is another type of heart failure (sometimes the terms "congestive heart failure" and "heart failure" are used interchangeably) that requires seeking timely medical attention.

Heart failure causes blood to flow out of the heart at a slower rate. At the same time, this causes blood in the veins trying to return to the heart to slow down and congestion in the body tissues occurs. Patients with heart failure with this congestion have swelling in the legs, ankles, wrists, and hands. Fluid also collects in the lungs and the patient will experience shortness of breath, especially pronounced when the person is lying down. Physicians describe the pulmonary congestion as pulmonary edema that must be treated before it produces respiratory distress or respiratory failure. The kidneys ability to filter and dispose of waste is hampered by heart failure. The body retains water when the kidneys are not functioning properly and swelling occurs in other parts of the body than strictly the extremities.

The term heart failure is not synonymous with congestive heart failure. Many patients with heart failure do not manifest pulmonary or systemic congestion. ICD-10-CM category I50 includes codes that distinguish between congestive heart failure (I50.9), left ventricular failure (I50.1), systolic heart failure (I50.2-), diastolic heart failure (I50.3-), and combined systolic and diastolic heart failure (I50.4-.)

Diagnostic Tests

Several diagnostic tests are important in diagnosing heart failure in a patient. Typical remarks on a chest x-ray indicating heart failure include hilar congestion, "butterfly" or "batwing" appearance of vascular markings, bronchial edema, Kerley B lines signifying chronic elevation of left atrial pressure, and heart enlargement. An echocardiograph measures the amount of blood pumped from the heart with each beat. This measurement is known as the ejection fraction. A normal heart pumps one half (50 percent) or more of the blood in the left ventricle with each heartbeat. With heart failure, the weakened heart may pump 40 percent or less, and less blood is pumped with less force to all parts of the body.

Urinalysis results show slight albuminuria, increased concentration with specific gravity of 1.020, and decreased urine sodium. Laboratory findings may include blood urea nitrogen

(BUN) 60 mg/100 ml; acidosis –pH 7.35 due to increased CO_2 in blood from pulmonary insufficiency; and increased blood volume with decrease in chloride, albumin, and total protein.

For most patients, heart failure is a chronic condition, which means it can be treated and managed, but not cured. Usually the patient's management plan consists of medications, such as angiotensin-converting enzyme (ACE) inhibitors; diuretics and digitalis; low sodium diet; possibly some modifications in daily activities; regular exercise such as walking and swimming; and other changes in lifestyle and health habits such as reducing alcohol consumption and quitting smoking.

Cardiac Arrhythmias and Conduction Disorders (I44–I49)

Cardiac arrhythmias identify disturbances or impairments of the normal electrical activity of heart muscle excitation. ICD-10-CM classifies cardiac arrhythmias to several categories depending on the specific type. Without further specification as to the type of cardiac arrhythmia, code I49.9 may be reported. A discussion of common arrhythmias follows.

Atrial fibrillation (I48.0–I48.2, I48.9-) is commonly associated with organic heart diseases, such as coronary artery disease, hypertension and rheumatic mitral valve disease, thyrotoxicosis, pericarditis, and pulmonary embolism. Treatment includes pharmacologic therapy (verapamil, digoxin, or propranolol) and cardioversion. Distinctions are made between the types of atrial fibrillation, such as paroxysmal, perisistent, chronic, and unspecified types.

Atrial flutter (I48.3–I48.4) is associated with organic heart diseases, such as coronary artery disease, hypertension, and rheumatic mitral valve disease. Treatment is similar to that for atrial fibrillation. Typical and atypical atrial flutter are coded separately.

Ventricular fibrillation (I49.01) involves no cardiac output and is associated with cardiac arrest. Treatment is consistent with that for cardiac arrest.

Paroxysmal tachycardia (I47.0–I47.9) is associated with congenital accessory atrial conduction pathway, physical or psychological stress, hypoxia, hypokalemia, caffeine and marijuana use, stimulants, and digitalis toxicity. Treatment includes pharmacologic therapy (quinidine, propranolol, or verapamil) and cardioversion.

Sick sinus syndrome (SSS) (I49.5) is an imprecise diagnosis with various characteristics. SSS may be diagnosed when a patient presents with sinus arrest, sinoatrial exit block, or persistent sinus bradycardia. This syndrome is often the result of drug therapy, such as digitalis, calcium channel blockers, beta-blockers, sympatholytic agents, or antiarrhythmics. Another presentation includes recurrent supraventricular tachycardias associated with bradyarrhythmias. Prolonged ambulatory monitoring may be indicated to establish a diagnosis of SSS. Treatment includes insertion of a permanent cardiac pacemaker.

Various forms of conduction disorders may be classified in ICD-10-CM. Conduction disorders are disruptions or disturbances in the electrical impulses that regulate the heartbeats.

Wolff-Parkinson-White (WPW) syndrome (I45.6) is caused by conduction from the sinoatrial node to the ventricle through an accessory pathway that bypasses the atrioventricular node. Patients with WPW syndrome present with tachyarrhythmias, including supraventricular tachycardia, atrial fibrillation, or atrial flutter. Treatment includes catheter ablation following electrophysiologic evaluation.

Atrioventricular (AV) heart blocks are classified as first, second, or third degree.

- **First-degree AV block** is associated with atrial septal defects or valvular disease. ICD-10-CM classifies first-degree AV block to code I44.0.

- **Second-degree AV block** is further classified as follows:

○ Mobitz type I (Wenckebach) is associated with acute inferior wall myocardial infarction or with digitalis toxicity. Treatment includes discontinuation of digitalis and administration of atropine. ICD-10-CM classifies Mobitz type I AV block to code I44.1.

○ Mobitz type II is associated with anterior wall or anteroseptal myocardial infarction and digitalis toxicity. Treatment includes temporary pacing and, in some cases, permanent pacemaker insertion, as well as discontinuation of digitalis and administration of atropine. ICD-10-CM classifies Mobitz type II AV block to code I44.1.

• **Third-degree heart block**, also referred to as complete heart block, is associated with ischemic heart disease or infarction, postsurgical complication of mitral valve replacement, digitalis toxicity, and Stokes-Adams syndrome. Treatment includes permanent cardiac pacemaker insertion. ICD-10-CM classifies third-degree heart block to code I44.2. When this type of heart block is congenital in nature, code Q24.6 is reported rather than 426.0.

Without further specification, AV block is reported with code I44.30.

Supraventricular tachycardia is a heart rate over 90 beats per minute triggered by the sinoatrial node, usually in response to exogenous factors, such as fever, exercise, anxiety, stress, pain, thyroid hormone, hypoxia, and dehydration. It may also accompany shock, left ventricular failure, cardiac tamponade, anemia, hyperthyroidism, hypovolemia, pulmonary embolism, and anterior myocardial infarction. Tachycardia is also a response to stimulants such as caffeine, cocaine, or amphetamines. Treatment is geared toward correcting the underlying cause. ICD-10-CM classifies supraventricular tachycardia to code I47.1.

Cardiac Arrest (I46)

ICD-10-CM includes three codes for cardiac arrest: I46.2, Cardiac arrest due to underlying cardiac condition; I46.8, Cardiac arrest due to other underlying condition; and I46.9, Cardiac arrest, cause unspecified. Under codes I46.2 and I46.3, there is a "code first" note to code the underlying cardiac or other underlying condition as the first code. The specificity of the type of cardiac is arrest is essential for coding; is it due to a cardiac condition or another disease or is the cardiac arrest related to another medical condition or procedure.

There is an Exclude1 note under category I46, Cardiac arrest that cardiogenic shock, R57.0, cannot be assigned with a code from category I46. Other codes are available in other chapters of ICD-10-CM for cardiac arrest complicating abortion—see Abortion, by types, complicated by, cardiac arrest. Other cardiac arrest codes exist for when it occurs in a newborn or when cardiac arrest complicates anesthesia and complicating a delivery. Intraoperative and postprocedural cardiac arrest codes are also available.

Cerebrovascular Disease (I60–I69)

ICD-10-CM contains very specific codes to identify various forms of **cerebrovascular accidents (CVAs)**. The codes specify whether the condition is a cerebral hemorrhage or infarction due to a thrombosis, embolism, or unspecified occlusion or stenosis in the cerebral vessel. The cerebral infarction codes identify the specific cerebral artery involved and laterality (right or left). Category I69, Sequelae of cerebrovascular disease, contains a lot of codes for very specific conditions that remain after the acute CVA is treated.

The category for late effects of cerebrovascular disease, I69, is titled "Sequelae of cerebrovascular disease"; all subcategory codes are expanded. This expansion involves specifying laterality, changing subcategory titles, making terminology changes, adding sixth characters, and providing greater specificity in general. Late effects of cerebrovascular disease are differentiated by type of stroke (hemorrhage, infarction).

Cerebrovascular disease is an insufficient blood supply to a part of the brain and is usually secondary to atherosclerotic disease, hypertension, or a combination of both.

At the beginning of the "Cerebrovascular Disease" section, there is a "use additional code" to identify the presence of

Alcohol abuse and dependence (F10.-)
Exposure to environmental tobacco smoke (Z77.22-)
History of tobacco use (Z87.891)
Hypertension (I10–I15)
Occupational exposure to environmental tobacco smoke (Z57.31)
Tobacco dependence (F17.-)
Tobacco use (Z72.0)

ICD-10-CM classifies cerebrovascular disease according to the following types of conditions:

I60	Nontraumatic subarachnoid hemorrhage
I61	Nontraumatic intracerebral hemorrhage
I62	Other and unspecified nontraumatic intracranial hemorrhage
I63	Cerebral infarction
I65	Occlusion and stenosis of precerebral arteries, not resulting in cerebral infarction
I66	Occlusion and stenosis of cerebral arteries, not resulting in cerebral infarction
I67	Other cerebrovascular disease
I68	Cerebrovascular disorders in diseases classified elsewhere
I69	Sequelae of cerebrovascular disease

Carotid Artery Stenosis (I65.2-)

Occlusion and stenosis of precerebral arteries include the carotid artery. The condition may be unilateral or bilateral. The codes for occlusion and stenosis of the carotid artery not resulting in cerebral infarction are codes:

I65.21	Occlusion and stenosis of right carotid artery
I65.22	Occlusion and stenosis of left carotid artery
I65.23	Occlusion and stenosis of bilateral carotid arteries
I65.29	Occlusion and stenosis of unspecified carotid artery

Cerebral Infarction (I63)

Category I63 includes occlusion and stenosis of cerebral and precerebral arteries that results in a cerebral infarction. The default code for "stroke" or "CVA" is I63.9, **Cerebral infarction,** unspecified. More specific codes are available when the physician's documentation includes the cause of the stroke (thrombosis or embolism) and the location of the artery where the stroke occurred (vertebral, carotid, cerebral). Laterality is also included in the coding options: right and left or unspecified artery. The specificity of the cerebral infarction can be coded according to the following:

I63.0-	Cerebral infarction due to thrombosis of precerebral arteries
I63.1-	Cerebral infarction due to embolism of precerebral arteries
I63.2-	Cerebral infarction due to unspecified occlusion or stenosis of precerebral arteries

I63.3-   Cerebral infarction due to thrombosis of cerebral arteries

I63.4-   Cerebral infarction due to embolism of cerebral arteries

I63.5-   Cerebral infarction due to unspecified occlusion or stenosis of cerebral arteries

I63.6   Cerebral infarction due to cerebral venous thrombosis, nonpyogenic

I63.8   Other cerebral infarction

I63.9   Cerebral infarction, unspecified

Conditions resulting from the cerebral infarction or other cerebrovascular events, such as aphasia or hemiplegia, should be coded in addition to the code for the cerebrovascular disease as well.

EXAMPLE: Patient was admitted with aphasia and left nondominant side hemiplegia due to an acute CVA. The CVA and the resulting conditions were treated. On discharge, the aphasia had cleared; however, the hemiplegia is still present and will require outpatient physical therapy. Codes include I63.9, the default code for acute cerebrovascular accident (CVA); G81.94, Hemiplegia, unspecified affecting left nondominant side; and R47.01, Aphasia.

Sequelae of Cerebrovascular Disease (I69)

Category I69 codes identify sequelae or late effects of cerebrovascular disease, which is usually a cerebral infarction but could be due to any of the conditions classifiable to categories I60 through I67. These conditions are specified as due to the cerebral infarction or as residuals that may occur at any time after the onset of the cerebrovascular disease. In other words, the conditions identified by the I69 category codes describe the condition that remains in the patient after the acute episode of the cerebral infarction or cerebrovascular disease is over. These conditions may be permanent after the stroke or the condition may remain for a period of time after the acute phase of the illness is over.

The neurologic deficits caused by cerebrovascular disease may be present from the onset or may arise at any time after the onset of the condition classifiable to I60 through I67.

EXAMPLE: Patient is receiving physical therapy for monoplegia of the left leg affecting the nondominant side due to an old cerebral infarction. The code reported would be I69.344, Monoplegia of lower limb following other cerebrovascular disease affecting the left nondominant side.

The coder must be very careful in using the Index to Diseases to code the sequelae conditions because the type of cerebrovascular disease or condition is precise. The particular neurological deficit or remaining condition is specified under the identified cause of the remaining sequelae in the Index. For example, the Index to Diseases and Injuries entries include:

Sequelae (of)
        Disease, cerebrovascular
        Hemorrhage, intracerebral
        Infarction, cerebral
        Stroke, NOS
        Each of these subterms are followed with
                Alteration of sensation
                Aphasia
                Apraxia
                And more entries listed alphabetically

The codes under category of I69 for sequelae of cerebrovascular disease are a combination of two facts:

1. The cerebrovascular disease responsible for the deficit, such as:
   Nontraumatic subarachnoid hemorrhage, I69.0
   Nontraumatic intracerebral hemorrhage, I69.1
   Other nontraumatic intracranial hemorrhage, I69.2
   Cerebral infarction, I69.3
   Other cerebrovascular disease, I69.8
   Unspecified cerebrovascular disease, I69.9

and

2. The type of deficit present such as:
   Unspecified sequelae
   Cognitive deficits
   Speech and language deficits
   Monoplegia of upper limb
   Monoplegia of lower limb
   Hemiplegia and hemiparesis
   Other paralytic syndrome
   Apraxia
   Dysphagia
   Facial weakness
   Ataxia
   Other sequelae

When the health record documentation indicates the patient has a history of a cerebral infarction but no neurological deficits are present, the code Z86.73, Personal history of transient ischemic attack (TIA) and cerebral infarction without residual deficits, should be assigned. In this circumstance, it is incorrect to assign a code from category I69.

The code Z86.73 is located in the Index under "History (personal), stroke without residual deficits, Z86.73" and "History (personal), cerebral infarction, cerebral, without residual deficits Z86.73."

Codes from category I69 may be assigned on a healthcare record with codes from I60 through I67, if the patient has a current stroke and deficits from an old stroke.

> **EXAMPLE:** Patient was admitted with occlusion of cerebral arteries resulting in a cerebral infarction. Patient has a history of previous cerebral infarction 1 year ago with residual hemiplegia affecting the right dominant side. Codes for this episode of care would be
>
> I63.50, Cerebral artery occlusion, unspecified, with cerebral infarction
>
> I69.351, Hemiplegia and hemiparesis following cerebral infarction affecting right dominant side.

Venous Embolism and Thrombosis (I82)

Very specific codes exist in ICD-10-CM to describe acute and chronic deep and superficial vein thrombosis. The codes identify the specific vessel involved and the right or left side of the body. This same type of detail is also included in the thrombophlebitis and varicose vein codes.

Venous embolism and thrombosis, also referred to as **venous thrombo-embolism (VTE)**, is an occlusion within the venous system. The terms **deep vein thrombosis (DVT)** and VTE are commonly documented in health records. Venous embolism and thrombosis may occur in deep and superficial veins. These conditions may occur in the thorax, neck, and upper and lower extremities. The patient with new or acute venous embolism and thrombosis conditions requires the initiation of anticoagulant therapy. The patient with the diagnosis of chronic or old venous embolism and thrombosis continues to receive anticoagulant therapy over a period of time but is no longer in the acute phase of the illness.

Category code I82, Other venous embolism and thrombosis, contains four-, five- and six-character codes that distinguish between the location of the VTE and the acute versus chronic status of the condition. Under subcategory code I82.5, Chronic embolism and thrombosis of deep veins of lower extremity, is an Exclude1 note that personal history of venous thrombosis and embolism, Z86.718, which describes the VTE condition that has resolved or no longer exists, cannot be used with a code from I82.5-. Another note that appears under subcategory code I82.5 is a "use additional code" note to use, if applicable, Z79.01 for associated long-term (current) use of anticoagulants.

Deep veins in the lower extremity include the femoral, iliac, popliteal, tibial, and other specified and unspecified deep veins of the lower extremity. Superficial veins in the lower extremity include the greater and lesser saphenous vein. Deep veins in the upper extremity include the brachial, radial, and ulnar veins. Superficial veins in the upper extremity include the antecubital, basilica, and cephalic veins.

Specific diagnosis codes for VTEs are as follows:

Acute embolism and thrombosis of deep veins of lower extremity, I82.4-
Chronic embolism and thrombosis of deep veins of lower extremity, I82.5-
Acute embolism and thrombosis of veins of upper extremity, I82.6-
Chronic embolism and thrombosis of veins of upper extremity, I82.7-
Embolism and thrombosis of axillary vein, I82.A-
Embolism and thrombosis of subclavian vein, I82.B-
Embolism and thrombosis of internal jugular vein, I82.C-
Embolism and thrombosis of other specified veins, I82.8-
Embolism and thrombosis of unspecified vein, I82.9-

Intraoperative and Postprocedural Circulatory Complications (I97)

Intraoperative and postprocedural circulatory complications can be identified with greater specificity in ICD-10-CM. Instructional notes appear under certain codes to add detail by using an additional code to further describe the condition, for example, using an additional code to identify heart failure or to further specify the disorder. For example, different codes exist for intraoperative and postprocedural complications, such as the following:

* Postcardiotomy syndrome
* Other postprocedural and intraoperative cardiac functional disturbances
* Intraoperative versus postprocedural cardiac arrest
* Postmastectomy lymphedema syndrome

- Postprocedural hypertension

- Postprocedural heart failure

- Intraoperative and postprocedural cerebral infarction

- Accidental puncture or laceration during a circulatory system procedure

- Accidental puncture or laceration of a circulatory system organ during another body system procedure

ICD-10-PCS Procedure Coding for Circulatory System Procedures

This section highlights several cardiovascular procedures that are commonly performed to treat conditions in patients with acute and chronic forms of heart disease. Described in this section are invasive procedures that are performed by Percutaneous and Open approaches.

Measurement and Monitoring (4A0–4B0)

Technically, a **cardiac catheterization** is not a procedure. The catheterization of the heart represents a Percutaneous approach to gain access to the heart for diagnostic and therapeutic procedures. In ICD-10-PCS, the coder assigns codes for the actual root operations or root types that are performed inside the heart and/or through the catheter. For example, if an angioplasty is performed, the root operation is Dilation. If only images are taken of the coronary vessels and structure, the imaging is coded. If pressure measurement and sampling is performed, the procedure is measurement and monitoring in ICD-10-PCS.

Through the cardiac catheter, diagnostic tests are used to identify, measure, and verify almost every type of intracardiac condition. The technique includes the passage of a flexible catheter through the arteries or veins into the heart chambers and vessels. The diagnostic procedures determine the size and location of a coronary lesion, evaluate left and right ventricular function, and measure heart pressures.

In addition to serving as a diagnostic tool, therapeutic procedures can be performed through the cardiac catheters. For example, both PTCAs and intracoronary streptokinase injections can be performed via a cardiac catheter.

Cardiac catheterization is most commonly performed on the left side of the heart, using the Percutaneous approach via the antecubital and femoral vessels. In a right heart catheterization, a catheter is inserted through the femoral or antecubital vein, advanced first into the superior or inferior vena cava, then into the right atrium, the right ventricle, and, finally, into the pulmonary artery. In a left heart catheterization, a catheter enters the body through either the brachial artery or the femoral artery. The catheter is advanced into the aorta, through the aortic valve, and then into the left ventricle.

There are two ways to access the correct ICD-10-PCS table for coding cardiac catheterization. First, the coder can use the Index term "catheterization, heart." The coder will be directed to see the term "measurement, cardiac A402." The other approach is to access the main term in the ICD-10-PCS Index as "Measurement" with subterms of cardiac, sampling, and pressure for bilateral, left heart, and right heart. The first three characters given are "4A0" (see table 12.1).

Table 12.1. **ICD-10-PCS Table 4A0**

Body System	Approach	Function/Device	Qualifier
2 Cardiac	0 Open 3 Percutaneous	N Sampling and Pressure	6 Right Heart 7 Left Heart 8 Bilateral

4 Measurement and Monitoring
A Physiological Systems
0 Measurement
The ICD-10-PCS code for a left heart catheterization for oxygen sampling and pressure measurements taken on the left side of the heart, usually, the left ventricle is: 4A023N7

Diagnostic Procedures

The following procedures are often performed during a cardiac catheterization:

- Coronary angiography

- Coronary arteriography

- Ventriculography

Coronary Angiography

Coronary angiography can be performed on the right or left side of the heart, or in a combined process including both the right and left sides of the heart. Right-side cardiac angiography is useful in detecting pericarditis and congenital lesions, such as Ebstein's malformation of the tricuspid valve. Left-side cardiac angiography reveals congenital and acquired lesions affecting the mitral valve, including mitral stenosis and mitral regurgitation.

Coronary Arteriography

Coronary arteriography serves as a diagnostic tool in detecting obstruction within the coronary arteries. The following two techniques are used in performing a coronary arteriography:

- The Sones technique uses a single catheter inserted via a brachial arteriotomy.

- The Judkins technique uses two catheters inserted percutaneously through the femoral artery.

Ventriculography

Ventriculography measures stroke volume and ejection fraction. The ejection fraction is the amount of blood ejected from the left ventricle per beat; it is presented as a percentage of the total ventricular volume. The fraction is usually about 65 percent, plus or minus 8 percent. A fraction below 50 percent is usually a sign of severe ventricular dysfunction; a fraction below 35 percent signals profound ventricular dysfunction.

Coding the Procedures

The imaging modality used for the coronary angiograms, arteriograms, and ventriculograms is fluoroscopy with the root type Fluoroscopy with the appropriate body part for the number and type of coronary arteries imaged. The main term to use in the ICD-10-PCS Index is fluoroscopy. The subterms under fluoroscopy are as follows:

Artery
    Coronary
        Bypass Graft
        Multiple (B213)
            Laser, Intraoperative (B213)
            Single (B212)
            Laser, Intraoperative (B212)
            Multiple (B211)
            Laser, Intraoperative (B211)
            Single (B210)
            Laser, Intraoperative (B210)

The first three characters for the ICD-10-PCS code for the above entries are "B21." The coder locates Table "B21" to build the ICD-10-PCS code (see table 12.2).

Table 12.2. **ICD-10-PCS Table B21**

Body Part	Contrast	Qualifier	Qualifier
0 Coronary Artery, Single 1 Coronary Artery, Multiple 2 Coronary Artery Bypass Graft, Single 3 Coronary Artery Bypass Graft, Multiple 4 Heart, Right 5 Heart, Left 6 Heart, Right and Left 7 Internal Mammary Bypass Graft, Right 8 Internal Mammary Bypass Graft, left F Bypass Graft, Other	0 High Osmolar 1 Low Osmolar Y Other Osmolar	Z None	Z None

B Imaging
2 Heart
1 Fluoroscopy

The ICD-10-PCS procedure code for a multiple vessel native coronary artery angiography or arteriography using low osmolar contrast material is B2111ZZ. The ICD-10-PCS procedure code for a left ventriculogram using low osmolar contrast material is B2151ZZ.

Percutaneous Transluminal Coronary Angioplasty

Percutaneous transluminal coronary angioplasty (PTCA) is used to relieve obstruction of coronary arteries. PTCA is performed to widen a narrowed area of a coronary artery by employing a balloon-tipped catheter. The catheter is passed to the obstructed area, and the balloon is inflated one or more times to exert pressure on the narrowed area. A thrombolytic agent may be infused into the heart.

A PTCA procedure may also include the insertion of one or more coronary stents. It is possible to insert stents in several different vessels during the same operative episode. It is also possible to insert multiple adjoining or overlapping stents.

The objective of a PTCA is to open or dilate the coronary artery or bypass coronary graft. The root operation in ICD-10-PCS for this procedure is Dilation by definition. The main term in the ICD-10-PCS Index is Dilation with subterms artery, coronary and then the number

Diseases of the Circulatory System (I00–I99)

of vessels: one, two, three, four, or more. The Index gives the first three digits as "027." To construct the procedure code for the PTCA, the coder accesses Table 027. If the insertion of a coronary artery stent is performed with the angioplasty, the sixth character (device) is used to identify the type of stent: Intraluminal Device, Drug Eluting or Intraluminal Device, or Nondrug Eluting. If the PTCA is performed without the insertion of a stent, there is a value of Z for no device used for the sixth character. The number of codes assigned depends on the number of vessels treated by angioplasty and the number of vessels that have a stent or device inserted. For example, if an angioplasty is performed on one coronary artery and if an angioplasty with the insertion of a stent is performed on a different coronary artery, two codes are assigned because the device value would be different for the two vessels. On the other hand, if an angioplasty is performed on two coronary arteries and neither has a stent inserted, there would be one procedure code assigned. Table 027 is shown in table 12.3. For example, if an angioplasty is performed on the left anterior descending and the right coronary artery without any stent insertion in either vessel, the code assigned would be 02713ZZ. However, if an angioplasty is performed on the left anterior descending and an angioplasty with a plain stent inserted in the right coronary artery, two codes would be assigned: 02703ZZ and 02703DZ.

Table 12.3.   **ICD-10-PCS Table 027**

Body Part	Approach	Device	Qualifier
0 Coronary Artery, One site 1 Coronary Artery, Two sites 2 Coronary Artery, Three sites 3 Coronary Artery, Four or more sites	0 Open 3 Percutaneous 4 Percutaneous endoscopic	4 Intraluminal Device, drug eluting D Intraluminal Device T Radioactive Intraluminal Device Z No Device	6 Bifurcation Z No Qualifier

0 Medical and Surgical
2 Heart and Great Vessels
7 Dilation

Coronary Artery Bypass Graft (CABG)

The coronary circulation consists of two main arteries, the right and the left, that are further subdivided into several branches:

EXAMPLE: Right coronary artery
    Right marginal
    Right posterior descending
Left main coronary artery
    Left anterior descending branch
        Diagonal
        Septal
    Left circumflex
        Obtuse marginal
        Posterior descending
        Posterolateral

Aortocoronary Bypass or Coronary Artery Bypass Graft

Aortocoronary bypass brings blood from the aorta into the obstructed coronary artery using a segment of the saphenous vein or a segment of the internal mammary artery for the graft. The procedure is commonly referred to as coronary artery bypass graft(s) or by the abbreviation CABG, pronounced "cabbage."

215

The following three surgical approaches are used in coronary artery bypass graft procedures:

- Aortocoronary bypass uses the aorta to bypass the occluded coronary artery.

- Internal mammary-coronary artery bypass uses the internal mammary artery to bypass the occluded coronary artery.

- Abdominal-coronary artery bypass uses an abdominal artery.

Internal mammary-coronary artery bypass is accomplished by loosening the internal mammary artery from its normal position and using the internal mammary artery to bring blood from the subclavian artery to the occluded coronary artery. Codes are selected based on whether one or both internal mammary arteries are used, regardless of the number of coronary arteries involved.

An **abdominal-coronary artery bypass** procedure involves creating an anastomosis between an abdominal artery, commonly the gastro-epiploic, and a coronary artery beyond the occluded portion.

The root operation for coronary artery bypass procedures is Bypass. The body part value identifies the number of coronary arteries bypassed to and the qualifier identifies the vessel bypassed from or the vessel that is the source of the blood flow to the bypassed vessel. The device character identifies the tissue used as the bypass. If a saphenous vein is used as the bypass tissue, the harvesting of the saphenous vein is coded as an Excision procedure based on the side (left or right) where it was harvested. The main term used in the ICD-10-PCS Index is Bypass with subterms of artery, coronary, and one, two, three, or four or more sites. The three digit character is 021, as shown in table 12.4.

Table 12.4. **ICD-10-PCS Table 021**

Body Part	Approach	Device	Qualifier
0 Coronary Artery, One site 1 Coronary Artery, Two sites 2 Coronary Artery, Three sites 3 Coronary Artery, Four or more sites	0 Open 4 Percutaneous Endoscopic	9 Autologous Venous Tissue A Autologous Arterial Tissue J Synthetic Substitute K Nonautologous Tissue Substitute	3 Coronary Artery 8 Internal Mammary, Right 9 Internal Mammary, Left C Thoracic Artery F Abdominal Artery W Aorta
0 Coronary Artery, One site 1 Coronary Artery, Two sites 2 Coronary Artery, Three sites 3 Coronary Artery, Four or more sites	0 Open 4 Percutaneous Endoscopic	Z No Device	3 Coronary Artery 8 Internal Mammary, Right 9 Internal Mammary, Left C Thoracic Artery F Abdominal Artery

0 Medical and Surgical
2 Heart and Great Vessels
1 Bypass

For example, using table 12.4, if a triple coronary artery bypass is performed with two aortocoronary bypass grafts and one left internal mammary artery bypass using a left saphenous vein and cardiopulmonary bypass, the procedure is coded as

021109W for the double vessel aortocoronary bypass using saphenous vein grafts
02100Z9 for the single vessel left internal mammary artery bypass

Using other Index and Table entries, we get

06BQ0ZZ for Excision of greater left saphenous vein for bypass material
5A1221Z for Bypass, cardiopulmonary.

Cardiac Pacemakers

A cardiac pacemaker has the following three basic components:

- The **pulse generator** is the pacing system that contains the pacemaker battery (power source) and the electronic circuitry.

- The **pacing lead** carries the stimulating electricity from the pulse generator to the stimulating electrode.

- The **electrode** is the metal portion of the lead that comes in contact with the heart.

There are different types of pacemakers:

- Single-chamber pacemakers use a single lead that is placed in the right atrium or the right ventricle.

- Dual-chamber pacemakers use leads that are inserted into both the atrium and the ventricle.

- Rate-responsive pacemakers have a pacing rate modality that is determined by physiological variables other than the atrial rate.

- Cardiac resynchronization pacemakers without a defibrillator (CRT-P) is also known as a biventricular pacing device without internal cardiac defibrillator.

ICD-10-PCS Coding of Pacemakers

ICD-10-CM classifies cardiac pacemakers by coding the insertion of each lead into one or more of the chambers of the heart and the insertion of the generator in the subcutaneous tissue.

For example, the insertion of a dual chamber cardiac pacemaker with leads inserted into the right atrium and right ventricle and the generator implanted in left chest subcutaneous tissue is coded as follows.

The root operation Insertion is used to code all three procedures. Codes for all three procedures are required because the insertion of each lead is coded separately, and the insertion of the pacemaker generator is coded separately. Leads are inserted percutaneously into the right atrium and right ventricle. The device value for both leads is J, Cardiac Lead, Pacemaker. There is no qualifier value for either code. The body part value for the pacemaker generator insertion is Subcutaneous Tissue and Fascia, Chest. The approach for this procedure is Open. The device value is Pacemaker, Dual Chamber, and there is no qualifier for this code. For example, the codes for insertion of the pacemaker device are

1. 02H63JZ, Insertion of device in, Atrium, right (device is J for Cardiac Lead, Pacemaker)
2. 02HK3JZ, Insertion of device in Ventricle, right (device is J for Cardiac Lead, Pacemaker)
3. 0JH606Z, Insertion of device in, Subcutaneous Tissue and Fascia, Chest (device is 6 for Pacemaker, Dual Chamber)

Automatic Implantable Cardioverter-Defibrillators

The **automatic implantable cardioverter-defibrillator (AICD)** is a special type of pacemaker that proves effective for patients with recurring, life-threatening dysrhythmias, such as ventricular tachycardia or fibrillation.

The AICD is an electronic device consisting of a pulse generator and three leads. The pulse generator is implanted under the patient's skin, usually in the shoulder area. The first lead senses heart rate at the right ventricle; the second lead, sensing morphology and rhythm, defibrillates at the right atrium; the third lead defibrillates at the apical pericardium. The AICD can be programmed to suit each patient's needs, and it uses far less energy than an external defibrillator.

The insertion of an AICD is coded similarly to the coding of cardiac pacemaker, however, the device value is different. For an AICD the device value is K for Cardiac Lead, Defibrillator in ICD-10-PCS Table 02H for insertion of device in (location). The insertion of the AICD generator in the subcutaneous tissue such as the chest has device values of 8 or 9 for the type of defibrillator generator used.

ICD-10-CM and ICD-10-PCS Review Exercises: Chapter 12

Assign the correct ICD-10-CM diagnosis codes and ICD-10-PCS procedure codes to the following.

1. Cerebral infarction with left nondominant hemiparesis and dysphasia

2. Acute pericardial effusion

3. Chronic atrial fibrillation; essential hypertension

4. Coronary artery disease in autologous vein bypass graft

5. Venous thrombosis of greater saphenous vein, right leg

6. Thoracic aortic aneurysm

ICD-10-CM and ICD-10-PCS Review Exercises: Chapter 12 (Continued)

7. Mitral valve insufficiency

8. Acute myocardial infarction (STEMI) of posterolateral wall

9. Subacute bacterial endocarditis secondary to *Staphylococcus aureus*; ventricular tachycardia

10. Coronary artery disease with unstable angina, no history of coronary artery bypass surgery

11. Arteriosclerosis of the right lower extremity native arteries with rest pain

12. End-stage renal disease (ESRD) with hypertension

13. Inflamed varicose veins of the left lower extremity with development of calf ulcer

14. Occlusive disease of iliac artery right side.

15. PROCEDURE: Coronary artery bypass graft (CABG) using four saphenous veins for aortocoronary bypass with cardiopulmonary bypass

16. PROCEDURE: Replacement of mitral valve using porcine graft

17. PROCEDURE: Percutaneous transluminal coronary angioplasty, two vessels, no stents

18. PROCEDURE: Percutaneous insertion of central venous catheter infusion device, left subclavian vein

19. PROCEDURE: Ablation, right atrium, percutaneous (MAZE procedure)

20. PROCEDURE: PTCA, via femoral approach, two vessels with insertion of drug-eluting stent into same two vessels

Chapter 13

Diseases of the Respiratory System (J00–J99)

Learning Objectives

At the conclusion of this chapter, you should be able to:

1. Describe the organization of the conditions and codes included in Chapter 10 of ICD-10-CM, Diseases of the respiratory system (J00–J99)

2. Identify the ICD-10-CM codes used to describe bronchitis

3. Identify the ICD-10-CM codes used to describe asthma

4. Identify the various conditions that may be described as forms of chronic obstructive pulmonary disease

5. Understand the ICD-10-CM coding and sequencing rules for assigning respiratory failure codes

6. Assign ICD-10-CM codes for diseases of the respiratory system

7. Assign ICD-10-PCS codes for procedures related to diseases of the respiratory system

Key Terms

- Acute bronchitis
- Acute exacerbation
- Asthma
- Bronchiectasis
- Bronchiolitis
- Bronchitis
- Chronic bronchitis
- Chronic obstructive pulmonary disease (COPD)
- Emphysema
- Endoscopy
- Mechanical ventilation
- Respiratory failure

- Status asthmaticus
- Streptococcus pneumonia
- Viral Pneumonia

Overview of ICD-10-CM Chapter 10, Diseases of the Respiratory System

Chapter 10 includes categories J00–J99 arranged in the following blocks:

J00–J06	Acute upper respiratory infections
J09–J18	Influenza and pneumonia
J20–J22	Other acute lower respiratory infections
J30–J39	Other diseases of upper respiratory tract
J40–J47	Chronic lower respiratory diseases
J60–J70	Lung diseases due to external agents
J80–J84	Other respiratory diseases principally affecting the interstitium
J85–J86	Suppurative and necrotic conditions of the lower respiratory tract
J90–J94	Other diseases of the pleura
J95	Intraoperative and postprocedural complications and disorders of respiratory system, not elsewhere classified
J96–J99	Other diseases of the respiratory system

Code titles in the respiratory system chapter of ICD-10-CM have been updated with current terminology. For example, asthma codes were updated to include the descriptors of mild intermittent, mild persistent, moderate persistent, and severe persistent. Emphysema codes include descriptors for panlobular and centrilobular emphysema. Influenza and acute bronchitis codes include the manifestations of these diseases in one code.

For example, ICD-10-CM category J43, Emphysema, contains codes with panlobular emphysema and centrilobular emphysema in the titles. ICD-10-CM category J45, Asthma, classifies asthma as mild intermittent, mild persistent, moderate persistent, and severe persistent.

Other enhancements to Chapter 10 include classification changes that provide greater specificity in the codes. ICD-10-CM has individual codes for acute recurrent sinusitis for each sinus. Subcategory J10.8, Influenza due to other identified influenza virus with other manifestations, has been expanded to reflect the manifestations of the influenza. Category J20, Acute bronchitis, has been expanded to reflect the causes of the acute bronchitis.

Coding Guidelines and Instructional Notes for ICD-10-CM Chapter 10

At the beginning of Chapter 10, the following instructional guideline appears: "When a respiratory condition is described as occurring in more than one site and is not specifically indexed, it should be classified to the lower anatomic site" (CDC 2012). For example, tracheobronchitis is classified to bronchitis in J40, Bronchitis, not specified as acute or chronic.

An additional instructional note also appears at the beginning of Chapter 10 that instructs the coding professional to use an additional code, where applicable, to identify

- exposure to environmental tobacco smoke (Z77.22),

- exposure to tobacco smoke in the perinatal period (P96.81),

- history of tobacco use (Z87.891),

- occupational exposure to environmental tobacco smoke (Z57.31),

- tobacco dependence (F17.-), or

- tobacco use (Z72.0).

Since these instructional notes appear at the beginning of the chapter, they should be followed when assigning any code from this chapter.

Some of the codes in Chapter 10 have been expanded to include notes indicating that an additional code should be assigned or an associated condition should be sequenced first. The following are examples of the instructional notes:

- Use additional code to identify the infectious agent

- Use additional code to identify the virus

- Code first any associated lung abscess

- Code first the underlying disease

- Use additional code to identify other conditions such as tobacco use or exposure

Notes for code usage may also be category specific. Under ICD-10-CM category J10, Influenza, is a note to use an additional code to identify the virus.

In the Tabular, there is a note under category J44 to code also the type of asthma, if applicable (J45.-). There is also an Excludes2 note under category J45 for asthma with chronic obstructive pulmonary disease. By definition, when an Excludes2 note appears under a code, it is acceptable to use both the code and the excluded code together if the patient has both conditions at the same time.

The NCHS has published chapter-specific guidelines for Chapter 10 in the *ICD-10-CM Official Guidelines for Coding and Reporting.* The coding student should review all of the coding guidelines for Chapter 10 of ICD-10-CM, which appear in an ICD-10-CM code book or at the website http://www.cdc.gov/nchs/icd/icd10cm.htm, or in Appendix E.

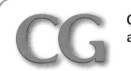

Guideline 1.C.10.a. Chronic Obstructive Pulmonary Disease [COPD] and Asthma

1. Acute exacerbation of chronic obstructive bronchitis and asthma

    The codes in categories J44 and J45 distinguish between uncomplicated cases and those in acute exacerbation.

    (Continued)

(Continued)

An acute exacerbation is a worsening or a decompensation of a chronic condition. An acute exacerbation is not equivalent to an infection superimposed on a chronic condition, though an exacerbation may be triggered by an infection.

Guideline I.C.10.b. Acute Respiratory Failure

1. Acute respiratory failure as principal diagnosis

   A code from subcategory J96.0, Acute respiratory failure, or subcategory J96.2, Acute and chronic respiratory failure, may be assigned as a principal diagnosis when it is the condition established after study to be chiefly responsible for occasioning the admission to the hospital, and the selection is supported by the Alphabetic Index and Tabular List. However, chapter-specific coding guidelines (such as obstetrics, poisoning, HIV, newborn) that provide sequencing direction take precedence.

2. Acute respiratory failure as secondary diagnosis

   Respiratory failure may be listed as a secondary diagnosis if it occurs after admission, or if it is present on admission, but does not meet the definition of principal diagnosis.

3. Sequencing of acute respiratory failure and another acute condition

   When a patient is admitted with respiratory failure and another acute condition, (e.g., myocardial infarction, cerebrovascular accident, aspiration pneumonia), the principal diagnosis will not be the same in every situation. This applies whether the other acute condition is a respiratory or nonrespiratory condition. Selection of the principal diagnosis will be dependent on the circumstances of admission. If both the respiratory failure and the other acute condition are equally responsible for occasioning the admission to the hospital, and there are no chapter-specific sequencing rules, the guideline regarding two or more diagnoses that equally meet the definition for principal diagnosis may be applied in these situations.

   If the documentation is not clear as to whether acute respiratory failure and another condition are equally responsible for occasioning the admission, query the provider for clarification.

Guideline I.C.10.c. Influenza due to certain identified influenza viruses

Code only confirmed cases of influenza due to certain identified influenza viruses (category J09), and due to other identified influenza virus (category J10). This is an exception to the hospital inpatient guideline Section II, H. (Uncertain Diagnosis).

In this context, "confirmation" does not require documentation of positive laboratory testing specific for avian or other novel influenza A or other identified influenza virus. However, coding should be based on the provider's diagnostic statement that the patient has avian influenza, or other novel influenza A, for category J09, or has another particular identified strain of influenza, such as H1N1 or H3N2, but not identified as novel or variant, for category J10.

If the provider records "suspected" or "possible" or "probable" avian influenza, or novel influenza, or other identified influenza, then the appropriate influenza code from category J11, Influenza due to unidentified influenza virus, should be assigned. A code from category J09, Influenza due to certain identified influenza viruses, should not be assigned nor should a code from category J10, Influenza due to other identified influenza virus.

Guideline I.C.10.d. Ventilator associated Pneumonia

1. Documentation of Ventilator associated Pneumonia

    As with all procedural or postprocedural complications, code assignment is based on the provider's documentation of the relationship between the condition and the procedure.

    Code J95.851, Ventilator associated pneumonia, should be assigned only when the provider has documented ventilator associated pneumonia (VAP). An additional code to identify the organism (e.g., Pseudomonas aeruginosa, code B96.5) should also be assigned. Do not assign an additional code from categories J12-J18 to identify the type of pneumonia.

    Code J95.851 should not be assigned for cases where the patient has pneumonia and is on a mechanical ventilator and the provider has not specifically stated that the pneumonia is ventilator-associated pneumonia. If the documentation is unclear as to whether the patient has a pneumonia that is a complication attributable to the mechanical ventilator, query the provider.

2. Ventilator associated Pneumonia Develops after Admission

    A patient may be admitted with one type of pneumonia (e.g., code J13, Pneumonia due to Streptococcus pneumonia) and subsequently develop VAP. In this instance, the principal diagnosis would be the appropriate code from categories J12–J18 for the pneumonia diagnosed at the time of admission. Code J95.851, Ventilator associated pneumonia, would be assigned as an additional diagnosis when the provider has also documented the presence of ventilator associated pneumonia.

225

Coding Diseases of the Respiratory System in ICD-10-CM Chapter 10

Chapter 10 of ICD-10-CM contains codes for a wide variety of pulmonary conditions, ranging from acute upper respiratory infections, pneumonia, influenza, as well as diseases of the lower respiratory tract including chronic lung diseases and diseases acquired from exposure to external substances. Intraoperative and postprocedural complications are also available to be coded in this chapter.

Acute Upper Respiratory Infections (J00–J06)

The codes in this section are used to describe acute infections of the sites within the upper respiratory tract including the nose, sinuses, pharynx, tonsils, larynx, and trachea. A "use additional code" note (B95–B97) to identify the infectious agent appears under the categories of acute sinusitis (J01), acute pharyngitis (J02), acute tonsillitis (J03), acute laryngitis and tracheitis (J04), and acute obstructive laryngitis and epiglottis (J05) to include the codes for such infectious organisms as Streptococcus, Staphylococcus, and other bacterial and viral organisms that can be identified as the cause of the acute upper respiratory conditions.

One three-character code, J00, is used to identify the classification of acute nasopharyngitis or the common cold, which may also be described as acute rhinitis. An Excludes1 listing of conditions under this category reminds the coder what conditions cannot be coded with acute nasopharyngitis. However, the Excludes2 note identifies conditions that can exist concurrently with acute nasopharyngitis and can be coded, for example, chronic pharyngitis and chronic rhinitis.

Influenza (J09–J11)

Influenza is classified with ICD-10-CM diagnosis codes to describe the type of influenza virus and the respiratory conditions it produces. The three categories of codes are as follows:

J09   Influenza due to identified novel influenza A virus
        Includes avian and bird influenza A/H5N1 and swine influenza viruses

J10   Influenza due to other identified influenza virus
        Includes novel (2009) H1N1 and novel influenza A/H1N1 viruses

J11   Influenza due to unidentified influenza virus
        Includes influenza when the type of virus is not or cannot be identified

Influenza due to Identified Novel Influenza A Virus (J09.X)

Avian influenza virus has not been reported in the United States. It has been identified in other parts of the globe with various body system complications. The subcategory codes included here are as follows:

J09.X1   Influenza due to identified novel influenza A virus with pneumonia.
        Code also, if applicable, associated lung abscess or other specified type of pneumonia

J09.X2   Influenza due to identified novel influenza A virus with other respiratory manifestations
        The respiratory manifestations coded here are laryngitis, pharyngitis and other upper respiratory symptoms.

J09.X3   The coder is reminded to use an additional code, if applicable, for associated pleural effusion and sinusitis.

J09.X3   Influenza due to identified novel influenza A virus with gastrointestinal manifestations

"Intestinal flu" or viral gastroenteritis would not be coded with J09.X3 according to the Excludes1 note that follows this code. Instead "intestinal flu" is coded as A08.-.

Influenza due to Identified Other Identified Influenza Virus (J10)

Novel H1N1 influenza virus can cause pneumonia, other respiratory conditions, and gastrointestinal manifestations. Outbreaks of identified H1N1 influenza virus with the accompanying complications occurred in 2009, hence the reason the virus may also be identified as the novel 2009 H1N1 virus.

Under the category heading is an instructional note to use an additional code to identify the virus from category B97, Viral agents as the cause of diseases classified elsewhere. The types of virus identified with the B97 category codes include adenovirus, enterovirus, coronavirus, and retroviruses.

The subcategory codes included here are as follows:

J10.00   Influenza due to other identified influenza virus with unspecified type of pneumonia

J10.01   Influenza due to other identified influenza virus with the same other identified influenza virus pneumonia

J10.08   Influenza due to other identified influenza virus with other specified type of pneumonia

Two instruction notes included here are "Code also associated lung abscess, if applicable (J85.1)" under subcategory J10.0, Influenza due to other identified influenza virus with pneumonia and "Code also other specified type of pneumonia" under code J10.08 for influenza with other specified type of pneumonia.

Other subcategory codes for the other identified influenza virus J10 codes are as follows:

J10.1   Influenza due to other identified influenza virus with other respiratory manifestations

J10.2   Influenza due to other identified influenza virus with gastrointestinal manifestations

J10.81–J10.89   Influenza due to other identified influenza virus with encephalopathy, myocarditis, otitis media and other manifestations

Two instruction notes appear with the J10.8x codes: "use additional code for any associated perforated tympanic membrane (H72.-)" with the code for influenzal otitis media and "use additional codes to identify the manifestations" to specify what other manifestations or conditions are caused by the influenza virus.

Influenza due to Unidentified Influenza Virus (J11)

The conditions coded to category J11 are respiratory, gastrointestinal, and other body system manifestations that are viral in nature but the exact type of influenza virus cannot be identified.

The subcategory codes of J11.0–J11.89 follow the pattern seen in the subcategories J10:

J11.0x   Influenza due to unidentified influenza virus with pneumonia

J11.1   Influenza due to unidentified influenza virus with other respiratory manifestations

J11.2   Influenza due to unidentified influenza virus with gastrointestinal manifestations

J11.8x   Influenza due to unidentified influenza virus with other manifestations

Pneumonia (J12–J18)

The category and subcategory codes in Chapter 10 of ICD-10-CM include codes for pneumonia with the following specific categories and subcategories identifying the underlying organisms or site:

J12   Viral pneumonia, not elsewhere classified

J13   Pneumonia due to Streptococcus pneumoniae

J14   Pneumonia due to Hemophilus influenzae

J15   Bacterial pneumonia, not elsewhere classified

J16   Pneumonia due to other infectious organisms, not elsewhere classified

J17   Pneumonia in diseases classified elsewhere

J18   Pneumonia, unspecified organism

Viral Pneumonia (J12)

Category J12, Viral pneumonia, is subdivided to fourth-character subcategories that identify the specific virus. When this condition is associated with influenza, a "code first" note appears under this category heading to direct the coder to code first the associated influenza if applicable with codes in the range of J09.x1, J10.0- and J11.0-. When this condition occurs with a lung abscess, the coder is reminded to code also associated abscess, if applicable, with J85.1.

Viral pneumonia is a highly contagious disease affecting both the trachea and the bronchi of the lungs. Inflammation destroys the action of the cilia and causes hemorrhage. Isolation of the virus is difficult, and x-rays do not reveal any pulmonary changes. The types of viruses causing pneumonia specified in this category include adenovirus, respiratory syncytial virus (RSV), parainfluenza virus, SARS-associated corona virus, and other specified viruses.

Pneumonia due to Streptococcus pneumoniae (J13)

Category J13, Pneumonia due to **Streptococcus pneumonia**, describes pneumonia caused by these specific pneumococcal bacteria. Physicians may document this disease as bronchopneumonia due to S. pneumoniae as well. The bacteria lodge in the alveoli and cause an inflammation. If the pleura are involved, the irritated surfaces rub together and cause painful breathing. On examination, pleural friction can be heard. A chest x-ray demonstrates a consolidation of the lungs that results from pus forming in the alveoli and replacing the air. Physicians may describe the same condition as pneumococcal pneumonia. When this condition is associated with influenza, a "code first" note appears under this category heading to direct the coder to code first the associated influenza if applicable with codes in the range of J09.x1, J10.0- and J11.0-. When this condition occurs with a lung abscess, the coder is reminded to code also associated abscess, if applicable, with J85.1.

Pneumonia due to Hemophilus influenza (J14)

Category J14, Pneumonia due to Hemophilus influenza or bronchopneumonia due to H. influenzae, is classified with this three-character code. When this condition is associated with influenza, a "code first" note appears under this category heading to direct the coder to code first the associated influenza if applicable with codes in the range of J09.x1, J10.0- and J11.0-. When this condition occurs with a lung abscess, the coder is reminded to code also associated abscess, if applicable, with J85.1.

Bacterial Pneumonia, Not Elsewhere Classified (J15)

Category J15, Bacterial pneumonia, not elsewhere classified, is subdivided to fourth- and fifth-character subcategories that identify specific bacteria, such as *Klebsiella pneumoniae* (J15.0), *Pseudomonas* (J15.1), *Staphylococcus* (J15.20–J15.212), *Streptococcus* B (J15.3, J15.4), and other specified types of pneumonia. Bacteria are the most common cause of pneumonia in adults. Gram staining is a rapid and cost-effective method for diagnosing bacterial pneumonia, if a good sputum sample is available.

Pneumonia due to Other Infectious Organisms, Not Elsewhere Classified (J16)

Category J16, Pneumonia due to other infectious organisms, not elsewhere classified, is used to identify organisms other than bacteria that cause pneumonia. For example, chlamydial pneumonia is coded with subcategory J16.0. When this type of pneumonia is associated with influenza, a "code first" note appears under this category heading to direct the codes to code first the associated influenza if applicable with codes in the range of J09.x1, J10.0- and J11.0-. When this condition occurs with a lung abscess, the coder is reminded to code also associated abscess, if applicable, with J85.1.

Pneumonia in Diseases Classified Elsewhere (J17)

Category J17, Pneumonia in diseases classified elsewhere, is a three-character code intended to identify that this type of pneumonia is the result or complication of another disease. This code is set in italic type and thus not meant to be listed first or as a single code. In addition, instructional notations in this category direct coders to code first the underlying disease, such as Q fever, rheumatic fever, or schistosomiasis. A lengthy Excludes1 note appears under category J17 to identify various types of pneumonia that have specific ICD-10-CM codes and cannot be used with category code J17.

Pneumonia, Unspecified Organism (J18)

Category J18, Pneumonia, unspecified organism, is subdivided at the fourth-character level to classify conditions that are not specified by the physician as being caused by a particular bacteria, virus, or other organism. Nonspecific diagnoses of pneumonia that are coded here are:

J18.0   Bronchopneumonia
J18.1   Lobar pneumonia
J18.2   Hypostatic pneumonia
J18.9   "Pneumonia"

A lengthy Excludes1 note appears under category J19 to identify various types of pneumonia that have specific ICD-10-CM codes and cannot be used with category code J19.

Other Acute Lower Respiratory Infections (J20–J22)

The conditions of the other part of the lower respiratory tract, the bronchus, is classified with codes from J20–J22 in ICD-10-CM.

Acute Bronchitis

Bronchitis is an inflammation of the bronchi and can be acute or chronic in nature. **Acute bronchitis** is an inflammation of the tracheo-bronchial tree with a short and more or less severe course. It is often due to exposure to cold, inhalation of irritant substances, or acute infections. **Chronic bronchitis** is a condition associated with prolonged exposure to nonspecific bronchial irritants and is accompanied by mucus hypersecretion and certain structural changes in the bronchi. Usually associated with cigarette smoking, one form of bronchitis is characterized clinically by a chronic productive cough. ICD-10-CM provides separate codes to describe acute and chronic bronchitis and acute bronchiolitis.

The following types of acute conditions of bronchitis are classified:

J20.0	Acute bronchitis due to Mycoplasma pneumoniae
J20.1	Acute bronchitis due to Hemophilus influenza
J20.2	Acute bronchitis due to streptococcus
J20.3	Acute bronchitis due to coxsackievirus
J20.4	Acute bronchitis due to parainfluenza virus
J20.5	Acute bronchitis due to respiratory syncytial virus
J20.6	Acute bronchitis due to rhinovirus
J20.7	Acute bronchitis due to echovirus
J20.8	Acute bronchitis due to other specified virus
J20.9	Acute bronchitis, unspecified

Acute bronchiolitis is classified according to the organisms that cause this disease. **Bronchiolitis** is an acute inflammatory disease of the bronchioles that is usually caused by a viral infection. Although it may occur in persons of any age, severe symptoms are usually only evident in young infants. The larger airways of older children and adults better accommodate mucosal edema associated with this condition.

Bronchiolitis most often affects children under the age of two years, with a peak occurrence in infants aged three to six months. Acute bronchiolitis is the most common cause of lower respiratory tract infection in the first year of life. It is generally a self-limiting condition and is most commonly associated with RSV (DeNicola 2012).

The following types of acute conditions of bronchiolitis are classified:

J21.0	Acute bronchiolitis due to respiratory syncytial virus
J21.1	Acute bronchiolitis due to human metapneumovirus
J21.8	Acute bronchiolitis due to other specified organisms
J21.9	Acute bronchiolitis, unspecified or stated as "bronchiolitis"

Other Diseases of the Upper Respiratory Tract (J30–J39)

This section identifies chronic conditions of body parts within the upper respiratory system. Almost all of the categories in this section include the instructional note "use additional code, where applicable" to direct the coder to assign an additional code for exposure to environmental tobacco smoke (Z77.22), exposure to tobacco smoke in the perinatal period (P96.81), history of tobacco use (Z87.891), occupational exposure to environmental tobacco smoke (Z57.31), tobacco dependence (F17.-), and tobacco use (Z72.0). The categories within this section include:

J30   Vasomotor and allergic rhinitis
Subcategories include allergic rhinitis due to pollen and food.

J31   Chronic rhinitis, nasopharyngitis and pharyngitis
Subcategories include chronic rhinitis and chronic pharyngitis.

J32   Chronic sinusitis
Codes in this category identify the sinus involved such as maxillary, frontal, ethmoidal sphenoidal and simple terminology such as chronic sinusitis.

J33   Nasal polyp
Polyp of the nasal cavity and the sinuses are included here.

J34   Other and unspecified disorders of nose and nasal sinuses
Conditions classified here include cyst and mucocele of nose and nasal sinuses, deviated nasal septum, and nasal mucositis among others.

J35   Chronic diseases of tonsils and adenoids
The most commonly occurring conditions coded here are chronic tonsillitis, chronic adenoiditis, and hypertrophy of tonsils and adenoids.

J36   Peritonsillar abscess
This three-character code is strictly for peritonsillar abscess with a note to "use additional code (B95–B97) to identify the infectious agent."

J37   Chronic laryngitis and laryngotracheitis
Only two subcategory codes are included here for chronic laryngitis and chronic laryngotracheitis.

J38   Diseases of vocal cords and larynx, not elsewhere classified
Frequently occurring conditions that would be classified with J38 category codes include vocal cord paralysis, vocal cord nodules, laryngeal spasm or cellulitis or abscess of vocal cords or larynx.

J39   Other diseases of upper respiratory tract
Every condition can be classified with an ICD-10-CM code. This category is intended to provide a code for all the other and unspecified diseases of the respiratory tract that are not appropriately coded to categories J30–J38.

Chronic Lower Respiratory Disease (J40–J47)

Conditions classified in this group of categories are chronic pulmonary conditions, such as chronic bronchitis, emphysema, asthma, chronic obstructive pulmonary disease (COPD), and bronchiectasis.

Chronic Bronchitis

Chronic bronchitis is a condition associated with prolonged exposure to nonspecific bronchial irritants and is accompanied by mucus hypersecretion and certain structural changes in the bronchi. Usually associated with cigarette smoking, one form of bronchitis is characterized clinically by a chronic productive cough.

Code J40, Bronchitis, not specified as acute or chronic, is assigned when the specific type of bronchitis is not documented in the health record. If the physician documented only "bronchitis" this is the code assigned. However it must be noted that code J40 is intended to reflect a chronic lung disease. When the primary care physician in her office or the emergency room physician writes "bronchitis" as a final diagnosis for an outpatient visit for a child, adolescent, or young adult, the physician probably means the patient has an acute type of bronchitis. However, the physician must be asked to clarify the type of bronchitis to assign a different code; no assumptions should be made based on the age of the patient.

Chronic bronchitis is included in the section titled "Chronic Obstructive Pulmonary Disease and Allied Conditions." Category J41, Simple and mucopurulent chronic bronchitis, contains subcategories including simple chronic bronchitis (J41.0), mucopurulent chronic bronchitis (J41.1), and mixed simple and mucopurulent chronic bronchitis (J41.8).

Emphysema

Emphysema is a specific type of chronic obstructive pulmonary disease (COPD). Emphysema is defined pathologically as an abnormal permanent enlargement of air spaces down to the terminal bronchioles, accompanied by the destruction of alveolar walls without obvious fibrosis. Emphysema frequently occurs in association with chronic bronchitis. Patients who have been diagnosed as having COPD have either an emphysema form of COPD or a chronic bronchitis type of COPD. There are at least two different morphological types of emphysema, that is, centriacinar or centrilobular and panacinar or panlobular (Demirjian 2012).

Centroacinar emphysema begins in the respiratory bronchioles and spreads peripherally. Also termed centrilobular emphysema, this form is associated with long-standing cigarette smoking and predominantly involves the upper half of the lungs.

Panacinar or panlobular emphysema destroys the entire alveolus uniformly and is predominant in the lower half of the lungs. Panacinar emphysema generally is observed in patients with homozygous alpha-1-antitrypsin (AAT) deficiency. In people who smoke, focal panacinar emphysema at the lung bases may accompany centriacinar emphysema.

The subcategory codes for emphysema are as follows:

J43.0   Unilateral pulmonary emphysema (MacLeod's syndrome)
J43.1   Panlobular emphysema
J43.2   Centrilobular emphysema
J43.8   Other emphysema
J43.9   Emphysema, unspecified

Chronic Obstructive Pulmonary Disease (COPD)

Chronic obstructive pulmonary disease (COPD) is a diffuse obstruction of the smaller bronchi and bronchioles that results in coughing, wheezing, shortness of breath, and disturbances of gas exchange. Exacerbations of COPD, such as episodes of increased shortness of breath and cough, often are treated on an outpatient basis. More severe exacerbations, such as an infection, usually result in admission to the hospital.

When acute bronchitis is documented with COPD, code J44.0, Obstructive chronic bronchitis with acute bronchitis, should be assigned. Code J44.1 is used when the medical record includes documentation of COPD with exacerbation or acute exacerbation, without mention of acute bronchitis.

Code J44.9 is an unspecified form of COPD. The diagnosis of COPD does not identify what type of chronic obstructive pulmonary disease the patient has. Sometimes physicians use COPD as a short-cut diagnosis, and other times the diagnosis of COPD is used because the patient has several forms of COPD, such as chronic bronchitis, obstructive asthma, or emphysema. Code J44.9 is an unspecified form of COPD and should not be used if the documentation from the provider is more specific as to what type of chronic obstructive pulmonary disease is present in the patient.

Instructional notes appear under category J44 to remind the coder to "code also" the type of asthma, if applicable, J45.-. There is another instruction to "use additional code" where applicable notes appear to direct the coder to assign an additional code for exposure to environmental tobacco smoke (Z77.22), history of tobacco use (Z87.891), occupational exposure to environmental tobacco smoke (Z57.31), tobacco dependence (F17.-), and tobacco use (Z72.0).

ICD-10-CM classifies COPD to the following codes:

J44.0 Chronic obstructive pulmonary disease with acute lower respiratory infection
Use additional code to identify the infection.

J44.1 Chronic obstructive pulmonary disease with (acute) exacerbation
This may be documented as decompensated COPD.

J44.9 Chronic obstructive pulmonary disease, unspecified
Chronic obstructive airway disease NOS
Chronic obstructive lung disease NOS

Asthma

Asthma is a condition marked by recurrent attacks of paroxysmal dyspnea, with wheezing due to spasmodic contraction of the bronchi. In some cases, it is an allergic manifestation in sensitized persons. The term reactive airway disease is considered synonymous with asthma.

The inclusion terms that appear under the category heading of J45, Asthma, include allergic asthma, allergic bronchitis, extrinsic allergic asthma, hay fever with asthma, intrinsic nonallergic asthma, and nonallergic asthma.

Conditions that are not classified to category J45, Asthma are included in the Excludes1 listing of codes such as detergent asthma, eosinophilic asthma, lung diseases due to external agents, miner's asthma, wheezing NOS, and wood asthma. The Excludes2 note includes conditions that can be coded with asthma J45 category codes, specifically:

Asthma with chronic obstructive pulmonary disease (J44.9)
Chronic asthmatic (obstructive) bronchitis (J44.9)
Chronic obstructive asthma (J44.9)

The terminology used to describe asthma in ICD-10-CM reflects the current clinical classification of asthma. The terms included in the codes to describe asthma are mild, intermittent, and three degrees of persistent—mild persistent, moderate persistent, and severe persistent (see table 13.1). Intrinsic asthma (nonallergic) and extrinsic (allergic) are both classified to J45.909, Unspecified asthma, uncomplicated, if not further specified.

Table 13.1. **Asthma severity terms**

Asthma Severity	Frequency of Daytime Symptoms
Intermittent	Less than or equal to 2 times per week
Mild Persistent	More than 2 times per week
Moderate Persistent	Daily. May restrict physical activity
Severe Persistent	Throughout the day. Frequent severe attacks limiting ability to breathe

Source: Li and Kaliner 2006.

233

Fourth- and Fifth-Character Subcategories

The following subcategories describe the specific types of asthma along with the clinical status:

J45.2		Mild intermittent asthma
	J45.20	Mild intermittent asthma, uncomplicated
	J45.21	Mild intermittent asthma with (acute) exacerbation
	J45.22	Mild intermittent asthma with status asthmaticus
J45.3		Mild persistent asthma
	J45.20	Mild persistent asthma, uncomplicated
	J45.21	Mild persistent asthma with (acute) exacerbation
	J45.22	Mild persistent asthma with status asthmaticus
J45.4		Moderate persistent asthma
	J45.20	Moderate persistent asthma, uncomplicated
	J45.21	Moderate persistent asthma with (acute) exacerbation
	J45.22	Moderate persistent asthma with status asthmaticus
J45.5		Severe persistent asthma
	J45.20	Severe persistent asthma, uncomplicated
	J45.21	Severe persistent asthma with (acute) exacerbation
	J45.22	Severe persistent asthma with status asthmaticus
J45.9		Other and unspecified asthma
	J45.90	Unspecified asthma
	J45.901	Unspecified asthma with (acute) exacerbation
	J45.902	Unspecified asthma with status asthmaticus
	J45.909	Unspecified asthma, uncomplicated
	J45.99	Other asthma
	J45.990	Exercise induced bronchospasm
	J45.991	Cough variant asthma
	J45.998	Other asthma

Fifth- and Sixth-Character Codes

The fifth-digit subclassifications describe whether the patient was in status asthmaticus or suffered what may be described as an exacerbation or acute exacerbation of the asthma.

An **acute exacerbation** or with exacerbation is an increase in the severity of the disease or any of its signs or symptoms, such as wheezing or shortness of breath.

Status asthmaticus is an acute asthmatic attack in which the degree of bronchial obstruction is not relieved by usual treatments such as epinephrine or aminophylline. A patient in status asthmaticus fails to respond to therapy administered during an asthmatic attack. This is a life-threatening complication that requires emergency care and, most likely, inpatient hospitalization.

Bronchiectasis

Bronchiectasis is a chronic, congenital, or acquired disease characterized by irreversible dilation of the bronchi with secondary infection. The incidence of bronchiectasis has decreased with the widespread use of antibiotics and immunizations in pediatrics. In adults, the condition may develop following a necrotizing pneumonia or lung abscess.

Category J47 codes are as follows:

J47.0   Bronchiectasis with acute lower respiratory infection
J47.1   Bronchiectasis with (acute) exacerbation
J47.9   Bronchiectasis, uncomplicated

Lung Diseases Due to External Agents (J60–J70)

Categories in this section describe lung diseases that are caused by external factors, chemical, organic, and inorganic substances. Numerous external agents cause lung disease; many of these are long-term conditions and may be incurable. Many of these conditions may be referred to as occupational lung disorders because the individuals acquire the conditions are part of their occupation or employment.

The categories of lung diseases due to external agents are as follows:

J60   Coalworker's pneumoconiosis
J61   Pneumoconiosis due to asbestos and other mineral fibers
J62   Pneumoconiosis due to dust containing silica
J63   Pneumoconiosis due to other inorganic dusts
       Includes aluminosis, bauxite fibrosis, berylliosis, graphite fibrosis, siderosis, stannosis
J64   Unspecified pneumoconiosis
J65   Pneumoconiosis associated with tuberculosis
J66   Airway disease due to specific organic dust
       Includes byssinosis, flax-dressers' disease, cannabinosis
J67   Hypersensitivity pneumonitis due to organic dust
       Includes farmer's lung, bagassosis, bird fancier's lung, suberosis, maltworker's lung, mushroom-worker's lung, maple-bark-stripper's lung and air-conditioner and humidifier lung
J68   Respiratory conditions due to inhalation of chemicals, gases, fumes and vapors
J69   Pneumonitis due to solids and liquids
       The most commonly coded condition from this category is aspiration pneumonia, J69.0.
J70   Respiratory conditions due to other external agents
       Instructional notes under this category's codes include "Use additional code (W88–W90, X93.0-) to identify the external cause" or "Use additional code for adverse effect, if applicable, to identify drug (T36–T50 with fifth or sixth characters 5)."

Other Categories to Classify Diseases of the Respiratory System

Other sections of ICD-10-CM codes included in Chapter 10, Diseases of the respiratory system are as follows:

J80–J84   Other respiratory diseases principally affecting the interstitium
           The more commonly coded conditions from this section include
           J80   Acute respiratory distress syndrome
           J81.0   Acute pulmonary edema

J81.1	Chronic pulmonary edema
J84.10	Pulmonary fibrosis
J85–J86	Suppurative and necrotic conditions of the lower respiratory tract

The conditions in this section that are coded frequently include

J85.1	Abscess of lung with pneumonia
J86.9	Pyothorax without fistula
J90–J94	Other diseases of the pleura

The commonly coded conditions in this section include

J90	Pleural effusion
J93.0	Spontaneous tension pneumothorax
J93.11	Primary spontaneous pneumothorax
J93.82	Other or persistent air leak
J94.2	Hemothorax and Hemopneumothorax

Intraoperative and Postprocedural Complications and Disorders of Respiratory System, Not Elsewhere Classified (J95)

Procedural complication codes are included in category J95 to identify specific respiratory complications such as the following:

J95.00–J95.09	Tracheostomy complications
J95.1–J95.3	Acute and chronic pulmonary insufficiency following thoracic surgery and nonthoracic surgery
J95.811–J95.812	Postprocedural pneumothorax and air leak
J95.851	Ventilator associated pneumonia

Other complications in this category include intraoperative and postprocedural hemorrhage, hematoma, and accidental puncture or laceration. Again, the complication can be identified as occurring during a respiratory system procedure or as complicating another body system procedure.

Other Diseases of the Respiratory System (J96–J99)

The commonly coded conditions in this section of codes include acute and chronic respiratory failure and acute bronchospasm.

Respiratory Failure (J96)

Respiratory failure is the inability of the respiratory system to supply adequate oxygen to maintain proper metabolism or to eliminate carbon dioxide (CO_2). ICD-10-CM classifies different forms of respiratory failure to the following codes in category J96, Respiratory failure, not elsewhere classified:

J96.0	Acute respiratory failure	
	J96.00	Acute respiratory failure, unspecified whether with hypoxia or hypercapnia
	J96.01	Acute respiratory failure with hypoxia
	J96.02	Acute respiratory failure with hypercapnia

J96.1   Chronic respiratory failure
    J96.10   Chronic respiratory failure, unspecified whether with hypoxia or hypercapnia
    J96.11   Chronic respiratory failure with hypoxia
    J96.12   Chronic respiratory failure with hypercapnia
J96.2   Acute and chronic respiratory failure
    J96.20   Acute and chronic respiratory failure, unspecified whether with hypoxia or hypercapnia
    J96.21   Acute and chronic respiratory failure with hypoxia
    J96.22   Acute and chronic respiratory failure with hypercapnia
J96.9   Respiratory failure, unspecified
    J96.90   Respiratory failure, unspecified, unspecified whether with hypoxia or hypercapnia
    J96.91   Respiratory failure, unspecified, with hypoxia
    J96.92   Respiratory failure, unspecified, with hypercapnia

Respiratory failure is assigned when documentation in the health record supports its use. It may be due to, or associated with, other respiratory conditions such as pneumonia, chronic bronchitis, or COPD. Respiratory failure also may be due to, or associated with, nonrespiratory conditions such as myasthenia gravis, congestive heart failure, myocardial infarction, or CVA.

Arterial blood gases may be useful in diagnosing respiratory failure; however, normal values may vary from person to person depending on individual health status. Coders should not assume the condition of respiratory failure exists based solely on laboratory and radiology test findings.

Coding and Sequencing of Acute Respiratory Failure

The coding and sequencing of acute respiratory failure presents many challenges to both the new and the experienced clinical coder. Various coding rules and guidelines must be considered.

Acute respiratory failure, codes J96.00–J96.02, may be assigned as a principal or secondary diagnosis depending on the circumstances of the inpatient admission. Chapter-specific coding guidelines (obstetrics, poisoning, HIV, newborn) provide specific sequencing direction. Respiratory failure may be listed as a secondary diagnosis. In addition, if respiratory failure occurs after admission, it may be listed as a secondary diagnosis.

When a patient is admitted in acute respiratory failure with another acute condition, the principal diagnosis will not be the same in every situation. There is not one respiratory failure coding rule. This is true whether or not the other acute condition is a respiratory or nonrespiratory condition. Selection of the principal diagnosis will depend on the circumstances of the admission. If both the respiratory failure and the other acute condition are equally responsible for the patient's admission to the hospital, and there are no chapter-specific sequencing rules, the guideline regarding two or more diagnoses that equally meet the definition for principal diagnosis may be applied. If the documentation is not clear as to whether the acute respiratory failure and another condition are equally responsible for occasioning the admission, the physician must be asked for clarification.

Respiratory failure is a life-threatening condition that is always caused by an underlying condition. It may be caused by diseases of the circulatory system, respiratory system, central nervous system, peripheral nervous system, respiratory muscles, and chest wall muscles.

The primary goal of the treatment of acute respiratory failure is to assess the severity of underlying disease and to correct the inadequate oxygen delivery and tissue hypoxia.

Bronchospasm (J98.01)

Acute bronchospasm is coded in ICD-10-CM with code J98.01. However, acute bronchospasm is frequently a symptom of another respiratory condition. The Excludes1 note under code J98.01 states that this code for bronchospasm is not coded if bronchospasm is specified as:

Acute bronchiolitis with bronchospasm (J21.-)
Acute bronchitis with bronchospasm (J20.-)
Bronchospasm with asthma (J45.-)
Exercise induced bronchospasm (J45.990)

ICD-10-PCS Procedure Coding for Respiratory System Procedures

Procedures performed on the sites in the respiratory system are included in the tables from 0B1–0BY with the root operations Bypass, Change, Destruction, Dilation, Drainage, Excision, Extirpation, Extraction, Fragmentation, Insertion, Inspection, Occlusion, Reattachment, Release, Removal, Repair, Reposition, Resection, Supplement, Restriction, Revision, and Transplantation.

Other procedures performed in the mouth and throat are included in the tables from 0C0–0CX with the root operations Alteration, Change, Destruction, Dilation, Drainage, Excision, Extirpation, Extraction, Fragmentation, Insertion, Inspection, Occlusion, Reattachment, Release, Removal, Repair, Replacement, Reposition, Resection, Supplement, Restriction, Revision, and Transfer.

Like procedures in other body systems, in order to code respiratory procedures, the coder needs to know the definition of root operations and the anatomy of the respiratory tract to identify the body parts.

This section describes the ICD-10-PCS coding of two respiratory procedures: closed endoscopic biopsy and other endoscopic procedures.

Closed Endoscopic Biopsy

Endoscopy means looking inside and typically refers to looking inside the body for medical reasons using an endoscope, an instrument used to examine the interior of a hollow organ or cavity of the body. Unlike most other medical imaging devices, endoscopes are inserted directly into the organ. An endoscope can consist of a rigid or flexible tube with a light delivery system to illuminate the organ or object under inspection. There is a lens attached to the tube transmitting the image from the lens to the viewer through an eyepiece. There is an additional tube to allow the entry of medical instruments. In the respiratory tract, two types of endoscopies are performed via the nose (rhinoscopy) and to the lower respiratory tract through the mouth (bronchoscopy) (NHLBI 2012).

A closed endoscopic biopsy is the excision of tissue for diagnostic purposes through a bronchoscope in the respiratory system. By ICD-10-PCS definition, a biopsy is an excision or cutting out or off, without replacement, a portion of a body part. For the respiratory system, excision procedures are coded according to table 13.2.

Table 13.2. **ICD-10-PCS Table 0BB**

Body Part	Approach	Device	Qualifier
1 Trachea 2 Carina 3 Main Bronchus, Right 4 Upper Lobe Bronchus, Right 5 Middle Lobe Bronchus, Right 6 Lower Lobe Bronchus, Right 7 Main Bronchus, Left 8 Upper Lobe Bronchus, Left 9 Lingula Bronchus B Lower Lobe Bronchus, Left C Upper Lung Lobe, Right D Middle Lung Lobe, Right F Lower Lung Lobe, Right G Upper Lung Lobe, Left H Lung Lingula J Lower Lung Lobe, Left K Lung, Right L Lung, Left M Lungs, Bilateral	0 Open 3 Percutaneous 4 Percutaneous Endoscopic 7 Via Natural or Artificial Opening 8 Via Natural or Artificial Opening Endoscopic	Z No Device	X Diagnostic Z No Qualifier
N Pleura, Right P Pleura, Left R Diaphragm, Right S Diaphragm, Left	0 Open 3 Percutaneous 4 Percutaneous Endoscopic	Z No Device	X Diagnostic Z No Qualifier

0 Medical and Surgical
B Respiratory System
B Excision

When coding closed endoscopic biopsies, the specific site where the excision is made including the laterality is required:

0BBK4ZX	Thoracoscopic lung biopsy, right
0BB78ZX	Closed [bronchoscopic] biopsy of left main bronchus
0BBG8ZX	Closed [bronchoscopic] biopsy of lung, upper lung lobe
0BBN4ZX	Thoracoscopic pleural biopsy, right

Endoscopic Procedures in the Respiratory System

Because many lesions in the respiratory tract can be removed by endoscopic means that do not require opening the chest, ICD-10-PCS provides codes for this type of procedure. For example:

0BB68ZZ	Bronchoscopic excision of lesion or tissue of bronchus, lower lobe bronchus, right
0BBG8ZZ	Bronchoscopic excision of lesion or tissue of lung, upper lung lobe, left
0BBG4ZZ	Thoracoscopic lobectomy of lung, upper lung lobe, left

The difference in the examples above is the type of endoscope used: bronchoscopy or thoracoscopy. The bronchoscope is performed with the Via Natural or Artificial Opening

Endoscopic approach (through mouth). The thoracoscopy is performed through a Percutaneous Endoscopic approach.

Mechanical Ventilation

Mechanical ventilation is clinically indicated for patients with apnea, acute respiratory failure, and impending acute respiratory failure. Invasive mechanical ventilation pumps air into the patient's lungs even when there is no attempt by the patient to breathe on his or her own.

Mechanical ventilation is coded to the Extracorporeal Assistance and Performance section in ICD-10-PCS. Insertion of the endotracheal tube as part of a mechanical ventilation procedure is not coded as a separate device insertion procedure, because it is merely the interface between the patient and the equipment used to perform the procedure, rather than an end in itself. On the other hand, insertion of an endotracheal tube in order to maintain an airway in patients who are unconscious or unable to breathe on their own is the central objective of the procedure. Therefore, insertion of an endotracheal tube as an end in itself is coded to the root operation Insertion and the device Endotracheal Airway (CMS 2012c, 122).

The ICD-10-PCS procedure codes for mechanical ventilation and related procedures are as follows:

5A1935Z	Mechanical ventilation for less than 24 consecutive hours
5A1945Z	Mechanical ventilation for 24 to 96 consecutive hours
5A1955Z	Mechanical ventilation for greater than 96 consecutive hours
0B110FA	Creation of tracheostomy for use with mechanical ventilation

ICD-10-CM and ICD-10-PCS Review Exercises: Chapter 13

Assign the correct ICD-10-CM diagnosis codes and ICD-10-PCS procedure codes to the following exercises.

1. Patient with a high fever, cough, and chest pain. Gram stain of the sputum showed numerous small gram-negative coccobacilli. Diagnosis: H. influenzae pneumonia.

2. Acute respiratory insufficiency due to acute exacerbation of COPD and tobacco dependence

3. Severe persistent asthma with acute exacerbation

4. Hypertrophy of tonsils and adenoids

5. Chronic simple bronchitis

6. Panlobular emphysema

ICD-10-CM and ICD-10-PCS Review Exercises: Chapter 13 (Continued)

7. Streptococcus pneumonia with associated lung abscess

8. Influenza with pneumonia

9. Hay fever due to pollen

10. Bilateral vocal cord paralysis

11. Tension pneumothorax

12. Chronic laryngotracheitis

13. Postprocedural pneumothorax

14. Black lung disease

15. PROCEDURE: Tracheostomy tube exchange

16. PROCEDURE: Thoracotomy with exploration of right pleural cavity

17. PROCEDURE: Laryngoscopy with endoscopic biopsy of larynx by excision

18. PROCEDURE: Bronchoscopic excision of lesion of right upper lobe of lung

19. PROCEDURE: Mechanical ventilation for 36 consecutive hours following endotracheal tube intubation

20. PROCEDURE: Thoracotomy with resection of left lower lobe of lung

Chapter 14

Diseases of the Digestive System (K00–K95)

Learning Objectives

At the conclusion of this chapter, you should be able to:

1. Describe the organization of the conditions and codes included in Chapter 11 of ICD-10-CM, Diseases of the digestive system (K00–K95)

2. Identify the ICD-10-CM codes for the various ulcers of the gastrointestinal tract

3. Identify the definitions of various types of hernia conditions that can be classified

4. Identify various types of noninfectious enteritis and colitis conditions that can be classified

5. Identify the ICD-10-CM codes for the various types of gallbladder disease and calculus

6. Understand the use of ICD-10-CM codes for gastrointestinal hemorrhage, and its relationship with other digestive conditions

7. Briefly describe the methods of repairing various digestive system hernias

8. Describe the types of procedures that can be performed endoscopically within the digestive system

9. Identify the ICD-10-PCS codes for various types of procedures performed for intestinal resection and anastomosis

10. Assign ICD-10-PCS codes for procedures related to diseases of the digestive system

Key Terms

- Anastomosis
- Bypass
- Cholecystitis
- Choledocholithiasis

- Cholelithiasis
- Colostomy
- Crohn's disease
- Duodenitis
- Excision
- Gastritis
- Gastroenteritis
- Gastrostomy
- Hematemesis
- Hernia
- Ileostomy
- Irreducible hernia
- Laparotomy
- Melena
- Mucositis
- Obstruction
- Occult blood
- Peritonitis
- Reducible
- Resection
- Stoma
- Strangulated hernia
- Supplement
- Ulcer

Overview of ICD-10-CM Chapter 11, Diseases of the Digestive System

Chapter 11 includes categories K00–K95 arranged in the following blocks:

K00–K14	Diseases of oral cavity and salivary glands
K20–K31	Diseases of esophagus, stomach and duodenum
K35–K38	Diseases of appendix
K40–K46	Hernia
K50–K52	Noninfective enteritis and colitis
K55–K64	Other diseases of intestines
K65–K68	Diseases of peritoneum and retroperitoneum
K70–K77	Diseases of liver
K80–K87	Disorders of gallbladder, biliary tract and pancreas
K90–K95	Other diseases of digestive system

This chapter contains commonly coded gastrointestinal (GI) conditions that occur in many patients from infections in the mouth and organs in the upper GI tract as well as in the appendix, small bowel, colon, gallbladder, and liver. There are combination codes to describe facts about digestive conditions, for example, if the condition is an acute versus a chronic disease, and whether bleeding is present. In ICD-10-CM, the term "hemorrhage" is used when referring to ulcers while the term "bleeding" is used when classifying gastritis, duodenitis, diverticulosis, and diverticulitis; note the following examples:

- K25.0 Acute gastric ulcer with hemorrhage

- K29.01 Acute gastritis with bleeding

- K57.31 Diverticulosis of large intestine without perforation or abscess with bleeding

Combination codes for specific sites of hernias in the digestive system also include whether the condition is present with gangrene or obstruction and whether the hernia is present on one side of the body or is a bilateral condition. Other codes identify whether complications exist, for example, whether rectal bleeding, intestinal obstruction, fistula, or abscess is present with ulcerative colitis or regional enteritis. Complications of artificial openings of the digestive system, including colostomy, enterostomy, and gastrostomy infections and malfunctions are included in the chapter. ICD-10-CM codes exist for intraoperative and postprocedural complications that are specific to the digestive system, such as postprocedural intestinal obstruction; there are also codes for hemorrhages, hematomas, accidental punctures, and lacerations that occur during procedures.

Coding Guidelines and Instructional Notes for ICD-10-CM Chapter 11

The NCHS has not published chapter-specific guidelines for Chapter 11 in the *ICD-10-CM Official Guidelines for Coding and Reporting* at time of this publication.

There are "use additional code to identify" instructional notes throughout the chapter to identify the use of substances that have an influence on the diseases of the digestive system. For example, under categories K05, Gingivitis and periodontal diseases and K12, Stomatitis and related lesions, there is a use additional code note to identify:

Alcohol abuse and dependence (F10.-)
Exposure to environmental tobacco smoke (Z77.22)
Exposure to tobacco smoke in the perinatal period (P96.81)
History of tobacco use (Z87.891)
Occupational exposure to environmental tobacco smoke (Z57.31)
Tobacco dependence (F17.-)
Tobacco use (Z72.0)

Other instructional notes appear under the ulcer of the stomach, duodenum, and other digestive system sites to "use additional code to identify" alcohol abuse and dependence (F10.-). Certain digestive conditions are the result of other diseases. For example, under code

K31.84, Gastroparesis, is a note stating "code first underlying disease, if known, such as anorexia nervosa, diabetes mellitus or scleroderma." For infections in the digestive tract, a "use additional code (B95–B97) to identify infectious agent" note appears with codes. For example, this note appears under category K65, Peritonitis, because the cause of the infection may be known and therefore should be coded. Other codes that identify infections that complicate the artificial openings of the digestive system include "use additional code to specify the type of infection." For example, this note appears under code K94.22, Gastrostomy infection, to instruct the coder to identify when cellulitis of the abdominal way (L03.311) or sepsis (A40-, A41-) is present.

There is an instructional note after the heading of Hernia (K40–K46). It states "hernia with both gangrene and obstruction is classified to hernia with gangrene." This applies to all conditions coded to categories K40 through K46. The "includes" note that follows states the codes K40–K46 includes acquired hernia, congenital hernia, and recurrent hernia.

Coding Diseases of the Digestive System in ICD-10-CM Chapter 11

Chapter 11 of ICD-10-CM, Diseases of the digestive system, (K00–K95) contains many commonly diagnosed problems that patients experience in their gastrointestinal tract. This section describes the coding of some of these digestive system conditions with ICD-10-CM diagnosis codes.

Diseases of Oral Cavity and Salivary Glands (K00–K14)

In the past, diagnosis coding was not widely used in dentistry. However, the need for dental diagnosis codes has become urgent with the advent of electronic health records and the desire of dentists to track patient conditions with their outcomes. The use of codes also supports the educational and research needs of dentistry. Codes describe types of dental caries, abrasions and erosions, gingival and periodontal disease, and other disorders of teeth and supporting structures. Other codes within this section include diseases of the salivary glands, mouth, lip, and tongue.

Mucositis can occur as an adverse effect of antineoplastic treatment and other medications. There is redness or ulcerative sores in the soft tissue of the mucosal surfaces throughout the body, resulting in severe pain as well as difficulty in eating, drinking, and taking oral medications. The most common location for mucosal toxicity is the oral cavity. The codes for oral mucositis due to antineoplastic therapy or other drugs are included in the digestive system chapter of ICD-10-CM with codes K12.31 and K12.32. Each code has a "use additional code for adverse effect" direction to identify antineoplastic and immunosuppressive drugs or other drugs (T36–T50) with fifth or sixth character 5.

Gastrointestinal Ulcers (K25–K28)

Ulcers of the gastrointestinal (GI) tract can be found in the following categories:

K25 Gastric ulcer
K26 Duodenal ulcer

K27 Peptic ulcer, site unspecified
K28 Gastrojejunal ulcer

The preceding categories are subdivided to fourth-digit subcategories that describe acute and chronic conditions and the presence of hemorrhage or perforation. An **ulcer** is a depressed lesion on the skin or mucous membrane of an internal organ or site (Melloni 2001). The bleeding ulcer or hemorrhage does not have to be actively bleeding at the time of the examination procedure, such as an endoscopy, to use the code for ulcer with hemorrhage. A statement by the physician that bleeding has occurred and it is attributed to the ulcer is sufficient. Each of these categories include the "use additional code" note to identify the concurrent condition, if applicable, for alcohol abuse and dependence (F10.-).

Gastritis and Duodenitis (K29)

Gastritis is the inflammation of the stomach lining, while **duodenitis** is the inflammation of the duodenal portion of the small intestine. ICD-10-CM classifies gastritis and duodenitis to category K29, which is subdivided to fourth- and fifth-digit subcategories that describe types of gastritis and duodenitis. The fourth-digit category identifies the severity or etiology of the gastritis, for example, alcoholic gastritis with and without bleeding or chronic atrophic gastritis with or without bleeding. Active bleeding during the current examination or procedure does not have to be present to use the specific code. It may be diagnosed clinically by the physician based on the patient's history or physical examination.

Hernia (K40–K46)

A **hernia** is the protrusion of a loop or knuckle of an organ or tissue through an abdominal opening. Many different types of hernias exist, including the following:

- An inguinal hernia is a hernia of an intestinal loop into the inguinal canal. An inguinal hernia may be referred to as "direct" or "indirect," which describes the anatomical location more precisely but cannot be coded as specifically with ICD-10-CM diagnosis codes.

- A femoral hernia is a hernia of a loop of intestine into the femoral canal.

- A hiatal hernia is the displacement of the upper part of the stomach into the thorax through the esophageal opening (hiatus) of the diaphragm.

- A diaphragmatic hernia is the protrusion of an abdominal organ into the chest cavity through a defect in the diaphragm.

- A ventral hernia, or abdominal hernia, is a herniation of the intestine or some other internal body structure through the abdominal wall.

- An incisional hernia is an abdominal hernia at the site of a previously made incision.

- An umbilical hernia is a type of abdominal hernia in which part of the intestine protrudes at the umbilicus and is covered by skin and subcutaneous tissue. This type may also be described as an omphalocele.

- A hernia may be described as **reducible.** This means the physician can manipulate the displaced structure(s) back into position.

Codes for different type of hernias of the abdominal cavity are included in the following categories:

K40 Inguinal hernia
K41 Femoral hernia
K42 Umbilical hernia
K43 Ventral hernia
K44 Diaphragmatic (hiatal) hernia
K45 Other abdominal hernia
K46 Unspecified abdominal hernia

A note appears under the category heading that hernia with both gangrene and obstruction is coded as a hernia with gangrene. Hernias are classified by the site or type of hernia, the clinical presentation of the presence of gangrene or obstruction, whether the hernia is unilateral, bilateral, or unspecified as to one- or two-sided, and whether it is recurrent condition.

ICD-10-CM uses the term **obstruction** to indicate that incarceration, irreducibility, or strangulation is present with the hernia.

- An **irreducible hernia** is also known as an incarcerated hernia. An incarcerated hernia is a hernia of intestine that cannot be returned or reduced by manipulation; it may or may not be strangulated.

- A **strangulated hernia** is an incarcerated hernia that is so tightly constricted as to restrict the blood supply to the contents of the hernial sac and possibly cause gangrene of the contents, such as the intestine. This represents a medical emergency requiring surgical correction.

Crohn's Disease [Regional Enteritis] (K50)

Crohn's disease, also known as regional enteritis, is defined as a chronic inflammatory disease commonly affecting the distal ileum and colon. Crohn's disease is characterized by chronic diarrhea, abdominal pain, fever, anorexia, weight loss, right lower quadrant mass or fullness, and lymphadenitis of the mesenteric nodes.

ICD-10-CM classifies Crohn's disease to category K50, with the fifth and sixth character identifying the specific site affected, such as the small or large intestine. The associated clinical manifestations of rectal bleeding, intestinal obstruction, fistula or abscess as well as other complications are identified with the sixth character under each site. Without further specification as to site and without complication, assign code K50.90 for Crohn's disease.

Gastroenteritis (K52)

Gastroenteritis, an inflammation of the stomach and intestine, is characterized by diarrhea, nausea and vomiting, and abdominal cramps. It can be caused by toxins and allergic and dietetic etiology, as well as bacteria, amoebae, parasites, viruses, reaction to drugs, or enzyme deficiencies. Allergic reactions as a response to food allergens may manifest as GI reactions, the most common of which are nausea, vomiting, diarrhea, and abdominal cramping. Codes exist in this category to identify the noninfectious origins of gastroenteritis in this category.

Gastroenteritis is classified by cause in Chapters 1 and 9 in the Tabular List in Volume 1 of ICD-10-CM.

A02.0 Salmonella gastroenteritis
A08.4 Viral gastroenteritis, NEC
A09   Infectious gastroenteritis
K52.1 Toxic gastroenteritis and colitis
K52.2 Allergic and dietetic gastroenteritis and colitis
K52.9 Noninfectious gastroenteritis and colitis, unspecified
      Includes colitis, enteritis, gastroenteritis, ileitis, jejunitis, and sigmoiditis, NOS

Toxic gastroenteritis and colitis, code K52.1, is followed by a "code first" note to identify the toxic agent with a code from the range T51–T66. Another possible cause of toxic gastro-enteritis and colitis is the side effect of a drug, which is the reason for the "use additional code for adverse effect" note that also appears under code K52.1.

Under code K52.2, Allergic and dietetic gastroenteritis and colitis, is a "use additional code" note to identify the type of food allergy (Z91.01-, Z91.02-) that caused the bowel inflammation.

Peritonitis, Other Disorders of Peritoneum and Disorders of Retroperitoneum (K65–K68)

Peritonitis is inflammation of the peritoneum, usually accompanied by abdominal pain and tenderness, constipation, vomiting, and moderate fever. It may be caused by a bacteria or a virus or caused by other factors, such as ruptured internal organs, trauma, or childbirth. Under the category heading K65, Peritonitis, there is an instructional note to use an additional code (B95–B97) to identify the infectious agent responsible for the infection.

Also appearing under the category heading is an Excludes1 note that identifies all the conditions that cannot be coded with a category K65 code. The codes listed here, such as acute appendicitis with generalized peritonitis or diverticulitis with peritonitis, already include the presence of peritonitis with the digestive and other disease.

ICD-10-CM codes distinguish between acute (generalized) peritonitis, code K65.0, and peritoneal abscess, code K65.1. Similarly, a retroperitoneal abscess (K68.19) is coded differently than other forms of retroperitoneal infections (such as K68.9). Spontaneous bacterial peritonitis is coded with K65.2. Choleperitonitis, code K65.3, occurs as the result of bile in the peritoneal cavity. Sclerosing mesenteritis, code K65.4, refers to a number of inflammatory processes involving the mesenteric fat, including fat necrosis and fibrosis. The generic diagnosis of peritonitis is presumed to be bacterial in origin and coded to the unspecified peritonitis code of K65.9. Each condition requires specific treatment. Another commonly occurring condition is peritoneal adhesions. The presence of adhesions could be due to infectious or developed after a procedure and is coded to K66.0 in the category K66 for other disorders of peritoneum. If the peritoneal adhesions cause an intestinal obstruction, use code K56.5, intestinal adhesions with obstruction.

Cholecystitis and Cholelithiasis (K80–K81)

Two categories are available to classify cholecystitis and cholelithiasis: K80, Cholelithiasis and K81, Cholecystitis.

Cholelithiasis is the presence of one or more calculi (gallstones) in the gallbladder. Gallstones tend to be asymptomatic. The most common symptom is biliary colic. More serious complications include cholecystitis, biliary tract obstruction (from stones in the bile ducts or choledocholithiasis), bile duct infection (cholangitis), and gallstone pancreatitis. A diagnosis is usually made by ultrasonography. If cholelithiasis causes symptoms or complications, a cholecystectomy may be necessary.

Choledocholithiasis is the presence of stones in the bile ducts. The stones can form in the gallbladder or in the bile ducts. The stones cause biliary colic, biliary obstruction, gallstone pancreatitis, or cholangitis. Cholangitis can lead to stricture, stasis, and choledocholithiasis. The diagnosis is usually made by magnetic resonance cholangiopancreatography (MRCP) or endoscopic retrograde cholangiopancreatography (ERCP). Frequently occurring with the stones is **cholecystitis** or inflammation of the gallbladder.

Category K80 is further divided into the following fifth-character subcategories to describe the existence of calculus or stones in the gallbladder or in the bile ducts or both locations with acute or chronic cholecystitis whether or not an obstruction is present:

K80.0- Calculus of gallbladder with acute cholecystitis
K80.1- Calculus of gallbladder with other cholecystitis
K80.2- Calculus of gallbladder without cholecystitis
K80.3- Calculus of bile duct with cholangitis
K80.4- Calculus of bile duct with cholecystitis
K80.5- Calculus of bile duct without cholangitis or cholecystitis
K80.6- Calculus of gallbladder and bile duct with cholecystitis
K80.7- Calculus of gallbladder and bile duct without cholecystitis
K80.8 Other cholelithiasis

The coder must be careful in following the Alphabetic Index directions when coding gallbladder disease. For example, if a patient had acute and chronic cholecystitis with cholelithiasis, the coder may access the Index using the diagnosis "cholecystitis." There is a connecting term "with" beneath the main term cholecystitis that is very important to read. The coder must follow the direction when reviewing the Index entry for "Cholecystitis" with "calculus, stones in gallbladder and follow the direction to see Calculus, gallbladder, with, cholecystitis." The coder must then go to the main term "calculus, gallbladder" and see the connecting term "with" and find codes following "cholecystitis, acute" and "cholecystitis, chronic." The code to be assigned for acute and chronic cholecystitis with cholelithiasis (without mention of obstruction) is K80.12.

Category K81 contains the following four codes relating to cholecystitis without mention of calculus or stones in the gallbladder or bile duct:

K81.0 Acute cholecystitis
K81.1 Chronic cholecystitis
K81.2 Acute cholecystitis with chronic cholecystitis
K81.9 Cholecystitis, unspecified

Gastrointestinal Hemorrhage (K92)

Category K92, Other diseases of the digestive system, includes subcategories for hematemesis (K92.0), melena (K92.1), and unspecified gastrointestinal hemorrhage (K92.2).

The use of category K92 is limited to cases where a GI bleed is documented, but no bleeding site or cause is identified. A hemorrhage in the GI tract may produce either dark black, tarry, clotted stools (also referred to as **melena**) or bright red blood in the stool or vomiting blood (**hematemesis**). This is not the same as occult blood, which is invisible and only detected by microscopic examination or by a guaiac test. **Occult blood** is a small amount of blood coming from the GI tract. Occult blood or guaiac-positive stool is reported with ICD-10-CM diagnosis code R19.5, Nonspecific abnormal findings in other body substances, stool contents.

Note the Excludes1 note under the code K92.2. This note identifies a number of GI conditions that can be coded based on the presence of hemorrhage. The use of the K92.2 code is not appropriate when one of the conditions listed under the Excludes1 note is present.

Even though ICD-10-CM includes the combination codes describing a gastrointestinal hemorrhage with a gastrointestinal condition (angiodysplasia, diverticulitis, gastritis, duodenitis, and ulcer), these codes should not be assigned unless the physician identifies a causal relationship. The coder should not assume a causal relationship between gastrointestinal bleeding and a single finding such as a gastric ulcer, gastritis, diverticulitis, and so on. The physician must identify the source of the bleeding and link the clinical findings from the colonoscopy or upper endoscopy because these findings may be unrelated to the bleeding. Active bleeding does not have to be occurring at the time of the examination or procedure, but it does have to be identified in the patient's history. Two codes should be assigned when the physician states that the GI hemorrhage is unrelated to a coexisting GI condition: one for the GI hemorrhage, and one for the GI condition without hemorrhage.

ICD-10-PCS Procedure Coding for Diseases of the Digestive System

Procedures performed on the digestive system are included in the tables from 0D1–0DY with the root operations Bypass, Change, Destruction, Dilation, Division, Drainage, Excision, Extirpation, Fragmentation, Insertion, Inspection, Occlusion, Reattachment, Release, Removal, Repair, Replacement, Reposition, Resection, Supplement, Restriction, Revision, Transfer, and Transplantation. Like procedures in other body systems, in order to code gastrointestinal procedures, the coder needs to know the definition of root operations and the anatomy to identify the body parts.

Gastrointestinal Procedures

This section highlights coding for GI procedures such as the following:

- Laparoscopic and open repair of hernia
- Closed endoscopic biopsies and endoscopic excisions of lesions
- Gastrointestinal stoma procedures
- Intestinal resection
- Laparotomy

Laparoscopic and Open Repair of Hernia

Surgery is the only treatment and cure for most hernias. Hernia repair is one of the most commonly performed surgeries in the United States. Hernia repair procedures are performed both by incision (open) and by the laparoscopic technique. Open hernia repairs are performed through an incision with sutured tissue repair. Using synthetic mesh materials to repair the hernia has become fairly standard technique. Laparoscopic hernia repair is a less invasive procedure, with a small incision made to allow a thin, lighted instrument called a laparoscope to be inserted through the incision. Laparoscopic procedures also use mesh that is fixated to the fascia with tacks or sutures to repair the hernia.

The main term "herniorrhaphy" is included in the Index with two root operations listed. Herniorrhaphy with synthetic substitute used for the repair directs the coder to see the root operation Supplement with subterms for anatomical regions for general and lower extremities. The second root operation listed under herniorrhaphy is Repair with subterms for anatomical regions for general and lower extremities. Use the main term "supplement" when synthetic substitute is used and "repair" for all other repairs, along with the subterm for the anatomic location where the hernia is being repaired. The subterms of abdominal wall, diaphragm, femoral region, or inguinal region under supplement give the first three characters 0WU, 0BU, and 0YU for coding. The root operation **Supplement** is defined as putting in or on biological or synthetic material that physically reinforces or augments the function of a portion of a body part. Using the Table 0YU (see table 14.1) for the repair of a laparoscopic right inguinal hernia repair using mesh, the procedure code 0YU54JZ is constructed.

Table 14.1.　**Excerpt from Table 0YU for the root operation Supplement**

Body Part	Approach	Device	Qualifier
5 Inguinal Region, Right 6 Inguinal Region, Left A Inguinal Region, Bilateral	0 Open 4 Percutaneous Endoscopic	7 Autologous Tissue Substitute J Synthetic Substitute K Nonautologous Tissue Substititue	Z No Qualifier

0 Medical and Surgical
Y Anatomical Regions, Lower Extremities
U Supplement: putting in or on biological or synthetic material that physically reinforces and/or augments the function of a portion of a body part

Closed Endoscopic Biopsies and Endoscopic Excision of Lesions

Closed endoscopic biopsies are common procedures performed on the gastrointestinal tract. A biopsy is taken to determine the pathology of a lesion in a digestive system organ. The main term of biopsy in the Index refers the coder to the terms "drainage" or "excision" with qualifier Diagnostic. The subterms under the main term "excision" identify the organ where the biopsy was taken. For example, the coding of an esophagoscopy with a biopsy of the middle esophagus would use the main term "excision" and subterm "esophagus, middle" in the Index and find 0DB2 listed. Table 14.2 contains an excerpt from table 0DB to show how code 0DB28ZX is constructed.

Table 14.2. Excerpt from Table 0DB for the root operation Excision

Body Part	Approach	Device	Qualifier
1 Esophagus, Upper 2 Esophagus, Middle 3 Esophagus, Lower 4 Esophagogastric Junction 5 Esophagus 7 Stomach, pylorus	0 Open 3 Percutaneous 4 Percutaneous Endoscopic 7 Via Natural or Artificial Opening 8 Via Natural or Artificial Opening Endoscopic	Z No Device	X Diagnostic Z No Qualifier

0 Medical and Surgical
D Gastrointestinal System
B Excision: Cutting out or off, without replacement, a portion of a body part

The same table 14.2 shows how an excision of a lesion performed endoscopically would be coded. For example, if an esophagogastroduodenoscopy is performed to excise a lesion of the pylorus of the stomach, the ICD-10-PCS code would be 0DB78ZZ. The qualifier is Z because the excision of a lesion is not a biopsy or diagnostic; instead is it a therapeutic procedure to remove the lesion.

Gastrointestinal Stoma

A **stoma** is an artificial opening between two cavities or channels or between a cavity or tube and the exterior (Melloni 2001). A stoma might also be called an "ostomy" to create a passage to allow for the contents of the gastrointestinal tract to move from the interior to the outside of the body through an opening in the skin.

A **gastrostomy** involves making an incision into the stomach to permit insertion of a synthetic feeding tube. This surgery is performed on patients who are unable to ingest food normally because of stricture or lesion of the esophagus. A **colostomy** is the creation of an artificial opening of the colon through the abdominal wall. It involves bringing a loop of the large intestine out through a small abdominal incision, suturing it to the skin, and opening it. This resulting colostomy provides a temporary channel for the emptying of feces. This procedure is performed to give the bowel a rest following a colon resection. When the bowel is able to return to normal functioning, the loop colostomy is closed. An **ileostomy** is the creation of an opening of the ileum through the abdominal wall. A loop ileostomy involves transposing a segment of the small intestine to the exterior of the body.

The root operation **Bypass** is defined as altering the route of passage of the contents of a tubular body part. The root operation Bypass is used to code gastrostomy, colostomy, ileostomy, and other enterostomy. Using either the term "bypass" in the Index or the title of the procedure (gastrostomy, colostomy, or ileostomy) leads the coder to Table 0D1 with the following characters to complete the code:

- The fourth character identifies the body part where the ostomy started, for example, the stomach, a part of the colon, or the ileum or other part of the digestive tract.

- The fifth character identifies the approach with the options of Open, Percutaneous Endoscopic, or Via Natural or Artificial Opening Endoscopic.

- The sixth character identifies if a synthetic or tissue substitute is used to create the bypass.

- The seventh character (the qualifier) is intended to identify where the new passage route is directed, for example, if the bypass ends through an opening in the skin, the seventh character is 4 for Cutaneous (skin).

Intestinal Resection

Colorectal surgery is often the treatment of colon cancer or other diseases of the colon, such as ulcerative colitis or Crohn's disease. Colectomy procedures or colon resections remove portions of the large intestine to treat the disease. The procedures can be performed through an incision (open procedure) or done with a laparoscope. Open surgeries can require six- to ten-inch incisions and are highly invasive procedures that require long recovery periods. Open and other partial excisions of the large intestine are reported with the ICD-10-PCS root operations Excision or Resection to classify such procedures.

The Index contains titles of gastrointestinal procedures and directional notes to see another term in the Index such as hemicolectomy (see Resection), colectomy (see Excision or Resection, gastrointestinal tract), sigmoidectomy (see Excision or Resection), and other similar procedures. The entries direct the coder to either 0DB or 0DT, as shown in table 14.3.

Table 14.3. **Excision and Resection**

Excision	Resection
0 Medical and Surgical	0 Medical and Surgical
D Gastrointestinal System	D Gastrointestinal System
B Excision: Cutting out or off, without replacement, a portion of a body part	**T Resection**: Cutting out or off, without replacement, all of a body part

The fourth character for both Excision and Resection is the body part excised or resected, such as Large Intestine, Right or Large Intestine, Left; Duodenum; Jejunum; Ileum; or Ascending, Descending, Transverse, or Sigmoid Colon, and such. The fifth character identifies the approach, specifically, Open, Percutaneous, Percutaneous Endoscopic, Via Natural or Artificial Opening, or Via Natural or Artificial Opening Endoscopic. A laparoscopic procedure would be the approach of Percutaneous Endoscopic. There is no option for the sixth character or seventh character other than Z, meaning there is no device and no qualifier.

An **anastomosis** is the surgical formation of a channel between tubular structures, such as blood vessels or intestines. The anastomosis performed as part of a colon resection would be coded separately with the root operation Bypass using Table 0D1, which identifies the two parts of the colon connected with the fourth character (body part) representing one end of the anastomosis and the seventh character identifying the other end where the two parts of the colon are connected.

Laparotomy

A **laparotomy** is an incision into the abdominal wall. If the laparotomy is for the purposes of opening the cavity, the definitive procedure performed in the cavity is coded with the approach Open. The definitive procedure may be a biopsy, control of postoperative bleeding, drainage, lysis of adhesions (release), or removal of a device. If the laparotomy is for exploratory purposes only, the root operation Inspection is coded with the approach Open.

ICD-10-CM and ICD-10-PCS Review Exercises: Chapter 14

Assign the correct ICD-10-CM diagnosis codes and ICD-10-PCS procedure codes to the following exercises.

1. Recurrent right inguinal hernia with gangrene and obstruction

    _____

2. Acute gastric ulcer with hemorrhage

    _____

3. Choledocholithiasis with acute cholangitis and obstruction

    _____

4. Leukoplakia of mouth and tongue

    _____

5. Chronic duodenal ulcer with hemorrhage; Chronic blood loss anemia

    _____

6. The patient is a 65-year-old woman who was admitted to the hospital for repair of an incisional hernia. During her pre-anesthesia evaluation, it was determined that she had both hypertension that was not well controlled and acute on chronic diastolic heart failure. The anesthesiologist and attending physician advised the patient that her surgery would be canceled in order to manage her medical conditions. The patient stayed in the hospital two days for treatment of the heart failure and hypertension and then was discharged with an appointment to see her attending physician in one week to evaluate if and when the hernia surgery can be rescheduled.

    _____

7. The patient is a 56-year-old man who was admitted with cellulitis of the abdominal wall due to an infection at the patient's colostomy site. It was determined that the infection was due to enterococcus and it was treated successfully with intravenous antibiotics.

    _____

8. Chronic alcoholic hepatitis with ascites; Chronic alcoholism

    _____

9. Acute and chronic cholecystitis with cholelithiasis

    _____

10. Irritable bowel syndrome with diarrhea

    _____

11. Rectal polyp

    _____

12. Acute and chronic pancreatitis

    _____

(Continued on next page)

ICD-10-CM and ICD-10-PCS Review Exercises: Chapter 14 (Continued)

13. Postgastrectomy malabsorption syndrome

_____

14. Diverticulitis of small intestine with abscess and perforation/rupture

_____

15. PROCEDURE: Laparoscopic cholecystectomy

_____

16. PROCEDURE: Colonoscopy with excision of colon polyp, descending colon

_____

17. PROCEDURE: Laparotomy with resection of a portion of the small intestine

_____

18. PROCEDURE: Open cholecystectomy with open choledocholithotomy

_____

19. PROCEDURE: Percutaneous needle biopsy of liver

_____

20. PROCEDURE: Left inguinal herniorrhaphy with mesh (synthetic material)

_____

Chapter 15

Diseases of the Skin and Subcutaneous Tissue (L00–L99)

Learning Objectives

At the conclusion of this chapter, you should be able to:

1. Describe the organization of the conditions and codes included in Chapter 12 of ICD-10-CM, Diseases of the skin and subcutaneous tissue (L00–L99)

2. Define and differentiate between the terms *cellulitis* and *abscess*

3. Describe the different stages of decubitus or pressure ulcers

4. Assign ICD-10-CM codes for diseases of the skin and subcutaneous tissue

5. Assign ICD-10-PCS codes for procedures related to diseases of the skin and subcutaneous tissue

Key Terms

- Abscess
- Actinic keratosis
- Cellulitis
- Debridement
- Decubitus ulcer
- Dermatitis
- Erythema
- Hyperhidrosis
- Lymphangitis
- Pressure ulcer
- Stage I pressure ulcer
- Stage II pressure ulcer
- Stage III pressure ulcer
- Stage IV pressure ulcer
- Stevens-Johnson syndrome (SJS)
- Toxic epidermal necrolysis (TEN)

- Unstageable pressure ulcer
- Urticaria

Overview of ICD-10-CM Chapter 12, Diseases of the Skin and Subcutaneous Tissue

Chapter 12 includes categories L00–L99 arranged in the following blocks:

L00–L08	Infections of the skin and subcutaneous tissue
L10–L14	Bullous disorders
L20–L30	Dermatitis and eczema
L40–L45	Papulosquamous disorders
L49–L54	Urticaria and erythema
L55–L59	Radiation-related disorders of the skin and subcutaneous tissue
L60–L75	Disorders of skin appendages
L76	Intraoperative and postprocedural complications of skin and subcutaneous tissue
L80–L99	Other disorders of the skin and subcutaneous tissue

Chapter 12 of ICD-10-CM is organized into blocks of codes for diseases of the skin and subcutaneous tissue that are grouped into similar types of conditions, for example, dermatitis and eczema is separated from urticaria and erythematous conditions. A block of codes for radiation-related disorders of the skin and subcutaneous tissue is included in ICD-10-CM that was not contained in previous classification systems.

The Chapter 12 codes contain specificity for the conditions at the fourth-, fifth-, and sixth-character levels. The specific site where the condition exists is included, for example, parts of the trunk are described as back, chest wall, groin, perineum, and umbilicus. Laterality is also part of the code's description, such as right upper limb, left lower limb, and such. Combination codes are included, for example, the codes for decubitus ulcers represent the site, the laterality, and the stage of the ulcer all in one code.

Coding Guidelines and Instructional Notes for ICD-10-CM Chapter 12, Diseases of the Skin and Subcutaneous Tissue

At the start of Chapter 12 in ICD-10-CM, a series of conditions listed under an Excludes2 note identifies conditions in other chapters that may be coded with diseases of the skin and subcutaneous tissue. As an example, diseases of the skin and subcutaneous tissue that are connective tissue disorders, viral conditions, or related to endocrine, nutritional, and metabolic diseases are classified to other chapters of ICD-10-CM.

An instruction "use additional code (B95–B97) to identify infectious agent" follows the heading for the block of codes for infections of the skin and subcutaneous tissue (L00–L08).

Instructions for coding dermatitis and eczema are included in Chapter 12. For example, the note "in this block the terms dermatitis and eczema are used synonymously and interchangeably" is included in the description of conditions classified to categories L20–L30. Additionally, the Excludes2 note for categories L20–L30 states:

Dermatitis and Eczema (L20–L30)

Excludes2   chronic (childhood) granulomatous disease (D71)

dermatitis gangrenosa (L08.0)

dermatitis herpetiformis (L13.0)

dry skin dermatitis (L85.3)

factitial dermatitis (L98.1)

perioral dermatitis (L71.0)

radiation-related disorders of skin and subcutaneous tissue (L55–L59)

stasis dermatitis (I83.1–I83.2)

Category L23, Allergic contact dermatitis, and category L24, Irritant contact dermatitis, include both Excludes1 and Excludes2 notes that identify what allergic or irritant contact dermatitis conditions can or cannot be coded with conditions classified in categories L23 and L24. For the conditions that are due to drugs in contact with the skin, a "use additional code for adverse effect, if applicable, to identify drug (T36–T50 with fifth or sixth character 5)" appears to direct the coder to use the additional code.

EXAMPLE: L23.3 Allergic contact dermatitis due to drugs in contact with skin

Use additional code for adverse effect, if applicable, to identify drug (T36–T50 with fifth or sixth character 5)

L24.4 Irritant contact dermatitis due to drugs in contact with skin

Use additional code for adverse effect, if applicable, to identify drug (T36–T50 with fifth or sixth character 5)

Other codes such as L25.1, Unspecified contact dermatitis due to drugs in contact with skin, L27.0 and L27.1 for generalized and localized skin eruption due to drugs and medicaments taken internally, and L43.2, Lichenoid drug reaction include a similar "use additional code" note relating to the adverse affect of drugs.

Skin and subcutaneous tissue conditions can be caused by other diseases and the underlying condition is significant in describing the total clinical situation. Within Chapter 12 of ICD-10-CM, there are codes identified as present "in diseases classified elsewhere." For these conditions, the coder is reminded to "Code first underlying disease" as shown with the following codes:

L14 Bullous disorders in diseases classified elsewhere

L45 Papulosquamous disorders in diseases classified elsewhere

L54 Erythema in diseases classified elsewhere

The NCHS has published chapter-specific guidelines for Chapter 12 in the *ICD-10-CM Official Guidelines for Coding and Reporting*. The coding student should review all of the coding guidelines for Chapter 12 of ICD-10-CM, which appear in an ICD-10-CM code book or at the website http://www.cdc.gov/nchs/icd/icd10cm.htm, or in Appendix E.

CG **Guideline 1.C.12.a. Pressure ulcer stage codes**

1. Pressure ulcer stages

   Codes from category L89, Pressure ulcer, are combination codes that identify the site of the pressure ulcer as well as the stage of the ulcer.

   The ICD-10-CM classifies pressure ulcer stages based on severity, which is designated by stages 1 to 4, unspecified stage and unstageable.

   Assign as many codes from category L89 as needed to identify all the pressure ulcers the patient has, if applicable.

2. Unstageable pressure ulcers

   Assignment of the code for unstageable pressure ulcer (L89.–0) should be based on the clinical documentation. These codes are used for pressure ulcers whose stage cannot be clinically determined (e.g., the ulcer is covered by eschar or has been treated with a skin or muscle graft) and pressure ulcers that are documented as deep tissue injury but not documented as due to trauma. This code should not be confused with the codes for unspecified stage (L89.–9). When there is no documentation regarding the stage of the pressure ulcer, assign the appropriate code for unspecified stage (L89.–9).

3. Documented pressure ulcer stage

   Assignment of the pressure ulcer stage code should be guided by clinical documentation of the stage or documentation of the terms found in the Alphabetic Index. For clinical terms describing the stage that are not found in the Alphabetic Index, and there is no documentation of the stage, the provider should be queried.

4. Patients admitted with pressure ulcers documented as healed

   No code is assigned if the documentation states that the pressure ulcer is completely healed.

5. Patients admitted with pressure ulcers documented as healing

   Pressure ulcers described as healing should be assigned the appropriate pressure ulcer stage code based on the documentation in the medical record. If the documentation does not provide information about the stage of the healing pressure ulcer, assign the appropriate code for unspecified stage.

If the documentation is unclear as to whether the patient has a current (new) pressure ulcer or if the patient is being treated for a healing pressure ulcer, query the provider.

6. Patient admitted with pressure ulcer evolving into another stage during the admission

If a patient is admitted with a pressure ulcer at one stage and it progresses to a higher stage, assign the code for the highest stage reported for that site.

Coding Diseases of Skin and Subcutaneous Tissue in ICD-10-CM Chapter 12

Chapter 12 of ICD-10-CM, Diseases of the skin and subcutaneous tissue (L00–L99), contains specific codes for infections of the skin and subcutaneous tissue, bullous disorders, dermatitis, eczema, papulosquamous disorders, urticaria, erythema, radiation-related skin disorders, pressure ulcers, and nonpressure chronic skin ulcers as well as intraoperative and postprocedural complications of skin and subcutaneous tissue.

Many codes include laterality, such as L02.522, Furuncle of the left hand, and L03.111, Cellulitis of the right axilla. Codes for unspecified sides of the body, such as L02.639, Carbuncle of unspecified foot, also exist.

Cutaneous Abscess and Cellulitis (L02–L03)

Cellulitis is an acute inflammation of a localized area of superficial tissue. Predisposing conditions are open wounds, ulcerations, tinea pedis, and dermatitis, but these conditions need not be present for cellulitis to occur. Physical findings of cellulitis reveal red, hot skin with edema at the site of the infection. The area is tender, and the skin surface has a *peau d'orange* (skin of an orange) appearance with ill-defined borders. Nearby lymph nodes often become inflamed.

A cutaneous or subcutaneous **abscess** is a localized collection of pus causing fluctuant soft-tissue swelling surrounded by erythema. These abscesses usually follow minor skin trauma, and the organisms isolated are typically bacterial infection indigenous to the skin of the involved area. Abscesses may occur internally in tissues, organs, and confined spaces. An abscess begins as cellulitis. Cellulitis will clear within a few days with antibiotic treatment. Although drainage of abscesses may occur spontaneously, some abscesses may require incision and drainage, and possibly antibiotic therapy.

Lymphangitis is the inflammation of lymph nodes. These lymph nodes are located superficially under the skin. Streptococcus bacteria are the common cause of lymphangitis. The bacteria usually invade the lymph nodes through openings in the skin caused by abrasions, lacerations, or skin infections. Symptoms of lymphangitis include warm, tender, red streaks on the affected area. The lymph nodes are warm, tender, and enlarged near the original injury, which could be a minor skin wound. It is important to treat lymphangitis quickly as there is the possibility that bacteria could spread quickly through the lymph system to other parts of the body.

ICD-10-CM classifies cellulitis and acute lymphangitis to the category code L03. The category code is subdivided to fourth-character subcategories that identify the site, such as finger and toe, other parts of limb, face and neck, trunk and other sites. Within the fourth-character, there are fifth-character codes that separate the two conditions—a set of codes for cellulitis and another set for lymphangitis. The sixth-character code identifies the condition, cellulitis or lymphangitis, and the anatomic site including laterality. An additional code should be assigned to identify the organism involved.

> **EXAMPLE:** Cellulitis of the left upper arm due to *Streptococcus*: L03.114, Cellulitis of left upper limb; B95.5, Unspecified *Streptococcus* as the cause of diseases classified elsewhere

Dermatitis and Eczema (L20–L30)

A note under block L20–L30, Dermatitis and eczema, indicates that in this block, the terms "dermatitis" and "eczema" are used synonymously and interchangeably. **Dermatitis** is an inflammation of the skin. There is no single test to diagnose dermatitis. The diagnosis is determined by the appearance of the skin and a thorough medical history. Treatment of the condition depends on the severity and identified cause. Medications may be prescribed to control the itchy nature of it, as well as drugs to control secondary infections. ICD-10-CM classifies dermatitis and eczema according to its cause or clinical type as follows:

L20—Atopic dermatitis
Atopic dermatitis is a noninfectious chronic skin inflammation characterized by itchy, inflamed skin usually in individuals who also have asthma or hay fever.

L21—Seborrheic dermatitis
Seborrheic dermatitis is an inflammation of unknown cause that appears on the scalp, eyebrows, and behind the ears as well as on the body that presents with varying degrees of redness, scaling and itchiness. In its mildest form it is known as dandruff.

L22—Diaper dermatitis
Diaper dermatitis is also known as diaper rash, which is skin irritation cause by prolonged dampness from urine, feces, and sweat in contact with the baby's skin.

L23—Allergic contact dermatitis
This is a skin inflammation or a localized reaction of redness, itching, and possibly blisters that is due to contact between the skin and an allergy-producing substance that may be a naturally occurring or manufactured substance. Common allergens are metals in jewelry or objects a person comes in contact with, adhesives, cosmetics, drugs in contact with the skin, dyes, certain chemical products like plastic or rubber, food in contact with the skin, plants, and animals.

L24—Irritant contact dermatitis
Irritant contact dermatitis is similar to allergic contact dermatitis in its presentation of redness, blisters, and itching but the substance is more likely chemical products that produce irritation such as detergents, oils, greasers, and solvents; it also can be caused by cosmetics, other chemical products, food, and plants that come in contact with the skin.

L25—Unspecified contact dermatitis
Category L25 is for use when the diagnosis of allergic or irritant contact dermatitis cannot be made but the cause may be specified as cosmetics, chemical products, dyes,

food, or plants in contact with the skin as well as the possibility that the substance is not identified but its presentation is consistent with contact dermatitis.

L26—Exfoliative dermatitis
This form of the disease produces a generalized exfoliation or shedding, pealing, or scaling of skin. Another exfoliative disease is exfoliative neonatorum dermatitis or Ritter's disease, a serious condition affecting young children and coded with L00.

L27—Dermatitis due to substances taken internally
The substances taken internally can be drugs and medications, ingested food, and other substances taken internally. An instructional note is included under the codes for generalized and localized skin eruptions due to drugs and medicaments to use an additional code for adverse effect, if applicable, to identify the drug (T36–T50 with fifth or sixth character 5).

Urticaria and Erythema (L49–L54)

Urticaria is the eruption of itchy patches of skin called wheals or a round raised area of skin. It is thought to be due to hypersensitivity to food or drugs and can also have an emotional component. It may be referred to as hives. Hives develop when natural chemicals including histamines are released in the skin as an allergic reaction to something but can also occur due to a nonallergic cause such as an autoimmune disease. Hives usually resolve quickly in less than 24 hours. The best treatment is to find the cause and eliminate contact with it. Persistent hives are usually treated with over-the-counter antihistamine topical ointments or creams. When hives are present with respiratory problems, emergency medical care is warranted.

Erythema is redness of the skin due to capillary dilation. Erythematous conditions are skin disorders relating to or marked by erythema. A number of distinct disorders are included in categories L51–L53. Erythema multiforme is an acute eruption of macules, papules, or subepidermal vesicles presenting in a multiform appearance. The characteristic lesions appear over the dorsal aspect of the hands and forearms. Its origin may be allergic, drug sensitivity, or it may be caused by herpes simplex infection. The eruption may be self-limited (erythema multiforme minor) or recurrent, or it could run a severe and possibly fatal course (erythema multiforme major).

Stevens-Johnson syndrome (SJS) is a bullous form of erythema multiforme that may be extensive over the body and produce serious subjective symptoms and possibly death. **Toxic epidermal necrolysis (TEN)** may also occur with SJS. TEN is a syndrome in which large portions of skin become intensely erythematous with epidermal necrolysis. The skin peels off the body in the manner of a second-degree burn. This condition may result from drug sensitivity but often its cause is unknown. Codes are available to describe SJS (code L51.1), SJS with TEN (L51.3), and TEN (L51.2).

If erythema multiforme is caused by an adverse effect of a drug, an instructional note reminds the coder to use additional code to identify the drug (T36–T50 with fifth or sixth character 5). Erythema multiforme produces other physical manifestations. An instructional note appears under the category L51 to use additional code(s) to assign codes for such conditions as arthropathy, conjunctivitis, corneal ulcer, and other conditions of eye that erythema multiforme can produce.

Erythema nodosum is the single condition classified with category code L52. Category L53, Other erythematous conditions, is separated at the fourth-character level into other forms of erythema. Toxic erythema (L53.0) may be caused by a drug or toxin poisoning or as a result of an adverse effect of a drug. A "code first" note for the poisoning and a "use additional code" note to identify the drug producing the adverse effect of toxic erythema remind the coder to assign the applicable codes.

Category code L49 identifies exfoliation due to erythematous conditions according to extent of body surface involved. Subcategory codes L49.0–L49.9 are used to describe the percentage of body surface that has the exfoliation. A "code first" note appears within the category to direct the coder to code first the erythematous condition causing the exfoliation, such as Ritter's disease, Staphylococcal scalded skin syndrome, SJS with or without TEN overlap, or toxic epidermal necrolysis.

Radiation-Related Disorders of the Skin and Subcutaneous Tissue (L55–L59)

Codes in this block of codes are skin conditions or skin damage that was caused by radiation such as solar factors, ultraviolet light, and nonionizing radiation. The sun is the major source of ultraviolet light damage to skin. But tanning bed lamps also produce ultraviolet light responsible for tanning and the resulting skin damage from overexposure.

Category L55, Sunburn, include four-character codes to identify first degree (L55.0), second degree (L55.1), and third degree sunburns (L55.2). An unspecified code for "sunburn" with no degree specified exists with L55.9.

Category L56 classifies other acute skin changes due to ultraviolet radiation. A "use additional" code note appears under the category heading to assign a code from W89 or X32 to identify the source of the ultraviolet radiation such as exposure to man-made visible and ultraviolet light or exposure to sunlight.

Conditions that are coded to this category are solar urticaria (L56.3) and disseminated superficial actinic porokeratosis (DSAP) (L56.5).

Skin damage can also be produced by chronic exposure to ultraviolet light radiation. Category code L37 contains codes for skin changes from this chronic exposure. The most common condition that is coded in this category is actinic keratosis (L57.0). **Actinic keratosis** is a precancerous growth on the skin that occurs on exposed areas of the body such as on the face and neck. These growths are the result of long-term sun exposure and have proven to progress to skin cancer if left untreated.

Disorders of Skin Appendages (L60–L75)

Categories L60–L75 contain some of the more commonly diagnosed and treated skin and nail conditions. Nail disorders such as ingrowing nail, oncolysis, and nail dystrophy are individual codes within category L60. Forms of alopecia and conditions involving hair loss are identified with codes in categories L65–L66. Hair color, hair shaft abnormalities, and excessive hair (hypertrichosis and hirsutism) are disorders coded with category codes L67–L68.

Some of the more frequently occurring and treated skin conditions that are treated in physicians' offices and ambulatory settings are contained in categories L70 for different types of acne, L71 for rosacea and rhinophyma, and L72 for follicular cysts of skin and subcutaneous tissue. Epidermal, pilar, trichodermal, and sebaceous cysts are examples of follicular cysts commonly excised in an outpatient setting when the cyst becomes enlarged or infected.

Eccrine sweat and apocrine sweat gland disorders are classified with codes from categories L74 and L75. Primary focal hyperhidrosis of the axilla, face, palms, and soles are coded with six-character codes L74.510–L74.513. **Hyperhidrosis** is excessive perspiration where the exact cause is unknown and can occur spontaneously. Topical preparations help reduce the sweating and botulinum toxin (Botox) injections also decrease sweat secretion.

Pressure (Decubitus) Ulcer (L89)

Category L89, Pressure ulcer, contains combination codes that identify the site, the laterality, as well as the stage of the pressure ulcer. Pressure ulcers may also be documented by a physician or a wound care provider as a decubitus ulcer or bed sore. No code is assigned in ICD-10-CM if the documentation states that the pressure ulcer is completely healed. For all the codes in category L89, Pressure ulcer, there is a note to "Code first any associated gangrene (I96)."

The codes for pressure ulcers are very specific:

- Individual codes are mostly six characters long with five-character codes for pressure ulcers of unspecified sites.

- Category L89 for pressure ulcers is a three-character category code.

- Each of the four-character codes identifies the anatomic site, such as elbow, back, hip, buttocks, contiguous sites of the back, ankle, heel, and other sites.

- Each of the five-character codes for each anatomic site identifies if the site is the right side of the body, left side, or unspecified side.

- Each of the six-character codes for each of the anatomic sites with its laterality identified includes the stage of the ulcer.

Examples of these codes follow:

L89.001	Pressure ulcer of unspecified elbow stage 1
L89.132	Pressure ulcer of right lower back, stage 2
L89.223	Pressure ulcer of left hip, stage 3
L89.314	Pressure ulcer of right buttock, stage 4
L89.520	Pressure ulcer of left ankle, unstageable

Pressure ulcers or **decubitus ulcers** are caused by tissue hypoxia secondary to pressure-induced vascular insufficiency, and they may become secondarily infected with components of the skin and gastrointestinal flora. The ulceration of tissue usually is at the location of a bony prominence that has been subjected to prolonged pressure against an external object, such as a bed, wheelchair, cast, or splint. Tissues over the elbows, sacrum, ischia, greater trochanters of the hip, external malleoli of the ankle, and heels are most susceptible. Other sites may be involved depending on the patient's positions. Patients may have more than one pressure ulcer, located at different sites on the body. Pressure ulcers may extend into deeper tissue including muscle and bone. The ulcers may also be referred to as pressure sores or bedsores.

The depth of the ulcer is identified by stages I through IV. According to the National Pressure Ulcer Advisory Panel the descriptions of the four stages are as follows:

Stage I   Intact skin with non-blanching erythema of a localized area usually over a bony prominence. This appears as a reddened area on the skin. It may be referred to as discoloration of the skin without ulceration.

Stage II   Abrasion, blister, shallow open ulcer or crater with a red pink wound bed, or other partial thickness skin loss

Stage III   Full-thickness skin loss involving damage or necrosis into subcutaneous soft tissues. Bone, tendon, and muscle are not exposed but slough may be present and may include undermining and tunneling.

Stage IV Full-thickness skin loss with necrosis of soft tissues through to the muscle, tendons, or tissues around underlying bone. The exposed bone, tendon, and muscle are visible in the wound. It often includes undermining and tunneling. Slough or eschar may be present on some parts of the wound bed (NPUAP 2012).

Pressure ulcers may also be described as "unstageable." This is a specific type of pressure ulcer, and should not be used when stages I through IV are not documented. When the documentation is absent, a code for pressure ulcer, stage unspecified is used. An **unstageable pressure ulcer** has full-thickness tissue loss in which the base of the ulcer is covered by slough or eschar in the wound bed or has been treated with a skin or muscle flap. Stages I and II may be described as superficial lesions, with more serious lesions being identified as stages III and IV.

Non-Pressure Chronic Ulcer of Lower Limb, Not Elsewhere Classified (L97)

A patient may have a chronic ulcer of the skin of the lower limbs as a sole problem or the ulcer may be the result of another condition. A code from L97 may be used as a principal or first-listed code if no underlying condition is documented as the cause of the ulcer. An important note under category L97 instructs the coder to "code first" any of the following underlying conditions:

Code first any associated underlying condition, such as:

- Atherosclerosis of the lower extremities (I70.23-, I70.24-, I70.33-, I70.34-, I70.43-, I70.44-, I70.53-, I70.54-, I70.63-, I70.64-, I70.73-, I70.74-)

- Chronic venous hypertension (I87.31-, I87.33-)

- Diabetic ulcers (E08.621, E08.622, E09.621, E09.622, E10.621, E10.622, E11.621, E11.622, E13.621, E13.622)

- Postphlebitic syndrome (I87.01-, I87.03-)

- Postthrombotic syndrome (I87.01-, I87.03-)

- Varicose ulcer (I83.0-, I83.2-)

Another note instructs the coder to "Code first any associated gangrene (I96)."

Individual codes in category L97 include (1) the site, (2) the laterality of (a) right, (b) left, or (c) unspecified, and (3) the severity of the ulcer identified as (a) limited to breakdown of skin, (b) fat layer exposed, (c) necrosis of muscle, (d) necrosis of bone, or (e) unspecified.

ICD-10-PCS Procedure Coding for Diseases of the Skin and Subcutaneous Tissues

Procedures that are performed on the skin and subcutaneous tissue are included in the two tables in ICD-10-PCS. Table 0H0–0HX includes the following root operations that are performed on the skin: Change, Destruction, Division, Drainage, Excision, Extirpation, Extraction, Inspection, Reattachment, Release, Removal, Repair, Replacement, Revision, and Transfer.

The same Table 0H0–0HX also include root operations that are performed on the breast, specifically Alteration, Change, Destruction, Drainage, Excision, Extirpation, Insertion,

Inspection, Reattachment, Release, Removal, Repair, Replacement, Reposition, Resection, Supplement, and Revision.

A different table is used to construct ICD-10-PCS procedure codes for root operations performed on subcutaneous tissue and fascia, 0J0–0JX. The root operations for these procedures are Alteration, Change, Destruction, Division, Drainage, Excision, Extirpation, Extraction, Insertion, Inspection, Release, Removal, Repair, Replacement, Supplement, Revision, and Transfer.

Like procedures in other body systems, in order to code procedures on the skin and subcutaneous tissue, the coder needs to know the definition of root operations and the anatomy and laterality to identify the body parts.

Operations on Skin and Subcutaneous Tissue

Commonly performed operations on skin and subcutaneous tissue includes excision of skin and subcutaneous lesions and skin grafting as well as the insertion of infusion pumps and totally implantable vascular access devices for chemotherapy or other long-term infusion.

Excision of skin lesions are coded using the root operation Excision or cutting out or off, without replacement, a portion of a body part from the root operation Table 0HB. An excision of skin is usually done for therapeutic purposes to remove a known diseased lesion. A skin biopsy is also a common procedure; however, a biopsy is a diagnostic procedure and would be identified with an Excision ICD-10-PCS code with the qualifier X for Diagnostic.

Table 0HT, for Resection or cutting out or off, without replacement, all of a body part does not contain the body part of Skin because it is not possible to perform a resection of skin as all of the skin could not possibly be performed. Body parts in the integumentary system that could be resected or completely removed are finger- and toenails, a breast, or a breast nipple. For example, the resection of the left breast would be coded 0HTU0ZZ in the Medical and Surgical section.

Excision of subcutaneous tissue and fascia is coded using the root operation Excision (0JB) but there is no table for Resection of subcutaneous tissue because it is not possible to cut out or off, without replacement, all of that body part, which is the definition of resection.

Skin grafting is described with the root operation Replacement when a full-thickness or partial-thickness graft is performed on skin. If a skin substitute is grafted into place on the skin, the root operation Supplement would describe the objective of the procedure, that is, putting in or on biological or synthetic material that physically reinforces or augments the function of a portion of a body part.

Insertion of infusion pumps and totally implantable vascular access devices is coded to the root operation of Insertion for subcutaneous tissue. There is no option to insert a device into skin. The type of device left in place is identified with the character 6 for the device. The choices for devices implanted in the subcutaneous tissue are an Infusion Pump device, Vascular Access Device Reservoir, and Vascular Access Device.

Debridement

Debridement is the removal of foreign material and contaminated or devitalized tissue from, or adjacent to, a traumatic or infected lesion until the surrounding healthy tissue is exposed. There is no root operation in ICD-10-PCS of simply the term "debridement."

ICD-10-PCS classifies debridement depending on whether it was identified as excisional or nonexcisional debridement. Following the main term "debridement" in the ICD-10-PCS Index, the entry of debridement, excisional sends the coder to the entry for the root operation Excision. If the debridement was described as nonexcisional debridement, the Index sends the coder to the entry for the root operation Extraction.

For excisional debridement, the entry in the Index is the main term "excision," with a sub-term of "skin" and it refers the coder to Table 0HB. The code is constructed based on where the excisional procedure is performed on the skin, that is, what body part's skin. Likewise, entries in the Index for excision of "subcutaneous tissue and fascia" procedures direct the coder to Table 0JB to select a code for the excision of subcutaneous tissue for the debridement according to the part body where the surgery is performed.

For nonexcisional debridement, the entry in the Index is the main term "extraction, skin" and it refers the coder to Table 0HD for skin and Table 0JD for subcutaneous tissue and fascia, respectively. Similar to the excisional procedures, the extraction procedures are constructed using the body part where the skin or subcutaneous tissue is removed with a nonexcision debridement procedure.

ICD-10-CM and ICD-10-PCS Review Exercises: Chapter 15

Assign the correct ICD-10-CM diagnosis and ICD-10-PCS procedure codes to the following exercises.

1. Actinic keratosis, right temple due to excessive exposure to sunlight (initial encounter)

2. Hidradenitis suppurativa, bilateral axilla

3. Localized primary hyperhidrosis of soles of both feet

4. Stage 4 pressure ulcer of sacrum

5. Chronic trophic ulcer of right calf with only skin breakdown

6. The patient was seen for initial treatment of a fine rash that had developed on the patient's trunk over the last three to four days. The patient was diagnosed with hypertension seven days ago and started on Ramipril 10 mg daily. The physician determined the rash to be dermatitis due to the Ramipril. The Ramipril was discontinued and the patient was prescribed a new antihypertensive medication, Captopril. In addition, the physician prescribed a topical cream for the localized dermatitis.

ICD-10-CM and ICD-10-PCS Review Exercises: Chapter 15 (Continued)

7. Irritant contact dermatitis due to cosmetics; Cystic acne

   The patient was seen with extensive inflammation and irritation of the skin of both upper eyelids and under her eyebrows that was spreading to her temples and forehead. Upon questioning the patient, the physician learned that she had recently used new eye cosmetics. The physician had examined the patient during a prior visit for cystic acne. During this visit, the physician also examined the patient's cystic acne on her forehead and jawline. The patient was advised to continue using the medication previously prescribed. The patient was also advised to immediately discontinue use of any makeup on the face and was given a topical medication to resolve the inflammation, which was an adverse effect of the cosmetics.

8. Cellulitis of the right anterior neck treated with intravenous antibiotics. The patient is also a known morphine drug abuser and exhibited considerable drug-seeking behavior, continuously requesting morphine. All narcotics were discontinued and the patient exhibited no drug withdrawal symptoms.

9. Pilonidal cyst with abscess

10. Erythema multiforme major nonbullous

11. Acute lymphadenitis bilateral lower limbs

12. Stevens-Johnson syndrome with toxic epidermal overlap syndrome, with skin exfoliation 10 percent of body surface

13. Pressure ulcer, stage 2, heel, left

14. Psoriatic juvenile arthropathy

15. PROCEDURE: Incision and drainage of abscess of pilonidal cyst, lower back

16. PROCEDURE: Excisional debridement of subcutaneous tissue and fascia, buttock by open approach

17. PROCEDURE: Skin biopsy, left cheek (face)

(Continued on next page)

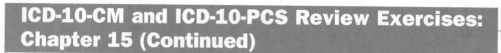

ICD-10-CM and ICD-10-PCS Review Exercises: Chapter 15 (Continued)

18. PROCEDURE: Excision of skin lesion, left cheek

_____

19. PROCEDURE: Cryoablation of multiple skin lesions on chest

_____

20. PROCEDURE: Cosmetic augmentation mammaplasty, bilateral with synthetic material implanted for the augmentation

_____

Chapter 16

Diseases of the Musculoskeletal System and Connective Tissue (M00–M99)

Learning Objectives

At the conclusion of this chapter, you should be able to:

1. Describe the organization of the conditions and codes included in Chapter 13 of ICD-10-CM, Diseases of the musculoskeletal system and connective tissue (M00–M99)

2. Describe the classification of rheumatoid arthritis and osteoarthritis

3. Describe the coding of various types of deforming dorsopathies

4. Define the two types of *compartment syndrome*

5. Describe the classification of different forms of osteoporosis

6. Define and differentiate between coding of *pathologic, malunion, nonunion,* and *stress* fractures

7. Describe the classification of different types of osteomyelitis

8. Describe the ICD-10-PCS coding of arthroscopic surgery and joint replacement procedures

9. Assign ICD-10-CM codes for diseases of the musculoskeletal system and connective tissue

10. Assign ICD-10-PCS codes for procedures related to diseases of the musculoskeletal system and connective tissue

Key Terms

- Ankylosis
- Arthroscope
- Compartment syndrome: traumatic and nontraumatic
- Direct infection of joint
- Felty's syndrome
- Indirect infection of joint
- Kyphosis

- Lordosis
- Malunion
- Nonunion
- Osteoarthritis
- Osteomyelitis
- Osteoporosis
- Pathologic fracture
- Polyosteoarthritis
- Primary osteoarthritis
- Rheumatism
- Rheumatoid arthritis
- Scoliosis
- Secondary osteoarthritis
- Spinal stenosis
- Spondylopathy
- Spondylosis
- Stress fracture
- Systemic lupus erythematosus (SLE)

Overview of ICD-10-CM Chapter 13, Diseases of the Musculoskeletal System and Connective Tissue

Chapter 13 of ICD-10-CM includes categories M00–M99 arranged in the following blocks:

M00–M02	Infectious arthropathies
M05–M14	Inflammatory polyarthropathies
M15–M19	Osteoarthritis
M20–M25	Other joint disorders
M26–M27	Dentofacial anomalies [including malocclusion] and other disorders of jaw
M30–M36	Systemic connective tissue disorders
M40–M43	Deforming dorsopathies
M45–M49	Spondylopathies
M50–M54	Other dorsopathies
M60–M63	Disorders of muscles
M65–M67	Disorders of synovium and tendon
M70–M79	Other soft tissue disorders
M80–M85	Disorders of bone density and structure
M86–M90	Other osteopathies

M91–M94	Chondropathies
M95	Other disorders of the musculoskeletal system and connective tissue
M96	Intraoperative and postprocedural complications and disorders of musculoskeletal system, not elsewhere classified
M99	Biomechanical lesions, not elsewhere classified

The codes in Chapter 13 of ICD-10-CM have been expanded to include greater anatomic specificity and laterality.

EXAMPLES: M23.011   Cystic meniscus, anterior horn of medial meniscus, right knee

M89.151   Complete physeal arrest, right proximal femur

Instructional notes have been expanded indicating that additional codes should be assigned for associated conditions and that underlying conditions should be coded first.

EXAMPLES: Arthritis of right hip due to staphylococcal infection

M00.051   Staphylococcal arthritis, right hip
Use additional code (B95.61–B95.8) to identify bacterial agent

B95.8   Unspecified staphylococcus as the cause of diseases classified elsewhere

Arthropathy of left hip due to erytherma multiforme

L51.9   Erythema multiforme, Unspecified
Use additional code to identify associated manifestation, such as:
Arthropathy associated with dermatological disorders (M14.8-)

M14.852   Arthropathies in other specified diseases classified elsewhere, left hip
Code first underlying disease, such as:
Erythema multiforme (L15.1-)

The type of osteoporosis including the site of a current pathological fracture is present in one combination code in Chapter 13. Category M80, Osteoporosis with current pathological fracture combines three facts into one code: the type of osteoporosis, the site of the fracture including laterality, and the episode of care to identify the status of the patient's treatment, for example, initial versus subsequent encounter.

EXAMPLE: Pathological fracture of right humerus due to age-related osteoporosis, initial encounter for fracture

M80.021A   Age-related osteoporosis with current pathological fracture, right humerus

Some categories and subcategories in diseases of the musculoskeletal system and connective tissue require the use of a seventh character to identify the episode of care, for example, initial encounter for fracture and subsequent encounter for fracture with routine healing, delayed healing, nonunion, or malunion in addition to sequelae of the disease.

> **EXAMPLE:** Patient seen in the doctor's office for a subsequent encounter to the stress fracture of the left tibia with routine healing
>
> M84.362D   Stress fracture, left tibia, subsequent encounter for fracture with routine healing

Coding Guidelines and Instructional Notes for ICD-10-CM Chapter 13

Chapter 13 begins with the a note to "use an external cause code following the code for the musculoskeletal condition, if applicable, to identify the cause of the musculoskeletal condition." An Excludes2 note identifies the other conditions such as certain infectious, parasitic, and neoplastic diseases that can be coded with diseases of the musculoskeletal system and connective tissue.

The first block codes in the chapter, M00–M02, are for infectious arthropathies, which include arthropathies due to microbiological agents. To assist coding professionals on the correct usage of categories M00–M02, new guidelines provide definitions for direct and indirect infection.

This block comprises arthropathies due to microbiological agents. The Guidelines define two types of etiological relationships:

- **Direct infection of joint**, where organisms invade synovial tissue and microbial antigen is present in the joint.

- **Indirect infection of joint**, which may be of two types: a reactive arthropathy, where microbial infection of the body is established but neither organisms nor antigens can be identified in the joint, and a postinfective arthropathy, where microbial antigen is present but recovery of an organism is inconstant and evidence of local multiplication is lacking (CMS 2012).

Instructional notes are also added to different categories or subcategories to explain how codes should be assigned.

> **EXAMPLE:** M21.7   Unequal limb length (acquired)
> Note: The site used should correspond to the shorter limb.
>
> M50   Cervical disc disorders
> Note: Code to the most superior level of disorder.

Includes notes have also been used to define terms.

> **EXAMPLE:** M66   Spontaneous rupture of synovium and tendon
> Note: A spontaneous rupture is one that occurs when a normal force is applied to tissues that are inferred to have less than normal strength.
>
> M70   Soft tissue disorders related to use, overuse and pressure
> Includes soft tissue disorders of occupational origin

M80   Osteoporosis with current pathological fracture
Includes osteoporosis with current fragility fracture

M87   Osteonecrosis
Includes avascular necrosis of bone

The NCHS has published chapter-specific guidelines for Chapter 13 in the *ICD-10-CM Official Guidelines for Coding and Reporting.* The coding student should review all of the coding guidelines for Chapter 13 of ICD-10-CM, which appear in an ICD-10-CM code book or at the website http://www.cdc.gov/nchs/icd/icd10cm.htm, or in Appendix E.

CG

Guideline I.C.13.a. Site and laterality: Most of the codes within Chapter 13 have site and laterality designations. The site represents the bone, joint or the muscle involved. For some conditions where more than one bone, joint or muscle is usually involved, such as osteoarthritis, there is a "multiple sites" code available. For categories where no multiple site code is provided and more than one bone, joint or muscle is involved, multiple codes should be used to indicate the different sites involved.

Guideline I.C.13.a.1 Bone versus joint: For certain conditions, the bone may be affected at the upper or lower end, (e.g., avascular necrosis of bone, M87, Osteoporosis, M80, M81). Though the portion of the bone affected may be at the joint, the site designation will be the bone, not the joint.

Guideline I.C.13.b. Acute traumatic versus chronic or recurrent musculoskeletal conditions: Many musculoskeletal conditions are a result of previous injury or trauma to a site, or are recurrent conditions. Bone, joint or muscle conditions that are the result of a healed injury are usually found in chapter 13. Recurrent bone, joint or muscle conditions are also usually found in chapter 13. Any current, acute injury should be coded to the appropriate injury code from chapter 19. Chronic or recurrent conditions should generally be coded with a code from chapter 13. If it is difficult to determine from the documentation in the record which code is best to describe a condition, query the provider.

Guideline I.C.13.c. Coding of Pathologic Fractures: 7th character A is for use as long as the patient is receiving active treatment for the fracture. Examples of active treatment are: surgical treatment, emergency department encounter, evaluation and treatment by a new physician. 7th character, D is to be used for encounters after the patient has completed active treatment. The other 7th characters, listed under each subcategory in the Tabular List, are to be used for subsequent encounters for treatment of problems associated with the healing, such as malunions, nonunions, and sequelae. Care for complications of surgical treatment for fracture repairs during the healing or

(Continued)

(Continued)

recovery phase should be coded with the appropriate complication codes.

See Section I.C.19. Coding of traumatic fractures.

Guideline I.C.13.d. Osteoporosis: Osteoporosis is a systemic condition, meaning that all bones of the musculoskeletal system are affected. Therefore, site is not a component of the codes under category M81, Osteoporosis without current pathological fracture. The site codes under category M80, Osteoporosis with current pathological fracture, identify the site of the fracture, not the osteoporosis.

Guideline I.C.13.d.1 Osteoporosis without pathological fracture: Category M81, Osteoporosis without current pathological fracture, is for use for patients with osteoporosis who do not currently have a pathologic fracture due to the osteoporosis, even if they have had a fracture in the past. For patients with a history of osteoporosis fractures, status code Z87.310, Personal history of (healed) osteoporosis fracture, should follow the code from M81.

Guideline I.C.d.2 Osteoporosis with current pathological fracture: Category M80, Osteoporosis with current pathological fracture, is for patients who have a current pathologic fracture at the time of an encounter. The codes under M80 identify the site of the fracture. A code from category M80, not a traumatic fracture code, should be used for any patient with known osteoporosis who suffers a fracture, even if the patient had a minor fall or trauma, if that fall or trauma would not usually break a normal, healthy bone.

Coding Diseases of the Musculoskeletal System and Connective Tissue in ICD-10-CM Chapter 13

Chapter 13 of ICD-10-CM, Diseases of the musculoskeletal system and connective tissue (M00–M99), describes many acute and chronic conditions of bones, joints, ligaments, muscles, and intervertebral discs. We also find another code alliteration in this chapter: M codes for Musculoskeletal.

Most of the codes in Chapter 13 include site and laterality. The site indicates the bone, joint, or muscle involved. For example, there are codes for stress fracture of right tibia (M84.361), rheumatoid bursitis of left shoulder (M06.212), and muscle spasm of back (M62.830).

Seventh Characters

Some current musculoskeletal conditions in Chapter 13 are the result of a previous injury or trauma to a site and others are recurrent conditions. Any acute injury is coded using a different chapter in ICD-10-CM. However, some fractures that are included in Chapter 13 are current events. Examples of exceptions are stress fractures (M84.3) and pathological fractures (M84.4–M84.6). These fracture codes require an appropriate seventh character to identify the episode of care.

The following seventh characters are used in Chapter 13:

- A indicates initial encounter for the fracture

- D indicates subsequent encounter for fracture with routine healing

- G indicates subsequent encounter for fracture with delayed healing

- K indicates subsequent encounter for fracture with nonunion

- P indicates subsequent encounter for fracture with malunion

- S indicates sequela

Seventh character A is for use as long as the patient is receiving active treatment for the fracture. Examples of active treatment are surgical treatment, emergency department encounter, and evaluation and treatment by a new physician.

Seventh character D is to be used for encounters after the patient has completed active treatment. Examples of subsequent treatment are cast change or removal, removal of external or internal fixation device, medication adjustment, and other aftercare and follow-up visits.

The use of these seventh characters for the episode of care in ICD-10-CM is also used for traumatic fractures coded in Chapter 19. Code extensions such as the seventh character letters are defined in the *ICD-10-CM Official Guidelines for Coding and Reporting* specifically in chapter-specific guidelines (Chapter 19) for injury, poisoning, and certain other consequences of external causes.

Rheumatoid Arthritis (M05–M06)

Rheumatoid arthritis is a chronic, crippling condition that affects the joints of the hands, wrists, elbows, feet, and ankles. Periods of remission and exacerbation occur in afflicted patients. Although the exact etiology is unknown, immunologic changes and tissue hypersensitivity, complicated by a cold and damp climate, may have a contributory effect. The synovial membranes are primarily affected. The joints become inflamed, swollen, and painful, as well as stiff and tender. A characteristic sign of rheumatoid arthritis is the formation of nodules over body surfaces. During an active period of rheumatoid arthritis, the patient suffers from malaise, fever, and sweating.

ICD-10-CM classifies rheumatoid arthritis to the following categories:

M05	Rheumatoid arthritis with rheumatoid factor
M06	Other rheumatoid arthritis
M08	Juvenile arthritis

Category M05 includes **Felty's syndrome**, that is, rheumatoid arthritis with splenoadenomegaly and leukopenia (M05.0-). Rheumatoid arthritis may also exist with rheumatoid lung disease (M05.1-). Rheumatoid lung disease is a group of lung conditions that may include any of the following: blockage of the small airways, pleural effusion, pulmonary hypertension, lung nodules, and pulmonary fibrosis (PubMed Health 2011). Other subcategories in M05 include rheumatoid arthritis with vasculitis, heart disease, myopathy, and polyneuropathy with and without involvement of other organs and systems.

Category M06 classifies rheumatoid arthritis without rheumatoid factor. This category includes bursitis, joint nodule, polyarthropathy, and other specified conditions that are caused by the rheumatoid condition. Juvenile rheumatoid arthritis is classified with category M08.

Subcategories for M08 include juvenile rheumatoid arthritis with systemic onset, which may also be documented as Still's disease. The codes within M06 and M08 include the specific joint and the laterality. Because juvenile arthritis is often associated with other conditions, a "code also" note appears under category M08 to advise the coder to code also any associate condition such as regional enteritis or ulcerative colitis.

The diagnosis of **rheumatism** can be classified in ICD-10-CM with code M79.0, Rheumatism, unspecified. The medical term of rheumatism is a popular name for any of a variety of disorders marked by inflammation, degeneration, or metabolic derangement of connective tissue structures of the body, especially the joints and related structures, including muscles, bursae, tendons, and fibrous tissue, with pain, stiffness, or limitation of motion. Rheumatism confined to the joints is more precisely called arthritis. While the code is valid, the code is nondescriptive of a patient's condition and the physician should be asked to be more specific if possible (Dorland 2007).

Osteoarthritis (M15–M19)

Osteoarthritis is the most common type of arthritis. It is a disease of the joints that mainly affects the cartilage in the joint. Cartilage is the tissue that covers the ends of the bones; it glides over each bone, allowing smooth movements and absorbing the shock of motion. However, the cartilage can break down and wear away. When the cartilage is thin or absent the bones under the cartilage rub together and create friction. The friction causes swelling, pain, and stiffness. This friction leads to deformity of the joint, which loses its normal shape. Bone spurs develop and pieces of bone or cartilage break off and float in the joint space. This creates more pain and joint damage. Osteoarthritis occurs over time as a person ages. But younger people can acquire osteoarthritis from joint injuries or the stress on joints from certain occupations or playing sports. Osteoarthritis can develop in any joint but the most common joints it occurs in are the hands, knees, hips, and spine, specifically the neck or low back (HHS 2010b).

Categories in this block of codes include **polyosteoarthritis** (M15), which is used to classify arthritis of multiple sites that may be described as generalized arthritis or osteoarthritis. Categories M16, M17, and M18 classify the common sites of the condition in the hip, knee, and carpometacarpal joints. Codes identify bilateral and unilateral conditions with laterality included. The osteoarthritis in these codes is described as primary, secondary, or posttraumatic.

Primary osteoarthritis is not caused by another disease; instead it is usually related to the aging process but could also be related to unrecognized congenital or developmental defects. Alternatively it may be idiopathic or have an unknown cause. **Secondary osteoarthritis** is a degenerative disease of the joints that results from a predisposing factor, usually trauma, that damages the cartilage or subchondral bone of the affected joints. Secondary osteoarthritis usually occurs in younger individuals (Stacy 2011).

Systemic Connective Tissue Disorders (M30–M36)

This block of codes includes autoimmune and collagen vascular disease. It does not include autoimmune disease of a single organ or cell type. The categories here include polyarteritis nodosa and related conditions (M30), other necrotizing vasculopathies (M31), systemic lupus erythematous (M32), dermatopolymyositis (M33), systemic sclerosis or scleroderma (M34), and other systemic involvement of connective tissue (M35).

Systemic Lupus Erythematosus (M32)

Systemic lupus erythematosus (SLE) is a chronic generalized connective tissue disorder ranging from mild to fulminating and marked by skin eruptions, arthralgia, fever, leukopenia, visceral lesions, and other constitutional symptoms, as well as many autoimmune phenomena, including hypergammaglobulinemia with the presence of antinuclear antibodies and lupus erythematosus (LE) cells. This is not the same condition as discoid lupus erythematosus (L93.0), which is a disease of the skin and subcutaneous tissue.

ICD-10-CM classifies SLE that is not specified further to code M32.9. When the diagnosis of SLE is more specific with the specific organ or diagnosis included, subcategory M32.1 is used. Codes to the fifth-character level identify when endocarditis, pericarditis, lung, and renal disease occurs as the result of the systemic lupus erythematosus.

Dorsopathies (M40–M54)

The dorsopathies section (M40–M545) contains codes describing deforming dorsopathies, spondylopathies, and other dorsopathies. The codes are specific to the regions of the cervical, thoracic, lumbar, and sacral spine.

Deforming Dorsopathies (M40–M43)

Conditions within this section of codes, as described by the title, are deformities of the back. Three common deformities of the spine are curvatures described in the following paragraph.

Kyphosis (M40.0–M40.2) is a rounding or outward curve of the thoracic spine that may be described as a hunchback or slouching posture. It can occur at any age but is not usually present at birth. A different form of the condition is adolescent kyphosis, also known as Scheuermann's disease, which is classified to M42.00–M42.19. In adults, kyphosis is usually caused by osteoporotic fracture, injuries to the spine, degenerative arthritis, disc diseases of the spine, or the slipping of one vertebra (spondylolisthesis). **Lordosis** (M40.4- to M40.5-) is the inward curvature of the lumbar spine. A layman's term for the condition is swayback. It is an anterior curvature where the abdomen appears to protrude and the buttocks appear more prominent. **Scoliosis** (M41.0- through M41.9) is a sideways curvature of the spine. In imaging views the curves may appear S-shaped or C-shaped. The diagnosis is frequently made in middle-school-age children and young teenagers and is known to occur in multiple generations of families. For an unknown reason, the curvature is more common in girls than it is in boys. Sometimes the curve is temporary and growth seems to straighten the spine. Other children benefit from wearing a brace to correct the curvature (MedlinePlus 2013).

Spondylopathies (M45–M49)

Spondylopathy is a disease of the spinal vertebrae (Melloni 2001). **Ankylosis** is an abnormal immobility and fixation of a joint (Melloni 2001). **Spondylosis** is an abnormal immobility and fixation of a vertebral joint (Melloni 2001). Ankylosing spondylitis is a common condition of the spine and is classified with category M45 according to the region of the spine that is involved. Spondylosis is classified by category M47 according to the region (cervical, thoracic, lumbar, lumbosacral) and whether or not it occurs with myelopathy or radiculopathy. Another common spondylopathy is spinal stenosis, which is classified in ICD-10-CM according to the location of the stenosis (M48.00–M48.08). **Spinal stenosis** is a narrowing of the spaces in between the vertebrae of the spine. This narrowing creates pressure on the spinal cord and the nerves and causes pain. Spinal stenosis usually occurs in individuals after the age of 50. Arthritis and scoliosis can cause spinal stenosis (MedlinePlus 2013).

Compartment Syndrome (M79.A-)

A compartment syndrome or compartmental syndrome is a condition in which increased pressure is within an enclosed tissue space. It most often occurs in an extremity but can occur in the abdomen and other sites. There are two types of **compartment syndrome—traumatic** and **nontraumatic**. Causes may be external compression or soft tissue swelling such as edema or hematoma. Some specific causes are burns, frostbite, snakebite, postsurgical edema or hemorrhage, hemophilia, and anticoagulant therapy. Compartments are covered by fascia and when pressure in the compartment is measured to be high or elevated, an emergency surgical procedure such as a fasciotomy is indicated. Exertional compartment syndrome, also known as nontraumatic compartment syndrome, is known to occur in individuals who exercise frequently, especially runners who suffer from compartment syndrome in their leg(s). It can also occur in the forearm. These nontraumatic types are usually considered a chronic form of the condition, but a patient can have an acute episode and may require emergency treatment. Nontraumatic compartment syndrome is coded based on its location in the body, that is, M79.A1- for upper extremity, M79.A2- for lower extremity, M79.A3 for abdomen, and M79. A8- for other sites. Traumatic compartment syndrome is recognized as an early complication of trauma and is coded within the injury section of ICD-10-CM. Specific codes exist in the range of T79.A- depending on the location of the compartment syndrome following trauma.

Osteoporosis (M80–M81)

Osteoporosis is a metabolic bone disease where bones gradually lose protein structure and mineral content and eventually deteriorate. The disease is an imbalance in the ongoing breakdown and renewal cycle of normal healthy bone formation (AMA 2003). Category M80, Osteoporosis with current pathological fracture, includes osteoporosis with current fragility fracture. Category M80.0- is age-related osteoporosis with current pathological fracture. Category M80.8- is other osteoporosis with current pathological fracture. Category M80 codes are combination codes that identify the type of osteoporosis such as age-related or other types including drug-induced, idiopathic, osteoporosis of disuse, postoophorectomy, postsurgical malabsorption, and posttraumatic osteoporosis. The individual codes include site and laterality of the pathological fracture that is present with the osteoporosis. These are pathological fractures as the bone breaks as a result of the osteoporotic nature of the bone. The sites of the fracture may occur at the shoulder, humerus, forearm, hand, femur, lower leg, or ankle and foot. If the patient has a major osseous defect occurring with the osteoporosis, an additional code is used from the series of codes in M89.7-. If there is a drug responsible for inducing the osteoporosis, an additional code for adverse effect to identify the drug (T36–T50 with fifth or sixth character 5) is used with the codes for drug-induced osteoporosis (M80.8-).

Codes in the M80 category require a seventh character to identify the episode of care and if there is another condition occurring with the osteoporosis and pathological fracture. The seventh character options are as follows:

A	Initial encounter for fracture
D	Subsequent encounter for fracture with routine healing
G	Subsequent encounter for fracture with delayed healing
K	Subsequent encounter for fracture with nonunion
P	Subsequent encounter for fracture with malunion
S	Sequela

Malunion of a fracture refers to a fracture that was reduced, but the bone ends did not align properly during the healing process. A malunion is often diagnosed during the healing stages and requires surgical intervention.

Nonunion of a fracture is the failure of the bone ends to align or heal. This usually requires a reopening of the fracture site, with some type of internal fixation and bone grafting performed. Nonunion fractures are often more difficult to treat than a malunion.

The condition of strictly osteoporosis with a current pathological fracture is classified with codes in category M81. The type of osteoporosis is identified at the fourth character level: age-related osteoporosis, localized osteoporosis, and other osteoporosis that may be drug-induced, idiopathic, osteoporosis of disuse, postoophorectomy, postsurgical malabsorption, and post-traumatic osteoporosis. The "use additional code" note that appears at the heading of M81 reminds the coder to use a code for any major osseous defect (M89.7-) or personal history of (healed) osteoporosis fracture (Z87.310) if applicable.

Pathologic and Stress Fractures (M84.3–M84.6)

Pathologic fractures and **stress fractures** are breaks in a bone as a result of disease or repetitive force. These are not traumatic fractures that are the result of an injury or trauma. Coders must be cautious not to confuse the pathologic and stress fractures with the traumatic injuries that cause bones to fracture, which are coded with the fracture injury codes in ICD-10-CM.

Stress fractures occur when bones develop fatigue or stress fractures from repetitive forces applied before the bone and its supporting structures have time to accommodate such force. When a stress fracture is first suspected, x-rays are often negative. Days or weeks may pass before the fracture line is visible. However, a presumptive diagnosis is necessary to begin prompt treatment. The terms stress reaction, fatigue fracture, and march fracture are synonymous with stress fracture. ICD-10-CM codes in the range of M84.30–M84.38 identify the site and laterality of the bone that has the stress fracture.

Codes in the M84.3- range require a seventh character to identify the episode of care and if there is another condition occurring with the osteoporosis and pathological fracture. The seventh character options are

A	Initial encounter for fracture
D	Subsequent encounter for fracture with routine healing
G	Subsequent encounter for fracture with delayed healing
K	Subsequent encounter for fracture with nonunion
P	Subsequent encounter for fracture with malunion
S	Sequela

Pathologic fractures are also classified to several subcategories of M84:

M84.4-	Pathological fracture, not elsewhere classified
M84.5-	Pathological fracture in neoplastic disease
M84.6-	Pathological fracture in other disease

These types of fractures occur in existing diseases such as cancer of the bone and other conditions that are capable of weakening the bone. Pathologic fractures are often spontaneous in nature; however, minor injuries can result in a fracture because the bone is already weakened. Pathologic fractures are reported with subcategory codes from M84.4-, M84.5-, and M84.6- depending on the known or unknown cause. The codes are used as long as the condition is treated and reported with the specific seventh character to indicate the episode of care and if there is a problem with a bone's healing.

Osteomyelitis (M86)

Osteomyelitis is an infection of the bone affecting the metaphyseal area of the long bones caused by bacteria, usually *Staphylococcus aureus* (Melloni 2001). The bacteria can enter the bone through the bloodstream and enter the bone at a weakened area. A puncture wound can allow bacteria to spread to a nearby bone. If the patient has a direct injury when the patient has an open fracture, bacteria can invade the bone. Finally direct contamination of the bone can occur during a joint replacement surgery or open repair of fractures. Most often osteomyelitis affects the long bones of the legs, the humerus, and vertebrae. Diabetic patients may develop osteomyelitis in the bones of their feet from foot ulcers (Mayo Clinic 2010).

Category M86, Osteomyelitis, is further subdivided to fourth-digit subcategories that describe acute, subacute, or chronic osteomyelitis. The fifth and sixth character subclassifications identify the bone involved and its laterality. Codes are also included for unspecified anatomic sites. Two "use additional code" notes appear at the heading of category M86 to remind the coder to use an additional code to identify an infectious agent (B95–B97) or major osseous defect (M89.7-).

ICD-10-PCS Procedure Coding for Musculoskeletal System Procedures

Operations on the many parts of the musculoskeletal systems are common procedures. ICD-10-PCS contains a large number of procedure codes based on the different parts of the system. The root operations for the various types of procedures that can be performed on bones, joints, muscles, tendons, and ligaments are shown in table 16.1.

Table 16.1. **Root operations for musculoskeletal procedures**

Site	Root Operations
Muscles 0K2–0KX	Change, Destruction, Division, Drainage, Excision, Extirpation, Insertion, Inspection, Reattachment, Release, Removal, Repair, Reposition, Resection, Supplement, Revision, Transfer
Tendons 0L2–0LX	Change, Destruction, Division, Drainage, Excision, Extirpation, Inspection, Reattachment, Release, Removal, Repair, Replacement, Reposition, Resection, Supplement, Revision, Transfer
Bursae and Ligaments 0M2–0MX	Change, Destruction, Division, Drainage, Excision, Extirpation, Extraction, Inspection, Reattachment, Release, Removal, Repair, Reposition, Resection, Supplement, Revision, Transfer
Head and Facial Bones 0N2–0NW	Change, Destruction, Division, Drainage, Excision, Extirpation, Insertion, Inspection, Release, Removal, Repair, Replacement, Reposition, Resection, Supplement, Revision

Site	Root Operations
Upper Bones 0P2–0PW	Change, Destruction, Division, Drainage, Excision, Extirpation, Insertion, Inspection, Release, Removal, Repair, Replacement, Reposition, Resection, Supplement, Revision
Lower Bones 0Q2–0QW	Change, Destruction, Division, Drainage, Excision, Extirpation, Insertion, Inspection, Release, Removal, Repair, Replacement, Reposition, Resection, Supplement, Revision
Upper Joints 0R2–0RW	Change, Destruction, Drainage, Excision, Extirpation, Fusion, Insertion, Inspection, Release, Removal, Repair, Replacement, Reposition, Resection, Supplement, Revision
Lower Joints 0S2–0SW	Change, Destruction, Drainage, Excision, Extirpation, Fusion, Insertion, Inspection, Release, Removal, Repair, Replacement, Reposition, Resection, Supplement, Revision

Arthroscopic Surgery

An **arthroscope** is a small, tubular instrument containing magnifying lenses, a light source, and a video camera. Very small instruments are used with the arthroscope to perform surgical procedures on a joint, such as repair or removal of tissue or to take a biopsy. Arthroscopic surgery is commonly performed on most joints, including the knee, shoulder, wrist, and ankle. Arthroscopic surgery is often performed on an outpatient basis, and these procedures cause less damage to the body, minimize pain and scarring, and allow a faster recovery than open joint procedures involving an arthrotomy.

The fifth character in a ICD-10-PCS code is the approach. An arthroscopic approach is identified by using the value of 4 for Percutaneous Endoscopic. If the procedure is strictly an arthroscopy with no additional procedure performed, the root operation is Inspection of the joint. According to the root operations defined in ICD-10-PCS, Inspection is "visually and/or manually exploring a body part" (CMS 2012b). When a more definitive procedure is performed through an arthroscope, only the definitive procedure code is assigned using the root operation that identifies the objective of the procedure. For example, if a patient had an arthroscopic excisional debridement of the right hip joint, the root operation would be Excision or cutting out or off, without replacement, a portion of a body part. This is coded with 0SB as shown in table 16.2.

Table 16.2.   **Arthroscopic excisional debridement of right hip joint**

Character	Code	Explanation
Section	0	Medical and Surgical
Body System	S	Lower Joints
Root Operation	B	Excision
Body Part	9	Hip Joint, Right
Approach	4	Percutaneous Endoscopic
Device	Z	No Device
Qualifier	Z	No Qualifier

Joint Replacement

The removal and replacement of a diseased joint with a device is a joint replacement. This is coded in ICD-10-PCS with the root operation Replacement, defined as "putting in or on biological or synthetic material that physically takes the place and/or function of all or a portion of a body part" (CMS 2012b). Lower joint replacement codes start with the three characters 0SR and upper joint replacement codes have the first three characters of 0RR. When coding a total hip replacement or when only the acetabular surface or the femoral surface is replaced, the body part replaced is identified with character 4 for the right or left-sided joint. The joint device left in place is identified with character 6 for the device.

The choices for hip joint replacement devices are the following values:

1—Synthetic Substitute, Metal
2—Synthetic Substitute, Metal on Polyethylene
3—Synthetic Substitute, Ceramic
4—Synthetic Substitute, Ceramic on Polyethylene
J—Synthetic Substitute

The only choice for the knee replacement device is the following value:

J—Synthetic Substitute

The two choices for the shoulder replacement device are the following values:

0—Synthetic Substitute, Reverse Ball and Socket
J—Synthetic Substitute

For both hip and knee joint replacements the seventh character (qualifier) identifies how the device is secured in place. The choices for lower joint replacement qualifiers are the following values:

9—Cemented
A—Uncemented
Z—No Qualifier (when there is no statement of cemented or uncemented)

For the shoulder joint replacement the seventh character (qualifier) identifies the surface of the joint replaced. The choices for upper joint replacement qualifiers are the following values:

6—Humeral Surface
7—Glenoid Surface
Z—No Qualifier

ICD-10-CM and ICD-10-PCS Review Exercises: Chapter 16

Assign the correct ICD-10-CM diagnosis codes or ICD-10-PCS procedure codes to the following exercises.

1. Bacterial septic arthritis, right knee

2. Juvenile rheumatoid arthritis, only occurring in both ankles

3. Patient has left upper lobe carcinoma, diagnosed over 5 years ago, but is seen now for a fracture of the shaft of the right femur. During this admission, the patient was diagnosed with metastatic bone cancer (from the lung) and this fracture is a result of the metastatic disease. This patient's lung cancer was treated with radiation and there is no longer evidence of an existing primary malignancy.

4. Patient with senile osteoporosis is seen with a complaint of severe back pain with no history of trauma. X-rays revealed pathological compression fractures of several lumbar vertebrae.

5. Displacement of intervertebral lumbosacral disc with radiculopathy

6. Bilateral primary osteoarthritis of hips

7. Spondylosis with myelopathy lumbar region

8. Chondromalacia of patella, right knee

9. Systemic lupus erythematosus with endocarditis

10. Acute osteomyelitis left femur due to *Staphylococcus aureus*

11. Postlaminectomy syndrome

12. Kyphosis due to age-related osteoporosis, thoracic region

13. Ruptured Baker's cyst of knee

(Continued on next page)

ICD-10-CM and ICD-10-PCS Review Exercises: Chapter 16 (Continued)

14. Internal derangement of right knee due to old medial meniscal tear

    _____

15. PROCEDURE: Right hip replacement using uncemented metal prosthesis

    _____

16. PROCEDURE: Left knee replacement using uncemented metal prosthesis

    _____

17. PROCEDURE: Open revision of left hip replacement metal prosthesis

    _____

18. PROCEDURE: Laminectomy of lumbosacral disc L5-S1

    _____

19. PROCEDURE: Arthroscopic partial medial meniscectomy right knee

    _____

20. PROCEDURE: Arthrotomy with removal of right hip metal prosthesis due to internal joint infection and insertion of spacer device in right hip for the next eight weeks of antibiotic therapy

    _____

Chapter 17

Diseases of the Genitourinary System (N00–N99)

Learning Objectives

At the conclusion of this chapter, you should be able to:

1. Describe the organization of the conditions and codes included in Chapter 14 of ICD-10-CM, Diseases of the genitourinary system (N00–N99)

2. Identify the types of conditions considered to be chronic kidney disease

3. Define the term cystitis and describe the various ICD-10-CM codes that are available to classify these conditions

4. Define the term enlarged prostate and identify the associated urinary conditions that can be coded

5. Review the types of female genital tract disorders that can be classified using ICD-10-CM codes

6. Define the abbreviations CIN I, CIN II, CIN III, and VIN I, VIN II, VIN III

7. Identify the options for coding various types of menopause states in ICD-10-CM

8. Assign ICD-10-CM codes for diseases of the genitourinary system

9. Assign ICD-10-PCS codes for procedures related to the diseases of the genitourinary system

Key Terms

- Acute kidney failure
- Benign bladder neck obstruction (BNO)
- Benign prostatic hypertrophy
- Cervical dysplasia
- Cervical intraepithelial neoplasia (CIN)
- Chronic kidney disease (CKD)
- Cystitis
- Endometriosis

- Enlarged prostate
- Female genital prolapse
- Gross hematuria
- Hematuria
- Lower urinary tract symptoms (LUTS)
- Menopause
- Microscopic hematuria
- Vulvar intraepithelial neoplasia (VIN)

Overview of ICD-10-CM Chapter 14, Diseases of the Genitourinary System

Chapter 14 includes categories N00–N99 arranged in the following blocks:

N00–N08	Glomerular diseases
N10–N16	Renal tubulo-interstitial diseases
N17–N19	Acute kidney failure and chronic kidney disease
N20–N23	Urolithiasis
N25–N29	Other disorders of kidney and ureter
N30–N39	Other diseases of the urinary system
N40–N53	Diseases of the male genital organs
N60–N65	Disorders of breast
N70–N77	Inflammatory diseases of female pelvic organs
N80–N98	Noninflammatory disorders of female genital tract
N99	Intraoperative and postprocedural complications and disorders of genitourinary system, not elsewhere classified

As indicated by the blocks of codes in Chapter 14, ICD-10-CM contains codes for urinary system, male and female reproductive systems, disorders of the breast, and complications occurring in the intraoperative and postoperative periods. When ICD-10-CM was developed, the terminology for genitourinary conditions was updated to reflect current medical practice. Specificity was added to the code descriptions including the identification of the patient's gender in order to correctly code posttraumatic urethral stricture.

Genitourinary disorders in diseases classified elsewhere have been placed in their own category at the end of each block of Chapter 14. For example, one category, N08, Glomerular disorders in diseases classified elsewhere, is used to identify glomerulonephritis, nephritis, and nephropathy in diseases classified elsewhere.

Changes have been necessary in some sections of Chapter 14 because of advances in medical treatment. For example, given what has been discovered since the last revision of ICD about male erectile dysfunction, ICD-10-CM includes category N52 for this condition with subcategories to identify the different causes of the dysfunction.

Coding Guidelines and Instructional Notes for ICD-10-CM Chapter 14

Throughout Chapter 14 are new Includes notes that help to clarify the types of disorders that are classified to the various categories.

EXAMPLES: N00 Acute nephritis syndrome
Includes: acute glomerular disease
        acute glomerulonephritis
        acute nephritis

N71 Inflammatory disease of uterus, except cervix
Includes: endo(myo)metritis
        metritis
        myometritis
        pyometra
        uterine abscess

Examples of instructional notes available throughout the chapter indicate that additional coding should be performed as follows:

- N00–N08, Glomerular diseases—Code also any associated kidney failure (N17–N19)

- N10 Acute tubulo-interstitial nephritis and many other infections—Use additional code (B95–B97) to identify infectious agent

- N17, Acute kidney failure—Code also associated underlying condition

- N18, Chronic kidney disease (CKD)—Code first any associated:

  ○ diabetic chronic kidney disease (E08.22, E09.22, E10.22, E11.22, E13.22)

  ○ hypertensive chronic kidney disease (I12.-, I13.-)

  ○ Use additional code to identify kidney transplant status, if applicable (Z94.0)

- N30, Cystitis—Use additional code to identify infectious agent (B95–B97)

- N31, Neuromuscular dysfunction of bladder, NEC—Use additional code to identify any associated urinary incontinence (N39.3–N39.4-)

- N33, Bladder disorders in diseases classified elsewhere—Code first underlying disease, such as: schistosomiasis (B65.0–B65.9)

  ○ This type of note appears with other categories in Chapter 14 for other disorders in diseases classified elsewhere.

- N40.1, Enlarged prostate with lower urinary tract symptoms (LUTS)—Use additional code for associated symptoms, when specified:

  ○ incomplete bladder emptying (R39.14)

  ○ nocturia (R35.1)

- ○ straining on urination (R39.16)

- ○ urinary frequency (R35.0)

- ○ urinary hesitancy (R39.11)

- ○ urinary incontinence (N39.4-)

- ○ urinary obstruction (N13.8)

- ○ urinary retention (R33.8)

- ○ urinary urgency (R39.15)

- ○ weak urinary stream (R39.12)

- N46.1, Oligospermia due to extratesticular causes

  - ○ Code also associated cause

- N99.0, Postprocedural (acute) (chronic) kidney failure

  - ○ Use additional code for type of kidney disease

ICD-10-CM includes a note stating menopausal and other perimenopausal disorders due to naturally occurring (age-related) menopause and perimenopause are classified to category N95. Other inclusion terms appear under Chapter 14 categories to explain the other diagnoses that would be classified with the category or the code, for example:

- N19, Unspecified kidney failure—includes uremia, NOS

- N28.0, Ischemia and infarction of kidney—includes renal artery embolism, obstruction, occlusion, thrombosis

- N40, Enlarged prostate—includes benign prostatic hypertrophy, BPH, nodular prostate

Includes notes appear throughout Chapter 14 to confirm all the terminology for diseases that are included in various categories. For example, the following sections and categories include the other terminology that may be more commonly seen in health records:

- N03, Chronic nephritic syndrome—includes chronic glomerulonephritis and chronic nephritis

- N10-N16, Renal tubulo-interstitial diseases—includes pyelonephritis

- N70, Salpingitis and oophoritis—includes tubo-ovarian abscess and pyosalpinx

- N97, Female infertility—includes female sterility

Excludes1 notes identify conditions that cannot be coded with category codes in Chapter 14, for example:

- N02, Recurrent and persistent hematuria with minor globular abnormality—excludes acute cystitis with hematuria or acute and chronic prostatitis with hematuria

- N43, Hydrocele and spermatocele—excludes congenital hydrocele

- N81, Female genital prolapse—excludes genital prolapse complicating pregnancy, labor or delivery, prolapse and hernia of ovary and fallopian tube or prolapse of vaginal vault after hysterectomy

- N92, Excessive, frequent and irregular menstruation—excludes postmenopausal bleeding and precocious puberty (menstruation)

Excludes2 notes identify other conditions that can be coded with category codes in Chapter 14, for example:

- N39, Other disorders of urinary system—excludes but can be coded with hematuria

- N83, Noninflammatory disorders of ovary, fallopian tube and broad ligament—excludes but can be coded with hydrosalpinx

The NCHS has published chapter-specific guidelines for Chapter 14 in the *ICD-10-CM Official Guidelines for Coding and Reporting.* The coding student should review all of the coding guidelines for Chapter 14 of ICD-10-CM, which appear in an ICD-10-CM code book or at the website http://www.cdc.gov/nchs/icd/icd10cm.htm, or in Appendix E.

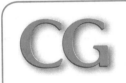

Guideline I.C.14.a.1. Stages of chronic kidney disease (CKD): The ICD-10-CM classifies CKD based on severity. The severity of CKD is designated by stages 1-5. Stage 2, code N18.2, equates to mild CKD; stage 3, code N18.3, equates to moderate CKD; and stage 4, code N18.4, equates to severe CKD. Code N18.6, End stage renal disease (ESRD), is assigned when the provider has documented end-stage-renal disease (ESRD).

If both a stage of CKD and ESRD are documented, assign code N18.6 only.

Guideline I.C.14.a.2. Chronic kidney disease and kidney transplant status: Patients who have undergone kidney transplant may still have some form of chronic kidney disease (CKD) because the kidney transplant may not fully restore kidney function. Therefore, the presence of CKD alone does not constitute a transplant complication. Assign the appropriate N18 code for the patient's stage of CKD and code Z94.0, Kidney transplant status. If a transplant complication such as failure or rejection or other transplant complication is documented, see section I.C.19.g for information on coding complications of a kidney transplant. If the documentation is unclear as to whether the patient has a complication of the transplant, query the provider.

Coding Guideline I.C.14.a.3. Chronic kidney disease with other conditions: Patients with CKD may also suffer from other serious

(Continued)

(Continued)

> conditions, most commonly diabetes mellitus and hypertension. The sequencing of the CKD code in relationship to codes for other contributing conditions is based on the conventions in the Tabular List.

Coding Diseases of the Genitourinary System in ICD-10-CM Chapter 14

A variety of common conditions in the urinary system and the reproductive systems of men and women are classified with Chapter 14 codes. The frequently coded diseases are discussed in this chapter.

Recurrent and Persistent Hematuria (N02)

Hematuria is the presence of blood or red blood cells in the urine. Hematuria can be a symptom of an undiagnosed disease or hematuria can be present with another condition in the genitourinary tract. If the cause of hematuria has not been identified, symptom codes are used. For example, **gross hematuria** (R31.0) is the presence of blood in the urine in sufficient quantity to be visible to the naked eye. **Microscopic hematuria** (R31.1–R31.2) is the presence of blood cells in the urine visible only under the microscope. The code R31.9 is used if only the symptom of hematuria is documented.

Hematuria can be caused by a number of underlying urinary conditions, including urinary tract infections, benign prostatic hypertrophy, and kidney and ureteral calculi. In patients with certain risk factors, hematuria is a cardinal sign of bladder cancer. These patients require more intensive workup than the primary hematuria patients. Patients presenting with hematuria who are at high risk for bladder cancer have other distinct risk factors: currently smoking or history of tobacco use, voiding dysfunction, personal history of urinary tract infections, and personal history of irradiation. Bladder cancer is generally associated with environmental or occupational factors and less often familial or inherited.

If the physician describes the patient's hematuria as recurrent, persistent, or idiopathic, the condition is classified to Chapter 14 category code N02, Recurrent and persistent hematuria. Upon investigation, the physician determines the hematuria is present with kidney disease. The subcategories of N02 identify whether glomerular lesions, glomerulonephritis, or other morphological changes are present in the kidney.

Acute Kidney Failure and Chronic Kidney Disease (N17–N19)

Renal failure and renal insufficiency represent a range of disease processes that occur when the kidneys have problems eliminating metabolic products from the blood. These problems can be caused by various underlying conditions such as hypertension and diabetes, or they may affect patients with a single kidney or those with a family history of kidney disease. There are both acute and chronic kidney diseases that are classified with different codes in ICD-10-CM.

Proper terminology, as used in ICD-10-CM, is **chronic kidney disease (CKD)**, rather than the vague terms of chronic renal failure and chronic renal insufficiency. CKD has five stages based on the glomerular filtration rate (GFR). Care of patients with stage IV and V CKD is intensive and complicated. For any patient, the goal is to slow the progression of CKD or better prepare the patient for renal replacement therapy. The determination of GFR is based on a well-established formula. Only patients in need of dialysis or receiving kidney transplants may be considered as having end-stage renal disease (ESRD). Code N18.6 is assigned when the provider has documented ESRD.

Chronic renal insufficiency is a form of CKD classified with code N18.9, Chronic kidney disease, unspecified. Also included in this unspecified code are the vague diagnoses of chronic renal disease and chronic renal failure. A specific form of CKD and chronic renal insufficiency should not be coded in the same record. Renal insufficiency or acute renal insufficiency, a vague but different condition from CKD, is classified to code N28.9, Disorder of kidney and ureter, unspecified, with other vague descriptions such as acute renal disease or renal disease unspecified. These forms of chronic kidney disease develop gradually in the patient over time, often associated with hypertension or diabetes. The condition may be controlled but generally is irreversible.

Acute kidney failure or acute renal failure, also described as nontraumatic acute kidney injury, occurs suddenly, usually as the result of physical trauma, infection, inflammation, or toxicity. Symptoms include oliguria or anuria with hyperkalemia and pulmonary edema. Physicians may identify acute kidney failure with more specificity by referring to it as prerenal, intrarenal, or postrenal, which more specifically identifies underlying causes such as congestive heart failure (prerenal), acute nephritis, or nephrotoxicity (intrarenal), or obstruction of urine flow out of the kidneys (postrenal). Acute kidney failure typically develops over a short period of time as part of another illness and is generally reversible; it is corrected as the underlying disease is treated or controlled. Acute kidney failure or acute renal failure is assigned to category N17, with the fourth character identifying the type of necrosis present.

Cystitis (N30)

Cystitis is a bacterial infection of the urinary bladder. Most common in women, this condition is often recurrent. Most cases are due to a vaginal infection that extends through the urethra to the bladder. Cystitis in men is due to urethral or prostatic infections or catheterizations. Symptoms include burning or painful urination, urinary urgency and frequency, nocturia, suprapubic pain, and lower back pain.

A diagnosis of cystitis is made by obtaining a urine specimen from the bladder by either catheterization or a clean-catch midstream sample. A bacterial colony count of greater than 1,000 colonies/mL in a catheterized specimen indicates cystitis, as does a bacterial count of greater than 100,000/mL in a midstream sample. Urine also may be positive for pyuria and hematuria. Therapy with antibiotics is prescribed for uncomplicated infections. The coder should not arbitrarily record an additional diagnosis on the basis of an abnormal laboratory finding alone, for example, bacteria present in a urine culture. If the specific diagnosis is not clearly stated in the health record, the physician should always be queried.

ICD-10-CM classifies cystitis to category N30, with the fourth-character subcategories describing type, severity, and location. The codes also identify whether or not hematuria is present with cystitis. An instruction at the beginning of this category advises that an additional code is used to identify the infectious agent (B95–B97). The options for coding cystitis in ICD-10-CM are as follows:

N30.00	Acute cystitis without hematuria
N30.01	Acute cystitis with hematuria
N30.10	Interstitial cystitis (chronic) without hematuria
N30.11	Interstitial cystitis (chronic) with hematuria
N30.10	Interstitial cystitis (chronic) without hematuria
N30.20	Other chronic cystitis without hematuria
N30.21	Other chronic cystitis with hematuria
N30.30	Trigonitis without hematuria
N30.31	Trigonitis with hematuria
N30.40	Irradiation cystitis without hematuria
N30.41	Irradiation cystitis with hematuria
N30.80	Other cystitis without hematuria
N30.81	Other cystitis with hematuria
N30.90	Cystitis, unspecified without hematuria
N30.91	Cystitis, unspecified with hematuria

Enlarged Prostate (N40)

The diagnosis of an **enlarged prostate** may also be stated as **benign prostatic hypertrophy**, benign prostatic hyperplasia, (BPH) or nodular prostate. The terminology of BPH is commonly found in health records in place of the diagnosis of enlarged prostate but the two descriptions are synonymous. It is a condition commonly occurring in men by the age of 60 years, as part of the normal aging process. The prostate gland, which encircles the urethra at the base of the bladder, becomes enlarged and presses on the urethra, obstructing the flow of urine from the bladder. This is known as **benign bladder neck obstruction (BNO)**. Symptoms of an enlarged prostate may be referred to as **lower urinary tract symptoms (LUTS)** and include incomplete bladder emptying, nocturia, straining on urination, frequency, hesitancy, incontinence, obstruction, retention, urgency, or weak urinary stream. Straining to void may rupture veins of the prostate, causing hematuria. The ICD-10-CM codes distinguish between enlarged prostate or nodular prostate with and without lower urinary tract symptoms.

A diagnosis of an enlarged prostate is made by a rectal examination that finds the prostate enlarged and with a rubbery texture. Urinalysis shows WBC, RBC, albumin, bacteria, and blood. Cystoscopy reveals the extent of enlargement. A postvoiding cystogram shows the amount of residual urine in the bladder.

ICD-10-CM classifies enlarged prostate or nodular prostate to category N40. Some forms of the disease may be indicative of the need for further testing due to the increased risk for prostatic cancer. The enlargement of the prostate often produces the symptom of urinary obstruction or the inability to urinate. The urinary obstruction is the problem that typically brings the patient to the physician or to the hospital emergency department.

Category N40 is expanded to the fourth-character subcategory level to describe the type of enlargement and whether or not lower urinary tract symptoms are present. For example:

N40.0	Enlarged prostate without urinary tract symptoms
N40.1	Enlarged prostate with lower urinary tract symptoms
N40.2	Nodular prostate without lower urinary tract symptoms
N40.3	Nodular prostate with lower urinary tract symptoms

Under each of the codes with lower urinary tract symptoms, a directional note states, "Use additional code for associated symptoms, when specified." Additional codes are used when the patient also has incomplete bladder emptying (R39.14), nocturia (R35.1), straining on urination (R39.16), urinary frequency (R35.0), urinary hesitancy (R39.11), urinary incontinence (N39.4-), urinary obstruction (N13.8), urinary retention (R33.8), urgency (R39.15), or weak urinary stream (R39.12) with the diagnosis of enlarged or nodular prostate.

Disorders of Breast (N60–N65)

Disorders such as gynecomastia, fibrocystic disease, inflammatory disease, and solitary cyst of the breast are included in this section. A breast lump or breast mass is classified to category code N63, Unspecified lump in breast.

Certain signs and symptoms of breast disease, such as mastodynia, induration of breast, and nipple discharge, are included in category N64, rather than in Chapter 18 of ICD-10-CM, with other symptoms, signs, and abnormal findings. Neoplasms of the breast are classified in Chapter 2, Neoplasms, in ICD-10-CM.

Specific codes describe conditions of the breast related to staged breast reconstruction following full or partial mastectomy due to breast disease or trauma. Codes identify the various stages for which a breast reconstruction encounter may occur or distinguish between the disorders of reconstructed breasts and native breasts. Specific conditions requiring reconstruction may be described with codes in the range of N64.81–N64.89 for ptosis, hypoplasia, capsular contracture, and other specified disorders of the breast. Deformity or disproportion of reconstructed breast is identified with ICD-10-CM codes N65.0–N65.1.

Inflammatory Disease of Female Pelvic Organs (N70–N77)

This section includes infections of the female pelvic organs. The note at the beginning of several category codes in this section states, "Use additional code (B95–B97) to identify infectious agent."

> **EXAMPLE:** Acute salpingitis; organism involved—*Streptococcus.*
>
> This can be classified with the codes N70.01, Acute salpingitis, and B95.5, Unspecified streptococcus as the cause of diseases classified elsewhere.

Codes in category N70, Salpingitis and oophoritis, distinguish between acute and chronic forms of the conditions. Acute salpingitis and ooporitis is classified to N70.0- and chronic salpingitis and oophoritis is classified to N70.1-. The unspecified form of salpingitis and oophoritis is classified with another set of subcategory codes.

Other categories exist in this block of codes to identify inflammatory diseases that are the result of another disease. For example, under category N74, Female pelvic inflammatory disorders in diseases classified elsewhere, there is a "code first underlying disease" note. This same direction also appears with codes N77.0, Ulceration of vulva in diseases classified elsewhere, and N77.1, Vaginitis, vulvitis and vulvovaginitis in diseases classified elsewhere.

Noninflammatory Disorders of Female Genital Tract (N80–N98)

This section includes conditions such as the following:

- **Endometriosis,** N80. This condition occurs when endometrial glands or stroma are present outside the uterine cavity. For example, endometriosis can be diagnosed in the ovary, fallopian tube, pelvic peritoneum, rectovaginal septum and vagina, intestine, and other sites. ICD-10-CM provides a specific code for the common sites of endometriosis as well as an unspecified code, N80.9. Many women suffer from the effects of endometriosis, and it is one of the most common causes of infertility in women.

- **Female genital prolapse**, N81. There are codes in this category for urethrocele, cystocele, uterovaginal prolapse, vaginal enterocele, rectocele and other weakening of tissue and pelvic muscle wasting.

- Fistulae involving female genital tract, N82

- Noninflammatory disorders of ovary, fallopian tube and broad ligament, N83. Commonly occurring conditions classified to this category are follicular cyst or ovary, corpus luteum cyst, torsion of ovary and fallopian tube, hematosalpinx, and hematoma of broad ligament. Ovarian cysts of a variety of types are the most common pelvic masses diagnosed in women.

- Polyp of female genital tract, N84. Polyps that occur in the corpus uteri, cervix uteri, vagina, vulva, and other parts of the female genital tract are classified here.

- Other inflammatory disorders of uterus, except cervix, N85. The more commonly occurring conditions that would be coded with category N85 codes are benign endometrial hyperplasia and endometrial hyperplasia neoplasia or that with atypia. These conditions frequently make a hysterectomy a medical necessity.

Other gynecological conditions described in this chapter of ICD-10-CM include:

- Other noninflammatory disorders of the cervix uteri, vagina, vulva, and perineum

- Disorders of menstruation

- Infertility

- Complications associated with artificial fertilization

Dyplasia of Cervix Uteri (N87) and Vulva (N90.0–N90.4)

Codes N87.0 through N87.9 describe mild dysplasia of the cervix or cervical intraepithelial neoplasia. Mild **cervical dyplasia** or **cervical intraepithelial neoplasia** I (CIN I) as a diagnosis is assigned code N87.0. Likewise, the diagnosis of moderate dysplasia of cervix (CIN II) is assigned code N87.1. There is a code available, N87.9, for an unspecified form of cervical dysplasia. However, if the condition is described as carcinoma in situ of the cervix, severe cervical dysplasia, or cervical intraepithelial neoplasia III (CIN III), it is classified in category D06, Carcinoma in situ of cervix.

Codes N90.0 through N90.1 describe **vulvar intraepithelial neoplasia** I and II (VIN I and VIN II). These conditions are also known as N90.0, mild dysplasia of vulva, N90.1, moderate dysplasia of vulva, N90.3, unspecified form of dysplasia, and N90.4, other leukoplakia of vulva. If the condition is described as carcinoma in situ of the vulva, severe dysplasia of vulva, or vulvar intraepithelial neoplasia III (VIN III), code D07.1 is used to classify the disease. The Alphabetic Index entry used to locate the codes for these conditions is the term "dysplasia, cervix" or "dysplasia, vulva."

Menopause

The diagnosis given by a healthcare provider of **menopause** or menopausal syndrome often needs to be more specific. ICD-10-CM includes several options for coding. Codes exist for both symptomatic menopausal syndrome and asymptomatic menopausal status. The symptoms a woman may experience with menopause are flushing, sleeplessness, headache, and a lack of concentration among other complaints. Subcategory code N95.1, Menopausal and female climacteric states, includes a "use additional code for associated symptoms" note to direct the coder to assign other codes to describe the menopausal symptoms the woman is experiencing.

A crucial factor is whether the menopause is the result of the natural aging process or whether surgical intervention or other treatment such as radiation has created artificially induced menopause. In addition, the fact that the woman is experiencing symptoms as a result of the menopausal process or is asymptomatic is required to code the status correctly.

The patient who has a menopausal disorder or symptoms associated with artificial or postsurgical menopause may be coded with the following:

E89.41 Symptomatic postprocedural ovarian failure
N95.1   Menopause and female climacteric states

The patient who is menopausal as a result of having her ovaries removed surgically but who is asymptomatic may be coded with either:

E89.40 Asymptomatic postprocedural ovarian failure
Z90.721 or Z90.722 Acquired absence of ovaries (unilateral)(bilateral)

The patient who has a menopausal disorder or symptoms associated with age-related or naturally occurring menopause may be coded with the following:

E28.39 Other primary ovarian failure
N95.1   Menopausal and female climacteric states

The patient who has premature menopause, that is, earlier in life than typically experienced by most women but not due to a procedure, may or may not have symptoms. This person would be diagnosed with a form of ovarian failure and coded with the following:

E28.310   Symptomatic premature menopause
E28.319   Asymptomatic premature menopause

The patient who is postmenopausal as a result of the natural or age-related process and is asymptomatic is coded with the following:

Z78.0 Asymptomatic menopausal state

Intraoperative and Postprocedural Complications and Disorders of Genitourinary System, Not Elsewhere Classified (N99)

The chapter ends with the intraoperative and postprocedural complications of the genitourinary system like those found in the preceding chapters. Examples of the conditions that are classified with category N99 codes are:

N99.0	Postprocedural (acute) (chronic) kidney failure
N99.1	Postprocedural urethral stricture
N99.4	Postprocedural pelvic peritoneal adhesions
N99.7	Accidental puncture and laceration of a genitourinary system organ or structure during a procedure

Complications of cystostomy and other external stoma of the urinary system are found in the range of codes N99.510–N99.538. The types of complications of the cystostomy or other external stoma that could be coded are hemorrhage or infection at the site or malfunction of the stoma.

ICD-10-PCS Procedure Coding for Genitourinary System Procedures

Procedures related to the genitourinary system would include procedures on the urinary system, female reproductive system, and the male reproductive system. ICD-10-PCS contains a large number of procedure codes based on the different parts of these body systems. The root operations for the various types of procedures that can be performed are shown in table 17.1. Like procedures in other body systems, in order to code genitourinary procedures, the coder needs to know the definition of root operations and the anatomy to identify the body parts.

Table 17.1.   **Genitourinary system root operations**

Root Operations and (3rd) Character Root Operation Value	Root Operations and (3rd) Character Root Operation Value	Root Operations and (3rd) Character Root Operation Value
Urinary System	**Female Reproductive System**	**Male Reproductive System**
Bypass (1) Change (2) Destruction (5) Dilation (7) Division (8) Drainage (9) Excision (B) Extirpation (C) Extraction (D) Fragmentation (F) Insertion (H) Inspection (J) Occlusion (L) Reattachment (M) Release (N) Removal (P)	Bypass (1) Change (2) Destruction (5) Dilation (7) Division (8) Drainage (9) Excision (B) Extirpation (C) Extraction (D) Fragmentation (F) Insertion (H) Inspection (J) Occlusion (L) Reattachment (M) Release (N)	Bypass (1) Change (2) Destruction (5) Dilation (7) Drainage (9) Excision (B) Extirpation (C) Insertion (H) Inspection (J) Occlusion (L) Reattachment (M) Release (N) Removal (P) Repair (Q) Replacement (R)

Repair (Q) Replacement (R) Reposition (S) Resection (T) Supplement (U) Restriction (V) Revision (W) Transplantation (Y)	Removal (P) Repair (Q) Reposition (S) Resection (T) Supplement (U) Restriction (V) Revision (W) Transplantation (Y)	Resection (T) Supplement (U) Revision (W)

Body parts include laterality, for example right and left kidney and bilateral for such organs as ovary, fallopian tube, seminal vesicle, spermatic cord, epididymis, vas deferens, and such. The approach for these procedures is frequently endoscopic through a natural orifice, such as vagina and urethra, as well as percutaneous (for example, laparoscopic). Robotic assisted prostatic and uterine procedures are becoming more common. An additional code is used to designate the procedure was robotic assisted. The Index entry for robotic assisted procedure directs the coder to Table 8E0. A code is constructed based on the relevant body region; the sixth character designates the method as a robotic assisted procedure.

ICD-10-CM and ICD-10-PCS Review Exercises: Chapter 17

Assign the correct ICD-10-CM diagnosis codes or ICD-10-PCS procedure codes to the following exercises.

1. Chronic nephritic syndrome with diffuse membranous glomerulonephritis with symptoms of proteinuria and hematuria

2. Patient complained of frequent urination with pain and was diagnosed with acute suppurative cystitis, with hematuria due to E. coli

3. Menometrorrhagia that the physician further documented as excessive and frequent menstruation with irregular menstrual cycles.

4. This male patient complained of lower abdominal pain and the inability to urinate over the past 24 hours. After study, the patient was diagnosed as having acute kidney failure due to acute tubular necrosis, caused by a urinary obstruction. The urinary obstruction was a result of the patient's benign prostatic hypertrophy. The patient was treated with medications and the acute kidney failure was resolved prior to discharge.

5. The patient has end stage renal disease (ESRD) and requires renal dialysis three days a week

6. Infection of nephrostomy site/external stoma

(Continued on next page)

ICD-10-CM and ICD-10-PCS Review Exercises: Chapter 17 (Continued)

7. Uterine and tubo-ovarian endometriosis. Mucous polyp of cervix

8. Moderate dysplasia of cervix (CIN II)

9. Fibrocystic disease of breast, bilateral

10. Left ureteral stone

11. Female midline cystocele with prolapse of uterus

12. Acute pyelonephritis due to pseudomonas

13. Postmenopausal bleeding with symptomatic menopause

14. Subacute salpingo-oophoritis

15. Female infertility due to uterine anomaly

16. PROCEDURE: Transurethral resection of prostate (TURP). The documentation in the operative report describes the procedure as an excision of prostate tissue and not a complete removal of the prostate.

17. PROCEDURE: Total abdominal hysterectomy with bilateral salpingo-oophorectomy

18. PROCEDURE: Total left laparoscopic nephrectomy

19. PROCEDURE: Anterior colporrhaphy by vaginal approach

20. PROCEDURE: Lithotripsy (ESWL) to destroy right renal pelvis small calculus

Chapter 18

Pregnancy, Childbirth and the Puerperium (O00–O9A)

Learning Objectives

At the conclusion of this chapter, you should be able to:

1. Describe the organization of the conditions and codes included in Chapter 15 of ICD-10-CM, Pregnancy, childbirth and the puerperium (O00–O9A)

2. Identify the different ICD-10-CM categories used to classify the diagnosis of abortion

3. Identify the difference between *missed abortion* and *threatened abortion*

4. Define the term *pregnancy* and describe the guidelines for determining preterm, term, and postterm pregnancies

5. Define the term *ectopic pregnancy* and explain how the condition is classified

6. Define the term *normal delivery* and describe the procedures that can be performed with a normal delivery

7. Identify the ICD-10-CM category Z37 codes and describe the circumstances in which these codes are used with a delivery code

8. Briefly describe the ICD-10-PCS procedure codes used to identify delivery procedures

9. Assign diagnosis codes for Chapter 15 of ICD-10-CM

10. Assign ICD-10-PCS procedure codes for obstetric conditions

Key Terms

- Abortion (procedure)
- Complete abortion
- Delivery (procedure)
- Drainage (procedure)
- Ectopic pregnancy

- Elderly pregnant female
- Elective termination of pregnancy
- Failed attempted termination of pregnancy
- First trimester
- Hyperemesis gravidarum
- Incomplete abortion
- Insufficient antenatal care
- Missed abortion
- Normal delivery
- Outcome of delivery
- Preterm labor
- Preterm pregnancy
- Postpartum
- Postterm pregnancy
- Pregnancy
- Pregnancy state, incidental
- Prolonged pregnancy
- Puerperium
- Recurrent pregnancy loss
- Second trimester
- Spontaneous abortion
- Term pregnancy
- Third trimester
- Threatened abortion
- Weeks of gestation
- Young pregnant female

Overview of ICD-10-CM Chapter 15, Pregnancy, Childbirth and the Puerperium

Chapter 15 includes categories O00–O9A arranged in the following blocks:

O00–O08	Pregnancy with abortive outcome
O09	Supervision of high risk pregnancy
O10–O16	Edema, proteinuria and hypertensive disorders in pregnancy, childbirth and the puerperium
O20–O29	Other maternal disorders predominantly related to pregnancy
O30–O48	Maternal care related to the fetus and amniotic cavity and possible delivery problems
O60–O77	Complications of labor and delivery
O80, O82	Encounter for delivery
O85–O92	Complications predominantly related to the puerperium
O94–O9A	Other obstetric conditions, not elsewhere classified

In ICD-10-CM Chapter 15, terminology is descriptive of what obstetric condition is intended to be represented by the obstetric code. Codes for elective (legal or therapeutic) abortions are classified with the abortion codes in Chapter 15. Complications of induced termination of pregnancy are found in category O04. In comparison, the elective abortion without complication code Z33.2 is included in Chapter 21 of ICD-10-CM that includes factors influencing health status and contact with health services. Chapter 15 also identifies the trimester of pregnancy in which the condition occurred at the fifth- and sixth-character level.

ICD-10-CM requires the use of a seventh character to identify the fetus to which certain complication codes apply.

> **EXAMPLE:** O32 Maternal care for malpresentation of fetus
> One of the following seventh characters is to be assigned to each code under category O32.
> 0 not applicable or unspecified
> 1 fetus 1
> 2 fetus 2
> 3 fetus 3
> 4 fetus 4
> 5 fetus 5
> 9 other fetus

Coding Guidelines and Instructional Notes for ICD-10-CM Chapter 15

At the beginning of Chapter 15 are notes that provide instructions for coding professionals. Codes from this chapter are for use only on maternal records, never on newborn records. For example, Z37.0, Single live birth, is the only outcome of delivery code appropriate for use with O80.

The **postpartum** period begins immediately after delivery and continues for six weeks following delivery. A postpartum complication is any complication occurring within the six-week period.

Trimesters are counted from the first day of the last menstrual period. They are defined as follows:

- **First trimester**—less than 14 weeks 0 days
- **Second trimester**—14 weeks 0 days to less than 28 weeks 0 days
- **Third trimester**—28 weeks 0 days until delivery

Another note appears at the start of Chapter 15 that instructs the coder to use an additional code from category Z3A, Weeks of gestation, to identify the specific week of the pregnancy.

The NCHS has published chapter-specific guidelines for Chapter 15 in the *ICD-10-CM Official Guidelines for Coding and Reporting*. The coding student should review all of the coding guidelines for Chapter 15 of ICD-10-CM, which appear in an ICD-10-CM code book or at the website http://www.cdc.gov/nchs/icd/icd10cm.htm, or in Appendix E.

CG

Guideline I.C.15.a. General Rules for Obstetric Cases

Guideline I.C.15.a.1. Codes from Chapter 15 and sequencing priority: Obstetric cases require codes from Chapter 15, codes in the range O00–O9A, Pregnancy, Childbirth, and the Puerperium. Chapter 15 codes have sequencing priority over codes from other chapters. Additional codes from other chapters may be used in conjunction with Chapter 15 codes to further specify conditions. Should the provider document that the pregnancy is incidental to the encounter, then code Z33.1, Pregnant state, incidental, should be used in place of any Chapter 15 codes. It is the provider's responsibility to state that the condition being treated is not affecting the pregnancy.

Guideline I.C.15.a.2. Chapter 15 codes used only on the maternal record: Chapter 15 codes are to be used only on the maternal record, never on the record of the newborn.

Guideline I.C.15.a.3. Final character for trimester: The majority of codes in Chapter 15 have a final character indicating the trimester of pregnancy. The timeframes for the trimesters are indicated at the beginning of the chapter. If trimester is not a component of a code it is because the condition always occurs in a specific trimester, or the concept of trimester of pregnancy is not applicable. Certain codes have characters for only certain trimesters because the condition does not occur in all trimesters, but it may occur in more than just one.

Assignment of the final character for trimester should be based on the provider's documentation of the trimester (or number of weeks) for the current admission/encounter. This applies to the assignment of trimester for pre-existing conditions as well as those that develop during or are due to the pregnancy. The provider's documentation of the number of weeks may be used to assign the appropriate code identifying the trimester.

Whenever delivery occurs during the current admission, and there is an "in childbirth" option for the obstetric complication being coded, the "in childbirth" code should be assigned.

Guideline I.C.15.a.4. Selection of trimester for inpatient admissions that encompass more than one trimester: In instances when a patient is admitted to a hospital for complications of pregnancy during one trimester and remains in the hospital into a subsequent trimester, the trimester character for the antepartum complication code should be assigned on the basis of the trimester when the complication developed, not the trimester of the discharge. If the condition developed prior to the current admission/encounter or represents a pre-existing condition, the trimester character for the trimester at the time of the admission/encounter should be assigned.

Guideline I.C.15.a.5. Unspecified trimester: Each category that includes codes for trimester has a code for "unspecified trimester." The "unspecified trimester" code should rarely be used, such as when the documentation in the record is insufficient to determine the trimester and it is not possible to obtain clarification.

Guideline I.C.15.a.6. Seventh (7th) character for Fetus Identification: Where applicable, a 7th character is to be assigned for certain categories (O31, O32, O33.3 - O33.6, O35, O36, O40, O41, O60.1, O60.2, O64, and O69) to identify the fetus for which the complication code applies.

Assign 7th character "0":

- For single gestations

- When the documentation in the record is insufficient to determine the fetus affected and it is not possible to obtain clarification.

- When it is not possible to clinically determine which fetus is affected.

Guideline I.C.15.b. Selection of OB Principal or First-listed Diagnosis

Guideline I.C.15.b.1. Routine outpatient prenatal visits: For routine outpatient prenatal visits when no complications are present, a code from category Z34, Encounter for supervision of normal pregnancy, should be used as the first-listed diagnosis. These codes should not be used in conjunction with Chapter 15 codes.

Guideline I.C.15.b.2. Prenatal outpatient visits for high-risk patients: For routine prenatal outpatient visits for patients with high-risk pregnancies, a code from category O09, Supervision of high-risk pregnancy, should be used as the first-listed diagnosis. Secondary Chapter 15 codes may be used in conjunction with these codes if appropriate.

Guideline I.C.15.b.3. Episodes when no delivery occurs: In episodes when no delivery occurs, the principal diagnosis should correspond to the principal complication of the pregnancy which necessitated the encounter. Should more than one complication exist, all of which are treated or monitored, any of the complications codes may be sequenced first.

Guideline I.C.15.b.4. When a delivery occurs: When a delivery occurs, the principal diagnosis should correspond to the main circumstances or complication of the delivery. In cases of

(Continued)

(Continued)

cesarean delivery, the selection of the principal diagnosis should be the condition established after study that was responsible for the patient's admission. If the patient was admitted with a condition that resulted in the performance of a cesarean procedure, that condition should be selected as the principal diagnosis. If the reason for the admission/encounter was unrelated to the condition resulting in the delivery, the condition related to the reason for the admission/encounter should be selected as the principal diagnosis.

Guideline I.C.15.b.5. Outcome of delivery: A code from category Z37, Outcome of delivery, should be included on every maternal record when a delivery has occurred. These codes are not to be used on subsequent records or on the newborn record.

Guideline I.C.15.c. Pre-existing conditions versus conditions due to the pregnancy: Certain categories in Chapter 15 distinguish between conditions of the mother that existed prior to pregnancy (pre-existing) and those that are a direct result of pregnancy. When assigning codes from Chapter 15, it is important to assess if a condition was pre-existing prior to pregnancy or developed during or due to the pregnancy in order to assign the correct code.

Categories that do not distinguish between pre-existing and pregnancy-related conditions may be used for either. It is acceptable to use codes specifically for the puerperium with codes complicating pregnancy and childbirth if a condition arises postpartum during the delivery encounter.

Guideline I.C.15.d. Pre-existing hypertension in pregnancy: Category O10, Pre-existing hypertension complicating pregnancy, childbirth and the puerperium, includes codes for hypertensive heart and hypertensive chronic kidney disease. When assigning one of the O10 codes that includes hypertensive heart disease or hypertensive chronic kidney disease, it is necessary to add a secondary code from the appropriate hypertension category to specify the type of heart failure or chronic kidney disease.

See Section I.C.9. Hypertension.

Guideline I.C.15.e. Fetal Conditions Affecting the Management of the Mother

Guideline I.C.15.e.1. Codes from categories O35 and O36: Codes from categories O35, Maternal care for known or suspected fetal abnormality and damage, and O36, Maternal care for other fetal problems, are assigned only when the fetal condition is actually responsible for modifying the management of the mother, i.e., by requiring diagnostic studies, additional observation, special care, or termination of pregnancy. The fact that the fetal condition exists does not justify assigning a code from this series to the mother's record.

Guideline I.C.15.e.2. In utero surgery: In cases when surgery is performed on the fetus, a diagnosis code from category O35, Maternal care for known or suspected fetal abnormality and damage, should be assigned identifying the fetal condition. Assign the appropriate procedure code for the procedure performed.

No code from Chapter 16, the perinatal codes, should be used on the mother's record to identify fetal conditions. Surgery performed in utero on a fetus is still to be coded as an obstetric encounter.

Guideline I.C.15.f. HIV Infection in Pregnancy, Childbirth and the Puerperium: During pregnancy, childbirth or the puerperium, a patient admitted because of an HIV-related illness should receive a principal diagnosis from subcategory O98.7-, Human immunodeficiency [HIV] disease complicating pregnancy, childbirth and the puerperium, followed by the code(s) for the HIV-related illness(es).

Patients with asymptomatic HIV infection status admitted during pregnancy, childbirth, or the puerperium should receive codes of O98.7- and Z21, Asymptomatic human immunodeficiency virus [HIV] infection status.

Guideline I.C.15.g. Diabetes mellitus in pregnancy: Diabetes mellitus is a significant complicating factor in pregnancy. Pregnant women who are diabetic should be assigned a code from category O24, Diabetes mellitus in pregnancy, childbirth, and the puerperium, first, followed by the appropriate diabetes code(s) (E08-E13) from Chapter 4.

Guideline I.C.15.h. Long term use of insulin: Code Z79.4, Long-term (current) use of insulin, should also be assigned if the diabetes mellitus is being treated with insulin.

Guideline I.C.15.i. Gestational (pregnancy induced) diabetes: Gestational (pregnancy induced) diabetes can occur during the second and third trimester of pregnancy in women who were not diabetic prior to pregnancy. Gestational diabetes can cause complications in the pregnancy similar to those of pre-existing diabetes mellitus. It also puts the woman at greater risk of developing diabetes after the pregnancy. Codes for gestational diabetes are in subcategory O24.4, Gestational diabetes mellitus. No other code from category O24, Diabetes mellitus in pregnancy, childbirth, and the puerperium, should be used with a code from O24.4.

The codes under subcategory O24.4 include diet controlled and insulin controlled. If a patient with gestational diabetes is treated with both diet and insulin, only the code for insulin-controlled is required.

(Continued)

(Continued)

Code Z79.4, Long-term (current) use of insulin, should not be assigned with codes from subcategory O24.4.

An abnormal glucose tolerance in pregnancy is assigned a code from subcategory O99.81, Abnormal glucose complicating pregnancy, childbirth, and the puerperium.

Guideline I.C.15.j. Sepsis and septic shock complicating abortion, pregnancy, childbirth and the puerperium: When assigning a Chapter 15 code for sepsis complicating abortion, pregnancy, childbirth, and the puerperium, a code for the specific type of infection should be assigned as an additional diagnosis. If severe sepsis is present, a code from subcategory R65.2, Severe sepsis, and code(s) for associated organ dysfunction(s) should also be assigned as additional diagnoses.

Guideline I.C.15.k. Puerperal sepsis: Code O85, Puerperal sepsis, should be assigned with a secondary code to identify the causal organism (e.g., for a bacterial infection, assign a code from category B95–B96, Bacterial infections in conditions classified elsewhere). A code from category A40, Streptococcal sepsis, or A41, Other sepsis, should not be used for puerperal sepsis. If applicable, use additional codes to identify severe sepsis (R65.2-) and any associated acute organ dysfunction.

Guideline I.C.15.l. Alcohol and tobacco use during pregnancy, childbirth and the puerperium

Guideline I.C.15.l.1. Alcohol use during pregnancy, childbirth and the puerperium: Codes under subcategory O99.31, Alcohol use complicating pregnancy, childbirth, and the puerperium, should be assigned for any pregnancy case when a mother uses alcohol during the pregnancy or postpartum. A secondary code from category F10, Alcohol related disorders, should also be assigned to identify manifestations of the alcohol use.

Guideline I.C.15.l.2. Tobacco use during pregnancy, childbirth and the puerperium: Codes under subcategory O99.33, Smoking (tobacco) complicating pregnancy, childbirth, and the puerperium, should be assigned for any pregnancy case when a mother uses any type of tobacco product during the pregnancy or postpartum. A secondary code from category F17, Nicotine dependence, or code Z72.0, Tobacco use, should also be assigned to identify the type of nicotine dependence.

Guideline I.C.15.m. Poisoning, toxic effects, adverse effects and underdosing in a pregnant patient: A code from subcategory O9A.2, Injury, poisoning and certain other consequences of external causes complicating pregnancy, childbirth, and the puerperium, should be sequenced first, followed by the appropriate injury, poisoning, toxic effect, adverse effect or underdosing code, and then the additional code(s) that specifies the condition caused by the poisoning, toxic effect, adverse effect or underdosing.

See Section I.C.19. Adverse effects, poisoning, underdosing and toxic effects.

Guideline I.C.15.n. Normal Delivery, Code O80

Guideline.I.C.15.n.1. Encounter for full term uncomplicated delivery: Code O80 should be assigned when a woman is admitted for a full-term normal delivery and delivers a single, healthy infant without any complications antepartum, during the delivery, or postpartum during the delivery episode. Code O80 is always a principal diagnosis. It is not to be used if any other code from Chapter 15 is needed to describe a current complication of the antenatal, delivery, or perinatal period. Additional codes from other chapters may be used with code O80 if they are not related to or are in any way complicating the pregnancy.

Guideline I.C.15.n.2. Uncomplicated delivery with resolved antepartum complication: Code O80 may be used if the patient had a complication at some point during the pregnancy, but the complication is not present at the time of the admission for delivery.

Guideline I.C.15.n.3. Outcome of delivery for O80 Z37.0, Single live birth, is the only outcome of delivery code appropriate for use with O80.

Guideline I.C.15.o. The Peripartum and Postpartum Periods

Guideline I.C.15.o.1. Peripartum and Postpartum periods: The postpartum period begins immediately after delivery and continues for six weeks following delivery. The peripartum period is defined as the last month of pregnancy to five months postpartum.

Guideline I.C.15.o.2. Peripartum and postpartum complication: A postpartum complication is any complication occurring within the six-week period.

Guideline I.C.15.o.3. Pregnancy-related complications after 6 week period: Chapter 15 codes may also be used to describe pregnancy-related complications after the peripartum or postpartum period if the provider documents that a condition is pregnancy related.

Guideline I.C.15.o.4. Admission for routine postpartum care following delivery outside hospital: When the mother delivers outside the hospital prior to admission and is admitted for routine postpartum care and no complications are noted, code Z39.0, Encounter for care and examination of mother immediately after delivery, should be assigned as the principal diagnosis.

Guideline I.C.15.o.5. Pregnancy associated cardiomyopathy: Pregnancy associated cardiomyopathy, code O90.3, is unique in

(Continued)

(Continued)

that it may be diagnosed in the third trimester of pregnancy but may continue to progress months after delivery. For this reason, it is referred to as peripartum cardiomyopathy. Code O90.3 is only for use when the cardiomyopathy develops as a result of pregnancy in a woman who did not have pre-existing heart disease.

Guideline I.C.15.p. Code O94, Sequelae of complication of pregnancy, childbirth, and the puerperium

Guideline I.C.15.p.1. Code O94: Code O94, Sequelae of complication of pregnancy, childbirth, and the puerperium, is for use in those cases when an initial complication of a pregnancy develops a sequelae requiring care or treatment at a future date.

Guideline I.C.15.p.2. After the initial postpartum period: This code may be used at any time after the initial postpartum period.

Guideline I.C.15.p.3. Sequencing of Code O94: This code, like all sequela codes, is to be sequenced following the code describing the sequelae of the complication.

Guideline I.C.15.q. Abortions

Guideline I.C.15.q.1. Abortion with Liveborn Fetus: When an attempted termination of pregnancy results in a liveborn fetus, assign a code from subcategory O60.1, Preterm labor with preterm delivery, and a code from category Z37, Outcome of Delivery. The procedure code for the attempted termination of pregnancy should also be assigned.

Guideline I.C.15.q.2. Retained Products of Conception following an abortion: Subsequent encounters for retained products of conception following a spontaneous abortion or elective termination of pregnancy are assigned the appropriate code from category O03, Spontaneous abortion, or codes O07.4, Failed attempted termination of pregnancy without complication and Z33.2, Encounter for elective termination of pregnancy. This advice is appropriate even when the patient was discharged previously with a discharge diagnosis of complete abortion.

Guideline I.C.15.r. Abuse in a pregnant patient: For suspected or confirmed cases of abuse of a pregnant patient, a code(s) from subcategories O9A.3, Physical abuse complicating pregnancy, childbirth, and the puerperium, O9A.4, Sexual abuse complicating pregnancy, childbirth, and the puerperium, and O9A.5, Psychological abuse complicating pregnancy, childbirth, and the puerperium, should be sequenced first, followed by the appropriate codes (if applicable) to identify any associated current injury due to physical abuse, sexual abuse, and the perpetrator of abuse.

See Section I.C.19. Adult and child abuse, neglect and other maltreatment.

Coding Pregnancy, Childbirth and the Puerperium in ICD-10-CM Chapter 15

Codes in Chapter 15, Pregnancy, childbirth and the puerperium are in the range of O00 (letter O, digit zero, digit zero) to O9A, an interesting coding coincidence given these letter O codes are for Obstetrics. As the note specifies at the beginning of Chapter 15, codes from Chapter 15 are used only on maternal records and never on newborn infant records. The note also specifies that codes from this chapter are for use for conditions related to or aggravated by the pregnancy, childbirth, or by the puerperium (maternal causes or obstetric causes).

The majority of codes in Chapter 15 have a final character indicating the trimester of pregnancy. The time frames for the trimesters are as follows

- **First Trimester:** less than 14 weeks, 0 days

- **Second Trimester:** 14 weeks, 0 days to less than 28 weeks, 0 days

- **Third Trimester:** 28 weeks, 0 days until delivery

Assignment of the final character for trimester should be based on the trimester for the current admission or encounter. Whenever delivery occurs during the current admission and there is an "in childbirth" option for the obstetric complication being coded, the "in childbirth" code should be assigned.

Pregnancy-Related Codes in ICD-10-CM Chapter 21

Codes from other chapters in ICD-10-CM are used to describe conditions and factors related to reproduction. One block of codes in Chapter 21, Factors influencing health status and contact with health services includes Z30–Z39, Persons encountering health services in circumstances related to reproduction. These codes are used to describe reasons for healthcare services for the pregnant female or for services for men and women seeking reproductive health services. The categories are described in the following sections.

Z30 Encounter for contraceptive management

Codes in this category are used to describe encounters of care for initial prescription of contraceptives, natural family planning, and other general counseling and advice on contraception. Other codes represent visits for surveillance of contraceptives and other contraceptive management visits, including for the male for an encounter for postvasectomy sperm count.

Z31 Encounter for procreative management

Codes in this category identify when procreative management services are provided. These services include encounters for fertility testing, genetic testing for men and women seeking procreative services, and genetic counseling. Code Z31.83 is used for the visit when an assisted reproductive fertility procedure is performed.

Z32 Encounter for pregnancy test and childbirth and childcare instruction

The codes in this category identify an encounter for a pregnancy test and encounters for childbirth education and child care education. The codes for the pregnancy testing identify if the test result was positive, negative, or the result unknown.

Z33 Pregnant state

The ICD-10-CM code for an uncomplicated elective termination of pregnancy (Z33.2) is found in Chapter 21, Factors influencing health status and contact with health services, not with the OB codes found in Chapter 15. An **elective termination of pregnancy**, or an elective abortion, is the intentional ending of a pregnancy by a medical or surgical procedure. In the United States, abortion is legal during the first trimester or first 12 weeks of pregnancy (Merck 2012).

Code Z33.1, **Pregnant state, incidental**, would be assigned as an additional code only if a pregnant patient was seen for a reason unrelated to the pregnancy. It is the physician's responsibility to document that the pregnancy is in no way complicating the reason for the visit or the nonobstetrical condition currently being treated. However, it is not a common occurrence for the physician to state the pregnancy is unaffected, no matter how minor the injury or condition. For this reason, a code from Chapter 15 in ICD-10-CM is more frequently used than the Z33.1. Code Z33.1 is indexed under the main term "Pregnancy" in the Alphabetic Index.

> **EXAMPLE:** The patient is seen in the emergency department for the initial visit for a sprained left wrist; the doctor documents that the patient is pregnant, but specifically states the pregnancy is incidental to the encounter: S63.502A, Sprains and strains of unspecified site of wrist; Z33.1, Pregnant state, incidental.

Z34 Encounter for supervision of normal pregnancy

For routine prenatal outpatient visits when there is no complication present, a code from category Z34 for the encounter for supervision of normal pregnancy is used as the first-listed code. If the prenatal outpatient visit is to manage a high-risk pregnancy, a code from Chapter 15 category O09, Supervision of high-risk pregnancy, is used as the first-listed code. The high-risk pregnancy supervision codes are in the obstetric code chapter and not in the equivalent Z code chapter, where the Z34 codes are located.

A category Z34 code is assigned for supervision of a pregnancy. Code Z34.0, Supervision of normal first pregnancy, uses a fifth character identifying the first, second, third, or unspecified trimester. Z34.8 is a similar code but it is for supervision of other normal pregnancy than the first pregnancy. The trimester of the pregnancy is identified by the fifth character. Supervision of normal subsequent pregnancies is generally used in outpatient settings and for routine prenatal visits.

When a complication of the pregnancy is present, the code for that condition is assigned rather than a code from category Z34. These codes are not used with any other pregnancy code in Chapter 15 of ICD-10-CM because the Z34 code indicates the patient is pregnant and healthy, whereas the Chapter 15 codes indicate an obstetrical problem or condition exists. Codes in category Z34 are indexed under "Pregnancy, supervision (of) (for)" in the Index to Diseases and Injuries.

Z36 Encounter for antenatal screening of mother

One single code, Z36, is used to describe the encounter for antenatal or prenatal screening of the pregnant female. Screening tests are performed for preventive measures and not because the mother is experiencing symptoms or problems.

Z3A Weeks of Gestation

A code from category Z3A is for use only on the maternal record. The Z3A code is used to indicate the **weeks of gestation** of the pregnancy. The gestation period is the duration of the pregnancy. The weeks of gestation indicate the length of the pregnancy measured in completed weeks. The average pregnancy extends for 266 days or 38 weeks from the time of fertilization of the oocyte or egg until the birth of the infant. In obstetrics, the gestation period is also considered to be the first day of the woman's last menstrual prior to fertilization to the birth of the infant thus lasting an average of 280 days or 40 weeks (Dorland 2007). This code for the weeks of gestation is used in addition to a code from Chapter 15 to identify the condition or complication of the pregnancy, childbirth, and the puerperium. The fifth-character level of the code identifies the individual specific week of gestation starting at 8 weeks through 42 weeks of gestation with other codes for shorter or longer periods of gestation. The following is an example of some of the relevant codes:

Z3A.01	Less than 8 weeks gestation of pregnancy
Z3A.08	8 weeks of gestation of pregnancy
Z3A.20	20 weeks of gestation of pregnancy
Z3A.38	38 weeks of gestation of pregnancy
Z3A.49	Greater than 42 weeks of gestation of pregnancy

Z37 Outcome of delivery

Outcome of delivery codes (Z37.0–Z37.9) are intended for use as an additional code to identify the outcome of delivery on the mother's record. It is not for use on the newborn record. These codes exclude stillbirth (P95), which would be assigned to the record of a stillborn infant if a record was created for the stillborn. The **outcome of delivery** codes identify the status of the infant, single, twin, or other multiple births, and whether the infant was liveborn or stillborn.

Z39 Encounter for maternal postpartum care and examination

Code Z39.0 is assigned when the pregnant female delivers a baby outside the hospital and is admitted for care and observation in uncomplicated cases. Two other frequently used codes in this category are Z39.1, Encounter for care and examination of the lactating mother (which is also applicable to supervision of lactation), and code Z39.2, which is used for an encounter for a routine postpartum follow-up visit for a woman who delivered in the previous six weeks.

Pregnancy with Abortive Outcome (O00–O08)

Codes within this block of codes represent the disease and conditions of the woman who experiences a pregnancy that does not produce a liveborn or stillborn infant. The pregnancies described by these codes end before the completion of 20 weeks of gestation.

Ectopic Pregnancy (O00)

An **ectopic pregnancy** is a pregnancy arising from implantation of the ovum outside the uterine cavity. About 98 percent of ectopic pregnancies are tubal (occurring in the fallopian tube). Other sites include the peritoneum or abdominal viscera, ovary, or cervix. ICD-10-CM classifies ectopic pregnancy to category O00, with fourth digits identifying the site of the ectopic pregnancy: abdominal, tubal, ovarian, or other site. An unspecified code O00.9 is used for the rare occasions when the site of the ectopic pregnancy is not specified. A "use additional code" note appears under the category heading to use a code from category O08, Complication following ectopic and molar pregnancy, to identify any associated complication. Complications that may occur with an ectopic pregnancy are infection, hemorrhage, embolism, shock, renal failure, metabolic disorders, damage to pelvic organs, or other specified conditions.

Missed Abortion (O02.1)

A **missed abortion** occurs when the fetus has died before completion of 20 weeks' gestation, with retention in the uterus. The American Congress of Obstetricians and Gynecologists (ACOG) states a missed abortion is usually diagnosed when a pregnant woman has a closed cervix and a uterus that does not increase in size over time or after an ultrasound of the uterus shows embryonic or fetal demise (ACOG 2012). The ICD-10-CM Tabular includes a description of a missed abortion under code O02.1 as early fetal death before completion of 20 weeks of gestation with retention of dead fetus.

A woman with a missed abortion may develop disseminated intravascular coagulation (DIC) and progressive hypofibrinogenemia. Massive bleeding may occur when delivery is finally completed. During this time, symptoms of pregnancy disappear. A brownish vaginal discharge may occur, but no bleeding.

Missed abortions should be completed by physician intervention as soon as a diagnosis with Doppler ultrasound or other methods is certain. A common method of terminating the pregnancy involves the insertion of laminaria stents to dilate the cervix followed by aspiration.

Spontaneous Abortion (O03)

The diagnosis of **spontaneous abortion** is defined as the expulsion or extraction from the uterus of all or part of the products of conception: an embryo or a nonviable fetus weighing less than 500 grams. The spontaneous abortion occurs without a medical or surgical intervention to cause it. When a fetus's weight cannot be determined, an estimated gestation of less than 20 completed weeks is considered an abortion in ICD-10-CM. The procedure also known as abortion is more precisely described as a dilation and curettage, dilation and evacuation, or aspiration curettage.

Coders frequently confuse the clinical condition of missed abortion with a different clinical state: spontaneous abortion. A missed abortion is the retention in the uterus of a fetus that has died. The death is indicated by cessation of growth, hardening of the uterus, loss of size of the uterus, and absence of fetal heart tones after they have been heard on previous examinations. In contrast to a spontaneous abortion, no products of conception, fetal parts, or tissue is expelled from the uterus when the patient has a missed abortion. All of the uterine contents remain in the uterus. When a spontaneous abortion occurs, the woman experiences one or more of the classic symptoms, such as uterine contractions, uterine hemorrhage, dilation of the cervix, and presentation or expulsion of all or part of the products of conception.

The fourth characters used with category O03 indicate the presence or absence of a complication arising during an admission or an encounter for a spontaneous abortion. The fourth-digit subcategories are classified as follows:

O03.0   Genital tract and pelvic infection following incomplete spontaneous
         abortion
         Endometritis
         Oophoritis
         Parametritis
         Pelvic peritonitis
         Salpingitis
         Salpingo-oophoritis
O03.1   Delayed or excessive hemorrhage following incomplete spontaneous
         abortion
         Afibrinogenemia
         Defibrination syndrome
         Hemolysis
         Intravascular hemolysis
O03.2   Embolism following incomplete spontaneous abortion
         Air embolism
         Amniotic fluid embolism
         Blood-clot embolism
         Embolism NOS
         Fat embolism
         Pulmonary embolism
         Pyemic embolism
         Septic or septicopyemic embolism
         Soap embolism
O03.3   Other and unspecified complications following incomplete spontaneous
         abortion
         Circulatory collapse
         Shock
         Renal failure
         Metabolic disorders
         Damage to pelvic organs
         Other venous complication
         Cardiac arrest
         Sepsis
         Urinary tract infection
O03.4   Incomplete spontaneous abortion without complication
O03.5   Genital tract and pelvic infection following complete or unspecified spontaneous abortion
O03.6   Delayed or excessive hemorrhage following complete or unspecified spontaneous abortion
O03.7   Embolism following complete or unspecified spontaneous abortion
O03.8   Other and unspecified complications following complete or unspecified spontaneous abortion
O03.9   Complete or unspecified spontaneous abortion without complication

ICD-10-CM uses the following definitions for complete and incomplete spontaneous abortions:

- A **complete abortion** is the expulsion of all of the products of conception from the uterus prior to the episode of care.

- An **incomplete abortion** is the expulsion of some, but not all, of the products of conception from the uterus. If placenta or secundines remain, the abortion is considered incomplete. A subsequent admission for retained products of conception following a spontaneous or legally induced abortion is assigned the appropriate code from category 634, Spontaneous abortion, or 635, Legally induced abortion, with a fifth digit of 1 for incomplete. This advice is appropriate even when the patient was discharged previously with a discharge diagnosis of complete abortion. A review of the pathology report will confirm a complete or an incomplete abortion.

Complications Following (Induced) Termination of Pregnancy (O04)

Category O04, Complications following (induced) termination of pregnancy is used when a complication occurs after the abortion itself was completed during a previous admission. According to the Excludes1 note that appears in category O04, these codes are not used during an encounter for elective termination of pregnancy that is uncompleted or during an encounter when a failed attempted termination of pregnancy occurs. The subcategories classify the complications classifiable to the fourth-digit level.

O04.5   Genital tract and pelvic infection following (induced) termination of pregnancy
O04.6   Delayed or excessive hemorrhage following (induced) termination of pregnancy
O04.7   Embolism following (induced) termination of pregnancy
O04.8   (Induced) termination of pregnancy with other and unspecified complications
        Shock
        Renal failure
        Metabolic disorder
        Damage to pelvic organs
        Other venous complication
        Cardiac arrest
        Urinary tract infection
        Other complications
        Unspecified complications

Failed Attempted Termination of Pregnancy (O07)

Category O07, **Failed attempted termination of pregnancy**, is used when an attempted abortion fails and the pregnancy continues. The failed termination may not produce any complications (O07.4). However, other fourth-character subcategory codes are used when a complication occurs. According to the Excludes1 note that appears in category O07, these codes are not used during an encounter for treatment of an incomplete spontaneous abortion (O03.0-). The subcategories classify the complications classifiable to the fourth-digit level.

O07.0   Genital tract and pelvic infection following failed attempted termination of pregnancy

O07.1   Delayed or excessive hemorrhage following failed attempted termination of pregnancy

O07.2   Embolism following failed attempted termination of pregnancy

O07.3   (Induced) termination of pregnancy with other and unspecified complications
Shock
Renal failure
Metabolic disorder
Damage to pelvic organs
Other venous complication
Cardiac arrest
Sepsis
Urinary tract infection
Other complications

O07.4   Failed attempted termination of pregnancy without complication

Complications Following Ectopic and Molar Pregnancy (O08)

Category O08, Complications following ectopic and molar pregnancy, is used when a complication occurs with an ectopic and molar pregnancy. According to the note that appears in category O08, these codes are used with categories O00–O02 to identify any associated complications. The subcategories classify the complications classifiable to the fourth-digit level.

O08.0   Genital tract and pelvic infection following ectopic and molar pregnancy
Endometritis
Oophoritis
Parametritis
Pelvic peritonitis
Salpingitis
Salpingo-oophoritis

O08.1   Delayed or excessive hemorrhage following ectopic and molar pregnancy
Afibrinogenemia
Defibrination syndrome
Hemolysis
Intravascular hemolysis

O08.2   Embolism following ectopic and molar pregnancy
Air embolism
Amniotic fluid embolism
Blood-clot embolism
Embolism NOS
Fat embolism
Pulmonary embolism
Pyemic embolism
Septic or septicopyemic embolism
Soap embolism

O08.3   Shock following ectopic and molar pregnancy
Circulatory collapse
Shock

O08.4   Renal failure following ectopic and molar pregnancy

O08.5   Metabolic disorders following ectopic and molar pregnancy

O08.6   Damage to pelvic organs and tissues following ectopic and molar pregnancy

O08.7   Other venous complications following an ectopic and molar pregnancy

O08.8   Other complications following an ectopic and molar pregnancy
Cardiac arrest
Sepsis
Urinary tract infection
Other complications

O08.9   Unspecified complications following an ectopic and molar pregnancy

Supervision of High Risk Pregnancy (O09)

Category O09 provides information on conditions that may add risk to a present pregnancy. A code from O09 can be assigned as a principal or first-listed diagnosis or as an additional code. A code from Chapter 15 in ICD-10-CM can be assigned with a code from category O09. Typically, these codes are used for prenatal outpatient visits. Code O09.3-, Supervision of pregnancy with **insufficient antenatal care**, may be assigned to patients who had little or no prenatal care. Healthcare providers must define "insufficient" prenatal care and consistently capture this code for the information to be valuable. Codes within the O09.5- (**elderly pregnant females**, 35 years or older at the expected date of delivery) and O09.6- (**young pregnant females**, younger than 16 years old at expected date of delivery) subcategories identify patients whose age and current pregnancies put them at a high risk for problems and thus make them worthy of close monitoring. Codes O09.81- and O09.82- identify the fact that the patient is pregnant as a result of assisted reproductive technology or is pregnant with a history of an in utero procedure during a previous pregnancy. The sixth-character level identifies the first, second, third or unspecified trimester of pregnancy when the supervision occurred.

The O09 category codes are indexed under the main terms "Pregnancy, supervision (of) (for)" in the Alphabetic Index.

> **EXAMPLE:**   Pregnancy, first trimester with history of infertility: O09.01, Supervision of pregnancy with history of infertility, first trimester

> **EXAMPLE:**   Full term with intrauterine death, spontaneous delivery; no prenatal care received during pregnancy: O36.4xx0, Maternal care for intrauterine death; O09.33, Supervision of pregnancy with insufficient prenatal care; Z37.1, Single stillborn

Threatened Abortion (O20.0)

A **threatened abortion** is characterized by bleeding of intrauterine origin occurring before the 20th completed week of gestation, with or without uterine colic, without expulsion of the products of conception, and without dilation of the cervix. ICD-10-CM category O20 states hemorrhage occurs before completion of 20 weeks. The physician may also document the condition as an intrauterine hemorrhage due to a threatened abortion. When a physician describes the patient's condition as a threatened abortion it means the loss of the pregnancy is prevented and the patient remains pregnant at the end of the admission or encounter.

Recurrent Pregnancy Loss (O26.20–O26.23 and N96)

A **recurrent pregnancy loss**, also known as a habitual or recurrent abortion, is the spontaneous expulsion of a dead or nonviable fetus in two or more pregnancies at any gestational age. Coding guidelines for this condition include the following:

- If the recurrent spontaneous abortion is current, that is, the patient's admission or encounter is for an abortion, ICD-10-CM offers direction to the spontaneous abortion code (category O03).

- If the current hospital admission or encounter involves a pregnancy, assign code O26.20–O26.23, Pregnancy care for patient with recurrent pregnancy loss, with the trimester of pregnancy identified if known.

- If the current hospital admission or encounter does not involve a pregnancy, assign code N96, Recurrent pregnancy loss. During an admission or encounter that does not involve pregnancy care there is likely an investigation or care of a nonpregnant woman with a history of recurrent pregnancy loss.

Pregnancy

Pregnancy is the state of a female after conception until the birth (delivery) of the child. Normal pregnancies are intrauterine and the duration of pregnancy from conception to delivery is about 266 days. The following guidelines may be used in determining preterm, term, and postterm pregnancies:

- **Preterm**: Delivery before 37 completed weeks of gestation (patient is in her 37th or earlier week of pregnancy)

- **Term**: Delivery between 38 and 40 completed weeks of gestation (patient is in her 38th, 39th, or 40th week of pregnancy)

- **Postterm**: Delivery between 41 and 42 completed weeks of gestation (patient is in her 41st or 42nd week of pregnancy)

- **Prolonged**: Delivery for a pregnancy that has advanced beyond 42 completed weeks of gestation (patient is in her 43rd or later week of pregnancy)

The postpartum period, or **puerperium**, begins immediately after delivery and continues for six weeks. In the Alphabetic Index to Diseases and Injuries, long listings of conditions appear under the following main terms: Pregnancy, Delivery, and Puerperium/Puerperal/Postpartum.

Indentations are often used in the Alphabetic Index under these main terms, so extreme care should be taken in locating and selecting the appropriate code.

Encounter for Delivery (O80 and O82)

Two categories are available to describe an uncomplicated **normal delivery** and an encounter for cesarean delivery when there is no mention of the reason for the cesarean delivery.

Encounter for Full-Term Uncomplicated Delivery (O80)

Category O80 is used when the pregnant female has a

- Full-term, single, live-born infant

- Spontaneous, cephalic, vaginal delivery

- Delivery requiring minimal or no assistance, with or without episiotomy, without fetal manipulation (that is, rotation version) or instrumentation (forceps)

Code O80 is used as a single diagnosis code and is not to be used with any other code from Chapter 15. This code must be accompanied by a delivery code from the appropriate procedure classification. For example, an ICD-10-PCS procedure code would be used for an inpatient admission and a CPT procedure code would be used for an outpatient health care encounter or for a provider's professional fee billing. An additional code to indicate the outcome of delivery, Z37.0, Single live birth, must be used with code O80.

Encounter for Cesarean Delivery without Indication (O82)

Code O82 is used when the pregnant female has a cesarean delivery without the indication or the reason for the cesarean delivery documented in the health records. This is not necessarily the preferred diagnosis code to be used with all encounters for a cesarean delivery. When the reason for the surgical delivery is documented in the health record the condition must be coded instead of code O82. When code O82 is used, an additional code Z37.0 is used to indicate the outcome of delivery.

Outcome of Delivery (Z Codes)

The outcome of delivery, as indicated by a code from category Z37, should be included on all maternal delivery records. This is always an additional, not a principal, diagnosis code used to reflect the number and status of babies delivered. Many hospitals rely on these codes to provide more information on obstetrical outcomes. Code Z37 is referenced in the Alphabetic Index to Diseases and Injuries under the main term "Outcome of delivery."

> **EXAMPLE:** Encounter for full-term uncomplicated delivery: O80, Normal delivery; Z37.0, Outcome of delivery, single live birth

Obstetrical and Nonobstetrical Complications

Many preexisting conditions, including diabetes, hypertension, and anemia, may affect or complicate the pregnancy or its management. In addition, the pregnancy may aggravate the preexisting condition.

For this reason, if the pregnancy aggravates the preexisting or nonobstetrical condition or vice versa, the condition is reclassified to Chapter 15 of ICD-10-CM. The categories representing such conditions are as follows:

- Edema, proteinuria and hypertensive disorders in pregnancy, childbirth and the puerperium (O10–O16)

- Other maternal disorders predominantly related to pregnancy (O20–O29)

- Maternal care related to the fetus and amniotic cavity and possible delivery problems (O30–O48)

- Complications of labor and delivery (O60–O77)

- Complications predominantly related to the puerperium (O85–O92)

- Other obstetric conditions, not elsewhere classified (O94–O9A)

Preexisting Hypertension (O10)

Category O10, Preexisting hypertension complicating pregnancy, childbirth, and the puerperium, provides specific subcategories for the type of hypertensive disease:

O10.0   Preexisting essential hypertension complicating pregnancy, childbirth and the puerperium
This code represents any condition in I10, Essential (primary) hypertension specified as a reason of obstetric care during pregnancy, childbirth or the puerperium. No additional code is required to identify the hypertension.

O10.1   Preexisting hypertensive heart disease complicating pregnancy, childbirth and the puerperium
This code represents any condition in I11, Hypertensive heart disease specified as a reason of obstetric care during pregnancy, childbirth or the puerperium. An additional code from I11 is required to identify the type of hypertensive heart disease.

O10.2   Preexisting hypertensive chronic kidney disease complicating pregnancy, childbirth and the puerperium
This code represents any condition in I12, Hypertensive chronic kidney disease specified as a reason of obstetric care during pregnancy, childbirth or the puerperium. An additional code from I12 is required to identify the type of hypertensive chronic kidney disease.

O10.3   Preexisting hypertensive heart and chronic kidney disease complicating pregnancy, childbirth and the puerperium
This code represents any condition in I13, Hypertensive heart and chronic kidney disease specified as a reason of obstetric care during pregnancy, childbirth or the puerperium. An additional code from I13 is required to identify the type of hypertensive heart and chronic kidney disease.

O10.4   Preexisting secondary hypertension complicating pregnancy, childbirth and the puerperium
This code represents any condition in I15, Secondary hypertension specified as a reason of obstetric care during pregnancy, childbirth or the puerperium. An additional code from I15 is required to identify the type of secondary hypertension.

O10.9   Unspecified preexisting hypertension complicating pregnancy, childbirth and the puerperium

Other Forms of Hypertension, Pre-eclampsia and Eclampsia (O11–O16)

Other forms of hypertensive disease with pre-eclampsia as well as gestational hypertension, pre-eclampsia, eclampsia, and other material hypertension are classified with categories O11–O16. Specifically these categories are described in the following manner:

O11   Preexisting hypertension with pre-eclampsia
        This category requires an additional code from O10, Preexisting hypertension complicating pregnancy, childbirth and the puerperium.
O12   Gestational [pregnancy-induced] edema and proteinuria without hypertension
O13   Gestational [pregnancy-induced] hypertension without significant proteinuria
O14   Pre-eclampsia
O15   Eclampsia
O16   Unspecified maternal hypertension

Excessive Vomiting in Pregnancy (O21)

Hyperemesis is excessive vomiting. **Hyperemesis gravidarum** is severe morning sickness or excessive nausea and vomiting experienced during the early weeks of pregnancy by some women (Dorland 2007). Category O21, Excessive vomiting in pregnancy, provides specific subcategories; therefore, additional codes are not required unless ICD-10-CM notations instruct otherwise. For example, code O21.8, Other vomiting complicating pregnancy, has the note to "Use additional code to specify the cause." The codes in the category that do not require an additional code are the following:

O21.0   Mild hyperemesis gravidarum
         This code represents excessive vomiting in pregnancy starting before the end of the 20th week of gestation.
O21.1   Hyperemesis gravidarum with metabolic disturbance
         The metabolic disturbances included in this code with excessive vomiting are carbohydrate depletion, dehydration, or electrolyte imbalance starting before the end of the 20th week of gestation.
O21.2   Late vomiting of pregnancy
         This code represents excessive vomiting in pregnancy starting after the 20th completed week of pregnancy.
O21.9   Vomiting of pregnancy, unspecified

Late Pregnancy (O48)

Two codes exist to identify women who are beyond 40 completed weeks of gestation, as this may be the primary reason for the obstetrical services being rendered. A pregnancy is not considered a prolonged pregnancy until it extends after 42 completed weeks. Women in this group are considered potentially high risk for pregnancy complications.

Subcategory O48.0 is used to describe post-term pregnancy or pregnancy over 40 completed weeks to 42 completed weeks of gestation. Subcategory O48.1 is used to describe prolonged pregnancy or pregnancy that has advanced beyond 42 completed weeks of gestation.

Preterm Labor with or without Delivery (O60)

Category O60, **Preterm labor** is defined as the onset (spontaneous) of labor before 37 completed weeks of gestation. Even when the delivery of a liveborn infant occurs as the result of an attempted elective abortion, it is considered a preterm labor and delivery and not an abortion. If the infant was not liveborn, the elective abortion would have been the diagnosis provided by the physician. In addition to category O60, a code to describe the outcome of delivery (Z37) must be assigned.

A coder cannot assign *both* the diagnosis code for an early onset of delivery (O60) and an elective abortion (Z33.2) on the same patient's record for a woman whose pregnancy lasted for less than 20 completed weeks. If a woman delivers a liveborn infant at any time before 37 completed weeks of gestation it would not be an abortion but instead coded as an early onset of delivery (O60). If the woman's pregnancy ends before 20 completed weeks and there is a nonviable or dead infant expelled, it would be classified with code Z33.2. A Z37 code is also assigned for the single infant born.

> **EXAMPLE:** Spontaneous abortion, second trimester, resulting in liveborn fetus: O60.120, Preterm labor second trimester with preterm delivery; Z37.0, Outcome of delivery, single live birth.
>
> **EXAMPLE:** Elective termination of pregnancy resulting in liveborn, second trimester: O60.120, Preterm labor second trimester with preterm delivery; Z37.0, Outcome of delivery, single live birth.

Puerperal Sepsis (O85) and Other Puerperal Infection (O86)

Category O85, Puerperal sepsis, includes the most serious manifestations of major postpartum infection including postpartum sepsis, puerperal peritonitis, and puerperal pyemia. This condition occurs during the six weeks or 42 days following delivery. The coder should use an additional code (B95–B97) to identify the known infectious agent responsible for the infection. In addition, if the patient also has severe sepsis an additional code is used for severe sepsis without septic shock (R65.20) or severe sepsis with septic shock (R65.21). Any organ failure or other systemic complication that is present would also be coded with the severe sepsis and the puerperal sepsis codes.

Category O86, Other puerperal infection, identifies localized infections that occur during the postpartum period, such as the following:

O86.0	Infection of obstetric surgical wound
O86.1	Other infection of genital tract following delivery
O86.2	Urinary tract infection following delivery
O86.4	Pyrexia of unknown origin following delivery
O86.8	Other specified puerperal infections, such as puerperal septic thrombophlebitis

Venous Complications and Hemorrhoids in the Puerperium (O87)

Category O87, Venous complications and hemorrhoids in the puerperium, is subdivided to identify the types of venous conditions or complications. Under subcategory O87.1,

Deep phlebothrombosis in the puerperium, an additional code is required to identify the deep vein thrombosis that exists. In addition, a code for associated long-term (current) use of anti-coagulants is used with code O87.1 if applicable.

Coding Procedures in the Obstetrics Section

Procedure coding guidelines exist in the *Official ICD-10-PCS Coding Guidelines* and can be found at http://www.cms.gov/Medicare/Coding/ICD10/Downloads/pcs_2013_guidelines .pdf or at the CMS webpage for current year ICD-10-PCS and GEMS documents. Specific procedure coding guidelines exist for coding procedures in the Obstetrics section.

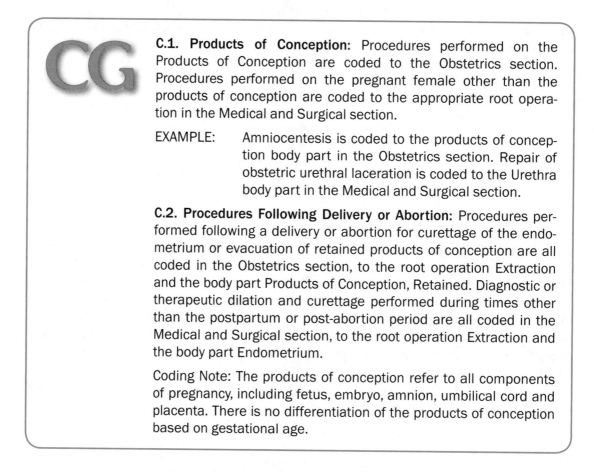

CG

C.1. Products of Conception: Procedures performed on the Products of Conception are coded to the Obstetrics section. Procedures performed on the pregnant female other than the products of conception are coded to the appropriate root operation in the Medical and Surgical section.

EXAMPLE: Amniocentesis is coded to the products of conception body part in the Obstetrics section. Repair of obstetric urethral laceration is coded to the Urethra body part in the Medical and Surgical section.

C.2. Procedures Following Delivery or Abortion: Procedures performed following a delivery or abortion for curettage of the endometrium or evacuation of retained products of conception are all coded in the Obstetrics section, to the root operation Extraction and the body part Products of Conception, Retained. Diagnostic or therapeutic dilation and curettage performed during times other than the postpartum or post-abortion period are all coded in the Medical and Surgical section, to the root operation Extraction and the body part Endometrium.

Coding Note: The products of conception refer to all components of pregnancy, including fetus, embryo, amnion, umbilical cord and placenta. There is no differentiation of the products of conception based on gestational age.

Assigning ICD-10-PCS Procedure Codes for Obstetrics

The Obstetrics section follows the same conventions established in the Medical and Surgical section with all seven characters retaining the same meaning.

The seven characters in the Obstetrics section codes are the following:

Character 1—Section: The first character is a digit "1" in the Obstetrics section.

Character 2—Body System: The second character for body system is one single body system, Pregnancy.

Character 3—Root Operation: There are a total of 12 root operations in the Obstetrics section. Ten of the root operations are found in other sections of ICD-10-PCS and two are unique to the Obstetrics section. The two unique root operations are Abortion and Delivery.

Character 4—Body Part: The fourth character for body part is a single part: Products of Conception

Character 5—Approach: The fifth character, depending on the root operation, identifies the approach, such as Open, Percutaneous, Percutaneous Endoscopic, Via Natural or Artificial Opening, Via Natural or Artificial Opening Endoscopic, and External.

Character 6—Device: The sixth character is used to identify the device involved, specifically a Monitoring Electrode or Other Device. Most of the procedure codes in the Obstetrics section do not include a device.

Character 7—Qualifier: The seventh character or qualifier values are dependent on the root operation, approach, and body system. The methods of extraction, methods of terminating pregnancy, and substances drained are examples of the qualifier in the Obstetrics section. The qualifier adds additional information depending on the procedure, such as the type of cesarean delivery (classical, low cervical, or extraperitoneal) or the body system involved with the repair of anatomic structures of the fetus in utero.

The two root operations unique to the Obstetrics section are Abortion and Delivery. **Abortion (procedure)** is defined as artificially terminating a pregnancy. This root operation is subdivided according to whether an additional device such as a lamineria or abortifacient is used, or whether the abortion was performed by mechanical means. If either a laminaria or abortifacient is used, the approach is Via Natural or Artificial Opening. All other abortion procedures are those done by mechanical means; that is, the products of conception are physically removed using instrumentation and the device value is Z, No Device. An example of an abortion procedure is a transvaginal abortion using vacuum aspiration.

Delivery (procedure) is defined as assisting the passage of the products of conception from the genital canal. This root operation applies only to manually assisted vaginal delivery. Cesarean deliveries are coded in this section to the root operation Extraction.

Another procedure that is frequently used as a root operation in the Obstetrics section is **drainage**. As in the Medical and Surgical section, drainage is defined as taking or letting out fluids or gases from a body part. In the Obstetrics section, the qualifier used with the root operation Drainage identifies the substance that is drained from the products of conception, specifically fetal blood, fetal spinal fluid, or amniotic fluid. Examples of procedures coded to the root operation Drainage in the Obstetrics section are amniocentesis and percutaneous fetal spinal tap.

ICD-10-CM and ICD-10-PCS Review Exercises: Chapter 18

Assign the correct ICD-10-CM diagnosis codes or ICD-10-PCS procedure codes to the following exercises.

1. The patient is a 40-year-old G2 P1 woman who is 26-weeks pregnant and being seen for gestational hypertension. Other than being an elderly, multigravida patient, she is not having any other problems during this pregnancy.

   _____

2. A 16-week pregnancy with mild hyperemesis and urinary tract infection, which grew out E. coli in the culture.

   _____

3. Patient returns to the office with breast pain. The patient is a 24-year-old woman who is three weeks postpartum. Final diagnosis documented as nonpurulent postpartum mastitis.

   _____

4. Delivery of single liveborn infant, full-term, vaginal delivery by cephalic presentation, 40 weeks of gestation

   _____

5. Normal full-term vaginal delivery by cephalic presentation, 38 weeks of gestation, elderly multigravida with gestational diabetes that is diet controlled, single liveborn infant

   _____

6. Full-term vaginal delivery, complicated by second-degree perineal laceration, 39 weeks of pregnancy, twin pregnancy, dichorionic/diamniotic, both liveborn infants

   _____

7. Postpartum office visit, 5 days after discharge, with partial lactation failure

   _____

8. False labor with Braxton Hicks contractions, 32 weeks of pregnancy, undelivered

   _____

9. Office visit for pregnant female, 19 weeks of gestation, with cervical incompetence complicating pregnancy. Surgical consent signed for cervical cerclage procedure to be performed the following day at the ambulatory surgery center.

   _____

10. Pregnancy delivered, single liveborn, vaginal delivery following prolonged second stage of labor, 38 weeks of gestation

    _____

11. Ectopic pregnancy, tubal, 10 weeks gestation

    _____

ICD-10-CM and ICD-10-PCS Review Exercises: Chapter 18 (Continued)

12. Spontaneous incomplete abortion, 11 weeks

13. Induced abortion, complicated by excessive hemorrhage, 8 weeks

14. Mild pre-eclampsia in pregnancy, second trimester, 26 weeks, undelivered

15. Pregnancy, 32 weeks, placenta previa without hemorrhage, undelivered

16. PROCEDURE: Low cervical cesarean delivery

17. PROCEDURE: Manually assisted delivery

18. PROCEDURE: Vacuum assisted delivery

19. PROCEDURE: Induced abortion by laminaria

20. PROCEDURE: Treatment of incomplete spontaneous abortion by dilation and curettage (extraction) of retained products of conception

Chapter 19

Certain Conditions Originating in the Perinatal Period (P00–P96)

Learning Objectives

At the conclusion of this chapter, you should be able to:

1. Describe the organization of the conditions and codes included in ICD-10-CM Chapter 16, Certain conditions originating in the perinatal period (P00–P96)

2. Describe the newborn or perinatal period

3. Describe the circumstances in which a code from Chapter 16 of ICD-10-CM can be assigned in terms of the age of the patient who has the condition

4. Briefly describe the newborn ICD-10-CM coding guidelines, including how to sequence the newborn and perinatal codes

5. Describe the types of conditions classified in ICD-10-CM categories P00–P04, Newborn affected by maternal factors and by complications of pregnancy, labor and delivery

6. Describe the circumstances in which codes from ICD-10-CM categories P05–P08 are used on a newborn or perinatal record, including weeks of gestation and birth weight

7. Define the term *meconium* and describe the conditions associated with the passage of meconium

8. Review the types of respiratory infections and cardiac dysrhythmias that can occur in newborn and perinatal infants

9. Assign ICD-10-CM codes for certain conditions originating in the perinatal period

10. Assign ICD-10-PCS procedure codes related to perinatal conditions

Key Terms

- Bacterial sepsis of newborn
- Exceptionally large baby
- Extreme immaturity
- Fetal growth retardation (FGR)
- Gestational age
- Heavy-for-dates
- Large baby
- Large-for-dates
- Late newborn
- Light-for-dates
- Low birth weight
- Meconium
- Meconium staining
- Meconium aspiration syndrome
- Neonatal aspiration
- Perinatal period
- Post maturity baby
- Post-term newborn
- Prematurity
- Respiratory distress syndrome (RDS)
- Short gestation
- Small-for-dates

Overview of ICD-10-CM Chapter 16, Certain Conditions Originating in the Perinatal Period

Chapter 16 includes categories P00–P96 arranged in the following blocks:

P00–P04	Newborn affected by maternal factors and by complications of pregnancy, labor and delivery
P05–P08	Disorders of newborn related to length of gestation and fetal growth
P09	Abnormal findings on neonatal screening
P10–P15	Birth trauma
P19–P29	Respiratory and cardiovascular disorders specific to the perinatal period
P35–P39	Infections specific to the perinatal period
P50–P61	Hemorrhagic and hematological disorders of newborn
P70–P74	Transitory endocrine and metabolic disorders specific to newborn
P76–P78	Digestive system disorders of newborn
P80–P83	Conditions involving the integument and temperature regulation of newborn
P84	Other problems with newborn
P90–P96	Other disorders originating in the perinatal period

The codes in this chapter describe conditions that begin before birth or develop during the first 28 days of life (the perinatal period). These are not congenital conditions. The conditions that develop in the perinatal period may continue to exist past the first 28 days of life and can be coded regardless of the patient's age.

Codes P00–P04 have the descriptor phrase "suspected to be" included in the code title as a nonessential modifier to indicate the codes are for use when the listed maternal condition is specified as the cause of confirmed or suspected newborn morbidity or potential morbidity. An example of this feature is code P00.3, Newborn (suspected to be) affected by other maternal circulatory and respiratory diseases.

EXAMPLES:	P00.3	Newborn (suspected to be) affected by other maternal circulatory and respiratory diseases
	P00.4	Newborn (suspected to be) affected by maternal nutritional disorders
	P00.5	Newborn (suspected to be) affected by maternal injury

The block of codes for the perinatal conditions are organized by type, for example, disorders related to length of gestation and fetal growth versus conditions produced by birth trauma. Other blocks of codes are grouped by the type of condition or body system where the disease is present. For example, there are blocks of codes for infections versus respiratory and cardiovascular system disorders.

Coding Guidelines and Instructional Notes for ICD-10-CM Chapter 16

Codes from Chapter 16, Certain conditions originating in the perinatal period, are only for use on the newborn or infant record, never on the maternal record. This note appears at the beginning of Chapter 16. Codes from this chapter are also only applicable for liveborn infants.

Further, the following Includes note appears on the first page of Chapter 16: "Conditions that have their origin in the fetal or **perinatal period** (before birth through the first 28 days after birth) even if morbidity occurs later."

This statement should be interpreted such that if a condition originated in the perinatal period and continued throughout the life of the child, the perinatal code should continue to be used regardless of the age of the patient.

Throughout Chapter 16 are notes that help to clarify how codes are to be sequenced. For example, the following note appears under P07: "When both birth weight and gestational age of the newborn are available, both should be coded with birth weight sequenced before gestational age."

The following note appears under P08.21 to define a **post-term newborn**: "Newborn with gestation period over 40 completed weeks to 42 completed weeks."

A note at block P00–P04, Newborn affected by maternal factors and by complications of pregnancy, labor, and delivery also provides guidance:

These codes (P00–P04) are for use when the listed maternal conditions are specified as the cause of confirmed morbidity or potential morbidity which has their origin in the perinatal period (before birth through the first 28 days after birth). Codes from these categories are also for use for newborns who are suspected of having an abnormal condition resulting from exposure from the mother or the birth process, but without signs or symptoms, and which after examination and observation, is found not to exist. These codes may be used even if treatment is begun for a suspected condition that is ruled out (CMS 2012).

The NCHS has published chapter-specific guidelines for Chapter 16 in the *ICD-10-CM Official Guidelines for Coding and Reporting.* The coding student should review all of the coding guidelines for Chapter 16 of ICD-10-CM, which appear in an ICD-10-CM code book or at the website http://www.cdc.gov/nchs/icd/icd10cm.htm, or in Appendix E.

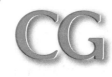

Chapter 16: Certain Conditions Originating in the Perinatal Period (P00–P96): For coding and reporting purposes the perinatal period is defined as before birth through the 28th day following birth. The following guidelines are provided for reporting purposes.

Guideline I.C.16.a. General Perinatal Rules

Guideline I.C.16.a.1. Use of Chapter 16 Codes: Codes in this chapter are never for use on the maternal record. Codes from Chapter 15, the obstetric chapter, are never permitted on the newborn record. Chapter 16 codes may be used throughout the life of the patient if the condition is still present.

Guideline I.C.16.a.2. Principal Diagnosis for Birth Record: When coding the birth episode in a newborn record, assign a code from category Z38, Liveborn infants according to place of birth and type of delivery, as the principal diagnosis. A code from category Z38 is assigned only once, to a newborn at the time of birth. If a newborn is transferred to another institution, a code from category Z38 should not be used at the receiving hospital.

A code from category Z38 is used only on the newborn record, not on the mother's record.

Guideline I.C.16.a.3. Use of Codes from other Chapters with Codes from Chapter 16: Codes from other chapters may be used with codes from Chapter 16 if the codes from the other chapters provide more specific detail. Codes for signs and symptoms may be assigned when a definitive diagnosis has not been established. If the reason for the encounter is a perinatal condition, the code from Chapter 16 should be sequenced first.

Guideline I.C.16.a.4. Use of Chapter 16 Codes after the Perinatal Period: Should a condition originate in the perinatal period, and continue throughout the life of the patient, the perinatal code should continue to be used regardless of the patient's age.

Guideline I.C.16.a.5. Birth process or community acquired conditions: If a newborn has a condition that may be either due to the birth process or community acquired and the documentation does not indicate which it is, the default is due to the birth process and the code from Chapter 16 should be used. If the condition is community-acquired, a code from Chapter 16 should not be assigned.

Guideline I.C.16.a.6. Code all clinically significant conditions: All clinically significant conditions noted on routine newborn examination should be coded. A condition is clinically significant if it requires:

clinical evaluation; or

therapeutic treatment; or

diagnostic procedures; or

extended length of hospital stay; or

increased nursing care and/or monitoring; or

has implications for future health care needs

Note: The perinatal guidelines listed above are the same as the general coding guidelines for "additional diagnoses", except for the final point regarding implications for future health care needs. Codes should be assigned for conditions that have been specified by the provider as having implications for future health care needs.

Guideline I.C.16.b. Observation and Evaluation of Newborns for Suspected Conditions not Found: Originally the Official Coding and Reporting Guidelines included a description of how to code for observation and evaluation of newborns for suspected conditions not found. However, in the 2013 version of the guidelines, the explanation of how to code this situation was removed and the statement of "reserved for future expansion" was included.

Guideline I.C.16.c. Coding Additional Perinatal Diagnoses

Guideline I.C.16.c.1. Assigning codes for conditions that require treatment: Assign codes for conditions that require treatment or further investigation, prolong the length of stay, or require resource utilization.

Guideline I.C.16.c.2. Codes for conditions specified as having implications for future health care needs: Assign codes for conditions that have been specified by the provider as having implications for future health care needs. Note: This guideline should not be used for adult patients.

Guideline I.C.16.d. Prematurity and Fetal Growth Retardation: Providers utilize different criteria in determining prematurity. A code for prematurity should not be assigned unless it is documented. Assignment of codes in categories P05, Disorders of newborn related to slow fetal growth and fetal malnutrition, and P07, Disorders of newborn related to short gestation and low birth weight, not elsewhere classified, should be based on the recorded birth weight and estimated gestational age. Codes from category P05 should not be assigned with codes from category P07.

(Continued)

(Continued)

When both birth weight and gestational age are available, two codes from category P07 should be assigned, with the code for birth weight sequenced before the code for gestational age.

Guideline I.C.16.e. Low birth weight and immaturity status: Codes from category P07, Disorders of newborn related to short gestation and low birth weight, not elsewhere classified, are for use for a child or adult who was premature or had a low birth weight as a newborn and this is affecting the patient's current health status.

See Section I.C.21. Factors influencing health status and contact with health services, Status

Guideline I.C.16.f. Bacterial Sepsis of Newborn: Category P36, Bacterial sepsis of newborn, includes congenital sepsis. If a perinate is documented as having sepsis without documentation of congenital or community acquired, the default is congenital and a code from category P36 should be assigned. If the P36 code includes the causal organism, an additional code from category B95, Streptococcus, Staphylococcus, and Enterococcus as the cause of diseases classified elsewhere, or B96, Other bacterial agents as the cause of diseases classified elsewhere, should not be assigned. If the P36 code does not include the causal organism, assign an additional code from category B96. If applicable, use additional codes to identify severe sepsis (R65.2-) and any associated acute organ dysfunction.

Guideline I.C.16.g. Stillbirth: Code P95, Stillbirth, is only for use in institutions that maintain separate records for stillbirths. No other code should be used with P95. Code P95 should not be used on the mother's record.

Coding Certain Conditions Originating in the Perinatal Period in ICD-10-CM Chapter 16

The introductory notes at the beginning of the chapter provide clarification. Codes from this chapter are for use on newborn records only, never on maternal records, and include conditions that have their origin in the fetal or perinatal period (before birth through the first 28 days after birth) even if morbidity occurs later. Coding Guideline I.C.16.a.1 further states that Chapter 16 codes may be used throughout the life of the patient if the condition is still present. Coding Guideline I.C.16.a.4 clarifies that conditions originating in the perinatal period, and continuing throughout the life of the patient, would have perinatal codes assigned regardless of the patient's age.

Although the perinatal period lasts through 28 days following birth, the codes within Chapter 15 may be assigned beyond that period when the condition still exists. However, the condition must have its origin in the perinatal period, even though it could continue to affect the patient beyond that time.

> **EXAMPLE:** Six-month-old was admitted to the hospital with acute respiratory failure due to bronchopulmonary dysplasia: J96.00, Acute respiratory failure; P27.1, Bronchopulmonary dysplasia originating in the perinatal period.

In the above example, the patient developed bronchopulmonary dysplasia (BPD) during the perinatal period while receiving prolonged and high concentrations of inspired O_2. Although this patient is no longer in the perinatal period, the BPD is still present and, as such, should be coded. BPD occurs commonly in infants who had respiratory distress syndrome at birth, as well as those who have required endotracheal intubation and a respirator for many days.

Codes in Chapter 16 identify newborns affected by maternal factors, disorders related to length of gestation and fetal growth, abnormal findings on neonatal screening, birth trauma, infections, and respiratory, cardiovascular, hemorrhagic, endocrine, and digestive conditions that originate in the perinatal period.

Newborn Affected by Maternal Factors and by Complications of Pregnancy, Labor, and Delivery (P00–P04)

Codes in this block of codes are used on the newborn or individual's record when a maternal condition is identified as the cause of the newborn or person's condition or possible condition and it originated in the perinatal period. These codes may be used when the condition is suspected to be the result of exposure from the mother or the birth process. The newborn or person may not have any signs or symptoms of the disease. The healthcare provider may describe the conditions as "suspected" and after an investigation it may be determined that the condition does not exist or the physician may state the condition is "ruled out." During the investigation the newborn or individual may receive treatment for the condition and these codes may still be used even though the condition is later ruled out. The titles of the categories include the word "suspected" in the title to recognize these conditions may or may not in the end prove to exist (for example, P01, Newborn (suspected to be) affected by the maternal complications of pregnancy). With the phrase "suspected to be" in parenthesis it is considered a nonessential modifier in ICD-10-CM, which means it may or may not be present in the description and it does not affect the use of the code.

A number of substances are known to have effects on the development of the fetus when the mother is exposed to the substance during pregnancy. Category P04, Newborn (suspected to be) affected by noxious substances transmitted via placenta or breast milk, identifies through the use of the fourth or fifth character the substance (suspected) found to have harmed the fetus or newborn. The substances include maternal anesthesia and analgesia, other maternal medication, maternal use of tobacco, maternal use of alcohol, and maternal use of drugs of addiction.

> **EXAMPLE:** Live born infant (vaginal birth in hospital) to an alcohol-dependent mother; the physician determines the infant has the effects of the mother's use of alcohol during pregnancy: Z38.00, Single liveborn infant, delivered vaginally in hospital; P04.3, Newborn (suspected to be) affected by maternal use of alcohol

> **EXAMPLE:** Delivery of a normal and healthy infant (in hospital) to a mother who occasionally uses cocaine: Z38.00, Single liveborn, delivered vaginally in hospital

In the first example, the use of alcohol by the mother was manifested in the infant; therefore, a code for newborn affected by maternal use of alcohol.

In the second example, however, the infant was healthy and normal despite the mother's occasional use of cocaine; therefore, the code for newborn (suspected to be) affected by maternal use of cocaine (P04.41) was not assigned. The P00–P04 codes are found in the Index under the main term "Newborn, affected by (suspected to be)" with subterms for the maternal condition affecting the newborn.

Disorders of Newborn Related to Length of Gestation and Fetal Growth (P05–P08)

Categories P05, P07, and P08 are classified in this block of codes for disorders related to length of gestation and fetal growth. The specific categories are as follows:

P05	Disorders of newborn related to slow fetal growth and fetal malnutrition
P07	Disorders of newborn related to short gestation and low birth weight, not elsewhere classified
P08	Disorders of newborn related to long gestation and high birth weight

Disorders of Newborn Related to Slow Fetal Growth and Fetal Malnutrition (P05)

Subcategories within P05 are used to classify an infant that the physician identifies as **light-for-dates** or light for gestational age. Other diagnoses written by the physician are **small-for-dates** for the babies. Another subcategory is used when the physician diagnoses fetal malnutrition. Other physicians may use a less specified diagnosis of **fetal growth retardation** (FGR). The coder must use the physician's terminology precisely and not substitute light-for-dates with small-for-dates and so on. These are infants who are born at a lighter weight or small size than expected at their full-term birth or at their gestational age.

Most physicians and hospital staff indicate a newborn's weight in grams. However, weight may also be recorded in pounds and ounces. One pound equals approximately 454 grams. A two-pound infant weighs about 907 grams, a five-pound infant weighs about 2,268 grams, and a ten-pound infant weighs about 4,536 grams.

The following fifth-characters are used with subcategories P05.0, Newborn light for gestational age and P05.1, Newborn small for gestational age:

0   unspecified weight
1   less than 500 grams
2   500–749 grams
3   750–999 grams
4   1,000–1,249 grams
5   1,250–1,499 grams
6   1,500–1,749 grams
7   1,750–1,999 grams
8   2,000–2,499 grams

These fifth digits are used to identify the weight of the infant at birth, not the weight at subsequent visits.

Disorders of Newborn Related to Short Gestation and Low Birth Weight, Not Elsewhere Classified (P07)

The codes from category P07, Disorders of newborn related to **short gestation** and **low birth weight**, not elsewhere classified, are to be used for a child or an adult who was premature at birth or who had a low birth weight as a newborn and this condition is affecting the patient's current health status.

The first two subcategories identify the low birth weight:

P07.0   Extremely low birth weight newborn
         Codes describe birth weight of 999 grams or less
P07.1   Other low birth weight newborn
         Codes describe birth weight of 1,000 to 2,499 grams

The last two subcategories identify short gestational age:

P07.2   Extreme immaturity of newborn
         Extreme immaturity is less than 28 completed weeks or less than 196 completed days of gestation
P07.3   Preterm (premature) newborn
         Prematurity is 28 completed weeks or more but less than 37 completed weeks (or 196 completed days but less than 259 completed days) of gestation

Physicians must document a newborn's prematurity and estimated gestational age. A coder should not assign an infant premature strictly based on the birth weight documented. A coder should not assign a code for prematurity unless the statement of prematurity has been made by the physician in the infant's health record. As is true in category P05, Disorders of newborn related to slow fetal growth and fetal malnutrition, the coder's assignment of codes from P07, Disorders of newborn related to short gestation and low birth weight, not elsewhere classified, should be based on the recorded birth weight and estimated gestational age. As the Excludes1 note under the category heading of P07 indicates, codes from category P05 should not be assigned with codes from category P07.

For a premature infant, the physician will likely document the baby's birth weight and estimated gestational age in the newborn's physical examination or other documentation. When both birth weight and gestational age are available, the codes should assign two codes from category P07, with the code for birth weight sequenced first. The code for **gestational age** is sequenced following the birth weight code. The code for the birth weight does not specify the gestational age and likewise for the gestational age codes. Both provide valuable information about the infant. Weeks of gestation may be predictive of the probability, but not a guarantee, of developmental problems for the infant in the future.

Disorders of Newborn Related to Long Gestation and High Birth Weight (P08)

Codes are also available for babies who have long gestational periods or have high birth weights. Physicians may describe the baby as a **large baby** or **exceptionally large baby**. Other phrases used by physicians are **heavy-for-dates** or **large-for-dates** to describe such a baby. The assignment of the code for the birth weight should take priority over the estimated gestational age code. Code P08.0, Exceptionally large newborn baby, is used for a baby who has a birth weight of 4,500 grams or more. The code P08.8 for heavy for gestational age is the code for a baby weighing between 4,000 and 4,499 grams. The physician's documentation of a large baby or heavy-for-dates baby is critical to assigning the codes as the coder cannot assume the codes are appropriate for an infant strictly based on a weight listed in the newborn record.

Another subcategory code, P08.2, is titled **Late newborn**, not heavy for gestational age. The coder will find here a code for a post-term newborn, P08.21, which is defined as a gestation period over 40 completed weeks to 42 completed weeks. Code P08.22, Prolonged gestation of newborn, includes a definition of over 42 completed weeks of gestational age. This code is the default code for the unspecified term of post maturity baby. The physician's documentation of gestational age is required for coding.

The main terms used in the Index to locate the codes in this category include premature newborn, preterm newborn, immaturity, small-for-dates, light-for-dates, low birth weight, heavy-for-dates, and large baby.

Conditions Associated with Meconium

Meconium is present in the baby's first intestinal discharge and may be referred to as a newborn's first stool, although technically it is not stool. **Meconium** is a thick substance that lines the infant's intestine during gestation and consists of a combination of swallowed amniotic fluid and mucus from the baby. The substance is usually not released in the baby's bowel movement until after birth. However a baby can pass meconium out of their bowel prior to birth, which excretes the meconium into the amniotic fluid. If this passage of meconium occurs in utero, the amniotic fluid will have **meconium staining** that will be seen when the baby is delivered. If the meconium is present during labor and delivery, the infant will be watched more closely for signs of fetal distress. The concern is when meconium is present in the amniotic fluid the baby will aspirate the meconium in the throat and possibly into the lungs.

The passage of meconium before birth can be an indication of fetal distress. It is seen in infants small for gestational age, post-term infants, or those with cord complications or other factors compromising placental circulation. **Meconium aspiration syndrome** occurs when meconium from amniotic fluid in the upper airway is inhaled into the lungs by the newborn with his or her first breath. This invokes an inflammatory reaction in the lungs, which can be fatal. Meconium staining is not meconium aspiration. Meconium aspiration is not meconium aspiration syndrome. ICD-10-CM provides distinct codes for the different conditions involving meconium:

P03.82	Meconium passage during delivery
P24.00	Meconium aspiration without respiratory symptoms
P24.01	Meconium aspiration with respiratory symptoms (aspiration syndrome)
P76.0	Meconium ileus (plug syndrome)
P78.0	Meconium peritonitis
P96.83	Meconium staining (of amniotic fluid)

Respiratory and Cardiovascular Disorders Specific to the Perinatal Period (P19–P29)

Conditions classified to categories P19–P29, Respiratory and cardiovascular disorders specific to the perinatal period, are unfortunately present in many infants. An example of one of these conditions is **respiratory distress syndrome (RDS)** of newborn. This condition or inflamed lungs with pulmonary edema occurs in infants born prematurely. It is caused by pulmonary surfactant deficiency because surfactant is not produced in inadequate amounts until later in pregnancy, usually after 37 weeks of gestation. The diagnosis is made when the infant exhibits grunting respirations, nasal flaring, and the use of accessory muscles in the chest. The infant is treated with surfactant therapy and supportive oxygen replacement because the infant is hypoxemic (Merck 2012).

Category P22, Respiratory distress of newborn, contains subcategories such as the following:

P22.0   Respiratory distress syndrome of newborn
       This code would also be used for diagnoses of hyaline membrane disease, cardio-respiratory distress syndrome of newborns, and idiopathic RDS or RDS type I.

P22.1   Transient tachypnea of newborn
       This code would be used for RDS type II, idiopathic tachypnea of newborn or wet lung syndrome.

In addition to RDS, other codes are available for respiratory arrest of newborn (P28.81) and respiratory failure of newborn (P28.5).

Category P24, **Neonatal aspiration**, includes aspiration in utero and during delivery, of different substances, for example, meconium, clear amniotic fluid, blood, milk and regurgitated food, and other specified substances. Each of the subcategory codes P24.0–P24.8 has two options for the fifth-character:

0—without respiratory symptoms
1—with respiratory symptoms

The respiratory symptoms are frequently pneumonia or pneumonitis. Each of the fifth-character codes has a "use additional" code note to identify any secondary pulmonary hypertension, I27.2, if applicable.

Category P29, Cardiovascular disorders originating in the perinatal period, contains neonatal cardiac conditions. Infants may have either bradycardia or tachycardia after birth that is unrelated to the stress of labor or delivery or other intrauterine complications. These symptoms are almost always a symptom of an underlying condition, but the cause may not be immediately known. Neonatal tachycardia is coded to P29.11 and neonatal bradycardia is coded to P29.12. Another code for persistent fetal circulation, P29.3, is available for conditions described as delayed closure of ductus arteriosus or persistent pulmonary hypertension of newborn.

Infections Specific to the Perinatal Period (P35–P39)

ICD-10-CM classifies perinatal infections to the block of codes from P35–P39, Infections specific to the perinatal period. According to the note that appears under the block heading of P35–P39, these infections can be acquired in utero, during birth via the umbilicus, or during the first 28 days after birth. The perinatal period is defined as before birth through the first 28 days after birth even if the illness occurs later in life.

Therefore, an infant who develops a urinary tract infection at the age of 20 days would be assigned code P39.3, Neonatal urinary tract infection. Newborn, neonatal, and perinatal refer to the time period of birth through 28 days of life. If the infection is acquired within the first 28 days of life, the perinatal code is used.

According to Guideline I.C.16.a.5, the coder has discretion on how to code conditions that are community acquired or due to the birth process. If a newborn has a condition that may be either community acquired or due to the birth process and the documentation does not indicate which it is, the default code should be assigned to the code associated to the birth process. The code from Chapter 16 should be used. If the condition is community acquired, a code from Chapter 16 should not be assigned.

Category P36, **bacterial sepsis of newborn**, contains codes used frequently to classify conditions in newborns with infections. Bacterial sepsis is the presence of bacteria in the blood of the infant. This produces an invasive infection, which is demonstrated in the infant having apnea, bradycardia, low temperature, respiratory distress, vomiting, diarrhea, abdominal distention, seizure, jaundice, and jitteriness. It is treated with intravenous antibiotics and is more common in low birth weight babies (Merck 2012). Unique codes exist for septicemia or sepsis of newborn due to various organisms such as streptococcus group B, other streptococci, staphylococcus aureus, as well as sepsis due to E. Coli and anaerobes. Because these codes include the causal organism, an additional code from categories B95–B96, Bacterial agents as the cause of diseases classified elsewhere, is not needed. However, if the P36 code does not include the causal organism, the coder should assign an additional code from category B96. If the infant has severe sepsis, the code should use additional codes to identify severe sepsis (R65.2-) and any associated acute organ dysfunction.

According to Guideline I.C.16.f, congenital sepsis is include in category B36, Bacterial sepsis of newborn. If the documentation in the infant's record does not identify the sepsis as congenital or if it was community acquired, the coder should assume the condition is congenital and the default code of P36 is used.

Liveborn Infants According to Place of Birth and Type of Delivery (Z38)

The principal diagnosis for coding the birth episode of a newborn is not included in Chapter 16. The birth episode is coded with a code from category Z38, Liveborn infants according to place of birth and type of delivery, from Chapter 21, Factors influencing health status and contact with health services. The Z38 category codes in ICD-10-CM identify the number of liveborn infants, where they are born (in hospital, outside hospital), and how they were delivered (vaginally or by cesarean). Other codes exist for twin, triplet, quadruplet, quintuplet, and other multiple liveborn infants. For example, the birth record for a single liveborn infant, born in the hospital, and delivered vaginally is code Z38.00. A twin liveborn infant, born in the hospital, delivered by cesarean, is code Z38.31. A code from category Z38 is assigned only once to a newborn at the time of birth. If the newborn is transferred to another institution or readmitted to the hospital, a code from category Z38 should not be used at the next hospital. The Z38 codes are located in the Index under the main term "newborn" with subterms of born in hospital, twin, triplet, quadruplet, and quintuplet.

ICD-10-PCS Procedure Coding for Certain Conditions Originating in the Perinatal Period

There are no procedures unique to treating certain conditions originating in the perinatal period. Instead the newborn or other patient may have procedures performed that relate to the cardiovascular system, respiratory system, digestive systems, and others as appropriate. Other supportive procedures are coded for infants in the extracorporeal assistance and performance section of ICD-10-PCS for mechanical ventilation, continuous positive airway pressure breathing, or insertion of an intra-aortic balloon pump in seriously ill infants.

ICD-10-CM and ICD-10-PCS Review Exercises: Chapter 19

Assign the correct ICD-10-CM diagnosis codes or ICD-10-PCS procedure codes to the following exercises.

1. A 20-day-old infant was admitted with *Staphylococcus aureus* sepsis.

2. Full-term newborn was delivered four days ago and discharged home. The infant was readmitted to the hospital and diagnosed with hyperbilirubinemia. Phototherapy was initiated and the baby will continue to have phototherapy provided at home after discharge.

3. Newborn, full term, born in hospital, vaginal birth with meconium peritonitis

4. Premature "crack" baby born in the hospital by cesarean section to a mother dependent on cocaine. The newborn did not show signs of withdrawal. Birth weight of 1,247 grams and 31 completed weeks of gestation. Dehydration was also diagnosed and treated.

5. Full-term newborn, Infant of diabetic mother syndrome. Baby was born by cesarean delivery in the hospital. Mother has preexisting diabetes.

6. Newborn transferred to Children's Hospital after birth at local community hospital. Reasons for transfer are premature infant, 32 weeks gestation, and birthweight of 1,800 grams with grade 1 intraventricular hemorrhage.

7. Full-term infant with omphalitis with mild hemorrhage, born in hospital by vaginal delivery

8. Premature infant, 35 weeks gestation, birthweight 2,000 grams with stage 1 necrotizing enterocolitis, born in hospital by vaginal delivery

(Continued on next page)

ICD-10-CM and ICD-10-PCS Review Exercises: Chapter 19 (Continued)

9. Single newborn, born in hospital, by cesarean delivery; birth injury of scalpel wound during cesarean delivery

10. Twin newborn, born in hospital, by cesarean delivery, full term; newborn with neonatal bradycardia

11. Full-term infant, born in hospital, vaginal delivery. Meconium staining was noted at the time of delivery. There were no complications in the infant as the result of it.

12. Full-term infant, born in hospital, vaginal delivery with respiratory distress syndrome, type I

13. Full-term infant, born in hospital, cesarean delivery, with transient neonatal neutropenia, cause unknown

14. A 10-day-old infant readmitted for sepsis due to E. coli

15. A 21-day-old infant readmitted with neonatal urinary tract infection due to E. coli bacteria

16. PROCEDURE: Mechanical ventilation, 112 consecutive hours following endotracheal intubation

17. PROCEDURE: Insertion of intra-aortic balloon pump (continuous)

18. PROCEDURE: CPAP (continuous positive airway pressure), 48 hours

19. PROCEDURE: Diagnostic audiology—hearing screening test using audiometer

20. PROCEDURE: Percutaneous endoscopic insertion of feeding tube into jejunum

Chapter 20

Congenital Malformations, Deformations and Chromosomal Abnormalities (Q00–Q99)

Learning Objectives

At the conclusion of this chapter, you should be able to:

1. Describe the organization of the conditions and codes included in ICD-10-CM Chapter 17, Congenital malformations, deformations and chromosomal abnormalities (Q00–Q99)

2. Briefly describe the types of common congenital anomalies classified in Chapter 17 of ICD-10-CM

3. Describe the circumstances in which a code from Chapter 17 of ICD-10-CM can be assigned in terms of the age of the patient who has the condition

4. Assign ICD-10-CM codes for congenital anomalies

5. Assign ICD-10-PCS codes for procedures related to these conditions

Key Terms

- Aortic valve stenosis (AS)
- Atrial septal defect (ASD)
- Bladder exstrophy
- Chromosome
- Chromosome abnormality
- Cleft lip
- Cleft palate
- Clubfoot
- Coarctation of aorta
- Congenital anomaly
- Cystic or polycystic kidney disease (PKD)
- Down syndrome
- Ebstein's anomaly
- Edward syndrome (trisomy 18)
- Endocardial cushion defect

- Epispadias
- Hypoplastic left heart syndrome
- Hypospadias
- Lung hypoplasia (dysplasia)
- Mullerian anomalies of the uterus
- Obstructive genitourinary defect
- Patau syndrome
- Patent ductus arteriosus (PDA)
- Persistent/patent truncus arteriosus (PTA)
- Pulmonary valve atresia
- Pyloric stenosis
- Renal agenesis or hypoplasia
- Spina bifida
- Stenosis
- Tetralogy of Fallot (TOF)
- Total anomalous pulmonary vein return (TAPVR)
- Transposition of great vessels (TGV)
- Tricuspic valve atresia (stenosis)
- Ventricular septal defect (VSD)

Overview of ICD-10-CM Chapter 17, Congenital Malformations, Deformations and Chromosomal Abnormalities

Chapter 17 includes categories Q00–Q99 arranged in the following blocks:

Q00–Q07	Congenital malformations of the nervous system
Q10–Q18	Congenital malformations of eye, ear, face and neck
Q20–Q28	Congenital malformations of the circulatory system
Q30–Q34	Congenital malformations of the respiratory system
Q35–Q37	Cleft lip and cleft palate
Q38–Q45	Other congenital malformations of the digestive system
Q50–Q56	Congenital malformations of genital organs
Q60–Q64	Congenital malformations of the urinary system
Q65–Q79	Congenital malformations and deformations of the musculoskeletal system
Q80–Q89	Other congenital malformations
Q90–Q99	Chromosomal abnormalities, not elsewhere classified

A **congenital anomaly**, malformation, or deformation is an irregularity, abnormality, or a combination of abnormalities that are present at, and existing from, the time of birth. In eukaryotic cells or cells with a true nucleus, a **chromosome** is the structure in the nucleus consisting of chromatin carrying the genetic information of the cell. A **chromosome abnormality** is an irregularity in the number or structure of chromosomes that may alter the course of the development of the embryo. The irregularity may be a duplicate of a chromosome, a deletion of loss of a chromosome, a translocation or exchange of a chromosome, or an alteration in the sequence of genetic material.

Chapter 17 of ICD-10-CM is organized by body system, beginning with the nervous system with a block of codes at the end of the chapter for chromosomal abnormalities. Because many conditions can be either congenital in origin or acquired, coders must carefully review the subterms in the Index to select the appropriate code to describe congenital conditions.

The congenital conditions are grouped into subcategories or blocks to make it easy to identify the type of condition included in Chapter 17. Updated terminology in the code descriptors in the chapter is specific as to the exact type of condition classified. An example of the ICD-10-CM codes for congenital conditions can be found in category Q61 with codes for specific forms of cystic kidney disease in addition to codes for less specified types of cystic kidney disease.

EXAMPLES:	Q61	Cystic kidney disease
	Q61.0	Congenital renal cyst
	Q61.1	Polycystic kidney, infantile type
	Q61.2	Polycystic kidney, adult type
	Q61.3	Polycystic kidney, unspecified
	Q61.4	Renal dysplasia
	Q61.5	Medullary cystic kidney
	Q61.8	Other cystic kidney disease
	Q61.9	Cystic kidney disease

Other changes to Chapter 17 include classification changes that provide greater specificity according to the anatomic site and the combination of congenital conditions that can be coded as follows.

EXAMPLES:	Q35.1	Cleft hard palate
	Q35.3	Cleft soft palate
	Q35.5	Cleft hard palate with cleft soft palate
	Q35.7	Cleft uvula
	Q35.9	Cleft palate, unspecified

Coding Guidelines and Instructional Notes for ICD-10-CM Chapter 17

At the start of Chapter 17, a note states codes from this chapter are not for use on maternal or fetal records. But this note should not be interpreted to state that the codes in this chapter cannot be used on infant or other records. When an infant is born with a congenital anomaly, an appropriate code from Chapter 17 should be used on the infant's record. During the admission when the infant is born, the appropriate code from category Z38 is sequenced first to identify the place of birth and the type of delivery. A secondary code is used to identify the congenital condition present at birth.

EXAMPLE: Liveborn male infant, born in the hospital via vaginal birth with tetralogy of Fallot: Z38.00, Single liveborn, delivered in hospital without mention of cesarean delivery; Q21.3, Tetralogy of Fallot

However, if the patient was transferred on the day of birth to another hospital for care of the congenital anomaly, the principal diagnosis at the second hospital would be the congenital anomaly.

EXAMPLE: Liveborn male infant transferred to another hospital for care of thoracic spina bifida with hydrocephalus: Q05.1, Thoracic spina bifida with hydrocephalus

An important guideline states that codes for the congenital condition can be used throughout the entire life of the patient as long as it is still present. Congenital condition codes are not restricted for use at the time of birth or during the perinatal period. However, if a congenital condition has been corrected, the congenital condition should no longer be coded. Instead the coder should indicate a personal history of a congenital condition, for example, from subcategory Z87.7, Personal history of (corrected) congenital malformation.

Instructions are included in Chapter 17 to direct the coder when additional codes are required. For example, a "use additional code for associated paraplegia, G82.2-" note appears with category Q05, Spina bifida. Another note appears with ICD-10-CM codes Q13.1 and Q13.81 to use an additional code for associated glaucoma, H42. Under section heading Q35–Q37, Cleft lip and cleft palate, a note appears to remind the coder to use an additional code to identify an associated malformation of the nose with code Q30.2. Another type of note appears under code Q55.3, Atresia of vas deferens, to code first any associated cystic fibrosis (E84.-). Coding guidelines also state that when a congenital condition does not have a unique code assignment, the coder should assign additional code(s) for any manifestations that may be present. An example of this guideline is shown. For example, a malformation may be described as a syndrome with various conditions present. Under category Q87, Other specified congenital malformation syndromes affecting multiple systems, a directional note states "use additional code(s) to identify all associated manifestations." A similar type of instruction is also used with chromosomal abnormality codes. For example, under section Q90–Q99, Chromosomal abnormalities, not elsewhere classified, a note appears to remind the coder to use additional codes to identify any associated physical condition or the degree of intellectual disabilities that are present with the chromosomal abnormality.

The NCHS has published chapter-specific guidelines for Chapter 17 in the *ICD-10-CM Official Guidelines for Coding and Reporting.* The coding student should review all of the coding guidelines for Chapter 17 of ICD-10-CM, which appear in an ICD-10-CM code book or at the website http://www.cdc.gov/nchs/icd/icd10cm.htm, or in Appendix E.

Official guidelines for the codes in Chapter 17, Congenital malformations, deformations, and chromosomal abnormalities (Q00–Q99) are as follows:

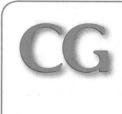 Assign an appropriate code(s) from categories Q00–Q99, Congenital malformations, deformations, and chromosomal abnormalities when a malformation/deformation or chromosomal abnormality is documented. A malformation/deformation/or chromosomal abnormality may be the principal/first-listed diagnosis on a record or a secondary diagnosis.

When a malformation/deformation/or chromosomal abnormality does not have a unique code assignment, assign additional code(s) for any manifestations that may be present.

When the code assignment specifically identifies the malformation/deformation/or chromosomal abnormality, manifestations that are an inherent component of the anomaly should not be coded separately. Additional codes should be assigned for manifestations that are not an inherent component.

Codes from Chapter 17 may be used throughout the life of the patient. If a congenital malformation or deformity has been corrected, a personal history code should be used to identify the history of the malformation or deformity. Although present at birth, malformation/deformation/or chromosomal abnormality may not be identified until later in life. Whenever the condition is diagnosed by the physician, it is appropriate to assign a code from codes Q00–Q99. For the birth admission, the appropriate code from category Z38, Liveborn infants, according to place of birth and type of delivery, should be sequenced as the principal diagnosis, followed by any congenital anomaly codes, Q00–Q99.

Coding Congenital Malformations, Deformation and Chromosomal Abnormalities in ICD-10-CM Chapter 17

Chapter 17 of ICD-10-CM, Congenital malformations, deformations and chromosomal abnormalities, contains codes in the range of Q00–Q99. Codes from Chapter 17 may be used throughout the life of the patient as long as the condition is present; the condition is not only coded at birth or when it is first diagnosed. If a congenital malformation or deformity has been corrected, a personal history code should be used to identify the history of the malformation or deformity.

Conditions included in Chapter 17 are organized by body system—for example, Q20–Q28, Congenital malformations of the circulatory system, and Q65–Q79, Congenital malformations and deformations of the musculoskeletal system—and include laterality for limbs and bones. Specific codes are included in ICD-10-CM to further describe the congenital condition. For example, there are four codes (Q90.0–Q90.9) to identify Down syndrome as trisomy 21, nonmosaicism, mosaicism, translocation, or unspecified. Updated terminology is also included. In place of Patau's syndrome and Edward's syndrome, the same conditions are coded with specific types of trisomy 18 and trisomy 13 codes in the range of Q91.0–Q91.7. The terminology of Patau's and Edward's syndrome does appear in the Alphabetic Index but directs the coder to the index entry for trisomy 18 or trisomy 13.

Many codes for congenital conditions and chromosomal abnormalities are included in ICD-10-CM. There are nine categories (Q90, Q91, Q92, Q93, Q95, Q96, Q97, Q98, and Q99) for chromosomal abnormalities, not elsewhere classified to distinguish between the nonmosaicism, mosaicism, and translocation types of the abnormalities. As more has become known about these complex chromosomal abnormalities, the ICD-10-CM codes were included to report the different types of conditions.

Common Congenital Anomalies

A congenital anomaly, also known as a birth defect, has been the leading cause of infant mortality in the United States over the past several years. Birth defects substantially contribute to childhood morbidity and long-term disability. More than 4,500 different birth defects have been identified. Congenital anomalies can affect almost every body system.

There are three major categories of known causes of congenital anomalies:

1. Chromosomal disorders (either hereditary or arising during conception)

2. Exposure to an environmental chemical (for example, medications, alcohol, cigarettes, solvents)

3. Mother's illness during pregnancy, exposing the infant to viral or bacterial infections

The stage of fetal development at the time of exposure to one of the two latter causes is critical. Fetal development is particularly vulnerable in the first trimester of pregnancy. The life expectancy and quality of life for individuals with many birth defects has improved greatly over the past 40 years. This is a result of pioneering surgery that can correct certain defects before the infant is born, as well as neonatal intensive care units that provide specialized care and advanced technology to treat the infant.

Central Nervous System Defects

Central nervous system (CNS) defects involve the brain, spinal cord, and associated tissue. These include neural tube defects (anencephaly, spina bifida, and encephalocele), microcephalous, and hydrocephalus.

One of the more common CNS defects is spina bifida. **Spina bifida** is a defective closure of the vertebral column. It ranges in severity from the occult type revealing few signs to a completely open spine (rachischisis). In spina bifida cystica, the protruding sac contains meninges (meningocele), the spinal cord (myelocele), or both (myelomeningocele). Commonly seen in the lumbar, low thoracic, or sacral region, spina bifida extends for three to six vertebral segments. When the spinal cord or lumbosacral nerve roots are involved, as is usually the case, varying degrees of paralysis occur below the involved level. This may result in orthopedic conditions such as clubfoot, arthrogryposis, or dislocated hip. The paralysis also usually affects the sphincters of the bladder and rectum. In addition, an excessive accumulation of cerebrospinal fluid within the ventricles, called hydrocephalus, is associated with the lumbosacral type of spina bifida in at least 80 percent of affected patients.

In ICD-10-CM, most types of spina bifida, excluding spina bifida occulta, are assigned to category Q05. This category is further subdivided to fourth-digit subcategories that describe the sites, such as cervical, thoracic, lumbar, or sacral with presence or absence of hydrocephalus. As indicated by the Excludes1 note, Spina bifida occulta (Q76.0) would not be coded with the Q05 category codes, as it is mutually exclusive to those conditions.

Cardiovascular System Defects

Cardiovascular system defects involve the heart and circulatory system and are the most common group of birth defects in infants. Surgical procedures repair defects and restore circulation to as normal as possible. Some defects can be repaired before birth, whereas others may require multiple surgical procedures after birth. Smaller defects may be repaired in a cardiac catheterization laboratory instead of an operating room. Some of the more commonly occurring cardiovascular defects are patent ductus arteriosus, atrial septal defect, ventricular septal defect, and pulmonary artery anomalies.

Descriptions of cardiovascular system defects and their common abbreviations are as follows:

- **Hypoplastic left heart syndrome** (Q23.4) is a condition in which the entire left half of the heart is underdeveloped. This condition may be repaired in a series of three procedures over one year. If not treated, the condition can be fatal within one month.

- **Persistent/patent truncus arteriosus (PTA)** (Q25.0) is a failure of the fetal truncus arteriosus to divide into the aorta and pulmonary artery. It can be corrected surgically.

- **Pulmonary valve atresia** (Q25.5) and **stenosis** (Q25.6) are conditions that obstruct or narrow the pulmonary heart valve. Mild forms are relatively well tolerated and require no intervention. More severe forms are surgically corrected.

- **Tetralogy of Fallot (TOF)** (Q21.3) is a defect characterized by four anatomical abnormalities within the heart that results in poorly oxygenated blood being pumped to the body. It can be corrected surgically.

- **Total anomalous pulmonary venous return (TAPVR)** (Q26.2) is a malformation of all of the pulmonary veins. In this condition, the pulmonary veins empty into the right atrium, or a systemic vein, instead of into the left atrium.

- **Transposition of great vessels** or great arteries **(TGV)** (Q20.3) is a defect in which the positions of the aorta and the pulmonary artery are transposed. Immediate surgical correction is required.

- **Tricuspid valve atresia and stenosis** (Q22.4) is the absence or narrowing of the valve between the right atrium and ventricle. Severe cases are surgically corrected.

- **Aortic valve stenosis (AS)** (Q23.0) is the congenital narrowing or obstruction of the aortic heart valve. This can be surgically repaired in some cases.

- **Atrial septal defect (ASD)** (Q21.1) is a hole in the wall between the upper chambers of the heart (the atria). The openings may resolve without treatment or require surgical intervention. This condition may also be referred to as patent foramen ovale.

- **Coarctation of the aorta** (Q25.1) is a defect in which the aorta is narrowed somewhere along its length. Surgical correction is recommended even for mild defects.

- **Endocardial cushion defect** is a spectrum of septal defects arising from imperfect fusion of the endocardial cushions in the fetal heart (Q21.1). This diagnosis may also be specified as atrioventricular septal defect. This condition is repaired surgically.

- **Patent ductus arteriosus (PDA)** is a condition in which the channel between the pulmonary artery and the aorta fails to close at birth (Q25.0). Many of these close spontaneously and cause no consequences. The condition can also be surgically and medically repaired.

- **Ventricular septal defect (VSD)** (Q21.0) is a hole in the lower chambers of the heart, or the ventricles. The openings may resolve without treatment; however, the condition can be surgically corrected.

- **Ebstein's anomaly** (Q22.5) is a deformation or displacement of the tricuspid valve with the septal and posterior leaflets being attached to the wall of the right ventricle. Only severe cases are corrected surgically.

Respiratory System Defects

Respiratory system congenital anomalies, mainly in the lungs, trachea, and nose, are life threatening, but less common than those involving other major organs. The major defect is **lung hypoplasia** or **dysplasia**, which is the failure to develop or underdevelopment of one or both lungs (Q33.6). Other unfortunate congenital malformations in the respiratory system are the underdevelopment or the lack or development of organs within the respiratory tract, such as the nose, trachea, bronchus, and lung. A web can be present in the larynx and cystic lesions develop in the mediastinum. All of these respiratory anomalies require immediate medical and surgical care to correct the malformation so that the infant regains adequate respiratory function.

Digestive System Defects

Digestive system defects include orofacial defects (for example, choanal atresia, or cleft palate and lip) and gastrointestinal defects (for example, esophageal atresia, rectal and intestinal atresia and stenosis, and pyloric stenosis).

Cleft Lip and Cleft Palate

Cleft lip, cleft palate, and combination of the two are the most common congenital anomalies of the head and neck. A cleft is a fissure or elongated opening of a specified site, usually occurring during the embryonic stage. A **cleft palate** is a split in the roof of the mouth (the palate) and a **cleft lip** is the presence of one or two splits in the upper lip. Cleft lips and palates are classified as partial or complete, and can occur either bilaterally or unilaterally. The most common clefts are left unilateral complete clefts of the primary and secondary palate, and partial midline clefts of the secondary palate involving the soft palate and part of the hard palate. The incisive foramen serves as the dividing point between the primary and the secondary palate.

In ICD-10-CM, cleft palate is classified to Q35 and cleft lip is classified to category Q36. The category Q35 for cleft palate is subdivided to describe cleft hard palate (Q35.1), cleft soft palate (Q35.2) or when both conditions are present, cleft hard palate with cleft soft palate (Q35.3). Category Q36 for cleft lip is subdivided to identify bilateral, median, or unilateral forms of the cleft lip. When both conditions exist, cleft palate with cleft lip, the fourth character codes identify which palate is involved (hard or soft) and whether the cleft lip is a bilateral or unilateral type. As is true with all medical documentation, the physician should be queried when the documentation is unclear.

Pyloric Stenosis

Pyloric stenosis is a narrowing of the outlet between the stomach and small intestine. It results from hypertrophy of the circular and longitudinal muscularis of the pylorus and distal antrum of the stomach. Typically, the infant feeds well from birth until two or three weeks after birth, at which time occasional regurgitation of food, or spitting up, occurs, followed several days later by projectile vomiting. Dehydration due to the vomiting is common. ICD-10-CM assigns code Q40.0 for congenital hypertrophic pyloric stenosis.

Genitourinary Tract Defects

Both male and female infants may be afflicted with defects of the reproductive organs and the urinary tract. Some are relatively minor and fairly common defects that can be repaired by surgery. Some of the genitourinary tract defects are as follows:

- Abnormalities of uterus codes (Q51.0–Q51.9) identify congenital anomalies such as agenesis and aplasia of uterus, doubling of uterus with doubling of cervix and vagina, septate uterus, unicornuate uterus, bicornuate uterus, arcuate uterus, and other anomalies of uterus. Collectively these conditions may be referred to as **Mullerian anomalies of the uterus**. Women are likely to be diagnosed with these conditions after seeking medical attention for infertility or repeated pregnancy loss.

- Different forms of **bladder exstrophy** (Q64.10–Q64.19) are conditions in which the bladder is turned inside out with portions of the abdominal and bladder walls missing. This must be surgically repaired.

- Male or female **epispadias** (Q64.0) is a relatively rare defect in which the urethra opens on the top surface of the penis and surgical correction is needed.

- Different forms of **hypospadias** (Q54.0–Q54.9) is a relatively common defect (1 in 250 male births) that appears as an abnormal urethral opening on the penis rather than at the end. The location of the abnormal condition is identified as anterior (balanic, glandular, coronal, or subcoronal) (Q54.0), middle (distal penile, midshaft, and proximal penile) (Q54.1), and posterior (penoscrotal or scrotal) (Q54.2). Another form of posterior hypospadias may be called perineal (Q54.3). A related condition also coded to this category is the condition known as congenital chordee or chordee without hypospadias. A chordee is a ventral curvature of the penis and may be present without hypospadias (Q54.4). Surgical correction may be needed for cosmetic, urologic, and reproductive reasons (Gatti 2011).

- **Obstructive genitourinary defect** is an obstruction of the ureter, renal pelvis, urethra, or bladder neck (Q62.0–Q62.8). Severity of the condition depends on the level of the obstruction. Urine accumulates behind the obstruction and produces organ damage. This condition can be corrected surgically while the fetus is in the uterus or after birth.

- **Renal agenesis or hypoplasia** (Q60.0–Q60.5) is the absence or underdevelopment of the kidneys and may be unilateral or bilateral. Newborns with bilateral renal atresia often expire due to respiratory failure within a few hours of birth. Unilateral renal atresia may not be detected for years.

- **Cystic or polycystic kidney disease (PKD)** is an inherited disorder characterized by multiple, bilateral, grapelike clusters of fluid-filled cysts that grossly enlarge the kidneys, compressing and eventually replacing functioning renal tissue. The infantile form of this condition reveals an infant with pronounced epicanthal folds, a pointed nose, a small chin, and floppy, low-set ears. Signs of respiratory distress and congestive heart failure also may be present. This condition eventually deteriorates into uremia and renal failure.

ICD-10-CM classifies cystic kidney disease to category Q61 with the following fourth-character subcategories:

Q61.00–Q61.02	Congenital renal cyst
Q61.11–Q61.19	Polycystic kidney, infantile type
Q61.2	Polycystic kidney, adult type
Q61.3	Polycystic kidney, unspecified
Q61.4	Renal dysplasia
Q61.5	Medullary cystic kidney
Q61.8	Other cystic kidney disease
Q61.9	Cystic kidney disease, unspecified

When there is no further specification as to type of polycystic kidney disease, assign code Q61.3. In addition, assign other complications that may be present, such as chronic kidney disease (N18.1–N18.9).

Musculoskeletal Defects

Musculoskeletal defects are relatively common disorders and range from minor problems to more serious conditions. Clubfoot is the most common musculoskeletal congenital anomaly.

Clubfoot

Clubfoot is a general term that is used to describe a variety of congenital structural foot deformities involving the lower leg, ankle, and foot joints, ligaments, and tendons. Clubfoot deformities include the following:

- Varus deformities, which are characterized by a turning inward of the feet (codes Q66.0–Q66.3)

- Valgus deformities, which are characterized by a turning outward of the feet (codes Q66.4, Q66.6)

- Talipes cavus, which is recognized by increased arch of the foot (code Q66.7)

- Talipes calcaneus or equinus, in which the entire foot exhibits an abnormal upward or downward misalignment (code Q66.89)

The generic term clubfoot is classified as talipes, not otherwise specified (code Q66.9).

Chromosomal Defects

Chromosomal abnormalities are disorders that arise from abnormal numbers of chromosomes or from defects in specific fragments of the chromosomes. Each disorder is associated with a characteristic pattern of defects that arises as a consequence of the underlying chromosomal abnormality. Congenital heart defects, especially septal defects, are common among these infants and are a major cause of death. Specific forms of chromosomal abnormalities are classified with categories Q90–Q99.

The more common chromosomal conditions include the following:

- **Down syndrome** is associated with the presence of a third number 21 chromosome. Another term for Down syndrome is trisomy 21. It results in mental retardation, distinctive malformations of the face and head, and other abnormalities. The severity of these problems varies widely among the affected individuals. Down syndrome is one of the more frequently occurring chromosomal abnormalities.

- **Edward's syndrome** or trisomy 18 is associated with the presence of a third number 18 chromosome. It causes major physical abnormalities and severe mental retardation. Many children with this disorder expire in the first year of life due to the abnormalities of the lungs and diaphragm, heart defects, and blood vessel malformations.

- **Patau syndrome** or trisomy 13 is associated with the presence of a third number 13 chromosome. The infants have many internal and external abnormalities, including profound retardation. Death may occur in the first few days of life due to the respiratory difficulties, heart defects, and severe defects in other organ systems.

ICD-10-PCS Procedure Coding to Correct Congenital Malformations and Deformations

Surgical procedures to correct congenital malformations, deformations, or congenital anomalies are coded based on the objective of the procedure. For example, if a hydrocephalus exists, the creation of a shunt may be necessary. The creation of a shunt is a Bypass within the central nervous system with the body part being the Cerebral Ventricle and the qualifier identifying the location where the bypass is directed to, for example, the Peritoneal Cavity for a ventriculo-peritoneal shunt.

Another example of a procedure to correct a congenital condition is a patient with spina bifida who requires surgical closure of the defect. The opening in the vertebral column is closed with the body part addressed as the Spinal Meninges. A closure as described in this type of procedure is Repair or the restoring, to the extent possible, a body part to its normal anatomic structure and function.

Surgical repair of cleft lips or palates may be immediately after birth or delayed for several weeks after birth depending on the individual patient. The root operation Repair is used for procedures in the mouth and throat to restore the lip and palate to the correct anatomic position. Other possible root operations to be used depending on the procedure would be Supplement or Transfer for a palatoplasty. Each body part repaired is coded separately, for example, Upper Lip, Hard Palate, or Soft Palate.

Congenital pyloric stenosis is a narrowing of the outlet between the stomach and small intestine. It results from hypertrophy of the circular and longitudinal muscularis of the pylorus and distal antrum of the stomach. Surgery is the treatment of choice. It is usually an open procedure to cut into the pylorus. The condition is marked by a thickening of the pylorus, which is the muscular band of tissue in the stomach that controls the exit of food and gastric juices from the stomach into the small bowel. By making an incision into the pylorus to divide the muscular band, the stenosis is relieved. Based on the specific description of the procedure, the root operation is likely Division in Table 0D8 with the body part Stomach, Pylorus. Other possible root operations for a pyloroplasty would be Dilation, Supplement, or Repair.

ICD-10-CM and ICD-10-PCS Review Exercises: Chapter 17

Assign the correct ICD-10-CM diagnosis codes and ICD-10-PCS procedure codes to the following exercises.

1. Spina bifida, lumbar region, without hydrocephalus

   _____

2. Coloboma of right eye iris

   _____

3. Full-term female infant was born in this hospital by vaginal delivery. Her mother has been an alcoholic for many years and would not stop drinking during her pregnancy. The baby was born with fetal alcohol syndrome and was placed in the NICU.

   _____

4. Fragile X Syndrome

   _____

5. Frontal encephalocele with hydroencephalocele

   _____

6. Cleft palate involving both the soft and hard palate, with bilateral cleft lip

   _____

7. Coronal hypospadias

   _____

8. Newborn was delivered by cesarean section. Congenital condition diagnosed was complete transposition of the great vessels with cyanosis.

   _____

9. Cri-du-chat syndrome

   _____

10. Polycystic kidney disease, autosomal recessive

    _____

11. Duplicate ureter, left kidney

    _____

12. Tetralogy of Fallot congenital defect with ventricular septal defect, pulmonary stenosis, dextroposition of aorta with hypertrophy of right ventricle

    _____

ICD-10-CM and ICD-10-PCS Review Exercises: Chapter 17 (Continued)

13. Hirschsprung's congenital megacolon disease

14. Acoustic neurofibromatosis

15. Patent ductus arteriosus

16. PROCEDURE: Open Blalock-Hanlon procedure with excision of the atrial septal opening for palliative treatment of transposition of great vessels

17. PROCEDURE: Laparoscopic Heller myotomy, which is described in the operative report as cutting into the muscle at the lower end of esophageal sphincter to release it.

18. PROCEDURE: Reopening of chest wall to control bleeding after thoracic surgery to correct congenital pulmonary abnormality, bleeding controlled and incision closed

19. PROCEDURE: Frenulotomy to treat ankyloglossia and speech dysfunction

20. PROCEDURE: Repair of congenital cerebral artery aneurysm by restriction with bioactive intravascular coil

Chapter 21

Symptoms, Signs and Abnormal Clinical and Laboratory Findings, Not Elsewhere Classified (R00–R99)

Learning Objectives

At the conclusion of this chapter, you should be able to:

1. Describe the organization of the conditions and codes included in Chapter 18 of ICD-10-CM, Symptoms, signs and abnormal clinical and laboratory findings, not elsewhere classified (R00–R99)

2. Describe the circumstances in which a coder should use a code from Chapter 18 of ICD-10-CM

3. Describe the guidelines for the assignment of a symptom code with an established disease code

4. Explain how symptom codes are organized in ICD-10-CM

5. Identify the Alphabetic Index entries for locating nonspecific abnormal findings in order to code them

6. Referring to the *ICD-10-CM Official Guidelines for Coding and Reporting*, briefly describe the use of sign and symptom codes for hospital inpatients as a principal or additional diagnosis

7. Describe the differences in coding of qualified diagnosis, such as possible or probable, when the patient is an inpatient in the hospital as opposed to an outpatient in any healthcare setting

8. Describe when the ICD-10-CM coma scale codes (R40.21–R40.24) are used

9. Assign ICD-10-CM codes for symptoms, signs, and abnormal findings

10. Assign ICD-10-PCS codes for procedures related to this chapter

Key Terms

- Abnormal findings
- Abnormal tumor markers
- Altered mental status
- Complex febrile seizure
- Glasgow coma scale
- Sign
- Simple febrile seizure
- Symptom

Overview of ICD-10-CM Chapter 18, Symptoms, Signs and Abnormal Clinical and Laboratory Findings, Not Elsewhere Classified

Chapter 18 includes categories R00–R99 arranged in the following blocks:

R00–R09	Symptoms and signs involving the circulatory and respiratory systems
R10–R19	Symptoms and signs involving the digestive system and abdomen
R20–R23	Symptoms and signs involving the skin and subcutaneous tissue
R25–R29	Symptoms and signs involving the nervous and musculoskeletal systems
R30–R39	Symptoms and signs involving the genitourinary system
R40–R46	Symptoms and signs involving cognition, perception, emotional state and behavior
R47–R49	Symptoms and signs involving speech and voice
R50–R69	General symptoms and signs
R70–R79	Abnormal findings on examination of blood, without diagnosis
R80–R82	Abnormal findings on examination of urine, without diagnosis
R83–R89	Abnormal findings on examination of other body fluids, substances and tissues, without diagnosis
R90–R94	Abnormal findings on diagnostic imaging and in function studies, without diagnosis
R97	Abnormal tumor markers
R99	Ill-defined and unknown cause of mortality

A **symptom** is any subjective evidence of disease reported by the patient to the physician. A **sign** is objective evidence of a disease observed by the physician (Shiel Jr. 2012).

Some symptoms, such as hives or urticaria (L50.9), gastrointestinal hemorrhage (K92.2), menstrual pain (N94.6), and low back pain (M54.5), have been classified elsewhere in ICD-10-CM. Such symptoms are associated with a given organ system and thus are assigned to the chapter in ICD-10-CM that deals with the corresponding organ system.

Other symptoms and signs are associated with different body systems or are of unknown cause; these are classified to Chapter 18. Examples of these types of symptoms and signs include tachycardia, epistaxis, dyspnea, chest pain, abdominal pain, nausea, vomiting, rash, dysuria, coma, fever, fatigue, syncope, anorexia, and dry mouth.

Abnormal findings include objective measurements documented in laboratory reports that are reported after examination of blood, urine, or other body fluids taken from the patient. Abnormal findings of imaging studies are the conclusions written by radiologists based on review of images collected during diagnostic x-rays, ultrasound, computed axial tomography, magnetic resonance imaging, positron emission tomography, and thermography studies of the various parts of the patient's body. Abnormal findings also include conclusions written by physicians in reports produced after the examination of body function with radioisotope studies or scans, electroencephalogram, electromyogram, electrocardiogram, and other function studies.

Abnormal tumor markers are objective measurements of biochemical substances that are indicative of the presence of tumors. Tumor makers are used to screen, diagnose, assess prognosis, follow response to treatment, and monitor for recurrence of neoplasia. Usually the measurement is an elevation in tumor associate antigens (TAA) or tumor specific antigens (TSA) such as carcinoembryonic antigen (CEA) or prostate specific antigen (PSA).

One category, R99, is provided to describe ill-defined and unknown cause of mortality; it is only for use in the situation when a patient arrives at the emergency department or other facility as dead on arrival (DOA) and pronounced dead by the examining physicians. It does not represent the discharge disposition of death and would not be used on every patient who has expired.

Coding Guidelines and Instructional Notes for ICD-10-CM Chapter 18

The following note appears at the beginning of Chapter 18 outlining the conditions classified to this chapter: "This chapter includes symptoms, signs, abnormal results of clinical or other investigative procedures, and ill-defined conditions regarding which no diagnosis classifiable elsewhere is recorded" (CMS 2012a).

Signs and symptoms that point rather definitely to a given diagnosis have been assigned to a category in other chapters of the classification. In general, categories in this chapter include the less well-defined conditions and symptoms that, without the necessary study of the case to establish a final diagnosis, point perhaps equally to two or more diseases or to two or more systems of the body. Practically all categories in the chapter could be designated "not otherwise specified," "unknown etiology," or "transient." The Alphabetical Index should be consulted to determine which symptoms and signs are to be allocated here and which to other chapters.

The conditions, signs, and symptoms included in Chapter 18 consist of the following:

- Cases for which no more specific diagnosis can be made even after all the facts bearing on the case have been investigated

- Signs or symptoms existing at the time of the initial encounter that proved to be transient and whose causes could not be determined

- Provisional diagnosis in a patient who failed to return for further investigation or care

- Cases referred elsewhere for investigation or treatment before the diagnosis was made

- Cases in which a more precise diagnosis was not available for any other reason

- Certain symptoms, for which supplementary information is provided, that represent important problems in medical care in their own right

Additionally, notes for code usage appear at the subchapter level. Many of the new blocks and categories in Chapter 18 have Excludes1 notes such as the one found under R09, Other symptoms and signs involving the circulatory and respiratory system, that directs the coder to locate diagnosis codes that appear in other chapters of ICD-10-CM. Guidelines that clarify code usage are also found under specific codes. Code R52, Pain unspecified, includes inclusive terms and Excludes1 notes.

The NCHS has published chapter-specific guidelines for Chapter 18 in the *ICD-10-CM Official Guidelines for Coding and Reporting*. The coding student should review all of the coding guidelines for Chapter 18 of ICD-10-CM, which appear in an ICD-10-CM code book or at the website http://www.cdc.gov/nchs/icd/icd10cm.htm, or in Appendix E.

CG

I.C.18. Chapter 18: Symptoms, signs, and abnormal clinical and laboratory findings, not elsewhere classified (R00–R99): Chapter 18 includes symptoms, signs, abnormal results of clinical or other investigative procedures, and ill-defined conditions regarding which no diagnosis classifiable elsewhere is recorded. Signs and symptoms that point to a specific diagnosis have been assigned to a category in other chapters of the classification.

I.C.18.a. Use of symptom codes: Codes that describe symptoms and signs are acceptable for reporting purposes when a related definitive diagnosis has not been established (confirmed) by the provider.

I.C.18.b. Use of a symptom code with a definitive diagnosis code: Codes for signs and symptoms may be reported in addition to a related definitive diagnosis when the sign or symptom is not routinely associated with that diagnosis, such as the various signs and symptoms associated with complex syndromes. The definitive diagnosis code should be sequenced before the symptom code.

Signs or symptoms that are associated routinely with a disease process should not be assigned as additional codes, unless otherwise instructed by the classification.

I.C.18.c. Combination codes that include symptoms: ICD-10-CM contains a number of combination codes that identify both the definitive diagnosis and common symptoms of that diagnosis. When using one of these combination codes, an additional code should not be assigned for the symptom.

I.C.18.d. Repeated falls: Code R29.6, Repeated falls, is for use for encounters when a patient has recently fallen and the reason for the fall is being investigated.

Code Z91.81, History of falling, is for use when a patient has fallen in the past and is at risk for future falls. When appropriate, both codes R29.6 and Z91.81 may be assigned together.

I.C.18.e. *Coma* scale: The coma scale codes (R40.2-) can be used in conjunction with traumatic brain injury codes, acute cerebrovascular disease or sequelae of cerebrovascular disease codes. These codes are primarily for use by trauma registries, but they may be used in any setting where this information is collected. The coma scale codes should be sequenced after the diagnosis code(s).

These codes, one from each subcategory, are needed to complete the scale. The 7th character indicates when the scale was recorded. The 7th character should match for all three codes.

At a minimum, report the initial score documented on presentation at your facility. This may be a score from the emergency medicine technician (EMT) or in the emergency department. If desired, a facility may choose to capture multiple coma scale scores.

Assign code R40.24, Glasgow coma scale, total score, when only the total score is documented in the medical record and not the individual score(s).

I.C.18.f. Functional quadriplegia: Functional quadriplegia (code R53.2) is the lack of ability to use one's limbs or to ambulate due to extreme debility. It is not associated with neurologic deficit or injury, and code R53.2 should not be used for cases of neurologic quadriplegia. It should only be assigned if functional quadriplegia is specifically documented in the medical record.

I.C.18.g. SIRS due to Non-Infectious Process: The systemic inflammatory response syndrome (SIRS) can develop as a result of certain non-infectious disease processes, such as trauma, malignant neoplasm, or pancreatitis. When SIRS is documented with a noninfectious condition, and no subsequent infection is documented, the code for the underlying condition, such as an injury, should be assigned, followed by code R65.10, Systemic inflammatory response syndrome (SIRS) of non-infectious origin without acute organ dysfunction, or code R65.11, Systemic inflammatory response syndrome (SIRS) of non-infectious origin with acute organ dysfunction. If an associated acute organ dysfunction is documented, the appropriate code(s) for the specific type of organ dysfunction(s) should be assigned in addition to code R65.11. If acute organ dysfunction is documented, but it cannot be determined if the acute organ dysfunction is associated with SIRS or due to another condition (e.g., directly due to the trauma), the provider should be queried.

I.C.18.h. Death NOS: Code R99, Ill-defined and unknown cause of mortality, is only for use in the very limited circumstance when a patient who has already died is brought into an emergency department or other healthcare facility and is pronounced dead upon arrival. It does not represent the discharge disposition of death.

Coding Symptoms, Signs, and Abnormal Clinical and Laboratory Findings in ICD-10-CM Chapter 18

Chapter 18 of ICD-10-CM, Symptoms, signs, abnormal clinical and laboratory findings, not elsewhere classified (R00–R99), includes symptoms, signs, and abnormal findings that relate to conditions in multiple body systems. Many of these codes are used for patients evaluated and treated in the outpatient settings, for example, in the physician's office, clinic, or emergency department. That does not mean a patient with a symptom could not be admitted to the hospital. It is possible to use a Chapter 18 code as a principal or secondary diagnosis for an inpatient if the reason for the symptom, sign, or finding could not be explained after inpatient studies were completed.

To help the coder locate the symptoms and signs without an established diagnosis, the ICD-10-CM Index to Diseases and Injuries contains such entries as "abnormal, abnormalities," "elevated, elevation," "findings, abnormal, inconclusive, without diagnosis," and "positive."

Symptoms and Signs by Body System (R00–R69)

Chapter 18 includes a variety of symptoms. In some cases, symptoms may be assigned in addition to a related definitive diagnosis when the symptoms or signs are not routinely associated with that diagnosis. The following discussion should be of assistance in determining when to assign a symptom as an additional diagnosis:

- Conditions that are routinely associated with a disease process: Symptoms and signs that are routinely associated with the disease process should not be assigned as additional codes unless otherwise instructed by the classification.

    EXAMPLE: Nausea and vomiting with gastroenteritis: K52.9, Noninfectious gastroenteritis and colitis, unspecified

    Only the code for gastroenteritis (K52.9) is assigned. The code for nausea and vomiting (R11.2) is not assigned because these are symptoms of gastroenteritis.

- Conditions that are not routinely associated with a disease process: Additional signs and symptoms that are not routinely associated with a disease process should be coded when present.

    EXAMPLE: Patient with metastases to brain admitted in comatose state: C79.31, Secondary malignant neoplasm of brain and spinal cord; R40.20, Coma

    The code for coma (R40.20) should be added as an additional diagnosis; coma is a significant condition that is not routinely associated with brain metastases.

Symptoms and signs are used frequently to describe reasons for service in outpatient settings. Outpatient visits do not always allow for the type of study that is needed to determine a diagnosis. Often the purpose of the outpatient visit is to relieve the symptom rather than to determine or treat the underlying condition. Coders must code the outpatient's condition to the highest level of certainty. The highest level of certainty is often an abnormal sign or symptom code that is assigned as the reason for the outpatient visit.

Most of the categories in the blocks of codes for symptoms and signs (R00–R69) are grouped by body systems, such as categories R00–R09, Symptoms and signs involving the circulatory and respiratory systems and categories R10–R19, Symptoms and signs involving the digestive system and abdomen.

Coma Scale (R40.2)

According to the *ICD-10-CM Official Coding and Reporting Guidelines*, subcategory R40.2, Coma, incorporates what may be documented in the health record as the **Glasgow coma scale** (R40.211–R40.236). The Glasgow coma scale (GCS) codes can be used in conjunction with traumatic brain injury or sequelae of cerebrovascular disease codes. They are primarily for use by trauma registries and research use, but they may be used in any setting where this information is collected. The coma scale codes are sequenced after the diagnosis code(s). These codes, one from each subcategory (R40.21, R40.22, R40.23), are needed to complete the scale. The seventh character indicates when the scale was recorded, and it should match for all three codes:

0—unspecified time
1—in the field [EMT or ambulance]
2—at arrival to emergency department
3—at hospital admission
4—24 hours or more after hospital admission

At a minimum, report the initial score documented on presentation at the facility. This may be a score from the emergency medicine technician (EMT) or in the emergency department. If desired, a facility may choose to capture multiple Glasgow coma scale scores.

Some emergency department personnel will document only one total Glasgow score. According to the coding guidelines, one code, R40.24, Glasgow coma scale, total score, may be the only coma scale code assigned instead of individual codes when only the total score is documented.

Altered Mental Status, Unspecified (R41.82)

Code R41.82, **Altered mental status**, unspecified, identifies a frequent clinical state that requires investigation. Altered mental status or a change in mental status can be a symptom of many different illnesses. Underlying etiologies may include trauma, infection, neoplasm, or alcohol and drug use, as well as endocrine disorders, neurological disorders, psychiatric disorders, and diseases of the kidney. Altered mental status is not to be confused with altered level of consciousness (R40.-) or delirium (R41.0). After workup, if a specific cause of the altered mental status is known, that condition should be coded, and the symptom code should not be used. An Excludes1 note appears under code R41.82 that states if the altered mental status is due to a known condition, the coder should code to that condition and not use this code.

General Symptoms and Signs (R50–R69)

The block of codes for general symptoms and signs (R50–R69), however, classifies general symptoms that are not related to one specific body system. Category R56, Convulsions, not elsewhere classified is subdivided to recognize different forms of seizures or convulsions not identified as epileptic. Two codes exist for febrile seizures. A **complex febrile seizure** (code R56.01) is defined as a fever-associated seizure that is focal, prolonged (lasting more than 15 minutes), or recurs within 24 hours in children between the ages of six months and five years. These may also be described as "atypical" or "complicated" febrile seizures. Any other fever-associated seizure that does not meet this definition is defined as a **simple febrile seizure** (code R56.00). A febrile seizure that is not specified as simple or complex will also be coded to the R56.00 code. Another code is included for posttraumatic seizures (code R56.1). The last code under this category, R56.9, includes other or recurrent convulsions that are not related to fever and may also be described as "convulsive seizure or fit" in the diagnostic statement.

Category R52, Pain, unspecified, is a symptom code for generalized pain or pain without specificity of site. This code would not be used if the pain is described as acute or chronic or if the patient has localized pain that would be coded to pain by anatomic site. This is a three-character code with no subdivisions.

Category R68, Other general symptoms and signs, is subdivided to include conditions that do not fit in other body system categories. Examples of conditions in this category are codes R68.12, Fussy infant (baby); R68.11, Excessive crying of infant (baby); R68.81, Early satiety; and R68.83, chills (without fever).

Other categories in this chapter include codes for symptoms involving different body systems:

R00	Abnormalities of heart beat
R06	Abnormalities of breathing
R10	Abdominal and pelvic pain
R11	Nausea and vomiting
R21	Rash and other nonspecific skin eruption
R26	Abnormalities of gait and mobility
R31	Hematuria
R40	Somnolence, stupor and coma
R42	Dizziness and giddiness
R50	Fever of other and unknown origin
R55	Syncope and collapse
R57	Shock, not elsewhere classified
R63	Symptoms and signs concerning food and fluid intake

As stated previously, symptom and sign categories are frequently used in outpatient settings to indicate that the patient has a physical complaint for which a definitive diagnosis has not been established. It is possible that a symptom code might be used for an inpatient diagnosis when a reason for the complaint cannot be determined. In addition, symptom codes may be used as additional codes with an established diagnosis to describe the complete story of the patient's illness if the symptom is not an integral or usual part of the disease.

Abnormal Findings (R70–R94)

Codes in this range contain descriptors for nonspecific abnormal findings from laboratory, x-ray, pathologic, and other diagnostic tests. These nonspecific findings may be referred to as signs or clinical signs. Codes for nonspecific abnormal test results or findings may be found under such Index entries as "abnormal, abnormality, abnormalities," "findings, abnormal, without diagnosis," "decreased," "elevation," "high," "low," or "positive."

Abnormal findings from laboratory, x-ray, pathologic, and other diagnostic results are not coded and reported unless the physician indicates their clinical significance. If the findings are outside the normal range and the physician has ordered other tests to evaluate the condition or has prescribed treatment, it is appropriate to ask the physician whether the diagnosis code(s) for the abnormal findings should be added.

Often abnormal findings are the reason for additional testing to be performed on patients in the outpatient setting. For example, elevated prostate specific antigen (PSA) (code R97.2) may be a reason for continued testing or monitoring of a patient. The code does not provide a specific diagnosis, but indicates an abnormal finding for a specific organ. Abnormal findings recorded in the record may or may not be appropriate to code. If the coder notes an abnormal laboratory finding that appears to have triggered additional testing or therapy, the coder should ask the physician whether the abnormal finding is a clinically significant condition.

On other occasions, the coder will notice abnormal findings on radiologic studies that may well be incidental to the patient's current condition. For example, an elderly patient with congestive heart failure is given a chest x-ray. A finding of degenerative arthritis is noted in the radiologist's conclusion, but no apparent treatment or further evaluation has occurred. It is unlikely that the arthritis should be coded as it is considered an incidental finding.

The radiologist's findings can be used to identify the specific site of a fracture when the attending or ordering physician's diagnosis statement is nonspecific. For example, the attending physician writes, "Fracture, left tibia." However, the radiologist describes the injury as a fracture of the shaft of the tibia. The coder may code S82.20-, Fracture, tibia, shaft, based on the specific findings of the radiologist.

The radiologist's findings may also be used to clarify an outpatient's diagnosis or reason for services. For example, a patient comes to the hospital for an outpatient x-ray. The physician's order for the x-ray is "possible kidney stones." The radiologist's statement on the radiology report is "bilateral nephrolithiasis." Based on the fact that the radiologist is a physician, it is appropriate to code the calculus of the kidney as the patient's diagnosis.

The title of category R92, Abnormal and inconclusive findings on diagnostic imaging of breast, includes the term "inconclusive." This category includes findings that are considered inconclusive and not necessarily abnormal. For example, a routine mammogram may be considered inconclusive due to what is termed "dense breasts." This is not an abnormal condition but a condition that may require further testing—for example, an ultrasound—to conclude that no malignant condition exists that cannot be found on the mammogram. The diagnosis of dense breast or inconclusive mammography is assigned code R92.2, Inconclusive mammogram.

Coding of Papanicolaou Test (Pap Smear) Findings

The coding of Papanicolaou tests (Pap smears) often involves the coding of nonspecific abnormal findings. Because the classification of abnormal Pap smears has become more specific in recent years, ICD-10-CM includes code options under subcategories R87.6–R87.9, Abnormal cytological, histological and other abnormal findings in specimens from female genital organs.

The Bethesda System of Cytologic Examination is used by most of the laboratories in the United States and has been endorsed by national and international societies as the preferred method of reporting the results of abnormal Pap smears. In ICD-10-CM, code R87.612 describes Pap smear of cervix with low-grade squamous intraepithelial lesion and code

R87.613 describes Pap smear of cervix with high-grade squamous intraepithelial lesion. Other codes describe Pap smear with cervical high-risk human papillomavirus (HPV) DNA test positive (R87.810), Pap smear of cervix with cytologic evidence of malignancy (R87.614), and Pap smear with cervical low-risk HPV DNA test positive (R87.820). Another code describes an unsatisfactory cytologic smear of cervix or an inadequate sample from cervix (R87.615).

The Excludes note for subcategory R87.61 refers the coder to other subcategories for confirmed dysplasia, CIN I–III, or carcinoma in situ conditions.

Abnormal Tumor Markers (R97)

Testing has become common practice for elevations in tumor-associated antigens (TAA), antigens that are relatively restricted to tumor cells, tumor-specific antigens (TSA), antigens unique to tumor cells, and in the diagnosis of and the follow-up care for many malignancies. A unique code for elevated PSA was created when this test became routine in the monitoring of prostate cancer. Many other TAA and TSA tests have become standard practice and other elevated tumor-associated antigen codes are available for use: R97.0, Elevated carcinoembryonic antigen (CEA); R97.1, Elevated cancer antigen 125 (CA 125); R97.2, Elevated prostate specific antigen (PSA); and R97.8, Other abnormal tumor marker.

Ill-Defined and Unknown Causes of Mortality (R99)

The ill-defined and unknown causes of mortality section of Chapter 18 includes death or unexplained death and other conditions that are unspecified causes of mortality. These codes should not be used when a more definitive diagnosis is available. Code R99 is likely to be used for the patient who is brought to the hospital emergency department or other facility but has appeared to die prior to arrival. There may or may not be resuscitation efforts depending on the individual circumstances. The reason for the death may not be known. The diagnosis in the record for this patient may be written as "dead on arrival" (DOA). The physician will pronounce the patient dead and document the date and time in the health record.

Otherwise, the terminology of "death" is not a diagnosis. It is considered the healthcare outcome or the discharge disposition. The code R99 is not to be used on every health record when a patient expires. Instead the cause of death and the underlying illness are coded on the health record. Code R99 is only used when the death is unexplained and there is no cause of death documented.

ICD-10-PCS Procedure Coding to Investigate Symptoms, Signs and Abnormal Clinical and Laboratory Findings

Diagnostic procedures may be performed to investigate symptoms, signs, and abnormal test findings. In the Medical and Surgical Section, procedures falling under the root operations Excision or Drainage may be performed as diagnostic studies or biopsies. The seventh character for these procedures would be X to distinguish this procedure as diagnostic when the procedure is identified as a biopsy. Other diagnostic procedures from the Medical and Surgical section are also possible tests that can be performed to investigate symptoms and signs, for example, inspection procedures such as bronchoscopy, cystoscopy, and colonoscopy that may be performed without a companion procedure such as a biopsy.

Diagnostic procedures also appear in other sections of the ICD-10-PCS classification system for example, procedures in the Administration, Measurement and Monitoring, Imaging, and Nuclear Medicine sections. It would be up to the institution or provider to decide what procedures outside the Medical and surgical Section would be coded; just because there is a code for a procedure does not mean it requires coding.

Administration

The codes in the Administration section identify procedures for putting in or on a therapeutic, prophylactic, protective, diagnostic, nutritional, or physiological substance. This section includes transfusions, infusions, and injections. The seven characters for the administration procedures are shown in table 21.1.

Table 21.1. **Administration procedures**

Character 1—Section	Administration procedure codes have the first-character value of 3
Character 2—Body System	Three values: Indwelling Device, Physiological Systems and Anatomical Regions, or Circulatory System
Character 3—Root Operation	Three values: Introduction, Irrigation, and Transfusion
Character 4—Body/System Region	Identifies the site where the substance is administered, not the site where the substance administered takes effect
Character 5—Approach	Approaches are External, Open, Percutaneous, Via Natural or Artificial Opening, and Via Natural or Artificial Opening Endoscopic
Character 6—Substance	Specifies the substance being introduced such as Anesthetic, Contrast, Dialysate, and Blood Products
Character 7—Qualifier	Indicates whether the substance is Autologous or Nonautologous

The main terms for procedures in the Administration section include such procedures as "transfusion" and "introduction of substance in or on." For example, the transfusion of nonautologous blood platelets through a peripheral vein is coded as 30233R1. The infusion of an electrolyte substance through a peripheral vein is coded as 3E0337Z.

Measurement and Monitoring

The codes in the Measurement and Monitoring section identify and describe procedures for determining the level of a physiological or physical function. A measurement is determining the level of a physiological or physical function at a point in time. Monitoring is determining the level of a physiological or physical function over a period of time. The seven characters for measurement and monitoring procedures are shown in table 21.2.

Examples of procedures coded to this section are electrocardiograms (EKG), electroencephalograms (EEG), and cardiac catheterization. An EKG is a measurement of cardiac electrical activity (4A02X4Z). An EEG is a measurement of the electrical activity of the central nervous system (4A00X4Z). A cardiac catheterization is a measurement of the sampling and pressures in the heart performed through a percutaneous approach. A left heart diagnostic cardiac catheterization is coded 4A023N7. The main terms used to locate the procedure codes are "measurement" and "monitoring" or the title of the procedure; for example, stress test is 4A12XM4.

Table 21.2. **Measurement and monitoring procedures**

Character 1—Section	Measurement and Monitoring procedure codes have the first-character value of 4
Character 2—Body System	Two values: Physiological Systems and Physiological Devices
Character 3—Root Operation	Two values: Measurement and Monitoring
Character 4—Body/System Region	Specifies the specific body system measured or monitored
Character 5—Approach	Approaches are External, Open, Percutaneous, Via Natural or Artificial Opening, Via Natural or Artificial Opening Endoscopic
Character 6—Function/Device	Specifies the physiological or physical function being measured or monitored, for example, Conductivity, Metabolism, Pulse, Temperature, and Volume. If a device is required and left in place, the insertion of the device is coded as a separate Medical and Surgical procedure
Character 7—Qualifier	Specific values to further identify the body part or the variation of the procedure performed

Imaging Section

The codes in the Imaging section include procedures such as plain radiography, fluoroscopy, CT, MRI, and ultrasound. The seven characters for the procedures in the Imaging section are shown in table 21.3.

Table 21.3. **Imaging procedures**

Character 1—Section	Imaging procedure codes have the first-character value of letter B
Character 2—Body System	Defines the body system such as Central Nervous System, Heart, Upper Arteries, Respiratory System, Digestive System, and such.
Character 3—Root Operation	Five values: Computerized Tomography, Fluoroscopy, Magnetic Resonance Imaging, Plain Radiology, and Ultrasonography
Character 4—Body Part	Defines the body part with different values for each of the body systems identified with character 2
Character 5—Contrast	Identifies whether the contrast material used in the imaging procedure is high or low osmolar when applicable
Character 6—Qualifier	Provides further details about the nature of the substance used or the technology involved
Character 7—Qualifier	Specifies the circumstances of the imaging performed, for example, Intraoperative, Intravascular, or Transesophageal

Examples of procedures coded to this section are the fluoroscopy performed on a single coronary artery using low osmolar contrast during a cardiac catheterization (B2101ZZ), CT of the abdomen (BW201ZZ), ultrasound of the bilateral breasts (BH42ZZZ), and plain x-ray of the right hip (BQ00ZZZ). The main terms used to locate the procedure codes are the root operations Computerized Tomography, Fluoroscopy, Magnetic Resonance Imaging, Plain Radiology, and Ultrasonography.

ICD-10-CM and ICD-10-PCS Review Exercises: Chapter 18

Assign the correct ICD-10-CM diagnosis codes or ICD-10-PCS procedure codes to the following exercises.

1. Right upper quadrant rebound abdominal tenderness

2. Assign the Glasgow coma scale code(s) when the patient had the following documented by the EMT: eyes do not open, no verbal response, with no motor response. The neurologist documented the following on day 2 of the hospital admission: eyes open to sound, verbal response produced inappropriate words, and motor response with flexion withdrawal.

3. Microcalcification found on breast mammography

4. The patient comes to the physician's office for an annual physical and two readings of elevated blood pressure are found. The physician requests the patient to return to the office in two weeks after the patient follows certain dietary and exercise instructions. The diagnosis recorded for the office visit is high blood pressure readings, rule out hypertension.

5. Malignant ascites due to carcinoma of the ovary, right side (primary site neoplasm)

6. Two-year-old child seen in emergency room with diarrhea, fever, and chills with a witnessed febrile seizure in the emergency room

7. The patient was seen in the physician's office complaining of chest pain and jaw pain with excessive sweating. An ambulance was summoned and the patient was taken to the hospital emergency room with the diagnosis of rule out acute myocardial infarction.

8. Shortness of breath, fatigue

9. Elevated PSA

10. At conclusion of physician office visit, doctor wrote the final diagnosis in the record as "Rule out diabetes." Patient complained of polydipsia and polyuria for several weeks

11. At the conclusion of the physician office visit, the physician documented "Postnasal drip, headache and localized lymphadenopathy, possible seasonal allergies."

(Continued on next page)

ICD-10-CM and ICD-10-PCS Review Exercises: Chapter 18 (Continued)

12. Elevated glucose tolerance test

13. Elevated CEA

14. Physician office visit conclusion: Radiology study finding of nonvisualization of gallbladder; possible chronic cholecystitis

15. Physician office visit conclusion: Radiology study of coin lesion of lung and chronic cough

16. PROCEDURE: Bronchoscopy with biopsy of left main bronchus

17. PROCEDURE: Control of epistaxis by electrocautery

18. PROCEDURE: EGD with mid-esophageal biopsy

19. PROCEDURE: Maxillary sinusoscopy

20. PROCEDURE: Cystoscopy with bladder biopsy

Chapter 22A

Injury (S00–T34)

Learning Objectives

At the conclusion of this chapter, you should be able to:

1. Describe the organization of the conditions and codes included in Chapter 19 of ICD-10-CM, with a focus on injuries, categories S00–T34

2. Identify the correct seventh character required for reporting certain injury codes in ICD-10-CM

3. Explain the ICD-10-CM coding guidelines related to the coding and reporting of injuries

4. Assign ICD-10-CM diagnosis codes for injuries

5. Assign ICD-10-PCS codes for procedures related to injuries

Key Terms

- Burn
- Closed fracture
- Comminuted fracture
- Contusion
- Corrosion
- Crush injury
- Dislocation
- Displaced fracture
- First-degree burn
- Frostbite
- Greenstick fracture
- Immobilization
- Impacted fracture
- Initial encounter
- Insertion
- Malunion

- Nondisplaced fracture
- Nonunion
- Oblique fracture
- Open fracture
- Open wound
- Pathological fracture
- Placeholder character
- Repair
- Reposition
- Second-degree burn
- Sequela
- Sprain
- Strain
- Stress fracture
- Subluxation
- Subsequent encounter
- Superficial injuries
- Third-degree burn
- Transverse fracture
- Traumatic amputation
- Traumatic fracture

Overview of the Injury Portion of ICD-10-CM Chapter 19

The Injury portion of Chapter 19 includes categories S00–T34 arranged in the following blocks:

S00–S09	Injuries to the head
S10–S19	Injuries to the neck
S20–S29	Injuries to the thorax
S30–S39	Injuries to the abdomen, lower back, lumbar spine, pelvis and external genitals
S40–S49	Injuries to the shoulder and upper arm
S50–S59	Injuries to the elbow and forearm
S60–S69	Injuries to the wrist, hand and fingers
S70–S79	Injuries to the hip and thigh
S80–S89	Injuries to the knee and lower leg
S90–S99	Injuries to the ankle and foot
T07	Injuries involving multiple body regions

T14	Injury of unspecified body region
T15–T19	Effects of foreign body entering through natural orifice
T20–T25	Burns and corrosions of external body surface, specified by site
T26–T28	Burns and corrosions confined to eye and internal organs
T30–T32	Burns and corrosions of multiple and unspecified body regions
T33–T34	Frostbite

This chapter will focus on the ICD-10-CM coding of injuries. The coding of drug-related illnesses such as poisoning, adverse effects, and underdosing of drugs will be addressed in Chapter 22B of this text.

Specific types of injuries found in categories S00–S99 of Chapter 19 of ICD-10-CM are arranged by body region beginning with the head and concluding with the ankle and foot. This results in the grouping of injury types together under the site where it occurred.

In addition, generally the listings of conditions that follow the anatomic site are as follows:

- Superficial injury
- Open wound
- Fracture
- Dislocation and sprain
- Injury of nerves
- Injury of blood vessels
- Injury of muscle and tendon
- Crushing injury
- Traumatic amputation
- Other and unspecified injuries

ICD-10-CM uses the terms "displaced" and "nondisplaced" in the code descriptor for fracture. Codes from blocks T20–T32 classify burns and corrosions. The burn codes identify thermal burns, except for sunburns, that come from a heat source. The burn codes are also for burns resulting from electricity and radiation. Corrosions are burns due to chemicals.

Coding Guidelines and Instructional Notes for the Injury Portion of ICD-10-CM Chapter 19

The following guideline appears at the beginning of ICD-10-CM Chapter 19: "Use secondary code(s) from ICD-10-CM Chapter 20, External causes of morbidity, to indicate cause of injury. Codes within the T code section that include the external cause do not require an additional external cause code."

Instructions for coding open wounds are included in ICD-10-CM. ICD-10-CM contains a note under the different categories for open wounds and directs the coding professional to code also any associated injuries or wound infection.

Most categories in ICD-10-CM Chapter 19 have seventh characters that identify the encounter:

A—Initial encounter
D—Subsequent encounter
S—Sequela

The fracture categories in Chapter 19 have different seventh characters that identify the fracture-care encounter:

A—Initial encounter for closed fracture
B—Initial encounter for open fracture or open fracture type I or II
C—Initial encounter for open fracture type IIIA, IIIB, or IIIC
D—Subsequent encounter for fracture with routine healing
E—Subsequent encounter for open fracture type I or II with routine healing
F—Subsequent encounter for open fracture type IIIA, IIIB, or IIIC with routine healing
G—Subsequent encounter for fracture with delayed healing
H—Subsequent encounter for open fracture type I or II with delayed healing
J—Subsequent encounter for open fracture type IIIA, IIIB, or IIIC with delayed healing
K—Subsequent encounter for fracture with nonunion
M—Subsequent encounter for open fracture type I or II with nonunion
N—Subsequent encounter for open fracture type IIIA, IIIB, or IIIC with nonunion
P—Subsequent encounter for fracture with malunion
Q—Subsequent encounter for open fracture type I or II with malunion
R—Subsequent encounter for open fracture type IIIA, IIIB, or IIIC with malunion
S—Sequela

The seventh characters for fractures are unique to each type of bone and type of fracture. Not all of these seventh characters are used with every fracture. It is necessary to review the fracture carefully before assigning a seventh character.

The NCHS has published chapter-specific guidelines for Chapter 19 in the *ICD-10-CM Official Guidelines for Coding and Reporting*. The coding student should review all of the coding guidelines for Chapter 19 of ICD-10-CM, which appear in an ICD-10-CM code book or at the website http://www.cdc.gov/nchs/icd/icd10cm.htm, or in Appendix E.

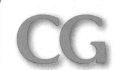
I.C.19.a. Application of 7th Characters in Chapter 19: Most categories in chapter 19 have a 7th character requirement for each applicable code. Most categories in this chapter have three 7th character values (with the exception of fractures): A, initial encounter, D, subsequent encounter and S, sequela. Categories for traumatic fractures have additional 7th character values.

7th character "A", initial encounter is used while the patient is receiving active treatment for the condition. Examples of active treatment are: surgical treatment, emergency department encounter, and evaluation and treatment by a new physician.

7th character "D" subsequent encounter is used for encounters after the patient has received active treatment of the condition and is receiving routine care for the condition during the healing or recovery phase. Examples of subsequent care are: cast change or removal, removal of external or internal fixation device, medication adjustment, other aftercare and follow up visits following treatment of the injury or condition.

The aftercare Z codes should not be used for aftercare for conditions such as injuries or poisonings, where 7th characters are provided to identify subsequent care. For example, for aftercare of an injury, assign the acute injury code with the 7th character "D" (subsequent encounter).

7th character "S", sequela, is for use for complications or conditions that arise as a direct result of a condition, such as scar formation after a burn. The scars are sequelae of the burn. When using 7th character "S", it is necessary to use both the injury code that precipitated the sequela and the code for the sequela itself. The "S" is added only to the injury code, not the sequela code. The 7th character "S" identifies the injury responsible for the sequela. The specific type of sequela (e.g. scar) is sequenced first, followed by the injury code.

I.C.19.b. Coding of Injuries: When coding injuries, assign separate codes for each injury unless a combination code is provided, in which case the combination code is assigned. Code T07, Unspecified multiple injuries should not be assigned in the inpatient setting unless information for a more specific code is not available.

Traumatic injury codes (S00–T14.9) are not to be used for normal, healing surgical wounds or to identify complications of surgical wounds.

The code for the most serious injury, as determined by the provider and the focus of treatment, is sequenced first.

I.C.19.b.1. Superficial injuries: Superficial injuries such as abrasions or contusions are not coded when associated with more severe injuries of the same site.

I.C.19.b.2. Primary injury with damage to nerves/blood vessels: When a primary injury results in minor damage to peripheral nerves or blood vessels, the primary injury is sequenced first with additional code(s) for injuries to nerves and spinal cord (such as category S04), and/or injury to blood vessels (such as category

(Continued)

(Continued)

S15). When the primary injury is to the blood vessels or nerves, that injury should be sequenced first.

IC.19.c. Coding of Traumatic Fractures: The principles of multiple coding of injuries should be followed in coding fractures. Fractures of specified sites are coded individually by site in accordance with both the provisions within categories S02, S12, S22, S32, S42, S49, S52, S59, S62, S72, S79, S82, S89, S92 and the level of detail furnished by medical record content.

A fracture not indicated as open or closed should be coded to closed. A fracture not indicated whether displaced or not displaced should be coded to displaced.

More specific guidelines are as follows:

I.C.19.c.1. Initial vs. Subsequent Encounter for Fractures: Traumatic fractures are coded using the appropriate 7th character for initial encounter (A, B, C) while the patient is receiving active treatment for the fracture. Examples of active treatment are: surgical treatment, emergency department encounter, and evaluation and treatment by a new physician. The appropriate 7th character for initial encounter should also be assigned for a patient who delayed seeking treatment for the fracture or nonunion.

Fractures are coded using the appropriate 7th character for subsequent care for encounters after the patient has completed active treatment of the fracture and is receiving routine care for the fracture during the healing or recovery phase. Examples of fracture aftercare are: cast change or removal, removal of external or internal fixation device, medication adjustment, and follow-up visits following fracture treatment.

Care for complications of surgical treatment for fracture repairs during the healing or recovery phase should be coded with the appropriate complication codes.

Care of complications of fractures, such as malunion and nonunion, should be reported with the appropriate 7th character for subsequent care with nonunion (K, M, N,) or subsequent care with malunion (P, Q, R).

A code from category M80, not a traumatic fracture code, should be used for any patient with known osteoporosis who suffers a fracture, even if the patient had a minor fall or trauma, if that fall or trauma would not usually break a normal, healthy bone.

See Section I.C.13. Osteoporosis.

The aftercare Z codes should not be used for aftercare for traumatic fractures. For aftercare of a traumatic fracture, assign the acute fracture code with the appropriate 7th character.

I.C.19.c.2. Multiple fractures sequencing: Multiple fractures are sequenced in accordance with the severity of the fracture.

I.C.19.d. Coding of Burns and Corrosions: The ICD-10-CM makes a distinction between burns and corrosions. The burn codes are for thermal burns, except sunburns, that come from a heat source, such as a fire or hot appliance. The burn codes are also for burns resulting from electricity and radiation. Corrosions are burns due to chemicals. The guidelines are the same for burns and corrosions.

Current burns (T20–T25) are classified by depth, extent and by agent (X code). Burns are classified by depth as first degree (erythema), second degree (blistering), and third degree (full-thickness involvement). Burns of the eye and internal organs (T26–T28) are classified by site, but not by degree.

I.C.19.d.1. Sequencing of burn and related condition codes: Sequence first the code that reflects the highest degree of burn when more than one burn is present.

I.C.19.d.1.a. When the reason for the admission or encounter is for treatment of external multiple burns, sequence first the code that reflects the burn of the highest degree.

I.C.19.d.1.b. When a patient has both internal and external burns, the circumstances of admission govern the selection of the principal diagnosis or first-listed diagnosis.

I.C.19.d.1.c. When a patient is admitted for burn injuries and other related conditions such as smoke inhalation and/or respiratory failure, the circumstances of admission govern the selection of the principal or first-listed diagnosis.

I.C.19.d.2. Burns of the same local site: Classify burns of the same local site (three-character category level, T20–T28) but of different degrees to the subcategory identifying the highest degree recorded in the diagnosis.

I.C.19.d.3. Non-healing burns: Non-healing burns are coded as acute burns.

Necrosis of burned skin should be coded as a non-healed burn.

I.C.19.d.4. Infected Burn: For any documented infected burn site, use an additional code for the infection.

I.C.19.d.5. Assign separate codes for each burn site: When coding burns, assign separate codes for each burn site. Category T30, Burn and corrosion, body region unspecified is extremely vague and should rarely be used.

(Continued)

(Continued)

I.C.19.d.6. Burns and Corrosions Classified According to Extent of Body Surface Involved: Assign codes from category T31, Burns classified according to extent of body surface involved, or T32, Corrosions classified according to extent of body surface involved, when the site of the burn is not specified or when there is a need for additional data. It is advisable to use category T31 as additional coding when needed to provide data for evaluating burn mortality, such as that needed by burn units. It is also advisable to use category T31 as an additional code for reporting purposes when there is mention of a third-degree burn involving 20 percent or more of the body surface.

Categories T31 and T32 are based on the classic "rule of nines" in estimating body surface involved: head and neck are assigned nine percent, each arm nine percent, each leg 18 percent, the anterior trunk 18 percent, posterior trunk 18 percent, and genitalia one percent. Providers may change these percentage assignments where necessary to accommodate infants and children who have proportionately larger heads than adults, and patients who have large buttocks, thighs, or abdomen that involve burns.

I.C.19.d.7. Encounters for treatment of *sequela* of burns: Encounters for the treatment of the late effects of burns or corrosions (i.e., scars or joint contractures) should be coded with a burn or corrosion code with the 7th character "S" for sequela.

I.C.19.d.8. Sequelae with a late effect code and current burn: When appropriate, both a code for a current burn or corrosion with 7th character "A" or "D" and a burn or corrosion code with 7th character "S" may be assigned on the same record (when both a current burn and sequelae of an old burn exist). Burns and corrosions do not heal at the same rate and a current healing wound may still exist with sequela of a healed burn or corrosion.

I.C.19.d.9. Use of an external cause code with burns and corrosions: An external cause code should be used with burns and corrosions to identify the source and intent of the burn, as well as the place where it occurred.

Coding of Injuries in Chapter 19 of ICD-10-CM

The Alphabetic Index to Diseases in ICD-10-CM classifies injuries according to their general type, such as a burn, dislocation, fracture, or wound. The subterms under the general type of injury identify the anatomical site.

Burn (electricity)(flame)(hot gas, liquid or hot object)(radiation)(steam)(thermal)
    abdomen, abdominal (muscle)(wall) T21.02
        first degree T21.12
        second degree T21.22
        third degree T21.32
Dislocation (articular)
    with fracture – see Fracture
    acromioclavicular (joint) S43.10-
        with displacement
        100%-200% S43.12-
        more than 200% S43.13-
Fracture, traumatic (abduction)(adduction)(separation)(see also Fracture,
pathological)
        acetabulum S32.40-
        column
           anterior (displaced) (iliopubic) S32.43-
           nondisplaced S32.436
Wound, open
    abdomen, abdominal
        wall S31.109
           with penetration into peritoneal cavity S31.609
           bite – see Bite, abdomen, wall
           epigastric region S31.102
               with penetration into peritoneal cavity S31.602

In ICD-10-CM, injuries are grouped by body part rather than by categories of injury, so that all injuries of the specific site (such as head and neck) are grouped together rather than groupings of all fractures or all open wounds. For example, categories are grouped by site, such as injuries to the head (S00–S09), injuries to the neck (S10–S19), injuries to the thorax (S20–S29), and so on.

Chapter 19 encompasses two alpha characters. The S section provides codes for the various types of injuries related to single body regions; the T section covers injuries to unspecified body regions as well as poisonings and certain other consequences of external causes.

Many codes, such as fractures, include specificity in ICD-10-CM. For example, some of the information that may be found in fracture codes includes the type of fracture, specific anatomical site, whether the fracture is displaced or not, laterality, routine versus delayed healing, nonunions, and malunions. Laterality and identification of type of encounter (initial, subsequent, sequela) are a significant component of the code expansion.

ICD-10-CM uses a **placeholder character** x for certain codes. The x is used as a placeholder at certain codes to allow for future expansion. For example, S01.01xA for an initial encounter for care of a laceration without foreign body of scalp requires the sixth character to have a placeholder x to allow the addition of the seventh character to indicate the initial encounter of care.

Separate ICD-10-CM codes are assigned for each injury unless there is a combination code available. However, some combination codes should not be assigned. For example, code T07, Unspecified multiple injuries, should not be assigned in an inpatient setting if at all possible. The only time a code like T07 should be used is when no more specific information is available from the provider.

The code for the most serious injury is sequenced. The physician determines what is the most serious injury in a patient with multiple injuries. If a patient has superficial injuries associated with a more serious injury at the same site, the code for the superficial injuries such as contusions and abrasions are not coded as the superficial injuries are expected to be present with a more serious injury.

Seventh Characters

Most categories in Chapter 19 of ICD-10-CM have a seventh character required for each applicable code. Most categories have three applicable codes. Three seventh character values are used for most of the categories with the exception of fractures, which have a most extensive list of seventh characters. The characters are as follows:

- The seventh character A for **initial encounter** is used while the patient is receiving active treatment for the injury, for example, surgical treatment, emergency department encounter, and evaluation and treatment by a new physician.

- The seventh character D for **subsequent encounter** is used for encounters after the patient has received active treatment of the injury and is receiving routine care for the injury during the healing or recovery phase. For example, cast change or removal, removal of an external or internal fixation device, medication adjustment, other aftercare, and follow-up visits following injury treatment are examples of the kind of encounters covered under this character.

- The seventh character S for **sequela** is used for complications or conditions that arise as a direct result of an injury, such as contracture formation after a burn. When using seventh character S, it is necessary to use both the injury code that precipitated the sequela and the code for the sequela itself. The S is added only to the injury code, not the sequela code. The seventh character S identifies the injury responsible for the sequela. The specific type of sequela (for example, contracture) is sequenced first, followed by the injury code.

The aftercare Z codes should not be used for aftercare for injuries according to the *ICD-10-CM Official Guidelines for Coding and Reporting*. For aftercare of an injury, the coder should assign the acute injury code with the seventh character D for subsequent encounter.

Fractures

A **traumatic fracture** is a break in the bone due to a traumatic injury. Tenderness and swelling develop at the site of the break, with a visible or palpable deformity, pain, and weakness. X-rays show a partial or an incomplete break at the site of the fracture.

In ICD-10-CM, traumatic fractures are coded to the specific sites of the fracture within categories S02, S12, S22, S32, S42, S49, S52, S59, S62, S72, S79, S82, S89, and S92. A fracture that is not indicated as an open fracture or a closed fracture is coded as a closed fracture. A fracture that is not indicated as a displaced fracture or a nondisplaced fracture is coded to a displaced fracture.

There are different types of fractures that may be described by physicians: closed, open, displaced, and nondisplaced. A **closed fracture** is when the bone breaks but there is no puncture or open wound in the skin. An **open fracture** is one in which the bone breaks through the skin even though it may fall back into the wound and may or may not be visible through the wound. A **displaced fracture** is described for a bone that breaks into two or more parts and the two ends of the bone are out of place and need to be realigned. This may also be called a comminuted fracture. In a **nondisplaced fracture**, the fracture of the bone occurs with a crack either part way or all the way through the bone but the bone remains in alignment. Some fractures are more severe than others based on its location and damage done to the bone and surrounding tissue. Fractures can damage blood vessels and nerves around the bone. A fractured bone can become infected or develop osteomyelitis. Healing time varies depending on the type of bone as well as the age and the overall health of a patient.

Physicians may use other terminology to describe a fracture:

- A **comminuted fracture** occurs when a bone breaks into several pieces.

- A **greenstick fracture** is an incomplete fracture in which the bone is bent and often occurs in children.

- An **impacted fracture** occurs when the bone breaks and the ends of the bone are pushed into each other or one end of the bone impacted into the other end of the bone at the site of the break. This type of fracture may also be referred to as a buckle fracture.

- An **oblique fracture** occurs when the bone breaks in a curved or sloped shape.

- A **pathological fracture** is one caused by disease that weakens the bone and breaks with minor trauma that otherwise would not break a healthy bone.

- **Stress fractures** are caused by overuse or repetitive force applied to a limb or bone, most commonly occurring in the bones of the lower leg and foot of athletes who run and jump in their sport. A stress fracture appears as small cracks in a bone that does not always appear on the first imaging or x-ray. Stress fractures can also occur with normal use of a bone when the bone is weakened by disease such as osteoporosis.

- A **transverse fracture** is one that breaks at a right angle to the bone's axis.

Traumatic fractures are coded with the appropriate seventh characters to identify the episode of care: initial treatment, subsequent treatment, or to identify an injury that is the cause of a sequela. Fracture seventh characters are expanded to include options for the initial care for a closed versus open fracture, subsequent care that includes routine and delayed healing, complications of nonunion and malunion, and identification of a sequela situation:

A—Initial encounter for closed fracture
B—Initial encounter for open fracture
D—Subsequent encounter for fracture with routine healing
G—Subsequent encounter for fracture with delayed healing
K—Subsequent encounter for fracture with nonunion
P—Subsequent encounter for fracture with malunion
S—Sequela

Some fracture categories provide for seventh characters to designate the specific type of open fracture. These seventh character designations are based on the Gustilo open fracture classification:

B—Initial encounter for open fracture type I or II (open NOS or not otherwise specified)
C—Initial encounter for open fracture type IIIA, IIIB, or IIIC
E—Subsequent encounter for open fracture type I or II with routine healing
F—Subsequent encounter for open fracture type IIIA, IIIB, or IIIC with routine healing
H—Subsequent encounter for open fracture type I or II with delayed healing
J—Subsequent encounter for open fracture type IIIA, IIIB, or IIIC with delayed healing
M—Subsequent encounter for open fracture type I or II with nonunion

N—Subsequent encounter for open fracture type IIIA, IIIB, or IIIC with nonunion
Q—Subsequent encounter for open fracture type I or II with malunion
R—Subsequent encounter for open fracture type IIIA, IIIB, or IIIC with malunion

There may be complications of fracture injuries and the care for these complications should be coded with the appropriate complication codes, such as postoperative wound infections. If there is a complication of the fracture healing such as malunion or nonunion, the code for the fracture should be reported with the seventh character for subsequent encounter for fracture with nonunion or malunion. A **malunion** fracture is a fractured bone that has healed in a poor alignment and may cause the bone to be shorter than it was before the break. A **nonunion** is a fracture that has failed to heal after several months of recovery. Both conditions cause significant impairment in the patient and usually require additional treatment including surgery.

Remember that pathologic fractures due to underlying bone disease are not considered traumatic and, as such, are not classified to Chapter 19 of ICD-10-CM with the traumatic fracture codes. A code from category M80, Age related osteoporosis with pathologic fracture, should be assigned when a patient with known osteoporosis acquires a fracture from a minor injury that normally would not cause a bone to break in a person without osteoporosis.

Multiple Fractures

When coding fractures, the coder should assign separate codes for each fracture unless a complication code is provided in the Alphabetic Index, in which case the combination code is assigned.

> **EXAMPLE:** Initial encounter for a patient who has a closed fracture of the distal radius and the first metacarpal bone of the right upper limb
>
> Closed fracture of the distal radius (radius, lower end): S52.501A, Unspecified fracture of the lower end of the right radius
>
> Closed fracture of the first metacarpal bone, right hand: S62.201A, Unspecified fracture of first metacarpal bone, right hand

Combination categories for multiple fractures are provided for use when the health record contains a description of multiple fractures at one site but without specific details.

> **EXAMPLE:** Initial encounter for multiple fractures of ribs right side is the only information provided in the health record: S22.41xA, Multiple fractures of ribs, right side
>
> **EXAMPLE:** Initial encounter for multiple pelvic fractures without disruption of the pelvic ring: S32.82xA, Multiple fractures of pelvic without disruption of pelvic ring

Dislocation and Subluxation

Dislocation is the displacement of a bone from its joint. The joints most commonly affected are in the fingers, thumbs, and shoulders. Pain and swelling occur, as well as the loss of use of the injured part. To promote healing, the dislocation can be reduced and the joint immobilized by applying a cast. A dislocation that occurs with a fracture is included in the fracture code. The reduction of the dislocation is included in the code for the fracture reduction.

A **subluxation** is an incomplete dislocation with the contact between the joint surfaces remaining in place. A subluxation commonly seen in children under the age of five is "nursemaid's elbow." This injury occurs when a small child is lifted, yanked, or swung by the hand or wrist or falls on an outstretched arm. The injury is a subluxation of the radial head from the annular ligament. The ligament is trapped in the elbow joint and causes acute pain. By manipulating the elbow joint to release the trapped tissue, the subluxation can be corrected, and the pain is immediately relieved.

In ICD-10-CM, traumatic dislocations and subluxations are coded to the specific sites of the dislocation within categories S03, S13, S23, S33, S43, S53, S63, S73, S83, and S93 with specific fourth characters to identify the dislocation and subluxation. The main term for dislocation and subluxation is "Dislocation" by site and "Subluxation" by site. Each of these codes requires a seventh character to identify whether the encounter of care for the condition is the initial (A) or a subsequent (D) encounter, or is for a sequela (S).

Dislocations may also be described as pathological or recurrent. These are not the same as traumatic dislocations. Codes for these conditions are contained in Chapter 13, Diseases of the musculoskeletal system and connective tissue, in subcategories M24.3-, Pathological dislocation of joint, not elsewhere classified and M24.4-, Recurrent dislocation of joint. The main term is dislocation, pathological or dislocation, recurrent, by site.

Once a dislocation of a joint has occurred, it takes less effort to produce another dislocation. Only the initial occurrence of the joint dislocation is coded to the injury code. All subsequent dislocations of the same joint are coded as recurrent dislocation. For example, a college athlete was brought to the emergency department with a dislocation of the right shoulder that occurred while he was wrestling at a sporting event. The athlete stated he has had a dislocated shoulder previously. The physician describes the dislocation as "recurrent." This is coded as M24.411, Recurrent dislocation of joint, right shoulder, from the ICD-10-CM chapter on musculoskeletal diseases. It is not coded with an acute dislocation code for the shoulder, S43.005-.

Sprains and Strains

A **sprain** is an injury of the supporting ligaments of a joint resulting from a turning or twisting of a body part. Sprains are extremely painful and are accompanied by swelling and discoloration. They require rest for the injury to heal. Whiplash is a specific type of sprain, usually due to a sudden throwing of the head forward and then backward. It results in a compression of the cervical spine that involves the bones, joints, and intervertebral discs.

A **strain** is simply an overstretching or overexertion of some part of the musculature. Strains usually respond to rest. Strains commonly occur in the musculature of the spine, especially in the neck (cervical strain) and in the low back (lumbar). A strain can be a partial tear in the muscle attached to a bone. The injury usually occurs when there is an unusual force applied to the muscle, for example in an accident or during an athletic exercise or sport activity. The treatment is usually rest of the site, application of ice and compression of the area with a wrap or supportive device (Merck 2007).

In ICD-10-CM, traumatic sprains are coded to the specific site within categories S03, S13, S23, S33, S43, S53, S63, S73, S83, and S93 with specific fourth characters to identify the sprain. The main term is "Sprain" by site. Each of these codes requires a seventh character to identify whether the encounter for care of the condition is the initial (A) or a subsequent (D) encounter, or is for a sequela (S).

A strain may also be a traumatic injury. The Alphabetic Index contains the main term "Strain" with subterms for a limited number of sites that direct the coder to the injury chapter for codes:

Strain
    back S39.012
    cervical S16.1
    low back S39.012
    muscle—see Injury, muscle, by site, strain
    neck S16.1
    tendon—see Injury, muscle, by site, strain

Injuries to muscles and tendons are coded to the specific site within categories S09, S16, S29, S29, S39, S46, S56, S66, S76, S86, and S96 with specific fourth characters to identify the strain. The main term is "Injury, muscle (and tendon)" or "Injury, tendon (see also Injury, muscle)" by site. Each of these codes requires a seventh character to identify whether the encounter for care for the condition is the initial (A) or a subsequent encounter (D), or is for a sequela (S).

Intracranial Injury, Excluding Those with Skull Fracture

Category S06, Intracranial injury, is used for various forms of traumatic brain injury excluding these injuries that occur with a skull fracture. The fourth-character subterms identify the specific intracranial injuries of concussion (S06.0), traumatic cerebral edema (S06.1), diffuse traumatic brain injury (S06.2), focal traumatic brain injury (S06.3), epidural hemorrhage (S06.4), traumatic subdural hemorrhage (S06.5), traumatic subarachnoid hemorrhage (S06.6), other specific intracranial injuries (S06.8), which includes injuries to carotid arteries, and unspecified intracranial injury (S06.9).

The sixth characters for the codes in category S06 identify whether the patient did or did not have a loss of consciousness:

0—without loss of consciousness
1—with loss of consciousness of 30 minutes or less
2—with loss of consciousness of 31 to 59 minutes
3—with loss of consciousness 1 hour to 5 hours 59 minutes
4—with loss of consciousness of 6 hours to 24 hours
5—with loss of consciousness of greater than 24 hours with return to preexisting conscious level
6—with loss of consciousness of greater than 24 hours without return to preexisting conscious level with patient surviving
7—with loss of consciousness of any duration with death due to brain injury prior to regaining consciousness

8—with loss of consciousness of any duration with death due to other cause prior to regaining consciousness

9—with loss of consciousness of unspecified duration

Category S06, Intracranial injury, includes two instructional notes so that the coder will recognize that a patient with both an intracranial injury with an open wound or with a skull fracture will require two codes:

Code also any associated:
Open wound of head (S01.1-)
Skull fracture (S02.-)

An Excludes1 note appears under category S06: "head injury NOS (S09.90)." If the coder finds the diagnosis of "head injury" without the specificity of an intracranial injury, the coder should access the Alphabetic Index under the main term of "injury, head." The entry of "injury, head" directs the coder to code S09.90. In addition, the Index entry of injury, head, with loss of consciousness provides the code S06.9-. This code identifies the condition as one classified to the intracranial injury category. A loss of consciousness is an indication that an intracranial injury has occurred. Another Index entry for "injury, head, specified type NEC" directs the coder to code S09.8. The diagnosis of "head injury" is a nonspecific description and should only be used if no further detail is provided in the health record documentation. Under code S09.90, Unspecified injury of head, an inclusion term of head injury NOS is provided to explain this is the code to use for the diagnosis of head injury when no further information is provided. The coder is reminded with an Excludes1 note that other specified descriptions of a head injury are coded elsewhere, for example, brain injury (S06.9-), head injury with loss of consciousness (S06.9-), and intracranial injury (S06.9-.) The Excludes1 note means that category S06 codes are not used with code S09.90 for unspecified head injury.

Injury to Internal Organs

ICD-10-CM classifies injuries to internal organs as well. The main term to use in the Alphabetic Index is injury with the subterms for the organ site or a region, for example, "injury, internal" with subterms for the anatomic sites of aorta, bladder, bronchus, cecum, and such. Other entries in the Index are Injury, internal, intra-abdominal, intracranial or intrathoracic for injuries to internal organs within the cavity. The following are examples of categories for injuries to internal organs with their instructional notes:

S26 Injury of heart
Code also any associated:
Open wound of thorax (S21.-)
Traumatic hemopneumothorax (S27.2)
Traumatic hemothorax (S27.1)
Traumatic pneumothorax (S27.0)
S36 Injury of intra-abdominal organs
Code also any associated open wound (S31.-)
S37 Injury to urinary and pelvic organs
Code also any associated open wound (S31.-)

Again, these codes require the use of the seventh characters A, D, or S to identify the encounter of care or the sequela of an injury.

Open Wound and Crush Injury

An **open wound** is an injury of the soft tissue parts associated with rupture of the skin. Open wounds may be animal bites, avulsions, cuts, lacerations, puncture wounds, and traumatic amputation. In addition, an open wound may be a penetrating wound, which involves the passage of an object through tissue that leaves an entrance and exit, as in the case of a knife or gunshot wound.

The seriousness of an open wound depends on its site and extent. If a major vessel or organ is involved, a wound may be life threatening. For example, the rupture of a large artery or vein may cause blood to accumulate in one of the body cavities, which is referred to as hemothorax, hemopericardium, hemoperitoneum, or hemarthrosis, depending on the body cavity involved. The significance of the hemorrhage rests on the volume of the blood loss, the rate of loss, and the site of hemorrhage. Large losses may induce hemorrhagic shock.

Open wounds in ICD-10-CM include such diagnoses as laceration, with and without foreign body; puncture wounds, with or without foreign body; and open bites as well as codes for unspecified open wounds. Animals or humans can cause the bites. The open wounds are classified by site, for example:

S01	Open wound of head
S11	Open wound of neck
S21	Open wound of thorax
S31	Open wound of abdomen, lower back, pelvis and external genitals
S41	Open wound of shoulder and upper arm
S51	Open wound of elbow and forearm
S61	Open wound of wrist, hand and fingers
S71	Open wound of hip and thigh
S81	Open wound of knee and lower leg
S91	Open wound of ankle, foot and toes

Instructional notes appear with the open wound categories to code also any associated injury to nerve, injury to muscle and tendon, intracranial injury, spinal cord injury, or associated wound infection. In addition, there are notes to code any associated injury, such as injury to the heart, intrathoracic organs, rib fractures, and such.

A **crush injury** occurs when a body part if caught or squeezed between two heavy objects usually by a high degree of pressure or force. Crushing injuries cause bruising, bleeding, compartment syndrome, fractures, lacerations, nerve injuries, and wound infections. Compartment syndrome is a serious condition that causes increased pressure in an extremity with serious muscle, tissue, nerve, and blood vessel damage. Crush injuries occur in motor vehicle accidents when a body part is caught for a short period of time, like a finger smashed in a car door to legs being trapped for a period of time between metal or heavy objects before the patient can be extricated from a vehicle. Crushing injuries can occur when part or all of an extremity is pulled into, and compressed by, rollers in a machine, such as those found in industrial plants. Avulsion of skin and fat or a friction burn of the tissues may result. Abrasion burns are often severe, including third degree. Vessels, nerves, and muscles may be avulsed, and bones may be dislocated or fractured. A common complication is secondary congestion, which can lead to paralysis and to severe muscle fibrosis and joint stiffness. Muscle compartments may need decompression, and muscles and ligaments may need to be sectioned. Often the overall circulation of the extremity is of greater concern than definitive management of specific structures. These types of injuries may also be called wringer or compression injuries in addition to crush, crushed, or crushing injuries.

Crushing wounds are classified to the following categories in Chapter 19 of ICD-10-CM:

S07	Crushing injury of head
S17	Crushing injury of neck
S28	Crushing injury of thorax, and traumatic amputation of part of thorax
S38	Crushing injury and traumatic amputation of abdomen, lower back, pelvis and external genitals
S47	Crushing injury of shoulder and upper arm
S57	Crushing injury of elbow and forearm
S67	Crushing injury of wrist, hand, and fingers
S77	Crushing injury of hip and thigh
S87	Crushing injury of lower leg
S97	Crushing injury of ankle and foot

Instructional notes with the categories for crushing injuries remind the coder to use additional codes for all associated injuries such as intracranial or spinal cord injuries, fractures, injury to blood vessels, and open wounds as applicable.

The main terms to be used in the Alphabetic Index are "crush, crushed, crushing," by site or injury, crushing—see Crush. These codes require the use of the seventh characters of A, D, or S to identify the encounter of care or the fact that the crushing injury is the sequel of an injury.

Burns and Corrosions

ICD-10-CM contains codes for burns and corrosions. **Burns** are caused by a heat source such as fire, electricity, radiation, or a hot appliance. **Corrosions** are burns due to a chemical. The same ICD-10-CM coding guidelines apply to both burns and corrosions. Current burns are coded to categories T20–T25 and classified by depth, extent, and by agent or external cause code. Burns of the eye and internal organs are coded by site, T26–T28, but are not classified by degree.

The burns coded by depth are classified as first degree (erythema), second degree (blistering), and third degree (full-thickness) described as follows:

- A **first-degree burn** is the least severe and includes damage to the epidermis or outer layer of skin alone. The burn may also be described as superficial. The skin appears pink to red and painful. There is some edema, but no blisters or eschar. Dead skin may peel away two to three days after the burn.

- A **second-degree burn** involves the epidermis and dermis. There is mild to moderate edema and the burn will blister but there is no eschar. The burn may also be described as either superficial partial thickness or deep partial thickness. Superficial partial thickness burns extend into the upper dermal layer and leave the skin pink to red. Because the nerve endings are exposed, any stimulation causes extreme pain. Deep partial thickness burns extend into the deeper layers of derma, leaving the skin red to pale with moderate edema. Blisters are infrequent but there will be soft, dry eschar. The patient will experience pain but not as severe as in a superficial partial thickness burn because some of the nerve endings have been destroyed.

- A **third-degree burn** is the most severe and includes all three layers of skin: epidermis, dermis, and subcutaneous. A third-degree burn is also known as a full-thickness burn. The skin may appear black, brown, yellow, white, or red. Edema is severe. The burn penetrates the derma and may reach the subcutaneous fat. Pain is minimal because nerve endings are almost completely destroyed. There are no blisters but there is hard eschar.

Burns often exist with other injuries from the same accident. When the reason for the encounter is for treatment of multiple external burns, the site of the burn with the highest degree is coded and sequenced first. Additional codes are used for additional sites with lesser degree burns. When a patient has both an external and internal burn, either type of burn could be coded and sequenced first depending on the circumstances of the admission or encounter. When the patient is admitted with burns and related injuries such as smoke inhalation or organ failure such as respiratory or renal failure, the circumstances of the admission will determine the sequencing of the principal diagnosis.

When a patient has burns of varying degrees on one site (a single category between T20–T28) one code is assigned for the highest degree for that site. If burns exist on multiple sites, multiple separate codes are assigned. The category code T30, Burn and corrosion, body region unspecified, should rarely be used as it is too vague and only appropriate if there is no possibility of getting more information to further specify the burn site.

Complications can exist with burns. If a burn is not healing, it is coded as an acute burn for each encounter in which it is treated. If the condition is described as necrosis of burned skin, it is equivalent to a nonhealing burn. Burns can also become infected. If a burn site is documented as infection, an additional code for the infection is also assigned.

Category T31, Burns classified according to extent of body surface involved, is used as the primary code when the site of the burn is unspecified. This category is used as an additional code with categories T20–T25 when the site is specified. The same rule applies for category T32, Corrosions classified according to extent of body surface involved, which is to be used as an additional code with categories T20–T25 when the site is specified. The use of category T31 can provide valuable data for evaluating burn care and the mortality that unfortunately results from burn injuries. Category T31 will be used as an additional code to report what extent of the body surface is covered and what percent of that body surface is a third-degree burn. For example, a patient that has 20 percent of the body surface burned with 10 percent of that surface covered with a third-degree burn would be coded with T31.21. The main term to locate these codes is "burn" or "corrosion," extent (percentage of body surface) followed by the percentage of third-degree burn.

Burns can cause long-term problems for patients. A patient may have a condition as the result of a healed burn that requires treatment. The condition the patient has for the long term is called the late effect of the sequela of the burn. The burn is healed but the secondary condition remains. Common sequela of burns are scars on the skin or joint contractures. The condition is coded as well as the code for the original burn with the seventh character of S. It is possible for a patient with multiple burns to have a healed burn and a current healing burn existing at the same time, as burns do not heal at the same rate.

An external cause of morbidity code should be used with burns or corrosions to identify the cause of the accident as well as the place where it occurred, information about what the patient was doing at the time of the accident, and their work or nonwork status.

Superficial Injury

Superficial injuries such as abrasions or contusions are not coded when associated with more severe injuries (for example, fracture or open wound) of the same site. The following subsections describe the conditions for coding superficial injuries.

Contusion

Contusions are injuries of the soft tissue. Although the skin is not broken, the small vessels or capillaries are ruptured and the result is bleeding into the tissue. When the blood becomes trapped in the interstitial spaces, the result is a hematoma. ICD-10-CM classifies contusions according to the body site with laterality for right, left, and unspecified site.

Superficial Injury

Superficial injuries include a variety of less serious conditions such as abrasion, blister, external constriction, superficial foreign body, insect bite, and other superficial bite of a specific location. These injuries are coded according to the body site where they exist and according to the specified laterality of the site with codes for right, left, and unspecified side.

The main terms to be used in the Alphabetic Index to locate these injuries are either "injury, superficial" followed by the body part or by the word for the injury, such as abrasion, contusion, or bite, by site and superficial. The appropriate seventh character is used with the superficial injury codes to identify whether the episode of care is the initial encounter (A) or a subsequent encounter (D), or for a sequela (S).

Injury to Blood Vessels, Nerves and Spinal Cord

This subsection describes the conditions for coding injury to blood vessels and the nerves and spinal cord.

When a primary injury results in minor damage to peripheral nerves or blood vessels, the coder must assign a code for the primary injury that is sequenced first with additional code(s) for injuries to nerves, spinal cord, or blood vessels. When the primary or major injury is to the blood vessel or nerve (for example, represented by codes from category S15 or category S04), the code for that injury to the blood vessel or nerve is sequenced first.

Injuries to blood vessels can be a minor laceration that may also be described as an incomplete transection of a vessel or a superficial laceration of a blood vessel. A blood vessel may also have a major laceration that would be a complete transection or traumatic rupture of the blood vessel. Injuries to regions of the spinal cord are classified as to the type of injury, such as complete lesion, central cord syndrome, anterior cord syndrome, Brown-Sequard syndrome, or other incomplete lesions. Injuries to nerves are classified by the specific nerve involved.

Some examples of Alphabetic Index entries for locating injuries to blood vessels, nerves, and spinal cord are as follows:

- Injury, blood vessel, by site, such as abdomen, laceration (S35.91)
- Injury, aorta, abdominal (S35.00)
- Injury, blood vessel, uterine, vein (S35.53-)
- Injury, nerve (by site) such as abducens, followed by the type of injury—contusion, laceration or specified type (S04.4-)
- Injury, nerve, cranial, fifth (trigeminal)—see Injury, nerve, trigeminal (S04.3-)
- Injury, spinal cord, by spinal region and then by level, for example,
  ○ Injury, spinal (cord), cervical, anterior cord syndrome, C1 level (S14.131)
  ○ Injury, spinal (cord), lumbar, complete lesion, L1 level (S34.111)

Each of these injuries requires a seventh character to identify the initial encounter of care (A), subsequent encounter of care (D), or sequel episode (S). Instructional notes appear throughout the chapter with categories for injuries to blood vessels, nerves and spinal cord. Examples of notes include the following:

- Code first any associated intracranial injury
- Code any associated open wound
- Code any associated fracture
- Code any associated transient paralysis

Codes for injuries of the cranial nerves are coded with the selection of the side or laterality based on the side of the body being affected. Codes for spinal cord injuries are coded to the highest level of spinal cord injury.

Traumatic Amputation

A traumatic amputation is another type of injury classified to codes within Chapter 19 of ICD-10-CM. A **traumatic amputation** is the loss of a body part as the result of an accident or injury, with the most common sites being finger, hand, toe, and foot. An amputation not identified as partial or complete is coded as a complete amputation. The categories for amputations of upper and lower extremities are as follows:

S48	Traumatic amputation of shoulder and upper arm
S58	Traumatic amputation of elbow and forearm
S68	Traumatic amputation of wrist, hand and fingers
S78	Traumatic amputation of hip and thigh
S88	Traumatic amputation of lower leg
S98	Traumatic amputation of ankle and foot

Each category requires the use of the appropriate seventh character to identify whether the treatment for the traumatic amputation is the initial encounter (A), a subsequent encounter (D), or is a sequela of the amputation (S). The codes for the traumatic amputations identify whether the right or left extremity is affected with other specificity as to the level of the amputation, such as between hip and knee, at knee level, between knee and ankle, and such.

Effects of Foreign Body Entering through Natural Orifice

The condition created in the body as a result of a foreign body entering through a natural orifice is coded with categories T15–T19. These codes do not include foreign body accidentally left in operative wound (T81.5-), foreign body in penetrating wound (see open wound by body region), residual foreign body in soft tissue (M79.5), or splinter without open wound (see superficial injury by body region).

Categories for the coding of foreign body are body systems, for example, respiratory tract, with fourth, fifth, and sixth character codes to identify the specific body part when the foreign body was located. The sixth character identifies a complication of the presence of the foreign body, for example, causing asphyxiation, compression, or other injury when this can occur based on the anatomic site.

Foreign objects often are found in various body openings in the pediatric population. Children sometimes put small items in their noses or ears or swallow coins or marbles. Foreign bodies also can lodge in the larynx, bronchi, or esophagus, usually during eating. Foreign bodies in the larynx may produce hoarseness, coughing, and gagging, and partially obstruct the airway, causing stridor. A grasping forceps through a direct laryngoscope can remove foreign bodies from the larynx.

Foreign bodies in the bronchi usually produce an initial episode of coughing, followed by an asymptomatic period before obstructive and inflammatory symptoms occur. Foreign bodies are removed from the bronchi through a bronchoscope. Foreign bodies in the esophagus produce immediate symptoms of coughing and gagging, with the sensation of something being "stuck in the throat," as well as causing difficulty in swallowing. Foreign bodies in the esophagus can be removed through an esophagoscope. Intraocular foreign bodies require removal by an ophthalmic surgeon.

These codes can be found in the Alphabetic Index by referencing the main term "Foreign body" and the subterm "entering through orifice." When the foreign body is associated with a laceration, this is located in the Index under "foreign body, in, laceration—see Laceration, by site, with foreign body." A foreign body accidentally left following a procedure is coded according to the type of procedure that was performed. The codes in categories T15–T19 require an appropriate seventh character to be added to indicate whether the episode of care was the initial encounter (A) or a subsequent encounter (D), or a sequela of the foreign body event (S).

Frostbite

Frostbite damages the skin and subcutaneous tissue when the skin is exposed to cold temperatures for a prolonged period of time or extreme cold for a short period of time. Patients with peripheral vascular disease and diabetes are more likely to develop frostbite when exposed to the cold. Symptoms of frostbite include varying sensations at the site, including the feeling of pins and needles followed by numbness, as well as a lack of sensation when the area is touched. The skin may appear hard and pale and after the area thaws, the body surface becomes red and painful. Severe cases of frostbite will have blisters, and damage to tendons, muscles, nerves, and bone. If frostbite affects blood vessels, the damage is likely to be permanent with possible gangrene developing that requires amputation of the affected site. If the blood vessels are not involved, the patient most likely will have a complete recovery. While frostbite can occur when any part of the body is exposed to cold temperatures, the most common sites of frostbite are hands, fingers, feet, toes, nose, and ears.

The injury of frostbite is classified in ICD-10-CM according to whether it is superficial frostbite (T33) or frostbite with tissue necrosis (T34). A superficial frostbite includes partial thickness skin loss. The more severe case of frostbite includes necrosis of tissue at the site where the frostbite occurred. Sites include head, ear, nose, neck, thorax, abdominal wall, arm, wrist, hand, finger, hip, thigh, knee, ankle, foot, and toe. The codes include the laterality of the site as well as an unspecified side. The categories for frostbite require the appropriate seventh character for the initial encounter (A) or a subsequent encounter (D), or for a sequela (S).

ICD-10-PCS Procedure Coding for Treatment of Injuries

Coding Fracture Treatment

The root operations typically used for coding fracture treatment are Reposition, Insertion, and Immobilization.

The definition of **Reposition** is moving to its normal location or other suitable location all or a portion of a body part. The body part is moved from an abnormal location or from a normal location where it is not functioning properly. The object of the procedure is to restore or establish normal function. The most common use of the root operation Reposition is to code a fracture or dislocation reduction. In a fracture reduction the physician moves the bone or bone fragments back into their proper location. For a dislocation reposition, the physician moves a dislocation joint back into the correct position for articulation or movement of the joint. The terminology used by the physician will likely be "reduction" and the coder needs to translate that term to the ICD-10-PCS root operation Reposition. The approach for a reposition procedure may be External or Closed, Percutaneous, Percutaneous Endoscopic, or Open.

The definition of **Insertion** is putting in a nonbiological device that monitors, assists, performs, or prevents a physiological function but does not physically take the place of a body part. In this procedure the sole objective is to put in a device without performing any other procedure. If the insertion of a device is a component of another procedure, the device is included in the device character for that procedure. Examples of an insertion procedure is putting in a pin to hold a nondisplaced fracture to allow it to heal properly or putting in a bone growth stimulator to promote healing of a fracture that is slow to heal.

The definition of **Immobilization** is limiting or preventing motion of a body region. An example of an immobilization procedure is the placement of cast or splint to promote healing of a nondisplaced fracture or a dislocation. The body region for an immobilization procedure for musculoskeletal procedures includes upper and lower extremity, upper and lower arm, upper and lower leg, hand, thumb, finger, foot and toe. The approach is always External. The device used for an immobilization may be a Splint, Cast, Brace, or another device. These devices are pre-made, out of the box items and do not require extensive adjustment or fitting. There is no qualifier used for immobilization procedures.

The reduction or manipulation of a displaced fracture is coded in ICD-10-PCS to the root operation Reposition. The application of a cast or splint with a fracture reduction is not coded separately. A nondisplaced fracture does not require a repositioning. Any treatment of a non-displaced fracture is coded to the procedure performed. For example, if a nondisplaced fracture is treated by putting in a fixation pin, the root operation is Insertion. If the nondisplaced fracture only requires the application of a cast or splint, the root operation is Immobilization.

Coding Repair of Lacerations

Repair is defined in ICD-10-PCS as a root operation to restore, to the extent possible, a body part to its normal anatomical structure and function. Repair is the root operation that is used if no other root operation applies. Repair is essentially the not elsewhere classifiable (NEC) root operation. Repair procedures include a variety of procedures such as suturing lacerations of skin or internal organs and herniorrhaphy that does not include mesh. If a fixation device is used to repair a bone or joint, it is included in the Repair root operation. If a Repair is performed on overlapping layers of the musculoskeletal system, the body part specifying the deepest layer is coded. The repair of skin lacerations is coded to 0HQ with the body part being skin of a specific location, such as skin of the scalp, face, right upper arm, left lower arm, right upper leg, left lower leg, right foot, and such. The approach is always External as the site can be accessed directly. There is no device included in the ICD-10-PCS code for repairs even though sutures remain in the body after the procedure but do not meet the definition of a device.

ICD-10-CM and ICD-10-PCS Review Exercises: Chapter 22A

Assign the correct ICD-10-CM diagnosis codes or ICD-10-PCS procedure to the following exercises.

Chapter 22A will provide practice coding ICD-10-CM Chapter 19 codes. External cause codes will be discussed and coded in Chapter 23. For Chapter 22A, assign only diagnosis and procedure codes, not external cause of morbidity V–Y codes.

1. Foreign body, cornea, right, initial encounter in emergency department

   _____

2. This patient is seen for increased pain in her ankle. She has a displaced trimalleolar fracture of the left ankle. During this subsequent evaluation for her fracture care, she was found to have a nonunion of her left trimalleolar fracture.

   _____

ICD-10-CM and ICD-10-PCS Review Exercises: Chapter 22A (Continued)

3. Displaced, compound comminuted fracture of the right radial shaft. It is a type II open fracture.

_____

4. Patient is a complete paraplegic due to a traumatic L2 vertebral fracture five years ago. At this time, she is experiencing no new problems.

_____

5. This is a follow-up visit for the healing of the patient's partial amputation of the right index finger through the metacarpophalangeal joint.

_____

6. Crushing injury of left hand sustained in an industrial accident when the patient's hand was caught in a piece of machinery. The crushing injury also produced an open fracture of the base of the first metacarpal bone of the left hand at the same time. This is the emergency room initial encounter for care of the injury.

_____

7. The patient was seen in the emergency room for the initial encounter. The patient was playing a high school football game and received a hard tackle by an opponent and complained of acute pain in his right side. Examination and imaging prove there is a small, less than 1 cm, laceration of the right kidney.

_____

8. Patient is seen in her physician's office complaining of acute low back pain. Based on her history of lifting heavy objects during a recent move from one apartment to another and the physical examination performed, the physician diagnosed the patient with an acute sacroiliac joint sprain.

_____

9. Patient came to the physician's office for follow up during the healing phase of the injury to the left index finger, specifically a laceration of the left index finger that was cut with a knife when the patient was preparing dinner one week ago. The physician also diagnosed a laceration to a digital nerve of the left index finger that occurred at the same time as the skin laceration. Both injuries are healing satisfactorily.

_____

10. Laceration of scalp with foreign body, initial encounter for care in emergency department.

_____

11. Patient is seen in the emergency department for treatment of a dislocation of left shoulder joint, specifically the anterior humerus.

_____

12. The patient is seen in the physician's office for a follow-up examination or subsequent visit during the recovery phrase for a sprain of the right lateral collateral ligament of the knee.

_____

ICD-10-CM and ICD-10-PCS Review Exercises: Chapter 22A

13. The patient is seen in the emergency department for the first time for a first- and second-degree burn of the right forearm.

   _____

14. The patient was brought to the emergency department and treated prior to transfer to a trauma center hospital with burns to multiple sites of the leg (lower limb) above the ankle and foot. The burns were diagnosed as first- and second-degree burns.

   _____

15. Gunshot injury, right upper arm producing an open wound with laceration injury to brachial artery and retained foreign body in wound. Initial encounter in emergency department prior to transfer to trauma center hospital.

   _____

16. PROCEDURE: Closed reduction, fracture distal radius, right with cast application

   _____

17. PROCEDURE: Open reduction with internal fixation, right femur shaft

   _____

18. PROCEDURE: Application of left lower arm cast for nondisplaced fracture of ulna

   _____

19. PROCEDURE: Suture laceration repair, laceration of forehead

   _____

20. PROCEDURE: Removal of foreign body, bullet from open wound, right neck muscle by incision

   _____

Chapter 22B

Poisoning and Certain Other Consequences of External Causes (T36–T88)

Learning Objectives

At the conclusion of this chapter, you should be able to:

1. Describe the organization of the conditions and codes included in Chapter 19 of ICD-10-CM, Injury, poisoning, and certain other categories of external causes, with a focus on poisoning and certain other consequences of external causes, categories T36–T88

2. Describe the organization of the ICD-10-CM Table of Drugs and Chemicals and identify which codes are used for which of the following circumstances: poisoning, adverse effect, and underdosing

3. Identify the correct seventh characters required for reporting certain codes in ICD-10-CM

4. Assign ICD-10-CM codes for adverse effects, poisonings, underdosing, and complications of surgical and medical care

5. Assign ICD-10-PCS codes for procedures for adverse effects, poisonings, underdosing, and complications of surgical and medical care

Key Terms

- Adverse effect
- Complications
- Dilation
- Extirpation
- Insertion
- Mechanical complications
- Poisoning
- Removal
- Replacement
- Revision
- Toxic effect

■ Transplant complications
■ Transplantation
■ Underdosing

Overview of Poisoning and Certain Other Consequences of External Causes in ICD-10-CM Chapter 19

Chapter 19 includes categories T36–T88 arranged in the following blocks for poisoning, adverse effect, underdosing, toxic effects, other consequences of external causes, and complications of surgical and medical care, not elsewhere classified:

T36–T50	Poisoning by, adverse effect of and underdosing of drugs, medicaments and biological substances
T51–T65	Toxic effects of substances chiefly nonmedicinal as to source
T66–T78	Other and unspecified effects of external causes
T79	Certain early complications of trauma, not elsewhere classified
T80–T88	Complications of surgical and medical care, not elsewhere classified

This chapter's discussion of Chapter 19 will focus on the poisoning and certain other consequences of external cause codes.

ICD-10-CM does not provide different category codes to identify poisonings versus adverse effect. Instead, under a single category for a specific drug, there is one code for each drug to identify poisoning, adverse effects, and underdosing by the drug (T36–T50). The sixth character of the code generally identifies the condition resulting from the use of the drug. The poisoning codes include the intent of the poisoning, if known, such as accidental, intentional self-harm, or assault as well as a code for undetermined when the facts are not known.

Underdosing is a term in ICD-10-CM defined as taking less of a medication than is prescribed by a provider or the manufacturer's instructions with a resulting negative health consequence. As a consequence, the patient suffers a negative health consequence, such as a worsening of the condition intended to be treated by the medication.

> **EXAMPLE:**   T46.1   Poisoning by, adverse effect of, and underdosing of calcium-channel blockers
>
> T46.1x1 Poisoning by calcium-channel blocker, accidental (unintentional)
>
> T46.1x2 Poisoning by calcium-channel blocker, intentional self-harm
>
> T46.1x3 Poisoning by calcium-channel blocker, assault

T46.1x4 Poisoning by calcium-channel blocker, undetermined

T46.1x5 Adverse effect of calcium-channel blocker

T46.1x6 Underdosing of calcium-channel blocker

Coding Guidelines and Instructional Notes for Chapter 19

A note at the start of the chapter states "Use secondary code(s) from Chapter 20, External causes of morbidity, to indicate cause of injury. Codes within the T section that include the external cause do not require an additional external cause code."

Under the block of codes T36–T50, Poisoning by, adverse effects of and underdosing of drugs, medicaments and biological substances, there is an Includes note that states the block of codes includes:

Adverse effect of correct substance properly administered

Poisoning by overdose of substance

Poisoning by wrong substance given or taken in error

Underdosing by (inadvertently)(deliberately) taking less substance than prescribed or instructed

Other instructions appear under the section heading for T36–T50 such as code first notes, directions, and use additional code notes.

1. Code first, for adverse effects, the nature of the adverse effect, such as:
   Adverse effect NOS (T88.7)
   Aspirin gastritis (K29-)
   Blood disorders (D56-D76)
   Contact dermatitis (L23–L25)
   Dermatitis due to substance taken internally (L27-)
   Nephropathy (N14.0–N14.2)

2. Note: The drug giving rise to the adverse effect should be identified by use of codes from categories T36–T50 with fifth or sixth character 5.

3. Use additional code(s) to specify:
   Manifestations of poisoning
   Underdosing or failure in dosage during medical and surgical care (Y63.6, Y63.8–Y63.9)
   Underdosing of medication regimen (Z91.12-, Z91.13-)

In ICD-10-CM a note is included stating to use an additional code (Y62–Y82) to identify devices involved and details of circumstances.

The NCHS has published chapter-specific guidelines for Chapter 19 in the *ICD-10-CM Official Guidelines for Coding and Reporting*. The coding student should review all of the coding guidelines for Chapter 19 of ICD-10-CM, which appear in an ICD-10-CM code book or at the website http://www.cdc.gov/nchs/icd/icd10cm.htm, or in Appendix E.

CG

Guideline I.C.19.e. Adverse Effects, Poisoning, Underdosing and Toxic Effects: Codes in categories T36–T65 are combination codes that include the substance that was taken as well as the intent. No additional external cause code is required for poisonings, toxic effects, adverse effects and underdosing codes.

Guideline I.C.19.e.1. Do not code directly from the Table of Drugs: Do not code directly from the Table of Drugs and Chemicals. Always refer back to the Tabular List.

Guideline I.C.19.e.2. Use as many codes as necessary to describe: Use as many codes as necessary to describe completely all drugs, medicinal or biological substances.

Guideline I.C.19.e.3. If the same code would describe the causative agent: If the same code would describe the causative agent for more than one adverse reaction, poisoning, toxic effect or underdosing, assign the code only once.

Guideline I.C.19.e.4. If two or more drugs, medicinal or biological substances: If two or more drugs, medicinal or biological substances are reported, code each individually unless a combination code is listed in the Table of Drugs and Chemicals.

Guideline I.C.19.e.5. The occurrence of drug toxicity is classified in ICD-10-CM as follows:

Guideline I.C.19.e.5(a). Adverse Effect: When coding an adverse effect of a drug that has been correctly prescribed and properly administered, assign the appropriate code for the nature of the adverse effect followed by the appropriate code for the adverse effect of the drug (T36–T50). The code for the drug should have a 5th or 6th character "5" (for example T36.0X5-) Examples of the nature of an adverse effect are tachycardia, delirium, gastrointestinal hemorrhaging, vomiting, hypokalemia, hepatitis, renal failure, or respiratory failure.

Guideline I.C.19.e.5(b). Poisoning: When coding a poisoning or reaction to the improper use of a medication (e.g., overdose, wrong substance given or taken in error, wrong route of administration), first assign the appropriate code from categories T36–T50. The poisoning codes have an associated intent as their 5th or 6th character (accidental, intentional self-harm, assault and undetermined.) Use additional code(s) for all manifestations of poisonings.

If there is also a diagnosis of abuse or dependence of the substance, the abuse or dependence is assigned as an additional code.

Examples of poisoning include:

i. Error was made in drug prescription

Errors made in drug prescription or in the administration of the drug by provider, nurse, patient, or other person.

ii. Overdose of a drug intentionally taken

If an overdose of a drug was intentionally taken or administered and resulted in drug toxicity, it would be coded as a poisoning.

iii. Nonprescribed drug taken with correctly prescribed and properly administered drug

If a nonprescribed drug or medicinal agent was taken in combination with a correctly prescribed and properly administered drug, any drug toxicity or other reaction resulting from the interaction of the two drugs would be classified as a poisoning.

iv. Interaction of drug(s) and alcohol

When a reaction results from the interaction of a drug(s) and alcohol, this would be classified as poisoning.

See Section I.C.4. if poisoning is the result of insulin pump malfunctions.

Guideline I.C.19.e.5(c). Underdosing: Underdosing refers to taking less of a medication than is prescribed by a provider or a manufacturer's instruction. For underdosing, assign the code from categories T36–T50 (fifth or sixth character "6").

Codes for underdosing should never be assigned as principal or first-listed codes. If a patient has a relapse or exacerbation of the medical condition for which the drug is prescribed because of the reduction in dose, then the medical condition itself should be coded.

Noncompliance (Z91.12-, Z91.13-) or complication of care (Y63.8–Y63.9) codes are to be used with an underdosing code to indicate intent, if known.

Guideline I.C.19.e.5(d). Toxic Effects: When a harmful substance is ingested or comes in contact with a person, this is classified as a toxic effect. The toxic effect codes are in categories T51–T65.

Toxic effect codes have an associated intent: accidental, intentional self-harm, assault and undetermined.

I.C.19.f. Adult and child abuse, neglect and other maltreatment: Sequence first the appropriate code from categories T74.- (Adult and child abuse, neglect and other maltreatment, confirmed) or T76.- (Adult and child abuse, neglect and other maltreatment,

(Continued)

(Continued)

suspected) for abuse, neglect and other maltreatment, followed by any accompanying mental health or injury code(s).

If the documentation in the medical record states abuse or neglect it is coded as confirmed (T74.-). It is coded as suspected if it is documented as suspected (T76.-).

For cases of confirmed abuse or neglect an external cause code from the assault section (X92–Y08) should be added to identify the cause of any physical injuries. A perpetrator code (Y07) should be added when the perpetrator of the abuse is known. For suspected cases of abuse or neglect, do not report external cause or perpetrator code.

If a suspected case of abuse, neglect or mistreatment is ruled out during an encounter code Z04.71, Encounter for examination and observation following alleged physical adult abuse, ruled out, or code Z04.72, Encounter for examination and observation following alleged child physical abuse, ruled out, should be used, not a code from T76.

If a suspected case of alleged rape or sexual abuse is ruled out during an encounter code Z04.41, Encounter for examination and observation following alleged physical adult abuse, ruled out, or code Z04.42, Encounter for examination and observation following alleged rape or sexual abuse, ruled out, should be used, not a code from T76.

See Section I.C.15. Abuse in a pregnant patient.

Guideline I.C.19.g. Complications of care

Guideline I.C.19.g.1. General guidelines for complications of care

a. Documentation of complications of care

See Section I.B.16. for information on documentation of complications of care.

Guideline I.C.19.g.2. Pain due to medical devices: Pain associated with devices, implants or grafts left in a surgical site (for example painful hip prosthesis) is assigned to the appropriate code(s) found in Chapter 19, Injury, poisoning, and certain other consequences of external causes. Specific codes for pain due to medical devices are found in the T code section of the ICD-10-CM. Use additional code(s) from category G89 to identify acute or chronic pain due to presence of the device, implant or graft (G89.18 or G89.28).

Guideline I.C.19.g.3. Transplant complications

Guideline I.C.19.g.3(a). Transplant complications other than kidney: Codes under category T86, Complications of transplanted organs and tissues, are for use for both complications and rejection of transplanted organs. A transplant complication code is only assigned if the complication affects the function of the transplanted organ. Two codes are required to fully describe a transplant complication: the appropriate code from category T86 and a secondary code that identifies the complication.

Pre-existing conditions or conditions that develop after the transplant are not coded as complications unless they affect the function of the transplanted organs.

See I.C.21. for transplant organ removal status

See I.C.2. for malignant neoplasm associated with transplanted organ.

Guideline I.C.19.g.3(b). Kidney transplant complications: Patients who have undergone kidney transplant may still have some form of chronic kidney disease (CKD) because the kidney transplant may not fully restore kidney function. Code T86.1- should be assigned for documented complications of a kidney transplant, such as transplant failure or rejection or other transplant complication. Code T86.1- should not be assigned for post kidney transplant patients who have chronic kidney (CKD) unless a transplant complication such as transplant failure or rejection is documented. If the documentation is unclear as to whether the patient has a complication of the transplant, query the provider.

Conditions that affect the function of the transplanted kidney, other than CKD, should be assigned a code from subcategory T86.1, Complications of transplanted organ, Kidney, and a secondary code that identifies the complication.

For patients with CKD following a kidney transplant, but who do not have a complication such as failure or rejection, *see section I.C.14. Chronic kidney disease and kidney transplant status.*

Guideline I.C.19.g.4. Complication codes that include the external cause: As with certain other T codes, some of the complications of care codes have the external cause included in the code. The code includes the nature of the complication as well as the type of procedure that caused the complication. No external cause code indicating the type of procedure is necessary for these codes.

Guideline I.C.19.g.5. Complications of care codes within the body system chapters: Intraoperative and postprocedural complication codes are found within the body system chapters with codes specific to the organs and structures of that body system. These codes should be sequenced first, followed by a code(s) for the specific complication, if applicable.

Coding Poisoning, Adverse Effects, Underdosing, and Certain Consequences of External Causes in ICD-10-CM Chapter 19

The coding of poisoning, adverse effect and underdosing of drugs is discussed in this section.

Alphabetic Index

The ICD-10-CM Alphabetic Index provides direction on how to code medical conditions caused by drugs used appropriately and inappropriately by a patient and causing a medical condition. Using the main term "Adverse effect" the coder is directed to see Table of Drugs and Chemicals, categories T36–T50, with the sixth character of S. The main term "Poisoning" or "Poisoning, drug" in the Index directs the coder to see also Table of Drugs and Chemicals. The third entry for underdosing states, "see also Table of Drugs and Chemicals, categories T36–T50, with final character of 6." The Table of Drugs and Chemicals follows the ICD-10-CM Neoplasm Table that appears after the ICD-10-CM Index to Diseases and Injuries.

Table of Drugs and Chemicals

The ICD-10-CM Table of Drugs and Chemicals is organized into seven columns with rows for the substances involved. The first, left-most column contains the name of the drug, chemical, or biologic substance. The next six columns contain ICD-10-CM codes for the following:

- Poisoning, accidental (nonintentional)
- Poisoning, intentional self-harm
- Poisoning, assault
- Poisoning, undetermined
- Adverse effect
- Underdosing

Not every row with a chemical name has a code in each of the six columns. This is because certain chemicals cannot produce an adverse effect or an underdosing because the substance is never used for therapeutic purposes. Codes that are found on the Table of Drugs and Chemicals are in the range of codes from T36–T50. These are combination codes that include the substance that was taken by the patient, appropriately or inappropriately, and describe the intent as well. For example, the codes differentiate between poisonings that are accidental, intentional, assault, or are of an undetermined nature. For this reason, there is no need for an additional external cause of morbidity code for poisonings, adverse effects, and underdosing codes.

Adverse Effects of Drugs

An **adverse effect** can occur in situations in which medication is prescribed correctly and administered properly in both therapeutic and diagnostic procedures. An adverse effect can occur when everything is done right—right drug, right dose, right patient receiving it, right route of administration—but a physical reaction is experienced. Common causes of adverse effects are as follows:

- Cumulative effects result when the inactivation or excretion of the drug is slower than the rate at which the drug is being administered. This is often documented as drug toxicity of a prescribed drug in the health record.

- Hypersensitivity or allergic reaction is a qualitatively different response to a drug acquired only after re-exposure to the drug.

- Synergistic reaction is enhancing the effect of a prior or concurrent administration of another drug.

- The effectiveness of a drug may change as the result of interaction with another pre-scribed medication.

- Side effects are the unwanted predictable pharmacologic effects that occur within therapeutic code ranges.

Instructions for Coding Adverse Effects

The following instructions apply when coding adverse effects:

1. Code first the manifestation or the nature of the adverse effects, such as urticaria, vertigo, gastritis, and so forth.

2. Locate the drug responsible for the adverse effect in the "Substance" column of the Table of Drugs and Chemicals in the Alphabetic Index to Diseases.

3. Assign the appropriate seventh character to the drug or chemical code to identify whether the healthcare was provided during the initial encounter, a subsequent encounter, or for a sequela.

4. If more than one drug or chemical is involved, the coder should use as many codes as necessary from the Table of Drugs and Chemicals to completely describe all the drugs or chemicals involved.

5. If the same drug produced more than one manifestation or adverse effect, the coder should assign the drug code only once.

6. If two or more drugs or chemicals are involved, each drug or chemical should be coded separately unless there is a combination code included in the Table of Drugs and Chemicals.

> **EXAMPLE:** Initial encounter to treat atrial tachycardia due to digitalis glycosides: I47.1, Supraventricular tachycardia; T46.0X5A, Adverse effect of cardiac-stimulant glycosides and drugs of similar action

7. If the patient has a current condition that is the late effect or sequela of an adverse effect of a correct substance properly administered, it is coded as follows:

- First code the residual or late effect, such as blindness or deafness.

- Assign the code for the drug that produced the adverse effect with the seventh character of S for sequela.

> **EXAMPLE:** Deafness in the right ear occurring as a result of previously administered streptomycin therapy: H91.91, Unspecified hearing loss, right ear; T36.5X5S, Adverse effect of aminoglycosides, sequela

See figure 22B.1 for assistance in coding adverse reactions to correct substances properly administered.

Figure 22B.1. **Coding adverse reactions to correct substances properly administered**

Current Condition		Sequela
Code effect: Coma, vertigo, and such	← Principal or First-Listed Diagnosis →	Code effect: Deafness, blindness, and such
And		**And**
Adverse effect of drug code from Table of Drugs and Chemicals with the fifth or sixth character 5 with the seventh character of A or D for initial or subsequent encounter	← Other Diagnosis →	Adverse effect of drug code from Table of Drugs and Chemicals with the fifth or sixth character 5 with the seventh character of S for sequela

Poisonings

Poisoning refers to conditions caused by drugs, medicinal substances, and other biological substances only when the substance involved is not used according to a physician's instructions. A poisoning occurs when something is done wrong—wrong drug, wrong dose, wrong route of administration, wrong person receiving the drug, or the drug should not have been used. A poisoning can occur with prescription drugs, over-the-counter purchased medications, illegal drugs, or when drugs are taken with alcohol beverages. Poisonings can occur in the following ways:

- There is an error made in the drug prescription. This includes errors made in drug prescription or in the administration of the drug by the provider, the nurse, the patient, or another person.

- An overdose of a drug is intentionally taken. If an overdose of a drug was intentionally taken or administered and resulted in drug toxicity, the situation would be classified as a poisoning.

- A nonprescribed drug is taken with a correctly prescribed and properly administered drug. If the nonprescribed drug or medicinal agent was taken in combination with a correctly prescribed and properly administered drug, any drug toxicity or other reaction resulting from the interaction of these two drugs would be classified as a poisoning.

- A drug is taken with alcohol. When a patient has a medical condition or reaction produced from the interaction of a drug or drugs and alcohol, the condition would be classified as a poisoning.

Instructions for Coding Poisonings

The following instructions apply when coding poisonings:

1. Use the Table of Drugs and Chemicals in the Alphabetic Index to Diseases to locate the drug or other agent.

2. Code first the code from the "Poisoning" column depending on the associated intent with the fifth or sixth character identifying it as accidental, intentional self-harm, assault, and undetermined.

3. Next code all the specified manifestation or effect of the poisoning, such as coma, vertigo, drowsiness, that might be experienced.

4. If there is also a diagnosis of drug abuse or dependence to the drug, the abuse or dependence is coded as an additional diagnosis.

    EXAMPLE: Overdosed on aspirin, suicide attempt, initial episode of care: T39.012A, Poisoning by aspirin, intentional self-harm, initial episode of care

5. If the patient has a current condition that is the late effect or sequela of an adverse effect of a poisoning or overdose, it is coded as follows:

    *   First code the residual condition or late effect, such as organ or nerve damage.

    *   Assign the code for the drug that produced the poisoning with the seventh character of S for sequela.

    EXAMPLE: Anoxic brain damage as a result of previously narcotic intentional overdose: G93.1, Anoxic brain damage, not elsewhere classified; T40.602S, Poisoning by unspecified narcotics, intentional self-harm, sequela

See figure 22B.2 for assistance in coding poisonings.

Figure 22B.2.   **Coding poisonings**

Current Injury		Sequela
Code from T36–T50 with fifth or sixth character for the associated intent (accidental, intentional self-harm, assault, or undetermined) with the seventh character for initial or subsequent encounter	← Principal or First-Listed Diagnosis →	Code for the residual condition first that is currently present
Plus		*Plus*
Specified effect— tachy-cardia, coma	← Other Diagnosis →	Code from T36–T50 with fifth or sixth character for the associated intent, accidental, intentional self-harm, assault or unde-termined with the seventh character for sequela

Underdosing

The concept of underdosing in ICD-10-CM refers to the situation when a patient takes less of a medication than is prescribed by the provider or a manufacturer's instruction. For this situation, the code from T36–T50 for the drug is assigned with the fifth or sixth character of 6. The code for the drug that was underdosed is never listed first or as the principal diagnosis. If the patient has a worsening of the medical condition that is being treated by the drug, then the medical condition is coded first. Noncompliance codes (Z91.12- or Z91.13-) or complication of care (Y63.6, Y63.8–Y63.9) codes are used with the underdosing code to intent if it is known.

> **EXAMPLE:** Hyperglycemia with type 2 diabetes as a result of the patient not taking his oral antidiabetic agents. The patient stated he cannot afford his prescriptions so he has not been taking his medications every day in order to make his prescription last longer: E11.65, Type 2 diabetes with hyperglycemia; T38.3x6A, Underdosing of insulin or oral hypoglycemic [antidiabetic] drugs, initial encounter; Z91.120, Patient's intentional underdosing of medication regimen due to financial hardship

Toxic Effects

A patient may come in contact with or ingest, accidentally or otherwise, a harmful substance that would be classified in ICD-10-CM as a **toxic effect**. The toxic effect code is included in categories T51–T65 and include the associated intent of accidental, intentional self-harm, assault, or undetermined. A note appears under the block of codes T51–T65 for toxic effects of substances chiefly nonmedicinal as to source that a code for accidental intent should be used if no intent is indicated. The undetermined intent is only for use when there is specific documentation in the record that the intent of the toxic effect cannot be determined.

> **EXAMPLE**: The patient came in contact with chloroform in the industrial plant where he worked and was brought to the emergency department with severe shortness of breath. This was the initial episode of care. T53.1X1A, Toxic effect of chloroform, accidental, initial encounter; R06.02, Shortness of breath.

Other and Unspecified Effects of External Cause (T66–T78)

The diagnoses represented by this block of codes represent injuries and conditions that are caused by an external agent, such as radiation, heat, light, cold, air, and water pressure as an example. The codes require the use of the appropriate seventh character to identify the episode of care, that is, the initial encounter (A), a subsequent encounter (D), or if the event represents a sequela (S).

Asphyxiation (T71)

Specific codes are provided to identify when a condition of asphyxiation is being treated. The diagnosis for this situation may also be described by the provider as a traumatic or mechanical suffocation. These are combination codes that identify the state of asphyxiation as well as the cause of it. For example, asphyxiation can be caused by smothering under a pillow, a plastic bag placed over the head, being trapped in bed linens, or smothering in furniture. Other external events that can cause asphyxiation are accidental or intentional hanging, being trapped in a car trunk, a cave-in, or otherwise being caught in a low-oxygen environment. The codes in this category require a seventh character to identify whether the care is provided in the initial encounter, a subsequent encounter, or as a sequela.

Adult and Child Abuse, Neglect and Other Maltreatment, Confirmed (T74) and Suspected (T76)

When an adult or child is treated for confirmed or suspected abuse, neglect, or other maltreatment, the appropriate code from categories T74 (Adult and child abuse, neglect and other maltreatment, confirmed) or T76 (Adult and child abuse, neglect and other maltreatment, suspected) is assigned as the principal or first-listed diagnosis code. Any injury or mental health condition that occurs as a result of the abuse, neglect, or maltreatment is coded as an additional diagnosis. The coder must examine the record for the provider's conclusion as to whether the abuse has been confirmed at the end of the encounter or is still suspected and unconfirmed. If the provider documents the patient's situation as abuse or neglect, it is coded as confirmed with category T74. If the documentation states the abuse or neglect is suspected, it is coded as suspected with category T76. A perpetrator code from category Y07 is added when the perpetrator of the abuse or neglect is known. If the patient's abuse or neglect is suspected, no code is assigned for the perpetrator identification.

Complications of Surgical and Medical Care, Not Elsewhere Classified (T80–T88)

Codes for intraoperative and postprocedureal complications and disorders are provided in specific body system chapters throughout ICD-10-CM, for example code N99.0, Postprocedural (acute)(chronic) kidney failure. These chapter specific codes are sequenced first when coding the condition but an additional code should be assigned for the specific complication, if applicable.

Specific **complications** are identified in this block of codes to represent all types of conditions that are unwanted but may not be entirely unavoidable in medical care. The coding guidelines direct the coder that the documentation of complications of care must be specific. The assignment of a complications code must be based on the provider's documentation and the fact that the provider has made a connection between the condition and the medical care or procedure that apparently caused it. As stated in the guidelines, not every condition that develops following medical care or a surgical procedure should be coded as a complication. The provider must indicate the condition is a complication and was caused by the care provided. It is the coder's responsibility to query the physician for this relationship if the documentation is not specific as to the cause of the condition the patient exhibits after medical care or a procedure has been provided.

Some of the complication codes in this chapter have the external cause as well as the condition included in the code. No external cause code is required when the code includes the nature of the complication as well as the type of procedure that caused the complication.

The conditions identified in this block of codes, T80–T88, identify complications of surgical and medical care that are not specific to a particular body system. A seventh character is required for these category codes to identify if the condition was treated in an initial encounter, subsequent encounter, or represents a sequela.

Three directional notes appear under the heading for these codes to remind the coder of the following:

1. Use additional code for adverse effect, if applicable, to identify drug (T36–T50) with fifth or sixth character of 5.

2. Use additional code(s) to identify the specified condition resulting from the complication.

3. Use additional code to identify devices involved and details of circumstances (Y62–Y83).

Complications of Procedures, Not Elsewhere Classified (T81)

Codes within this category include postprocedural shock, disruption of operative or surgical wound, infection following a procedure, complications of a foreign body accidentally left in the body following a procedure, acute reaction to foreign substance accidentally left during a procedure, and not elsewhere classified vascular complications.

Directional notes remind the coder to use an additional code for an adverse effect, if applicable, to identify a responsible drug from categories T36–T50 with a fifth or sixth character of 5. When a patient is diagnosed with an infection following a procedure, the coder should use an additional code to identify the infection by type or organism as well as use an additional code if the infection advances to severe sepsis. If the code is not specific, a use additional code note appears to remind the coder to specify the complication with an additional code.

Complications of Prosthetic Devices, Implants and Grafts (T82–T85)

Subcategory codes T82.0- to T82.5- identify **mechanical complications** of specific cardiac and vascular prosthetic devices, implants and grafts. Complications include the mechanical breakdown, displacement, leakage, or other mechanical complication of the device, implant, or graft. The types of devices identified in these codes are heart valves, cardiac electronic devices, coronary artery bypass grafts, other vascular grafts, vascular dialysis catheters, and surgically created arteriovenous fistula.

Subcategory codes T82.6–T82.7 identify an infection or inflammatory reaction to a specific cardiac and vascular prosthetic device, implant, or graft. Both of these subcategory codes would have an additional code to identify the infection if the documentation is provided. Subcategory codes T82.8–T82.9 identify other specified complications due to the presence of these devices. These complications include embolism, fibrosis, hemorrhage, pain, stenosis, thrombosis, or other specified condition that is due to the cardiac or vascular prosthetic device, implant, or graft.

Similar codes appear for complications of prosthetic devices, implants, and grafts in other body systems, for example, in category T83 for genitourinary devices, T84 for orthopedic devices, and T85 for other internal prosthetic devices, implants, and grafts. These codes also have subcategories including mechanical complications, infections, and inflammations as a result of the device and other specific conditions such as embolism, fibrosis, hemorrhage, pain, and such. All the codes in categories T82–T85 require the use of the seventh character to identify the initial or subsequent encounter or the sequela situation.

Complications of Transplanted Organs and Tissues (T86)

Three "use additional code" notes appear under the category heading for complications of transplanted organs and tissues. The notes remind the coder to use an additional code to identify other **transplant complications** such as graft-versus-host disease, malignancy associated with organ transplant, and post-transplant lymphoproliferative disorders.

It is important to note that patients may still have some form of chronic kidney disease after they have had a kidney transplant. The kidney transplant may not restore the kidney function completely. Code T86.1- should be assigned for a documented complication of a kidney transplant such as transplant failure or rejection. Chronic kidney disease in a kidney transplant patient is not assigned as a complication code unless the condition is documented as a complication. If the documentation is not clearly stated, the coder is obligated to ask the provider for clarification. Patients may have another condition that affects the function of the transplanted kidney. When a provider documents that another condition affects the transplanted kidney, a code from subcategory T86.1, Complications of kidney transplant, is assigned with an additional code for the specific complication.

Specific codes exist in category T86 for transplant rejection, failure, or infection for various types of organs and tissues that have been transplanted, for example, bone marrow, heart, lung, liver, skin, bone, corneal, intestine, and other transplanted tissue.

Complications Peculiar to Reattachment and Amputation (T87)

Specific codes are provided in this category to identify when there are complications related to a reattached (part of the) upper extremity, lower extremity, or other body part specified as right, left, or unspecified side. Other subcategory codes identify when there is a complication of an amputation stump, specifically a neuroma, infection, necrosis, or other specified and unspecified complication.

Other Complications of Surgical and Medical Care, Not Elsewhere Classified (T88)

The final category in Chapter 19 of ICD-10-CM contains less frequently occurring complications of surgical and medical care. Codes related to complications of anesthesia, such as shock, malignant hyperthermia, and other complications require the use of an additional code for the drug responsible for an adverse effect if it was applicable to this patient. The serious emergency of an anaphylactic reaction or shock due to an adverse effect of a drug is classified with code T88.6xx with the seventh character identifying the episode of care. The drug responsible for the adverse effect is identified with an additional code. If the specific adverse effect of a drug cannot be identified, the subcategory code T88.7xx is used with the seventh character to identify the episode of care. This code is used when the provider can only identify the condition as a "drug reaction" or "drug hypersensitivity."

ICD-10-PCS Procedure Coding for Poisoning and Certain Other Consequences of External Causes

There is no particular group of procedures that relate to coding of conditions addressed in this chapter. Surgical procedures are more commonly performed to treat complications of medical and surgical care. While any of the 31 root operations could be the objective of a procedure, there are a few root operations that should be addressed in this chapter.

One of the four root operations that involve procedures to alter the diameter or route of a tubular body part is **Dilation**. Solids, liquids, or gases pass through tubular body parts. These body parts are part of the circulatory system, digestive system, genitourinary, and respiratory system. Sometimes these tubular body parts become narrow or stenotic and can create problems as the solids, liquids, or gases cannot pass through it. The root operation Dilation is to expand the orifice or the lumen of the tubular body part to open it or make it larger. The dilation can be accomplished by intraluminal pressure to stretch the inner part of the tube as well as extraluminal methods to widen it. The objective of a Dilation procedure is to expand the tubular body part. It is also possible that dilation may be an approach for another procedure to achieve its objective, for example, dilation and curettage where the objective is to remove the lining of the uterus, that is, an extraction procedure. An example of a Dilation procedure is an angioplasty of a coronary or noncoronary vessel. A device can be used to perform the Dilation, such as a balloon catheter, and other devices can be left in place in the vessel to maintain the opening of the vessel, such as a stent or intraluminal device. Only a device left in place at the end of the procedure is considered in the sixth character of an ICD-10-PCS code.

An **Extirpation** procedure takes out or cuts out a solid matter from a body part. The solid matter may be a foreign body, such as piece of metal, or it may be a byproduct of a biological function, for example, a blood clot or a plaque deposit in a blood vessel. The medical term of "extirpation" is not commonly used in health record documentation. Instead the coder should trust the Alphabetic Index of ICD-10-PCS when the title of an operation, such as thrombectomy, directs the coder to the code tables for Extirpation. The removal of foreign objects from the body will also be coded as Extirpation procedures. The coder must realize that the likely procedure title of "removal" of a foreign body would not be the root operation when the objective of the procedure is to take a solid matter like a foreign body. A removal procedure in ICD-10-PCS always involves removing a device and a foreign body is not a device.

Other procedures that are often required to treat complications of disease all involve devices. These root operations are Insertion, Replacement, Removal, Revision, Supplement, and Change. Each of these procedures put in a device, remove a device, correct a device, or exchange a device. The root operation **Insertion** has the objective of putting in a nonbiological device that monitors, assists, performs, or prevents a physiological function but does not physically take the place of a body part. Commonly inserted devices include a central venous catheter for infusion or a cardiac pacemaker or cardioverter defibrillator. In a **Replacement** procedure, the original body part may be taken out before the Replacement is performed. The removal of the original body part is included in the Replacement procedure. However, if the Replacement is a repeat of a previous procedure, removing the device placed during the previous procedure is coded separately as a Removal. Examples of musculoskeletal Replacement procedures are joint replacements such as hips, knees, or shoulders. A **Removal** procedure takes out or off a device from any body part and does not involve putting in another device. Usually the patient's condition no longer requires the device to remain in place for therapy when a Removal procedure is performed. The removal of an infusion device, drainage device, internal fixation, or joint prosthetic device is an example of this root operation. A **Revision** procedure is the correction of a malfunctioning or displace device to the extent possible. The objective of a Revision procedure is to fix a device that remains in place at the end of the procedure. If the device is removed during the procedure, it is not a Revision. However, a part of the device may be taken out or put back in as part of a Revision procedure. Examples of Revision procedures are adjustment to catheters, cardiac devices, joint prostheses, or internal fixator.

Finally, a transplant procedure may be performed to treat complications of diseases. A **Transplantation** is putting in the body a portion or all of a living body part. The body part may be taken from another human or from an animal. The transplanted organ takes the place and function of the entire body part or a portion of the body part that is being replaced. The commonly replaced body parts are kidney, liver, heart, and lung. The seventh character for the root operation Transplantation identifies the type of transplant that is performed, that is, allogeneic, syngeneic, or zooplastic. An allogeneic transplant is an organ taken from different individuals of the same species or another human. A syngeneic transplant is an organ taken from an individual that has identical genetic composition as the recipient, such as an identical twin. A zooplastic transplant is an organ or tissue taken from an animal and place in a human. Some procedures that are commonly referred to as transplants are not coded with this root operation. For example, there is no code available for a corneal transplant, because the procedure performed in a corneal transplant does not involve a body part by ICD-10-PCS definition. In a corneal transplant a layer of tissue is placed in a body part. A corneal transplant is a replacement procedure by ICD-10-PCS definition. Other procedures also called transplants are bone marrow, stem cell, and pancreatic islet cell transplantations. These procedures are not coded to transplant either. Instead these procedures are coded to the root operation Administration because these procedures involve putting in autologous or nonautologous cells instead of organs or body parts.

ICD-10-CM and ICD-10-PCS Coding Exercises: Chapter 22B

Assign the correct ICD-10-CM diagnosis codes or ICD-10-PCS procedure codes to the following exercises (do not assign external cause codes).

1. Child is seen emergently for an accidental overdose of acetaminophen. He inadvertently ate several of these when he found an open bottle at home.

2. A patient has been taking Digoxin and is experiencing nausea and vomiting and profound fatigue. The patient indicates that he has been taking the drug appropriately. The evaluation and treatment was focused on adjustment of medication only.

3. This patient is seen in the hospital with a diagnosis of congestive heart failure due to hypertensive heart disease. Patient also has stage 5 chronic kidney failure. The patient had been prescribed Lasix previously but admits that he forgets to take his medication every day. This is due to his advanced age. What are the correct diagnosis codes?

(Continued on next page)

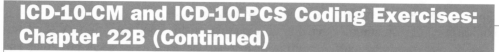

ICD-10-CM and ICD-10-PCS Coding Exercises: Chapter 22B (Continued)

4. The patient was in the Cardiac Cath Lab for insertion of a dual chamber pacemaker to treat his sick sinus syndrome. During the procedure the pacemaker electrode broke upon insertion. The procedure was abandoned and will be rescheduled.

   _____

5. The patient was seen in the emergency room complaining of right hip pain after falling at home. She stated that she had her right hip replaced six weeks ago and was walking fine before this fall. X-rays show the right hip prosthesis was dislocated. The patient was admitted for care by her orthopedic surgeon for possible surgery if a closed reduction is not successful.

   _____

6. A college-age male was brought to the emergency department by ambulance called by his friends after they were unable to wake him this morning. The patient now responds to commands but is very drowsy. Based on the history provided by friends that the patient was drinking heavily last night and was seen taking a couple of pills that were later determined to be naproxen because the patient said he had a headache. After receiving IV fluids and being placed on telemetry the patient became more alert and confirmed the history told by his friends. The ER physician discharged the patient with the final diagnosis of drowsiness due to the interaction of alcohol and naproxen.

   _____

7. The patient is seen in his internal medicine physician's office for the second time complaining of dizziness. This is a follow-up visit for both the patient's hypertension that was recently diagnosed and the dizziness he is experiencing. The patient stated he feels dizzier than his last visit and the dizziness started after he started taking his new antihypertensive medication, atenolol. The physician orders new antihypertensive medications to hopefully relieve the patient's side effect from the atenolol.

   _____

8. The patient is a 2-year-old female who had a heart transplant in the past year and was admitted to the hospital and diagnosed with a viral pericarditis due to parvovirus, which is a complication of her heart transplant status.

   _____

9. The patient is a 27-year-old male who was prescribed 14 days of amoxicillin for acute suppurative right otitis media. The patient felt better after taking the drug for 7 days and discontinued taking the pills that he then threw out in the trash. However, the right ear pain returned and the patient came back to the physician's office for another prescription. (This is the initial episode of care for the underdosing condition.)

   _____

10. Accidental overdose of oxytocin, initial encounter, emergency department treatment

    _____

11. Allergic reaction to contrast medium for radiology study exams. Patient experienced flushing of the face and neck and generalized itching.

    _____

ICD-10-CM and ICD-10-PCS Coding Exercises: Chapter 22B (Continued)

12. The 65-year-old male is an ESRD patient on renal dialysis. The patient's arteriovenous dialysis catheter is clogged with a thrombosis. The patient will have a revision of the dialysis catheter the next day in the outpatient surgery department.

    _____

13. The patient is a 45-year-old female who attempted suicide by taking a large amount of alcohol with a dozen Valium pills; she was found unconscious by her family, brought to the emergency department for treatment, and revived.

    _____

14. The patient is a 30-year-old male who works in a local zoo and was bitten by a venomous rattlesnake on his left arm while attempting to move the snake to a transportation container. A small open wound was treated on his left forearm that did not need sutures.

    _____

15. The patient was seen in the Pediatric Clinic of University Hospital as a follow-up or subsequent visit for a recent emergency department visit for suspected child abuse. The patient's Colles' fracture of the right arm is healing normally according to an x-ray exam taken during the clinic visit.

    _____

16. PROCEDURE: Open thrombectomy, right brachial artery

    _____

17. PROCEDURE: Right kidney transplant from living donor

    _____

18. PROCEDURE: Hemodialysis, single episode

    _____

19. PROCEDURE: Percutaneous removal of PICC venous catheter from upper arm

    _____

20. PROCEDURE: Angioplasty of left renal artery with insertion of a vascular stent

    _____

Chapter 23

External Causes of Morbidity (V00–Y99)

Learning Objectives

At the conclusion of this chapter, you should be able to:

1. Describe the organization of the codes included in Chapter 20 of ICD-10-CM, External causes of morbidity (V00–Y99)

2. Identify the types of entries found in the ICD-10-CM Index to External Causes that are used to locate the code for the external cause

3. Identify the correct seventh character required for reporting certain codes in ICD-10-CM

4. Be familiar with the separate ICD-10-CM Alphabetic Index to External Causes and identify the terminology used as main terms to access this Index

5. Explain the sequencing of ICD-10-CM external cause in comparison with diagnosis codes

6. Determine how many ICD-10-CM external cause codes may be assigned according to the general coding guidelines

7. Describe the ICD-10-CM multiple-cause coding guidelines for external cause codes, focusing on the priority given to particular external cause codes in terms of sequencing and reporting

8. Identify the way in which ICD-10-CM external cause codes should be used to report child or adult abuse according to the coding guidelines

9. Describe the ICD-10-CM "place of occurrence" codes and identify the circumstances in which the codes can be reported

10. Explain the types of ICD-10-CM external cause codes available to report a terrorism event

11. Describe the way in which ICD-10-CM external cause codes can be used to describe the late effect of an illness or injury

12. Assign ICD-10-CM codes for external causes of morbidity

Key Terms

- Activity codes
- External causes
- External cause status
- Intent of the event
- Never events
- Place of occurrence
- Sequela
- Seventh character

Overview of ICD-10-CM Chapter 20, External Cause of Morbidity

Chapter 20 includes categories V00–Y99 arranged in the following blocks:

V00–V99	Transport accidents
V00–V09	Pedestrian injured in transport accident
V10–V19	Pedal cycle rider injured in transport accident
V20–V29	Motorcycle rider injured in transport accident
V30–V39	Occupant of three-wheeled motor vehicle injured in transport accident
V40–V49	Car occupant injured in transport accident
V50–V59	Occupant of pick-up truck or van injured in transport accident
V60–V69	Occupant of heavy transport vehicle injured in transport accident
V70–V79	Bus occupant injured in transport accident
V80–V89	Other land transport accidents
V90–V94	Water transport accidents
V95–V97	Air and space transport accidents
V98–V99	Other and unspecified transport accidents
W00–X58	Other external causes of accidental injury
W00–W19	Slipping, tripping, stumbling and falls
W20–W49	Exposure to inanimate mechanical forces
W50–W64	Exposure to animate mechanical forces
W65–W74	Accidental non-transport drowning and submersion
W85–W99	Exposure to electric current, radiation and extreme ambient air temperature and pressure
X00–X08	Exposure to smoke, fire and flames
X10–X19	Contact with heat and hot substances

X30–X39	Exposure to forces of nature
X52–X58	Accidental exposure to other specified forces
X71–X83	Intentional self-harm
X92–Y08	Assault
Y21–Y33	Event of undetermined intent
Y35–Y38	Legal intervention, operations of war, military operations and terrorism
Y62–Y84	Complications of medical and surgical care
Y62–Y69	Misadventures to patients during surgical and medical care
Y70–Y82	Medical devices associated with adverse incidents in diagnostic and therapeutic use
Y83–Y84	Surgical and other medical procedures as the cause of abnormal reaction of the patient, or of later complication, without mention of misadventure at the time of the procedure
Y90–Y99	Supplementary factors related to causes of morbidity classified elsewhere

Chapter 20, External causes of morbidity (V00–Y99), contains codes that have the first character of V, W, X, and Y. It is helpful to review the Tabular List and read all the instructional notes to gain an understanding of the possible codes available.

This chapter permits the classification of **external causes,** defined as environmental events and circumstances as the cause of injury, and other adverse effects. External cause codes in Chapter 20 of ICD-10-CM capture the cause of the injury or health condition, the **intent of the event** (accidental or incidental), the place where the event occurred, the activity of the patient at the time of the event, and the patient's status (such as civilian or military). Coding external causes of injuries and other conditions provides valuable data for research and evaluation of injury prevention strategies. External cause codes provide information that is extremely useful to public health agencies and may assist healthcare planners in determining the kind of accidents a particular facility or physician treat.

An external cause code cannot be assigned as the principal, first-listed, or only listed diagnosis code. When a code from this section is applicable, it is intended that it will be used secondary to a code from another chapter of the classification indicating the nature of the condition. Most often, the condition will be classifiable to ICD-10-CM Chapter 19, Injury, poisoning and certain other consequences of external causes (S00–T88). Other conditions that may be stated to be due to external causes are classified in Chapters 1 to 18. For these conditions, the external cause codes from ICD-10-CM Chapter 20 should be used to provide additional information as to the cause of the condition.

The use of external cause codes is optional for many physicians and many healthcare facilities. Each provider or facility must decide whether it needs the information the external cause codes provide. Today, the information about accidents and other external causes of patients' injuries and illnesses may be of great value to hospital planning and to public health agencies. Because of the value of this information, many state governments have mandated the use of some or all of the types of external causes that can be reported. For example, some states have required the external cause of the injury and the place of occurrence. Other states have required reporting of external cause codes by certain providers, such as hospitals that are regional trauma centers. Each physician or hospital must consider the requirements of their state agencies in order to decide what reporting is mandated.

Coding Guidelines and Instructional Notes for ICD-10-CM Chapter 20

There are many notes in Chapter 20 to show which categories require the seventh character to indicate whether the episode of care being identified was the initial, subsequent, or a secondary encounter, or if the condition is a result of a past event (sequela). The category codes that require a seventh character include a note box that lists the instruction to it.
The appropriate seventh character is to be added to the code:

A—Initial encounter
D—Subsequent encounter
S—Sequela

In addition to the external cause code that identifies the event that cause the illness or injury, three other external cause codes identify other factors concerning the event. The additional facts that are available to be reported are:

Y92 Place of occurrence of the external cause
Y93 Activity codes
Y99 External cause status

The instructional note with category Y92, **Place of occurrence** of the external cause, states to use Y92 in conjunction with the activity code. A note under category Y92 states "The following category is for use, when relevant, to identify the place of occurrence of the external cause. Use in conjunction with an activity code. The place of occurrence should be recorded only at the initial encounter for treatment."

The instructional note with category Y93, **Activity codes** states "Category Y93 is provided for use to indicate the activity of the person seeking healthcare for an injury or health condition, such as a heart attack while shoveling snow, which resulted from, or was contributed to, by the activity." The activity code should be recorded only once at the initial encounter for treatment.

The third category used to provide additional facts about the event is category Y99, **External cause status.** The note that appears in the code book under category Y99 states "A single code from category Y99 should be used in conjunction with the external cause code(s) assigned to a record to indicate the status of the person at the time the event occurred." The external cause status code indicates the work status of the person at the time the event occurred. The external cause status code is used only once at the initial encounter for treatment.

The NCHS has published chapter-specific guidelines for Chapter 20 in the *ICD-10-CM Official Guidelines for Coding and Reporting*. The coding student should review all of the coding guidelines for Chapter 20 of ICD-10-CM, which appear in an ICD-10-CM code book or at the website http://www.cdc.gov/nchs/icd/icd10cm.htm, or in Appendix E.

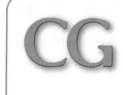

Guidelines for Chapter 20: External Causes of Morbidity (V01–Y99): Introduction: These guidelines are provided for the reporting of external causes of morbidity codes in order that there will be standardization in the process. These codes are secondary codes for use in any health care setting.

External cause codes are intended to provide data for injury research and evaluation of injury prevention strategies. These codes capture how the injury or health condition happened (cause), the intent (unintentional or accidental; or intentional, such as suicide or assault), the place where the event occurred, the activity of the patient at the time of the event, and the person's status (e.g., civilian, military).

Guideline I.C.20.a. General External Cause Coding Guidelines

Guideline I.C.20.a.1. Used with any code in the range of A00.0–T88.9, Z00–Z99: An external cause code may be used with any code in the range of A00.0–T88.9, Z00–Z99, classification that is a health condition due to an external cause. Though they are most applicable to injuries, they are also valid for use with such things as infections or diseases due to an external source, and other health conditions, such as a heart attack that occurs during strenuous physical activity.

Guideline I.C.20.a.2. External cause code used for length of treatment: Assign the external cause code, with the appropriate 7th character (initial encounter, subsequent encounter or sequela) for each encounter for which the injury or condition is being treated.

Guideline I.C.20.a.3. Use the full range of external cause codes: Use the full range of external cause codes to completely describe the cause, the intent, the place of occurrence, and if applicable, the activity of the patient at the time of the event, and the patient's status, for all injuries, and other health conditions due to an external cause.

Guideline I.C.20.a.4. Assign as many external cause codes as necessary: Assign as many external cause codes as necessary to fully explain each cause. If only one external code can be recorded, assign the code most related to the principal diagnosis.

Guideline I.C.20.a.5. The selection of the appropriate external cause code: The selection of the appropriate external cause code is guided by the Alphabetic Index of External Causes and by Inclusion and Exclusion notes in the Tabular List.

Guideline I.C.20.a.6. External cause code can never be a principal diagnosis: An external cause code can never be a principal (first-listed) diagnosis.

Guideline I.C.20.a.7. Combination external cause codes: Certain of the external cause codes are combination codes that identify sequential events that result in an injury, such as a fall which results in striking against an object. The injury may be due to either event or both. The combination external cause code used should correspond to the sequence of events regardless of which caused the most serious injury.

(Continued)

(Continued)

Guideline I.C.20.a.8. No external cause code needed in certain circumstances: No external cause code from Chapter 20 is needed if the external cause and intent are included in a code from another chapter (e.g. T36.0X1- Poisoning by penicillins, accidental (unintentional)).

Guideline I.C.20.b. Place of Occurrence Guideline: Codes from category Y92, Place of occurrence of the external cause, are secondary codes for use after other external cause codes to identify the location of the patient at the time of injury or other condition.

A place of occurrence code is used only once, at the initial encounter for treatment. No 7th characters are used for Y92. Only one code from Y92 should be recorded on a medical record. A place of occurrence code should be used in conjunction with an activity code, Y93.

Do not use place of occurrence code Y92.9 if the place is not stated or is not applicable.

Guideline I.C.20.c. Activity Code: Assign a code from category Y93, Activity code, to describe the activity of the patient at the time the injury or other health condition occurred.

An activity code is used only once, at the initial encounter for treatment. Only one code from Y93 should be recorded on a medical record. An activity code should be used in conjunction with a place of occurrence code, Y92.

The activity codes are not applicable to poisonings, adverse effects, misadventures or sequela.

Do not assign Y93.9, Unspecified activity, if the activity is not stated.

A code from category Y93 is appropriate for use with external cause and intent codes if identifying the activity provides additional information about the event.

Guideline I.C.20.d. Place of Occurrence, Activity, and Status Codes Used with other External Cause Code: When applicable, place of occurrence, activity, and external cause status codes are sequenced after the main external cause code(s). Regardless of the number of external cause codes assigned, there should be only one place of occurrence code, one activity code, and one external cause status code assigned to an encounter.

Guideline I.C.20.e. If the Reporting Format Limits the Number of External Cause Codes: If the reporting format limits the number of external cause codes that can be used in reporting clinical data, report the code for the cause/intent most related to the principal diagnosis. If the format permits capture of additional external cause codes, the cause/intent, including medical misadventures, of the additional events should be reported rather than the codes for place, activity, or external status.

Guideline I.C.20.f. Multiple External Cause Coding Guidelines: More than one external cause code is required to fully describe the external cause of an illness or injury. The assignment of external cause codes should be sequenced in the following priority:

If two or more events cause separate injuries, an external cause code should be assigned for each cause. The first-listed external cause code will be selected in the following order:

External codes for child and adult abuse take priority over all other external cause codes.

See Section I.C.19. Child and Adult abuse guidelines.

External cause codes for terrorism events take priority over all other external cause codes except child and adult abuse.

External cause codes for cataclysmic events take priority over all other external cause codes except child and adult abuse and terrorism.

External cause codes for transport accidents take priority over all other external cause codes except cataclysmic events, child and adult abuse and terrorism.

Activity and external cause status codes are assigned following all causal (intent) external cause codes.

The first-listed external cause code should correspond to the cause of the most serious diagnosis due to an assault, accident, or self-harm, following the order of hierarchy listed above.

Guideline I.C.20.g. Child and Adult Abuse Guideline: Adult and child abuse, neglect and maltreatment are classified as assault. Any of the assault codes may be used to indicate the external cause of any injury resulting from the confirmed abuse.

For confirmed cases of abuse, neglect and maltreatment, when the perpetrator is known, a code from Y07, Perpetrator of maltreatment and neglect, should accompany any other assault codes.

See Section I.C.19. Adult and child abuse, neglect and other maltreatment

Guideline I.C.20.h. Unknown or Undetermined Intent Guideline: If the intent (accident, self-harm, assault) of the cause of an injury or other condition is unknown or unspecified, code the intent as accidental intent. All transport accident categories assume accidental intent.

(Continued)

(Continued)

Guideline I.C.20.h.1. Use of undetermined intent: External cause codes for events of undetermined intent are only for use if the documentation in the record specifies that the intent cannot be determined.

Guideline I.C.20.i. Sequelae (Late Effects) of External Cause Guidelines

Guideline I.C.20.i.1. *Sequelae* **external cause codes:** Sequela are reported using the external cause code with the 7th character "S" for sequela. These codes should be used with any report of a late effect or sequela resulting from a previous injury.

Guideline I.C.20.i.2. *Sequela* **external cause code with a related current injury:** A sequela external cause code should never be used with a related current nature of injury code.

Guideline I.C.20.i.3. Use of *sequela* **external cause codes for subsequent visits:** Use a late effect external cause code for subsequent visits when a late effect of the initial injury is being treated. Do not use a late effect external cause code for subsequent visits for follow-up care (e.g., to assess healing, to receive rehabilitative therapy) of the injury when no late effect of the injury has been documented.

Guideline I.C.20.j. Terrorism Guidelines

Guideline I.C.20.j.1. Cause of injury identified by the Federal Government (FBI) as terrorism: When the cause of an injury is identified by the Federal Government (FBI) as terrorism, the first-listed external cause code should be a code from category Y38, Terrorism. The definition of terrorism employed by the FBI is found at the inclusion note at the beginning of category Y38. Use additional code for place of occurrence (Y92.-). More than one Y38 code may be assigned if the injury is the result of more than one mechanism of terrorism.

Guideline I.C.20.j.2. Cause of an injury is suspected to be the result of terrorism: When the cause of an injury is suspected to be the result of terrorism a code from category Y38 should not be assigned. Suspected cases should be classified as assault.

Guideline I.C.20.j.3. Code Y38.9, Terrorism, secondary effects: Assign code Y38.9, Terrorism, secondary effects, for conditions occurring subsequent to the terrorist event. This code should not be assigned for conditions that are due to the initial terrorist act.

It is acceptable to assign code Y38.9 with another code from Y38 if there is an injury due to the initial terrorist event and an injury that is a subsequent result of the terrorist event.

Guideline I.C.20.k. External cause status: A code from category Y99, External cause status, should be assigned whenever any other external cause code is assigned for an encounter, including an Activity code, except for the events noted below. Assign a code from category Y99, External cause status, to indicate the work status of the person at the time the event occurred. The status code indicates whether the event occurred during military activity, whether a non-military person was at work, whether an individual including a student or volunteer was involved in a non-work activity at the time of the causal event.

A code from Y99, External cause status, should be assigned, when applicable, with other external cause codes, such as transport accidents and falls. The external cause status codes are not applicable to poisonings, adverse effects, misadventures or late effects.

Do not assign a code from category Y99 if no other external cause codes (cause, activity) are applicable for the encounter.

An external cause status code is used only once, at the initial encounter for treatment. Only one code from Y99 should be recorded on a medical record.

Do not assign code Y99.9, Unspecified external cause status, if the status is not stated.

Coding External Cause of Morbidity in ICD-10-CM Chapter 20

An external cause code can never be a principal, first-listed, or only diagnosis code reported. An external cause code, with the appropriate seventh character (initial encounter, subsequent encounter, or sequela) is assigned for each encounter for which the injury or condition is being treated. This includes the initial encounter and all subsequent encounters when the condition being treated was caused by an external cause. Some of these healthcare encounters can be years later when the patient continues to suffer from the consequences of the original problem that was caused by an external event.

When it is applicable, an external cause code is used as an additional code with another code from other chapters in ICD-10-CM in the range of A00.0–T88.9, Z00–Z99 to identify when a health condition or injury is due to an external cause. External cause codes are used most commonly with codes for injuries. However, there may also be an external cause to be reported as the cause of other conditions such as infections or diseases, for example, when a musculoskeletal condition is produced as the result of overuse or repetitive motions.

The coder may use the full range of external cause codes to completely describe the cause, the intent, the place of occurrence, and if applicable, the activity of the patient at the time of the event, and the patient's status, for all injuries, and other health conditions due to an external cause. The coder may assign as many external cause codes as necessary to fully explain each cause. If only one external code can be recorded, the coder should assign the code most related to the principal diagnosis.

The coder must recognize that no external cause code from Chapter 20 is needed if the external cause and intent are included in a code from another chapter. For example, an external cause code is not used with a code for a poisoning. The code T36.0X1, Poisoning by penicillins, accidental (unintentional), includes the intent and therefore would not require the use of an external cause code.

Certain external cause codes are combination codes that identify sequential events that result in an injury, such as a fall that results in striking against an object. The injury may be due to either event or both. The combination external cause code used should correspond to the sequence of events regardless of which event caused the most serious injury.

If the reporting format limits the number of external cause codes that can be used in reporting clinical data, the coder should report the code for the cause or intent most relative to the principal diagnosis. If additional external cause codes are allowed, the cause or intent, including medical misadventures, of the additional events should be reported rather than the codes for place, activity, or external status.

Seventh Character to Identify the Encounter

ICD-10-CM indicates when one of the external cause codes in the range of V00–Y99 codes require a seventh character to indicate whether the healthcare encounter was the

A—Initial encounter,
D—Subsequent encounter, or
S—Sequela.

Because an external cause code is assigned for each encounter for which the injury or condition is being treated, the **seventh character** identifies the timing of the care for the condition. The encounter could be the first time the patient is treated, it could be a follow-up visit or subsequent encounter, or it could be a much later encounter. When the external cause is recognized as the cause of the **sequela**, or condition that the patient has today, and continues to receive treatment, the external cause is reported with the seventh character S for sequela. These later encounters identify when the long-term effect of an injury is being treated.

Certain external causes are only used once, at the initial encounter for treatment, such as the place of occurrence codes, the activity code, and the external status code(s). The actual external cause, such as a fall or transportation accident, continues to be reported with the appropriate seventh character for as long as the patient receives treatment.

The seventh character of an external cause code must always be the seventh character in the data field. If a code that requires a seventh character is not six characters, a placeholder X must be used to fill in the empty characters.

Alphabetic Index of External Causes

The selection of the appropriate external cause code is guided by the Alphabetic Index of External Causes and by inclusion and exclusion notes in the Tabular List. ICD-10-CM contains an Index to External Causes with main terms identifying the event with such entries as accident, drowning, exposure, force of nature, falling, slipping, and other events that can cause an injury. Other entries exist for assignment of the activity of the person, place of occurrence, and status of external cause, such as civilian activity, leisure activity, student activity, and such.

The external cause code is organized by the main term describing the accident, circumstance, event, or specific agent that caused the injury or illness, such as a car accident, earthquake, or dog bite.

Fall, falling (accidental) W19
building W20.1
  burning X00.3
down
  embankment W17.81
  escalator W10.0
  hill W17.81
  ladder W11
  ramp W10.2
  stairs, steps W10.9

Sequence of Place of Occurrence, Activity, and Status Codes

The place of occurrence, activity, and external cause status codes are sequenced after the main external cause code(s). Regardless of the number of external cause codes assigned, there should be only one place of occurrence code, one activity code, and one external cause status code assigned to the initial encounter. For example, if a patient was treated during an initial encounter for two injuries from two external causes that occurred at the same time, such as a burn from hot stove (X15.0XXA) and a fracture from a fall (W18.30XA), there is only one place of occurrence code used, for example, the kitchen in a single family residence (Y92.000), only one activity code, for example, baking and cooking (Y93.G3), and only one external cause status code, for example, this was a leisure activity for the patient (Y99.8). When the patient is treated during subsequent healthcare visits, only the external cause codes will be assigned with the seventh character D but no additional external cause codes will be assigned for the place of occurrence, activity, or external cause status.

Multiple External Cause Codes

The first-listed external cause code should correspond to the cause of the most serious diagnosis due to an assault, accident, or self-harm, following an established hierarchy. If two or more events cause separate injuries, an external cause code should be assigned for each cause. The first-listed external cause code will be selected in the following order:

1. External codes for child and adult abuse take priority over all other external cause codes.

2. External cause codes for terrorism events take priority over all other external cause codes except child and adult abuse.

3. External cause codes for cataclysmic events take priority over all other external cause codes except child and adult abuse and terrorism.

4. External cause codes for transport accidents take priority over all other external cause codes except cataclysmic events, child and adult abuse, and terrorism.

5. Activity and external cause status codes are assigned following all causal (intent) external cause codes.

External Cause Codes for Child and Adult Abuse

Adult and child abuse, neglect, and maltreatment are classified as assault. For cases of confirmed abuse or neglect is documented in the record, an external cause code from the assault section (X92–Y08) should be added to identify the cause of any physical injuries.

For confirmed cases of abuse, neglect, and maltreatment, when the perpetrator is known, a code from Y07, Perpetrator of maltreatment and neglect, should accompany any other assault codes. The relationship between the perpetrator and victim is identified with the Y07 code, for example, spouse or partner, parent, or sibling; the perpetrator may also be a nonfamily member, such as a daycare provider or teacher.

For suspected cases of abuse or neglect, the coder does not report an external cause of injury or perpetrator code for the encounter.

Identifying the Intent for External Cause Codes

All transport accident categories are assumed to be accidental and reported as having an accidental intent. In addition, if the intent of an event is unknown or unspecified, that is, it is not stated to be an accident, self-harm, or an assault, the coder can assume the intent of the event is accidental. The only time the coder uses the event codes that state there is an undetermined intent is when the documentation in the record specifically states the intent of the event cannot be determined.

Sequelae or Late Effect External Cause Codes

To identify that a patient's condition being treated today is from an event that occurred in the past, the external cause code is reported with the seventh character S for sequela. These external cause codes should be used with any report of a late effect or sequela resulting from a previous injury. A sequela external cause code should never be used with a related current nature of injury code. Typically, a patient with a sequela of a past injury or illness is coded as follows:

1. Residual effect or the condition the patient has at present, which is found in the Alphabetic Index to Diseases and Injuries

2. Sequela or late effect or the condition the patient originally had that produced the residual effect found in the Alphabetic Index to Disease and Injuries under the term "sequelae."

3. External cause code for the original accident or event, found in the Index to External Causes with the seventh character of "S" for sequelae.

Transport Accidents (V00–V99)

The transport accidents section (V00–V99) is structured in 12 groups:

1. Pedestrian injured in transport accident, V00–V09

2. Pedal cycle rider injured in transport accident, V10–V19

3. Motorcycle rider injured in transport accident, V20–V29

4. Occupant of three-wheeled motor vehicle injured in transport accident, V30–V39

5. Car occupant injured in transport accident, V40–V49

6. Occupant of pick-up truck or van injured in transport accident, V50–V59

7. Occupant of heavy transport vehicle injured in transport accident, V60–V69

8. Bus occupant injured in transport accident, V70–V79

9. Other land transport accidents, V80–V89

10. Water transport accidents, V90–V94

11. Air and space transport accidents, V95–V97

12. Other and unspecified transport accidents, V98–V99

Those relating to land transport accidents (V00–V89) reflect the victim's mode of transport and are subdivided to identify the victim's counterpart or the type of event. The vehicle of which the injured person is an occupant is identified in the first two characters since it is seen as the most important factor to identify for prevention purposes. A transport accident is one in which the vehicle involved must be moving or running or in use for transport purposes at the time of the accident. The definitions of transport vehicles are provided at the beginning of Chapter 20. A "use additional code" note appears under the heading for transport accidents (V00–V99) to use another code for airbag injury (W22.1-), type of street or road (Y92.4-), and use of cellular telephone or other electronic equipment at the time of the transport accident (Y93.C-).

Never Events or Serious Reportable Events

ICD-10-CM contains external cause codes to identify and track the occurrence of wrong site surgery, wrong surgery, and wrong patient having surgery to support the collection of data related to the National Quality Forum's **never events**. The federal government's Institute of Medicine (IOM) developed a comprehensive approach to improving patient safety in American healthcare organizations by identifying certain healthcare errors and particular events that were reported in a systemic manner. To accomplish this, the IOM worked with the National Quality Forum to identify a list of "serious reportable events" in healthcare that should never occur. This list of events has become known as "never events" as a result of the National Quality Forum's report "Serious Reportable Events in Healthcare: A Consensus Report" that was produced in 2002. A complete list of the never events and the work of the Department of Health and Human Services' Agency for Healthcare Research and Quality (AHRQ) can be found in table 23.1. A complete report of the "Serious Reportable Adverse Events in Health Care" written by Kenneth W. Kizer and Melissa B. Stegun can be found at http://www.ahrq.gov/downloads/pub/advances/vol4/Kizer2.pdf.

The wrong site, wrong surgery, and wrong patient never events or serious reportable events are among the list of adverse medical events that are serious, largely preventable, and of concern to patients and healthcare providers. The Joint Commission, the federal government, and state governments use the never events list as the basis for quality indicators and state-based reporting systems. Listed next are examples of external cause codes that can be used to describe the external cause of several of these factors.

Y65.51	Performance of wrong procedure (operation) on correct patient
Y65.52	Performance of procedure (operation) on patient not scheduled for surgery
Y65.53	Performance of correct procedure (operation) on wrong side or body part

Some of these events—such as stage 3 and 4 pressure ulcers acquired after admission to the healthcare facility and intravascular air embolism that occurs while being cared for in a healthcare facility—can be captured by ICD-10-CM diagnosis codes and present-on-admission indicators. Other events in this area cannot be captured using ICD-10-CM codes because the event is beyond the scope of the classification system. An example of a never event that cannot be coded is an infant discharged to the wrong patient or the abduction of a patient of any age.

Table 23.1. **List of serious reportable events or never events**

Event	Additional specifications
1. Surgical events	
A. Surgery performed on the wrong body part	Defined as any surgery performed on a body part that is not consistent with the documented informed consent for that patient. Excludes emergent situations that occur in the course of surgery and/or whose exigency precludes obtaining informed consent.
B. Surgery performed on the wrong patient	Defined as any surgery on a patient that is not consistent with the documented informed consent for that patient.
C. Wrong surgical procedure performed on a patient	Defined as any procedure performed on a patient that is not consistent with the documented informed consent for that patient. Excludes emergent situations that occur in the course of surgery and/or whose exigency precludes obtaining informed consent. Surgery includes endoscopies and other invasive procedures.
D. Retention of a foreign object in a patient after surgery or other procedure	Excludes objects intentionally implanted as part of a planned intervention and objects present prior to surgery that were intentionally retained.
E. Intraoperative or immediately post-operative death in an ASA Class I patient	Includes all ASA Class I patient deaths in situations where anesthesia was administered; the planned surgical procedure may or may not have been carried out. Immediately post-operative means within 24 hours after induction of anesthesia (if surgery not completed), surgery, or other invasive procedure was completed.
2. Product or device events	
A. Patient death or serious disability associated with the use of contaminated drugs, devices, or biologics provided by the health care facility	Includes generally detectable contaminants in drugs, devices, or biologics regardless of the source of contamination and/or product.
B. Patient death or serious disability associated with the use or function of a device in patient care, in which the device is used for functions other than as intended	Includes, but is not limited to, catheters, drains and other specialized tubes, infusion pumps, and ventilators.
C. Patient death or serious disability associated with intravascular air embolism that occurs while being cared for in a health care facility	Excludes deaths associated with neurosurgical procedures known to be a high risk of intravascular air embolism.

3.	Patient protection events	
A.	Infant discharged to the wrong person	
B.	Patient death or serious disability associated with patient elopement (disappearance) for more than four hours	Excludes events involving competent adults.
C.	Patient suicide, or attempted suicide resulting in serious disability, while being cared for in a health care facility	Defined as events that result from patient actions after admission to a health care facility. Excludes deaths resulting from self inflicted injuries that were the reason for admission to the health care facility.
4.	Care management events	
A.	Patient death or serious disability associated with a medication error (e.g., errors involving the wrong drug, wrong dose, wrong patient, wrong time, wrong rate, wrong preparation, or wrong route of administration)	Excludes reasonable differences in clinical judgment on drug selection and dose.
B.	Patient death or serious disability associated with a hemolytic reaction due to the administration of ABO-incompatible blood or blood products	
C.	Maternal death or serious disability associated with labor or delivery in a low-risk pregnancy while being cared for in a healthcare facility	Includes events that occur within 42 days post-delivery. Excludes deaths from pulmonary or amniotic fluid embolism, acute fatty liver of pregnancy or cardiomyopathy.
D.	Patient death or serious disability associated with hypoglycemia, the onset of which occurs while the patient is being cared for in a health care facility	
E.	Death or serious disability (kernicterus) associated with failure to identify and treat hyperbilirubinimia in neonates	Hyperbilirubinimia is defined as bilirubin levels >30 mg/dl. Neonates refers to the first 28 days of life.
F.	Stage 3 or 4 pressure ulcers acquired after admission to a health care facility	Excludes progression from Stage 2 to Stage 3 if Stage 2 was recognized upon admission.
G.	Patient death or serious disability due to spinal manipulative therapy	
5.	Environmental events	
A.	Patient death or serious disability associated with an electric shock while being cared for in a healthcare facility	Excludes events involving planned treatments such as electric countershock
B.	Any incident in which a line designated for oxygen or other gas to be delivered to a patient contains the wrong gas or is contaminated by toxic substances	
C.	Patient death or serious disability associated with a burn incurred from any source while being cared for in a health care facility	
D.	Patient death associated with a fall while being cared for in a health care facility	

(Continued)

Table 23.1.   List of serious reportable events or never events (*Continued*)

E. Patient death or serious disability associated with the use of restraints or bedrails while being cared for in a health care facility	
6. Criminal events	
A. Any instance of care ordered by or provided by someone impersonating a physician, nurse, pharmacist, or other licensed health care provider	
B. Abduction of a patient of any age	
C. Sexual assault on a patient within or on the grounds of the health care facility	
D. Death or significant injury of a patient or staff member resulting from a physical assault (i.e., battery) that occurs within or on the grounds of the health care facility	

Source: Kizer, K.W. and M.B. Stegun 2012

Military Operations

The US Department of Defense initiated the addition and expansion of external cause codes for the identification of the causes of injuries among the military population to assist with the prevention of such injuries. Two categories of ICD-10-CM external cause codes are available to report the cause of an injury or illness.

Operations of War (Y36)

The Includes note under category Y36 states these codes describe the cause of injuries to military personnel and civilians caused by war, civil insurrections, and peacekeeping missions. The Excludes1 note states this category is not to be used with category Y37, Military operations, which identify the cause of injuries to military personnel occurring during peacetime operations.

Military Operations (Y37)

The Includes note under category Y37 states these codes describe the cause of injuries to military personnel and civilians occurring during peacetime on military property and during routine military exercises and operations. The Excludes1 note states that military aircraft accidents, military vehicles transport accidents, and military watercraft transport accidents with civilian aircraft, vehicles, or watercrafts are coded to other categories. In addition, war operations that caused an injury are not reported with these external cause codes in category Y37. Examples of external cause codes to identify injuries from military operations are as follows:

Y37.010-	Military operations involving explosion of depth-charge, military personnel
Y37.210-	Military operations involving explosion of aerial bomb, military personnel
Y37.320-	Military operations involving incendiary bullet, military personnel

Y37.421-	Military operations involving firearms pellets, civilian
Y37.6x1-	Military operations involving biological weapons, civilian
Y37.92x-	Military operations involving friendly fire

Terrorism External Cause Codes

When the cause of an injury is identified by the Federal Bureau of Investigation (FBI) as terrorism, the first-listed external cause code should be a code from category Y38, Terrorism. The definition of terrorism employed by the FBI is found at the inclusion note at the beginning of category Y38. The note reads, "These codes are for use to identify injuries resulting from the unlawful use of force or violence against persons or property to intimidate or coerce a government, the civilian population, or any segment thereof, in furtherance of a political or social objective." Use an additional code for place of occurrence (Y92.-). More than one Y38 code may be assigned if the injury is the result of more than one mechanism of terrorism. When the cause of an injury is suspected to be the result of terrorism a code from category Y38 should not be assigned. Suspected cases should be classified as assault. Assign code Y38.9, Terrorism, secondary effects, for conditions occurring subsequent to the terrorist event. This code should not be assigned for conditions that are due to the initial terrorist act. It is acceptable to assign code Y38.9 with another code from Y38 if there is an injury due to the initial terrorist event and an injury that is a subsequent result of the terrorist event.

Place of Occurrence

The code for the place of occurrence is used to identify, when documented, where the event occurred. Category Y92 codes, Place of occurrence of the external cause, are used in conjunction with an activity code if the activity is stated by the healthcare provider. Place of occurrence should be recorded only at the initial encounter for treatment to identify the location of the patient at the time when the injury or other condition occurred. Only one code from Y92 should be recorded on a medical record. The coder should not use the unspecified place of occurrence code Y92.9 if the place is not stated in the record or is not applicable.

Activity Code

A code from category Y93, Activity code, is used to describe the activity of the patient at the time the injury or other health condition occurred. An activity code is used only once, at the initial encounter for treatment. Only one code from Y93 should be recorded on a medical record. An activity code should be used in conjunction with a place of occurrence code, Y92. The activity codes are not applicable to poisonings, adverse effects, misadventures, or sequela. The coder should not assign code Y93.9 for an unspecified activity if the activity is not stated.

A code from category Y93 is appropriate for use with external cause and intent codes if identifying the activity provides additional information about the event. A note at the beginning of category Y93 in the Tabular states the activity code is provided to indicate the activity of the person seeking healthcare for an injury or health condition that resulted from the activity or was contributed to by the activity, such as a heart attack while shoveling snow. These codes are appropriate for use for both acute injuries, such as those from Chapter 19, and conditions that are due to the long-term, cumulative effects of an activity, such as those from Chapter 13.

They are also appropriate for use with external cause codes for cause and intent if identifying the activity provides additional information on the event. These codes should be used in conjunction with codes for external cause status (Y99) and place of occurrence (Y92). The activity code is used only once, at the initial encounter for treatment.

This section contains the following broad activity categories:

Y93.0	Activities involving walking and running
Y93.1	Activities involving water and water craft
Y93.2	Activities involving ice and snow
Y93.3	Activities involving climbing, rappelling, and jumping off
Y93.4	Activities involving dancing and other rhythmic movement
Y93.5	Activities involving other sports and athletics played individually
Y93.6	Activities involving other sports and athletics played as a team or group
Y93.7	Activities involving other specified sports and athletics
Y93.a	Activities involving other cardiorespiratory exercise
Y93.b	Activities involving other muscle strengthening exercises
Y93.c	Activities involving computer technology and electronic devices
Y93.d	Activities involving arts and handcrafts
Y93.e	Activities involving personal hygiene and interior property and clothing maintenance
Y93.f	Activities involving caregiving
Y93.g	Activities involving food preparation, cooking, and grilling
Y93.h	Activities involving exterior property and land maintenance, building and construction
Y93.i	Activities involving roller coasters and other types of external motion
Y93.j	Activities involving playing musical instrument
Y93.k	Activities involving animal care
Y93.8	Activities, other specified
Y93.9	Activity, unspecified

External Cause Status Codes

A code from category Y99, External cause status, should be assigned whenever any other external cause code is assigned for an encounter, including an activity code, except for the events noted below. A code from category Y99, External cause status, should be assigned to indicate the work status of the person at the time the event occurred. The status code indicates whether the event occurred during military activity, whether a nonmilitary person was at work, or whether an individual including a student or volunteer was involved in a nonwork activity at the time of the causal event.

A code from Y99, External cause status, should be assigned, when applicable, with other external cause codes, such as transport accidents and falls. The external cause status codes are not applicable to poisonings, adverse effects, misadventures, or late effects. The coder should not assign a code from category Y99 if no other external cause codes (cause, activity) are applicable for the encounter.

An external cause status code is used only once, at the initial encounter for treatment. Only one code from Y99 should be recorded on a medical record. The coder should not assign code Y99.9, Unspecified external cause status, if the status is not stated in the record.

ICD-10-CM Review Exercises: Chapter 23

Assign the appropriate external cause codes only and not the injury or illness codes.

1. Assign external cause codes for this case: An 18-year-old driver of a car that collided with a pickup truck on the interstate highway. The driver confessed to using his cell phone to send a text message to his girlfriend.

2. Assign external cause only codes for this case: An army officer was injured while on patrol on the military base in Afghanistan by an explosion of an IED.

3. Assign external cause only codes for this case: The patient was bitten by a dog while attempting to rescue it from a barn while performing his job at animal control.

4. Assign initial encounter for this case: The patient was burned on his face by a fireworks accident that occurred in the neighborhood park. The patient is a high school student and was at the park as part of a student outing from his school.

5. Assign initial encounter for this case: The patient was injured while playing in a college football game at his college stadium. He was injured when he was tackled by an opposing team player.

6. Assign initial encounter for this case: The patient was injured when he was burned by hot food spilled on him while he was eating at a local restaurant during a business lunch. The patient is employed as a company executive.

7. Assign initial encounter for this case: The patient was hit by a falling tree while hiking in a forest. The patient was on vacation at the time.

8. Assign initial treatment for this case: The patient was injured when he was thrown off a horse as a student at a riding school; there was no collision with another object. The patient is a student in college.

9. Assign initial encounter for this case: The patient was hit by a water ski while waterskiing. The patient was on vacation at a lake.

(Continued on next page)

ICD-10-CM Review Exercises: Chapter 23 (Continued)

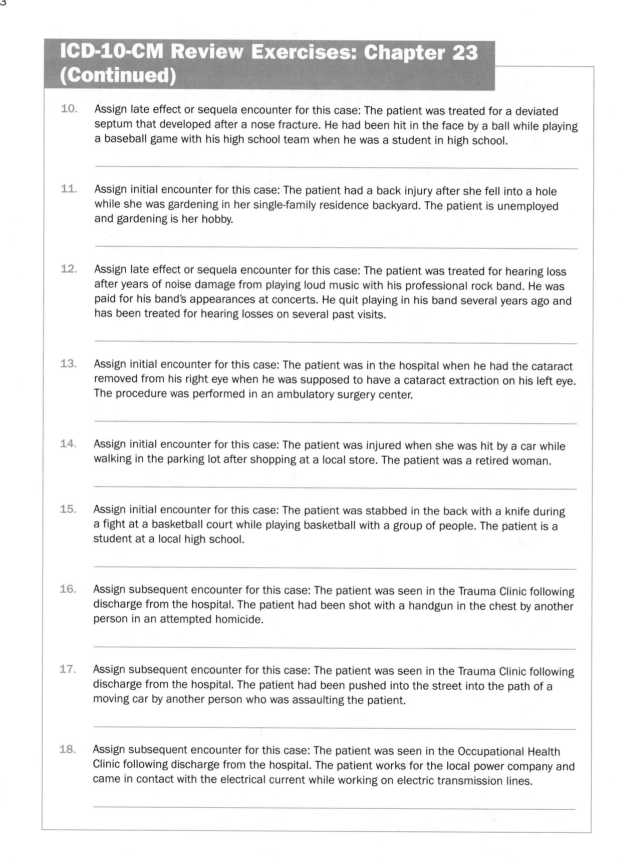

10. Assign late effect or sequela encounter for this case: The patient was treated for a deviated septum that developed after a nose fracture. He had been hit in the face by a ball while playing a baseball game with his high school team when he was a student in high school.

    _____

11. Assign initial encounter for this case: The patient had a back injury after she fell into a hole while she was gardening in her single-family residence backyard. The patient is unemployed and gardening is her hobby.

    _____

12. Assign late effect or sequela encounter for this case: The patient was treated for hearing loss after years of noise damage from playing loud music with his professional rock band. He was paid for his band's appearances at concerts. He quit playing in his band several years ago and has been treated for hearing losses on several past visits.

    _____

13. Assign initial encounter for this case: The patient was in the hospital when he had the cataract removed from his right eye when he was supposed to have a cataract extraction on his left eye. The procedure was performed in an ambulatory surgery center.

    _____

14. Assign initial encounter for this case: The patient was injured when she was hit by a car while walking in the parking lot after shopping at a local store. The patient was a retired woman.

    _____

15. Assign initial encounter for this case: The patient was stabbed in the back with a knife during a fight at a basketball court while playing basketball with a group of people. The patient is a student at a local high school.

    _____

16. Assign subsequent encounter for this case: The patient was seen in the Trauma Clinic following discharge from the hospital. The patient had been shot with a handgun in the chest by another person in an attempted homicide.

    _____

17. Assign subsequent encounter for this case: The patient was seen in the Trauma Clinic following discharge from the hospital. The patient had been pushed into the street into the path of a moving car by another person who was assaulting the patient.

    _____

18. Assign subsequent encounter for this case: The patient was seen in the Occupational Health Clinic following discharge from the hospital. The patient works for the local power company and came in contact with the electrical current while working on electric transmission lines.

    _____

ICD-10-CM Review Exercises: Chapter 23 (Continued)

19. Assign external cause code to describe the original event for the sequel the patient has: The patient is seen in the Dermatology Clinic for evaluation of scars on her skin from years of radiation damage from ultraviolet light from tanning beds.

   _____

20. Assign initial encounter for this case: The patient, a 16-year-old high school student, fell out of his bed in the apartment he shared with his family and injured his face when he hit his head on the wall next to the bed.

   _____

Chapter 24

Factors Influencing Health Status and Contact with Health Services (Z00–Z99)

Learning Objectives

At the conclusion of this chapter, you should be able to:

1. Describe the organization of the codes included in Chapter 21 of ICD-10-CM, Factors influencing health status and contact with health services (Z00–Z99)

2. Identify the healthcare settings and scenarios when Z code classifications are available for use

3. Understand the intent of the codes in Chapter 21 and assign ICD-10-CM codes for factors influencing health status and contact with health services

4. Assign ICD-10-CM diagnosis codes for factors influencing health status and contact with health services

Key Terms

- Aftercare
- Antenatal screening
- Body mass index (BMI)
- Do not resuscitate (DNR)
- Family history
- Follow-up codes
- Genetic carrier
- Genetic susceptibility
- Noncompliance
- Outcome of delivery
- Personal history
- Resistance
- Ruled out
- Screening
- Underimmunization

Overview of ICD-10-CM Chapter 21, Factors Influencing Health Status and Contact with Health Services

Chapter 21 includes categories Z00–Z99 arranged in the following blocks:

Z00–Z13	Persons encountering health services for examinations
Z14–Z15	Genetic carrier and genetic susceptibility to disease
Z16	Resistance to antimicrobial drugs
Z17	Estrogen receptor status
Z18	Retained foreign body fragment
Z20–Z28	Persons with potential health hazards related to communicable diseases
Z30–Z39	Persons encountering health services in circumstances related to reproduction
Z40–Z53	Encounters for other specific health care
Z55–Z65	Persons with potential health hazards related to socioeconomic and psychosocial circumstances
Z66	Do not resuscitate status
Z67	Blood type
Z68	Body mass index (BMI)
Z69–Z76	Persons encountering health services in other circumstances
Z77–Z99	Persons with potential health hazards related to family and personal history and certain conditions influencing health status

Codes included in Chapter 21, Factors influencing health status and contact with health services (Z00–Z99), represent reasons for encounters. Z codes are diagnosis codes. If a procedure is performed, a corresponding procedure code must be used with the Z code that identifies the reason for the encounter. Z codes are provided for encounters when circumstances other than a disease or injury are recorded in the health record as the diagnosis—the problem or reason for the encounter.

Some categories in Chapter 21 have titles to clearly describe the situations the code will classify. For example, the description for Z08 is "Encounter for follow-up examination after completed treatment for malignant neoplasm" to identify the reason for the visit for the patient who is being seen after having completed treatment for cancer. Another example of a clear description of the reason for the patient's examination is subcategory Z00.0, Encounter for general adult medical examination. Code Z00.00 identifies a general adult medical examination without abnormal findings and code Z00.01 identifies a general adult medical examination with abnormal findings. These codes distinguish between the encounter when a patient is found to be completely healthy and when an abnormal finding has been identified in the patient who presented for a medical examination. Under code Z00.01 is a "use additional code" note to identify the abnormal finding so that the patient's situation can be fully described.

However some conditions are not specifically identified. In ICD-10-CM there is category, Z16, to represent infection with antimicrobial drug-resistant microorganisms. For example, if a patient had an infection that did not respond to treatment by the usual penicillin medication, code Z16.11 would identify the resistance of the condition to this antimicrobial drug. Another example of a nonspecific situation is code Z23, Encounter for immunization. This code does not identify the types of immunizations that were administered.

Coding Guidelines and Instructional Notes for ICD-10-CM Chapter 21

Instructional notes are available in the different categories to explain how codes should be assigned. For example, under category Z01, Encounter for other special examination without complaint, suspected or reported diagnosis, is the following note: "Codes from category Z01 represent the reason for the encounter. A separate procedure code is required to identify any examination or procedure performed." Also, under category Z85, Personal history of malignant neoplasm, is the following note: "Code first any follow-up examination after treatment of malignant neoplasm (Z08)."

The NCHS has published chapter-specific guidelines for Chapter 21 in the *ICD-10-CM Official Guidelines for Coding and Reporting*. The coding student should review all of the coding guidelines for Chapter 21 of ICD-10-CM, which appear in an ICD-10-CM code book or at the website http://www.cdc.gov/nchs/icd/icd10cm.htm, or in Appendix E.

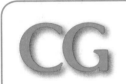

Chapter 21: Factors influencing health status and contact with health services (Z00–Z99): Note: The chapter specific guidelines provide additional information about the use of Z codes for specified encounters.

Guideline I.C.21.a. Use of Z codes in any healthcare setting: Z codes are for use in any healthcare setting. Z codes may be used as either a first-listed (principal diagnosis code in the inpatient setting) or secondary code, depending on the circumstances of the encounter. Certain Z codes may only be used as first-listed or principal diagnosis.

Guideline I.C.21.b. Z Codes indicate a reason for an encounter: Z codes are not procedure codes. A corresponding procedure code must accompany a Z code to describe any procedure performed.

Guideline I.C.21.c. Categories of Z Codes

Guideline I.C.21.c.1. Contact/Exposure: Category Z20 indicates contact with, and suspected exposure to, communicable diseases. These codes are for patients who do not show any sign or symptom of a disease but are suspected to have been exposed to it by close personal contact with an infected individual or are in an area where a disease is epidemic.

Category Z77, indicates contact with and suspected exposures hazardous to health.

(Continued)

(Continued)

Contact/exposure codes may be used as a first-listed code to explain an encounter for testing, or, more commonly, as a secondary code to identify a potential risk.

Guideline I.C.21.c.2. Inoculations and vaccinations: Code Z23 is for encounters for inoculations and vaccinations. It indicates that a patient is being seen to receive a prophylactic inoculation against a disease. Procedure codes are required to identify the actual administration of the injection and the type(s) of immunizations given. Code Z23 may be used as a secondary code if the inoculation is given as a routine part of preventive health care, such as a well-baby visit.

Guideline I.C.21.c.3. Status: Status codes indicate that a patient is either a carrier of a disease or has the sequelae or residual of a past disease or condition. This includes such things as the presence of prosthetic or mechanical devices resulting from past treatment. A status code is informative, because the status may affect the course of treatment and its outcome. A status code is distinct from a history code. The history code indicates that the patient no longer has the condition.

A status code should not be used with a diagnosis code from one of the body system chapters, if the diagnosis code includes the information provided by the status code. For example, code Z94.1, Heart transplant status, should not be used with a code from subcategory T86.2, Complications of heart transplant. The status code does not provide additional information. The complication code indicates that the patient is a heart transplant patient.

For encounters for weaning from a mechanical ventilator, assign a code from subcategory J96.1, Chronic respiratory failure, followed by code Z99.11, Dependence on respirator [ventilator] status.

The status Z codes/categories are:

Z14 Genetic carrier
Genetic carrier status indicates that a person carries a gene, associated with a particular disease, which may be passed to offspring who may develop that disease. The person does not have the disease and is not at risk of developing the disease.

Z15 Genetic susceptibility to disease
Genetic susceptibility indicates that a person has a gene that increases the risk of that person developing the disease.

Codes from category Z15 should not be used as principal or first-listed codes. If the patient has the condition to which he/she is susceptible, and that condition is the reason for the encounter, the code for the current condition should be sequenced first.

If the patient is being seen for follow-up after completed treatment for this condition, and the condition no longer exists, a follow-up code should be sequenced first, followed by the appropriate personal history and genetic susceptibility codes. If the purpose of the encounter is genetic counseling associated with procreative management, code Z31.5, Encounter for genetic counseling, should be assigned as the first-listed code, followed by a code from category Z15. Additional codes should be assigned for any applicable family or personal history.

Z16 Resistance to antimicrobial drugs
This code indicates that a patient has a condition that is resistant to antimicrobial drug treatment. Sequence the infection code first.

Z17 Estrogen receptor status

Z18 Retained foreign body fragments

Z21 Asymptomatic HIV infection status
This code indicates that a patient has tested positive for HIV but has manifested no signs or symptoms of the disease.

Z22 Carrier of infectious disease
Carrier status indicates that a person harbors the specific organisms of a disease without manifest symptoms and is capable of transmitting the infection.

Z28.3 Underimmunization status

Z33.1 Pregnant state, incidental
This code is a secondary code only for use when the pregnancy is in no way complicating the reason for visit. Otherwise, a code from the obstetric chapter is required.

Z66 Do not resuscitate
This code may be used when it is documented by the provider that a patient is on do not resuscitate status at any time during the stay.

Z67 Blood type

Z68 Body mass index (BMI)

Z74.01 Bed confinement status

Z76.82 Awaiting organ transplant status

Z78 Other specified health status
Code Z78.1, Physical restraint status, may be used when it is documented by the provider that a patient has been put in restraints during the current encounter. Please note that this code should not be reported when it is documented by the provider that a patient is temporarily restrained during a procedure.

(Continued)

(*Continued*)

Z79 Long-term (current) drug therapy

Codes from this category indicate a patient's continuous use of a prescribed drug (including such things as aspirin therapy) for the long-term treatment of a condition or for prophylactic use. It is not for use for patients who have addictions to drugs. This subcategory is not for use of medications for detoxification or maintenance programs to prevent withdrawal symptoms in patients with drug dependence (e.g., methadone maintenance for opiate dependence). Assign the appropriate code for the drug dependence instead.

Assign a code from Z79 if the patient is receiving a medication for an extended period as a prophylactic measure (such as for the prevention of deep vein thrombosis) or as treatment of a chronic condition (such as arthritis) or a disease requiring a lengthy course of treatment (such as cancer). Do not assign a code from category Z79 for medication being administered for a brief period of time to treat an acute illness or injury (such as a course of antibiotics to treat acute bronchitis).

Z88 Allergy status to drugs, medicaments and biological substances

Except: Z88.9, Allergy status to unspecified drugs, medicaments and biological substances status

Z89 Acquired absence of limb

Z90 Acquired absence of organs, not elsewhere classified

Z91.0- Allergy status, other than to drugs and biological substances

Z92.82 Status post administration of tPA (rtPA) in a different facility within the last 24 hours prior to admission to a current facility

Assign code Z92.82, Status post administration of tPA (rtPA) in a different facility within the last 24 hours prior to admission to current facility, as a secondary diagnosis when a patient is received by transfer into a facility and documentation indicates they were administered tissue plasminogen activator (tPA) within the last 24 hours prior to admission to the current facility. This guideline applies even if the patient is still receiving the tPA at the time they are received into the current facility. The appropriate code for the condition for which the tPA was administered (such as cerebrovascular disease or myocardial infarction) should be assigned first. Code Z92.82 is only applicable to the receiving facility record and not to the transferring facility record.

Z93 Artificial opening status

Z94 Transplanted organ and tissue status

Z95 Presence of cardiac and vascular implants and grafts

Z96 Presence of other functional implants

Z97 Presence of other devices

Z98 Other postprocedural states
Assign code Z98.85, Transplanted organ removal status, to indicate that a transplanted organ has been previously removed. This code should not be assigned for the encounter in which the transplanted organ is removed. The complication necessitating removal of the transplant organ should be assigned for that encounter.

See section I.C19. for information on the coding of organ transplant complications.

Z99 Dependence on enabling machines and devices, not elsewhere classified
Note: Categories Z89–Z90 and Z93–Z99 are for use only if there are no complications or malfunctions of the organ or tissue replaced, the amputation site or the equipment on which the patient is dependent.

Guideline I.C.21.c.4. History (of): There are two types of history Z codes, personal and family. Personal history codes explain a patient's past medical condition that no longer exists and is not receiving any treatment, but that has the potential for recurrence, and therefore may require continued monitoring.

Family history codes are for use when a patient has a family member(s) who has had a particular disease that causes the patient to be at higher risk of also contracting the disease.

Personal history codes may be used in conjunction with follow-up codes and family history codes may be used in conjunction with screening codes to explain the need for a test or procedure. History codes are also acceptable on any medical record regardless of the reason for visit. A history of an illness, even if no longer present, is important information that may alter the type of treatment ordered.

The history Z code categories are:

Z80 Family history of primary malignant neoplasm

Z81 Family history of mental and behavioral disorders

Z82 Family history of certain disabilities and chronic diseases (leading to disablement)

Z83 Family history of other specific disorders

(Continued)

(Continued)

Z84 Family history of other conditions

Z85 Personal history of malignant neoplasm

Z86 Personal history of certain other diseases

Z87 Personal history of other diseases and conditions

Z91.4- Personal history of psychological trauma, not elsewhere classified

Z91.5 Personal history of self-harm

Z91.8- Other specified personal risk factors, not elsewhere classified

Exception:

Z91.83, Wandering in diseases classified elsewhere

Z92 Personal history of medical treatment

Except: Z92.0, Personal history of contraception

Except: Z92.82, Status post administration of tPA (rtPA) in a different facility within the last 24 hours prior to admission to a current facility

Guideline I.C.21.c.5. Screening: Screening is the testing for disease or disease precursors in seemingly well individuals so that early detection and treatment can be provided for those who test positive for the disease (e.g., screening mammogram).

The testing of a person to rule out or confirm a suspected diagnosis because the patient has some sign or symptom is a diagnostic examination, not a screening. In these cases, the sign or symptom is used to explain the reason for the test.

A screening code may be a first-listed code if the reason for the visit is specifically the screening exam. It may also be used as an additional code if the screening is done during an office visit for other health problems. A screening code is not necessary if the screening is inherent to a routine examination, such as a pap smear done during a routine pelvic examination.

Should a condition be discovered during the screening then the code for the condition may be assigned as an additional diagnosis.

The Z code indicates that a screening exam is planned. A procedure code is required to confirm that the screening was performed.

The screening Z codes/categories:

Z11 Encounter for screening for infectious and parasitic diseases

Z12 Encounter for screening for malignant neoplasms

Z13 Encounter for screening for other diseases and disorders

Except: Z13.9, Encounter for screening, unspecified

Z36 Encounter for antenatal screening for mother

Guideline I.C.21.c.6. Observation: There are two observation Z code categories. They are for use in very limited circumstances when a person is being observed for a suspected condition that is ruled out. The observation codes are not for use if an injury or illness or any signs or symptoms related to the suspected condition are present. In such cases the diagnosis/symptom code is used with the corresponding external cause code.

The observation codes are to be used as principal diagnosis only. Additional codes may be used in addition to the observation code but only if they are unrelated to the suspected condition being observed.

Codes from subcategory Z03.7, Encounter for suspected maternal and fetal conditions ruled out, may either be used as a first-listed or as an additional code assignment depending on the case. They are for use in very limited circumstances on a maternal record when an encounter is for a suspected maternal or fetal condition that is ruled out during that encounter (for example, a maternal or fetal condition may be suspected due to an abnormal test result). These codes should not be used when the condition is confirmed. In those cases, the confirmed condition should be coded. In addition, these codes are not for use if an illness or any signs or symptoms related to the suspected condition or problem are present. In such cases the diagnosis/symptom code is used.

Additional codes may be used in addition to the code from subcategory Z03.7, but only if they are unrelated to the suspected condition being evaluated.

Codes from subcategory Z03.7 may not be used for encounters for antenatal screening of mother. *See Section I.C.21. Screening.*

For encounters for suspected fetal condition that are inconclusive following testing and evaluation, assign the appropriate code from category O35, O36, O40 or O41.

The observation Z code categories:

Z03 Encounter for medical observation for suspected diseases and conditions ruled out

Z04 Encounter for examination and observation for other reasons

Except: Z04.9, Encounter for examination and observation for unspecified reason

(Continued)

(Continued)

Guideline I.C.21.c.7. Aftercare: Aftercare visit codes cover situations when the initial treatment of a disease has been performed and the patient requires continued care during the healing or recovery phase, or for the long-term consequences of the disease. The aftercare Z code should not be used if treatment is directed at a current, acute disease. The diagnosis code is to be used in these cases. Exceptions to this rule are codes Z51.0, Encounter for antineoplastic radiation therapy, and codes from subcategory Z51.1, Encounter for antineoplastic chemotherapy and immunotherapy. These codes are to be first-listed, followed by the diagnosis code when a patient's encounter is solely to receive radiation therapy, chemotherapy, or immunotherapy for the treatment of a neoplasm. If the reason for the encounter is more than one type of antineoplastic therapy, code Z51.0 and a code from subcategory Z51.1 may be assigned together, in which case one of these codes would be reported as a secondary diagnosis.

The aftercare Z codes should also not be used for aftercare for injuries. For aftercare of an injury, assign the acute injury code with the appropriate 7th character (for subsequent encounter).

The aftercare codes are generally first-listed to explain the specific reason for the encounter. An aftercare code may be used as an additional code when some type of aftercare is provided in addition to the reason for admission and no diagnosis code is applicable. An example of this would be the closure of a colostomy during an encounter for treatment of another condition.

Aftercare codes should be used in conjunction with other aftercare codes or diagnosis codes to provide better detail on the specifics of an aftercare encounter visit, unless otherwise directed by the classification. Should a patient receive multiple types of antineoplastic therapy during the same encounter, code Z51.0, Encounter for antineoplastic radiation therapy, and codes from subcategory Z51.1, Encounter for antineoplastic chemotherapy and immunotherapy, may be used together on a record. The sequencing of multiple aftercare codes depends on the circumstances of the encounter.

Certain aftercare Z code categories need a secondary diagnosis code to describe the resolving condition or sequelae. For others, the condition is included in the code title.

Additional Z code aftercare category terms include fitting and adjustment, and attention to artificial openings.

Status Z codes may be used with aftercare Z codes to indicate the nature of the aftercare. For example code Z95.1, Presence of aortocoronary bypass graft, may be used with code Z48.812,

Encounter for surgical aftercare following surgery on the circulatory system, to indicate the surgery for which the aftercare is being performed. A status code should not be used when the aftercare code indicates the type of status, such as using Z43.0, Encounter for attention to tracheostomy, with Z93.0, Tracheostomy status.

The aftercare Z category/codes:

Z42 Encounter for plastic and reconstructive surgery following medical procedure or healed injury

Z43 Encounter for attention to artificial openings

Z44 Encounter for fitting and adjustment of external prosthetic device

Z45 Encounter for adjustment and management of implanted device

Z46 Encounter for fitting and adjustment of other devices

Z47 Orthopedic aftercare

Z48 Encounter for other postprocedural aftercare

Z49 Encounter for care involving renal dialysis

Z51 Encounter for other aftercare

Guideline I.C.21.c.8. Follow-up: The follow-up codes are used to explain continuing surveillance following completed treatment of a disease, condition, or injury. They imply that the condition has been fully treated and no longer exists. They should not be confused with aftercare codes, or injury codes with a 7th character for subsequent encounter, that explain ongoing care of a healing condition or its sequelae. Follow-up codes may be used in conjunction with history codes to provide the full picture of the healed condition and its treatment. The follow-up code is sequenced first, followed by the history code.

A follow-up code may be used to explain multiple visits. Should a condition be found to have recurred on the follow-up visit, then the diagnosis code for the condition should be assigned in place of the follow-up code.

The follow-up Z code categories:

Z08 Encounter for follow-up examination after completed treatment for malignant neoplasm

Z09 Encounter for follow-up examination after completed treatment for conditions other than malignant neoplasm

Z39 Encounter for maternal postpartum care and examination

(Continued)

(Continued)

Guideline I.C.21.c.9. Donor: Codes in category Z52, Donors of organs and tissues, are used for living individuals who are donating blood or other body tissue. These codes are only for individuals donating for others, not for self-donations. They are not used to identify cadaveric donations.

Guideline I.C.21.c.10. Counseling: Counseling Z codes are used when a patient or family member receives assistance in the aftermath of an illness or injury, or when support is required in coping with family or social problems. They are not used in conjunction with a diagnosis code when the counseling component of care is considered integral to standard treatment.

The counseling Z codes/categories:

Z30.0- Encounter for general counseling and advice on contraception

Z31.5 Encounter for genetic counseling

Z31.6- Encounter for general counseling and advice on procreation

Z32.2 Encounter for childbirth instruction

Z32.3 Encounter for childcare instruction

Z69 Encounter for mental health services for victim and perpetrator of abuse

Z70 Counseling related to sexual attitude, behavior and orientation

Z71 Persons encountering health services for other counseling and medical advice, not elsewhere classified

Z76.81 Expectant mother prebirth pediatrician visit

Guideline I.C.21.c.11. Encounters for Obstetrical and Reproductive Services: *See Section I.C.15. Pregnancy, Childbirth, and the Puerperium, for further instruction on the use of these codes.*

Z codes for pregnancy are for use in those circumstances when none of the problems or complications included in the codes from the Obstetrics chapter exist (a routine prenatal visit or postpartum care). Codes in category Z34, Encounter for supervision of normal pregnancy, are always first-listed and are not to be used with any other code from the OB chapter. Codes in category Z3A, Weeks of gestation, may be assigned to provide additional information about the pregnancy.

The outcome of delivery, category Z37, should be included on all maternal delivery records. It is always a secondary code. Codes in category Z37 should not be used on the newborn record.

Z codes for family planning (contraceptive) or procreative management and counseling should be included on an obstetric record either during the pregnancy or the postpartum stage, if applicable.

Z codes/categories for obstetrical and reproductive services:

Z30 Encounter for contraceptive management

Z31 Encounter for procreative management

Z32.2 Encounter for childbirth instruction

Z32.3 Encounter for childcare instruction

Z33 Pregnant state

Z34 Encounter for supervision of normal pregnancy

Z36 Encounter for antenatal screening of mother

Z3A Weeks of gestation

Z37 Outcome of delivery

Z39 Encounter for maternal postpartum care and examination

Z76.81 Expectant mother prebirth pediatrician visit

Guideline. I.C.21.c.12. Newborns and Infants: *See Section I.C.16. Newborn (Perinatal) Guidelines, for further instruction on the use of these codes.*

Newborn Z codes/categories:

Z76.1 Encounter for health supervision and care of foundling

Z00.1- Encounter for routine child health examination

Z38 Liveborn infants according to place of birth and type of delivery

Guideline I.C.21.c.13. Routine and administrative examinations: The Z codes allow for the description of encounters for routine examinations, such as, a general check-up, or, examinations for administrative purposes, such as, a pre-employment physical. The codes are not to be used if the examination is for diagnosis of a suspected condition or for treatment purposes. In such cases the diagnosis code is used. During a routine exam, should a diagnosis or condition be discovered, it should be coded as an additional code. Pre-existing and chronic conditions and history codes may also be included as additional codes as long as the examination is for administrative purposes and not focused on any particular condition.

Some of the codes for routine health examinations distinguish between "with" and "without" abnormal findings. Code assignment depends on the information that is known at the time the

(Continued)

encounter is being coded. For example, if no abnormal findings were found during the examination, but the encounter is being coded before test results are back, it is acceptable to assign the code for "without abnormal findings." When assigning a code for "with abnormal findings," additional code(s) should be assigned to identify the specific abnormal finding(s).

Pre-operative examination and pre-procedural laboratory examination Z codes are for use only in those situations when a patient is being cleared for a procedure or surgery and no treatment is given.

The Z codes/categories for routine and administrative examinations:

Z00 Encounter for general examination without complaint, suspected or reported diagnosis

Z01 Encounter for other special examination without complaint, suspected or reported diagnosis

Z02 Encounter for administrative examination
Except: Z02.9, Encounter for administrative examinations, unspecified

Z32.0- Encounter for pregnancy test

Guideline I.C.21.c.14. Miscellaneous Z codes: The miscellaneous Z codes capture a number of other health care encounters that do not fall into one of the other categories. Certain of these codes identify the reason for the encounter; others are for use as additional codes that provide useful information on circumstances that may affect a patient's care and treatment.

Prophylactic Organ Removal: For encounters specifically for prophylactic removal of an organ (such as prophylactic removal of breasts due to a genetic susceptibility to cancer or a family history of cancer), the principal or first-listed code should be a code from category Z40, Encounter for prophylactic surgery, followed by the appropriate codes to identify the associated risk factor (such as genetic susceptibility or family history).

If the patient has a malignancy of one site and is having prophylactic removal at another site to prevent either a new primary malignancy or metastatic disease, a code for the malignancy should also be assigned in addition to a code from subcategory Z40.0, Encounter for prophylactic surgery for risk factors related to malignant neoplasms. A Z40.0 code should not be assigned if the patient is having organ removal for treatment of a malignancy, such as the removal of the testes for the treatment of prostate cancer.

Miscellaneous Z codes/categories:

Z28 Immunization not carried out
Except: Z28.3, Underimmunization status

Z40 Encounter for prophylactic surgery

Z41 Encounter for procedures for purposes other than remedying health state
Except: Z41.9, Encounter for procedure for purposes other than remedying health state, unspecified

Z53 Persons encountering health services for specific procedures and treatment, not carried out

Z55 Problems related to education and literacy

Z56 Problems related to employment and unemployment

Z57 Occupational exposure to risk factors

Z58 Problems related to physical environment

Z59 Problems related to housing and economic circumstances

Z60 Problems related to social environment

Z62 Problems related to upbringing

Z63 Other problems related to primary support group, including family circumstances

Z64 Problems related to certain psychosocial circumstances

Z65 Problems related to other psychosocial circumstances

Z72 Problems related to lifestyle

Z73 Problems related to life management difficulty

Z74 Problems related to care provider dependency

Except: Z74.01, Bed confinement status

Z75 Problems related to medical facilities and other health care

Z76.0 Encounter for issue of repeat prescription

Z76.3 Healthy person accompanying sick person

Z76.4 Other boarder to healthcare facility

Z76.5 Malingerer [conscious simulation]

Z91.1- Patient's noncompliance with medical treatment and regimen

Z91.83 Wandering in diseases classified elsewhere

Z91.89 Other specified personal risk factors, not elsewhere classified

(Continued)

(Continued)

Guideline I.C.21.c.15. Nonspecific Z codes: Certain Z codes are so non-specific, or potentially redundant with other codes in the classification, that there can be little justification for their use in the inpatient setting. Their use in the outpatient setting should be limited to those instances when there is no further documentation to permit more precise coding. Otherwise, any sign or symptom or any other reason for visit that is captured in another code should be used.

Nonspecific Z codes/categories:

Z02.9 Encounter for administrative examinations, unspecified

Z04.9 Encounter for examination and observation for unspecified reason

Z13.9 Encounter for screening, unspecified

Z41.9 Encounter for procedure for purposes other than remedying health state, unspecified

Z52.9 Donor of unspecified organ or tissue

Z86.59 Personal history of other mental and behavioral disorders

Z88.9 Allergy status to unspecified drugs, medicaments and biological substances status

Z92.0 Personal history of contraception

Guideline I.C.21.c.16. Z Codes That May Only be Principal/First-Listed Diagnosis: The following Z codes/categories may only be reported as the principal/first-listed diagnosis, except when there are multiple encounters on the same day and the medical records for the encounters are combined:

Z00 Encounter for general examination without complaint, suspected or reported diagnosis

Z01 Encounter for other special examination without complaint, suspected or reported diagnosis

Z02 Encounter for administrative examination

Z03 Encounter for medical observation for suspected diseases and conditions ruled out

Z04 Encounter for examination and observation for other reasons

Z33.2 Encounter for elective termination of pregnancy

Z31.81 Encounter for male factor infertility in female patient

Z31.82 Encounter for Rh incompatibility status

Z31.83 Encounter for assisted reproductive fertility procedure cycle

Z31.84 Encounter for fertility preservation procedure

Z34 Encounter for supervision of normal pregnancy

Z39 Encounter for maternal postpartum care and examination

Z38 Liveborn infants according to place of birth and type of delivery

Z42 Encounter for plastic and reconstructive surgery following medical procedure or healed injury

Z51.0 Encounter for antineoplastic radiation therapy

Z51.1- Encounter for antineoplastic chemotherapy and immunotherapy

Z52 Donors of organs and tissues

Except: Z52.9, Donor of unspecified organ or tissue

Z76.1 Encounter for health supervision and care of foundling

Z76.2 Encounter for health supervision and care of other healthy infant and child

Z99.12 Encounter for respirator [ventilator] dependence during power failure

Coding Factors Influencing Health Status and Contact with Health Services in ICD-10-CM Chapter 21

Z codes are intended to provide reasons for healthcare encounters in different types of settings: ambulatory, inpatient, and post-acute care. Z codes are diagnosis codes. If a procedure is performed during the encounter, a procedure code is required. The Z code for the reason for the visit does not state that a procedure was performed. Z codes are used for patients who may or may not be sick but the person needs healthcare services for a particular reason. Patients may need care for a current condition. The patient may be receiving prophylactic vaccination or immunization. An organ or tissue donor is identified with a Z code. A patient may need counseling or other services to address a problem that is not a disease or illness. The patient may be at risk for a disease that is identified with a Z code. Many times a coder will use a Z code to describe a condition or problem that has an impact on the patient's health status and need for health services but the situation described by the Z code is not a current illness or injury. An outline of the Z codes is as follows:

Z00–Z13 Persons encountering health services for examinations

EXAMPLES: Z00.00 Encounter for general adult medical examination without abnormal findings
Z00.01 Encounter for general adult medical examination with abnormal findings

Z14–Z15   Genetic carrier and genetic susceptibility to disease

      EXAMPLES: Z14.01   Asymptomatic hemophilia A carrier
                                 Z15.01   Genetic susceptibility to malignant neoplasm of breast

Z16   Resistance to antimicrobial drugs
Z17   Estrogen receptor status
Z20–Z28   Persons with potential health hazards related to communicable diseases

      EXAMPLES: Z21   Asymptomatic human immunodeficiency virus (HIV) infection
                                 Z23   Encounter for immunization

Z30–Z39   Persons encountering health services in circumstances related to reproduction

      EXAMPLES: Z30.011 Encounter for initial prescription of contraceptive pills
                                 Z34.81   Encounter for supervision of other normal pregnancy, first trimester
                                 Z37   Outcome of delivery
                                 Z38   Liveborn infants according to place of birth and type of delivery
                                 Z3A   Weeks of gestation

Z40–Z53   Encounters for other specific health care

      EXAMPLES: Z48.22   Encounter for aftercare following kidney transplant
                                 Z51.11   Encounter for antineoplastic chemotherapy

Z55–Z65   Persons with potential health hazards related to socioeconomic and psychosocial circumstances

      EXAMPLES: Z59.5   Extreme poverty
                                   Z62.0   Inadequate parental supervision and control

Z66   Do not resuscitate (DNR) status
Z67   Blood type
Z68   Body mass index
Z69–Z76   Persons encountering health services in other circumstances

      EXAMPLES: Z71.42   Counseling for family member of alcoholic
                                 Z72.0   Tobacco use

Z77–Z99   Persons with potential health hazards related to family and personal history and certain conditions influencing health status

      EXAMPLES: Z79.4   Long term (current) use of insulin
                                 Z85.3   Personal history of malignant neoplasm of breast

There is an explanation of the use of the codes with a note at the beginning of the chapter:

Z codes represent reasons for encounters. A corresponding procedure code must accompany a Z code if a procedure is performed. Categories Z00–Z99 are provided for occasions when circumstances other than a disease, injury or external cause classifiable to categories A00–Y89 are recorded as "diagnoses" or "problems." This can arise in two main ways:

1. When a person who may or may not be sick encounters the health services for some specific purpose, such as to receive limited care or service for a current condition, to donate an organ or tissue, to receive prophylactic vaccination (immunization), or to discuss a problem which is in itself not a disease or injury.

2. When some circumstance or problem is present which influences the person's health status but is not in itself a current illness or injury (NCHS 2012).

Z code classifications are available for the following situations:

• When a person who is currently not sick uses health services for some purpose, such as acting as a donor, receiving prophylactic care such as an inoculation or vaccination, or receiving counseling on health-related issues.

> **EXAMPLE:** Patient was admitted to donate bone marrow for another patient: Z52.3, Bone marrow donor

• When a person with a resolving disease or injury or one with a chronic long-term condition requiring continuous care encounters the healthcare system for specific aftercare of that disease or injury (for example, chemotherapy for malignancy). A diagnosis or symptom code should be used whenever a current, acute diagnosis is being treated or a sign or symptom is being studied.

> **EXAMPLE:** Patient is admitted for antineoplastic radiation therapy, Z51.0

• When circumstances or problems influence a person's health status but are not in themselves a current illness or injury.

> **EXAMPLE:** Patient visits physician's office with a complaint of chest pain with an undetermined cause; patient is status post open-heart surgery for mitral valve replacement, 6 months ago: R07.9, Chest pain, unspecified; Z95.2, Presence of prosthetic heart valve

• For newborns, to indicate birth status.

> **EXAMPLE:** Single newborn delivered via cesarean section: Z38.01, Single live-born delivered by cesarean delivery

Z codes are assigned more frequently in hospital ambulatory care departments and other primary care sites, such as physicians' offices, than in acute inpatient facilities. Z codes may be used as either a first-listed (principal diagnosis code in the inpatient setting) or secondary code depending on the circumstances of the encounter. Certain Z codes may only be used as first listed, others only as secondary codes.

Main Terms

Z codes are indexed in the Alphabetic Index to Diseases along with codes for diseases, conditions, and symptoms. It is necessary, however, to become familiar with the main terms in the Alphabetic Index to Diseases that are related to Z codes. First, look for terms that describe the reason for the encounter or admission. The terms documented in the health record will often not lead to the appropriate code.

Then ask: Why is the patient receiving services?

> **EXAMPLE:** The health record states closure of colostomy: Z43.3, Encounter for attention to colostomy

The statement in the preceding example requires a Z code (Z43.3) because the patient was admitted for attention to an artificial opening. In addition, a procedure code must be assigned for the actual surgical closure.

Figure 24.1 shows how the main terms in the Alphabetic Index to Diseases lead to Z codes.

Figure 24.1   Main terms leading to Z codes

Admission (encounter)	Donor	Pregnancy
Aftercare	Encounter for	Problem
Attention to	Examination	Prophylactic
Boarder	Exposure	Replacement by artificial or
Care (of)	Fitting (of)	mechanical device or prosthesis of
Carrier (suspected) of	Follow-up	Resistance, resistant
Checking	Healthy	Screening
Chemotherapy	History (personal) of	Status (post)
Contact	Maintenance	Supervision (of)
Contraception, contraceptives	Maladjustment	Test(s)
Counseling	Newborn	Therapy
Dependence	Observation	Transplant(ed)
Dialysis	Outcome of delivery	Unavailability of medical facilities
		Vaccination

Persons Encountering Health Services for Examination (Z00–Z13)

The codes from this section are used for patients who may not be acutely ill but require or request an examination by a healthcare provider for routine physical examinations and other administrative purposes such as examinations for pre-employment, entrance into the military, sports participation, and insurance reasons. Other codes here identify patients who must be observed for suspected conditions that later were proven not to exist or for follow-up examinations following the completed treatment of malignant neoplasms and other health conditions.

Category Z00, Encounter for General Examination without Complaint, Suspected or Reported Diagnosis

The codes in category Z00 describe reasonably healthy adults and children who seek healthcare services for routine examinations, such as a general physical examination. Generally, the codes are only used as first-listed diagnoses. If a diagnosis or condition is identified during the course of the general medical examination, it should be reported as an additional diagnosis code. Preexisting or chronic conditions, as well as history codes, may also be used as additional diagnoses as long as the examination was for an administrative purpose and not focused on treatment of the medical condition. Nonspecific abnormal findings found at the time of these examinations are classified to categories R70–R94. These codes are indexed in the Alphabetic Index under "Admission (encounter), for, examination" and "Examination."

In subcategory Z00.0, Encounter for general adult medical examination, there are two specific codes to distinguish between the examination without abnormal findings and an examination when abnormal findings are identified. In this case, the coder would use an additional code to identify the abnormal finding or disease.

> **EXAMPLE:** A 55-year-old man has an appointment at his primary care physician's office for his annual physical examination. The patient has mild eczema that is treated with over-the-counter lotions, and he had an inguinal hernia repaired during the past year.
>
> Z00.01, Encounter for general adult medical examination with abnormal findings; Eczema, L30.9. The hernia is not coded because it no longer exists.

Subcategory Z00.1, Encounter for newborn, infant and child health examination identifies outpatient clinic or doctor office encounters with newborns and young children. Z00.12, Encounter for routine infant or child health examination, identifies a child over 28 days old who the physician may identify as a "well baby" or "well child" visit in the office or clinic when the infant or child does not have an illness but is seen for developmental testing, immunizations, or routine health checkups. Two specific codes, Z00.110, Health examination for newborn under eight days old and Z00.111, Health examination for newborn 8 to 28 days old, were created for specific post-hospital newborn care visits in the doctor's office or clinic. Most healthy newborns are discharged from the hospital less than 48 hours after birth. Pediatric care standards recommend an examination by the physician within two days of that discharge or no later than 28 days after birth. During this encounter the infant is evaluated for feeding, jaundice, hydration, and elimination problems; the clinician also assesses how well mother and infant are interacting, reviews the newborn's laboratory and screening tests, and communicates the plan for healthcare maintenance, future immunizations, and periodic examinations.

Other subcategory codes under Z00 identify examinations for a period of rapid growth in childhood, for adolescent development state, for a potential donor of organ and tissue, and for normal comparison and control in a clinical research program, along with examinations during periods of delayed growth in childhood. Finally, one code, Z00.8, Encounter for other general examination, is used for a health examination in a population survey, for example, a public health study.

Category Z01, Encounter for Other Special Examination without Complaint, Suspected or Reported Condition

Category Z01, Encounter for other special examination without complaint, suspected, or reported condition is used to identify the reason for another type of encounter. A separate procedure code is used to identify the examination or procedure actually performed. Subcategory codes under Z01 are used to code visits for eye and vision examinations, ear and hearing examinations, dental examinations and cleanings. and blood pressure examinations. There are specific codes under subcategory Z01 that state whether or not an abnormal finding was identified during the examination. If there was an abnormal finding, a note reminds the coder to use an additional code to identify the abnormal finding. A frequently used set of codes here will be used for "encounter for routine gynecological examination." The coder is reminded with a "use additional code" note to add a code for screening for human papillomavirus, if applicable (Z11.51), for screening vaginal pap smear, if applicable (Z12.72), and to identify acquired absence of uterus, if applicable (Z90.71-). Again there are options to report the routine gynecological examination with and without abnormal findings.

Another subcategory code, Encounter for other specified special examination, Z01.8-, will be used for preprocedural cardiovascular and respiratory examinations provided to the patient, which include physical examinations as well as visits specifically for radiological examinations, laboratory examinations, and preoperative examinations. Coding guidelines state for encounters for routine laboratory or radiology testing in the absence of any signs, symptoms, or associated diagnosis, the coder should assign a code from subcategory Z01. If routine testing is performed during the same encounter as a test to evaluate a sign, symptom, or diagnosis, it is appropriate to assign both the Z code and the codes describing the reason for the nonroutine test. For patients receiving preoperative evaluations only, the coder should sequence first a code from subcategory Z01.81 to describe the pre-op consultation. Then the coder should assign a code for the condition to describe the reason for the surgery as an additional diagnosis. The coder would also assign an additional code for any diagnosis or problem for which the service is being performed.

> **EXAMPLE:** Patient is examined in the cardiologist's office for a preprocedural cardiovascular examination prior to scheduled surgery for a right hip replacement for osteoarthritis of the right hip. The patient is known to have essential hypertension as well. The codes to be assigned are:
>
> Z01.810, Encounter for preprocedural cardiovascular examination
> M16.11, Osteoarthritis of right hip
> I10, Essential hypertension

The codes in category Z01 are not used for examinations for administrative purposes (Z02.-), for suspected conditions proven not to exist (Z03.-), for laboratory or radiology examinations as a component of general medical examinations (Z00.0-), or for encounters for laboratory, radiology, and imaging examinations for signs and symptoms. In those circumstances when a sign or symptom exists, the code for the sign or symptom should be used instead of the Z01 category codes.

Category Z03, Encounter for Medical Observation for Suspected Diseases and Conditions Ruled Out

Category Z03, Encounter for medical observation for suspected diseases and conditions ruled out, is used when a person without a diagnosis is suspected of having an abnormal condition. The patient does not have any signs or symptoms. However, the patient requires study for the suspected condition. However, test results and examinations prove the condition does not exist or is **ruled out**. Again, if the patient has signs and symptoms of a suspected disease, the coder should assign a code for the sign or symptom instead of the Z03 category codes. Conditions that are were ruled out and reported with the Z03 category codes include toxic effect from ingested substance, problem with amniotic fluids in the pregnant female, suspected fetal anomaly, and suspected exposure to biological agents.

Category Z04, Encounter for Examination and Observation for Other Reasons

Category Z04, Encounter for examination and observation for other reasons, includes encounters primarily for medical legal reasons. This category is used when a person is suspected of having an abnormal condition but does not have signs or symptoms of the condition. The patient is examined and tests may be done and after study it is proven the condition does not exist or it is ruled out. Codes from this category would be assigned to patients who were seen for examination and observation following various events, such as a work accident, other accident, alleged rape, or requested psychiatric examination by authority (usually a court system), and following alleged physical abuse.

Encounter for Follow-up Examination after Completed Treatment for Malignant Neoplasm (Z08) and Encounter for Follow-up Examination after Completed Treatment for Conditions Other Than Malignant Neoplasm (Z09)

Together, Z08 and Z09 category codes are called follow-up codes. The **follow-up codes** are used to explain medical surveillance following completed treatment of a disease, condition, or injury. The code means the patient has been fully treated for the condition that no longer exists. These codes are not the same as the aftercare codes in ICD-10-CM or the injury codes with a seventh character for subsequent encounter, which explain ongoing care of a healing condition or its sequelae. Follow-up codes may be used in conjunction with history codes to provide the full picture of the healed condition and its treatment. The follow-up code is sequenced first, followed by the history code. A patient may have multiple visits for follow-up for these conditions and the codes may be used each time. If a condition is found to have recurred during the follow-up visit, a diagnosis code for the condition would be assigned instead of the Z08 or Z09 follow-up code. Two notes appear under category code Z08 to remind the coder to use an additional code for any acquired absence of organ (Z90.-) and an additional code for a personal history of malignant neoplasm (Z85.-). Under category code Z09, a "use additional code" note appears to remind the coder to assign any applicable history of disease code (Z86.-, Z87.-). The coder must be aware that these codes are intended to represent the visit of a patient who has completed treatment for a condition and is being "followed" to assure the patient remains disease free. The coder must also be aware the term follow-up as it is intended in ICD-10-CM can be different from what a physician intends to describe when he uses the same phrase. When a physician documents follow-up, the physician may be describing ongoing medical treatment or a recovery phase of the illness or recent surgery. Categories Z08 and Z09 are to be used only to describe an encounter where the treatment of the condition is completed, and the patient is undergoing surveillance or a checkup to determine if his or her disease-free status continues. When a physician states follow-up for hypertension that remains under treatment or follow-up after recent cardiac surgery, the Z09 category is unlikely to be the appropriate set of codes to use. In these circumstances described by the physician, the hypertension under treatment is likely to be coded or a surgical aftercare code may be more appropriate to describe the healing or recovery phase after surgery. Codes in this category are indexed "Examination, follow-up" in the Alphabetic Index.

EXAMPLE: Patient admitted for follow-up cystoscopy to rule out recurrence of malignant neoplasm of the urinary bladder; patient had a transurethral resection of the bladder 1 year ago and has been cancer-free to date; cystoscopy revealed no recurrence: Z08, Follow-up examination after completed treatment for malignant neoplasm; Z85.51, History of malignant neoplasm of the urinary bladder. A procedure code would be assigned for the cystoscopy.

Encounter for Screening for Malignant Neoplasms, Z12

Category Z12 is used to describe when a patient is being examined by a screening examination. **Screening** is defined in ICD-10-CM as testing for a disease in asymptomatic patients. These patients do not have signs of symptoms of a disease. Instead the screening is intended to detect an unidentified condition so that it can be treated promptly. A note appears with category Z12 codes to use an additional code to identify any family history of malignant neoplasm (Z80.-) as patients with a family history of malignancy puts the patient at higher risk of having the same or related condition. Codes in this category that will be used frequently are Z12.11, Encounter for screening for malignant neoplasm of colon or otherwise described as an encounter for a screening colonoscopy and Z12.31, Encounter for screening mammogram for malignant neoplasm of breast. Two other commonly used codes are Z12.4, Encounter for screening for malignant neoplasm of cervix when the physician performs a screening Pap smear on an asymptomatic female patient and Z12.72, Encounter for screening for malignant neoplasm of vagina when the physician performs a vaginal Pap smear on a patient who has had a hysterectomy that included the removal of the cervix. If the patient had any signs or symptoms, category codes from Z12 would not be used but rather the diagnosis codes for the signs or symptoms are assigned for the encounter.

Encounter for Screening for Other Diseases and Disorders, Z13

Category Z13 is used to describe a screening procedure on an asymptomatic patient for a condition other than malignant neoplasms. If a patient had signs or symptoms, these conditions would be coded instead of a Z13 category code. A screening procedure is performed on an asymptomatic patient. The commonly used codes in this category are encounter for screening for certain developmental disorders in childhood (Z13.4), encounter for screening for osteoporosis (Z13.820), and encounter for screening of traumatic brain injury (Z13.850).

Genetic Carrier and Genetic Susceptibility to Disease (Z14–Z15)

Codes in category Z14, **Genetic carrier**, are intended to describe a patient who is known to carry a particular gene that could cause a disease to be passed on to his or her children. The code does not mean the patient has this particular disease. It also does not mean there is 100 percent certainty that the disease would be passed on genetically to the next generation. The code could be used to explain why a patient is receiving additional monitoring or testing. The codes in this category identify patients who are asymptomatic and symptomatic hemophilia A carriers, cystic fibrosis carriers, and genetic carriers of another disease.

Codes in category Z15, **Genetic susceptibility** to disease, are intended to describe a patient who has a confirmed abnormal gene that makes the patient more susceptible to a particular disease. Subcategory Z15.0, Genetic susceptibility to malignant neoplasm, is used with an additional code for any personal history of malignant neoplasm (Z85.-) if applicable. If the patient has a current malignant neoplasm (C00–C75, C81–C96), the code for the current neoplasm is sequenced first before the genetic susceptibility code. Genetic susceptibility to malignant neoplasms of breast, ovary, prostate, endometrium, and other specified sites are reported with these subcategory codes.

Resistance to Antimicrobial Drugs (Z16)

Category Z16, Resistance to antimicrobial drugs, should be used as an additional code to indicate the **resistance** and nonresponsiveness of a condition to an antimicrobial drug. An important note,

"Code first the infection," appears here to identify the type and site of the current infection present in the patient that is known to be resistant to these drugs. If the patient has a methicillin resistant Staphylococcus infection, other codes in ICD-10-CM should be used in place of the Z16 codes, for example, A49.02, Methicillin resistant Staphylococcus aureus infection, unspecified site; J15.212, Pneumonia due to Methicillin resistant Staphylococcus aureus; and A41.02, Sepsis due to Methicillin resistant Staphylococcus aureus. The coder should sequence the infection code first and then the Z16 code. Z16 codes are to be used when the documentation in the health record indicates that a patient's infection has a known causative bacteria or other organism that is resistant to the medication therapy administered. Subcategory Z16.1 is used to identify patients with resistance to beta lactam antibiotics, such as pencillins and cephalosporins. Subcategory Z16.2 is used to identify patients with resistance to other antibiotics, such as vancomycins, vancomycin related antibiotics, quinolones, or other multiple or single specified antibiotics. Subcategory Z16.3 is used to identify resistance in a patient to such drugs as antiparasitic, antifungal or antimycobacterial preparations. The organism resistance codes are indexed under the main term "Resistance, resistant, organism (to) drug, followed by the drug" type or name.

EXAMPLE: Sepsis (A41.9) with infection resistant to vancomycin (Z16.21)

Estrogen Receptor Status (Z17)

The status codes Z17.0, Estrogen receptor positive status [ER+] or Z17.1, Estrogen receptor negative status [ER–] are used as an additional code for patients who have been diagnosed with breast cancer, both females and males, and have had their estrogen receptor status determined. About two-thirds of breast cancer patients have an estrogen receptor positive [ER+] tumor. The incidence is greater among postmenopausal women. These patients are more likely to benefit from endocrine therapies, so knowledge of their receptor status is important in the selection of adjuvant or palliative therapy. Oral hormones, such as tamoxifen, and estrogen ablation by oophorectomy have proven effective to prolong the duration of disease-free survival, as well as for palliation in the patient with advanced disease when the patient's tumor was estrogen receptor positive.

Retained Foreign Body Fragment (Z18)

Category Z18 contains codes created for embedded foreign body fragment status to identify the type of embedded material. The codes were requested primarily to identify military personnel who have had an injury, most likely from an explosion that resulted in embedded fragments remaining in the body because the location of the fragment makes it too difficult to remove. Any embedded object has the potential to cause infection due to the object itself or any organism present on it when it entered the body. An embedded magnetic object is a contraindication to certain imaging studies and can pose long-term toxicological hazards. Codes in the range of Z18.0–Z18.9 identify radioactive, metal, plastic, organic, and other types of foreign body fragments. Another code, Z87.821, identifies the personal history of a retained foreign body having been removed. An Excludes1 note appears under category Z18 to direct the coder to other ICD-10-CM diagnosis codes that describe other types of foreign body that may be present in the patient.

Persons with Potential Health Hazards Related to Communicable Diseases (Z20–Z28)

Codes from categories Z20–Z28 are assigned when a patient has come in contact with, or has been exposed to, a communicable disease. The person does not show any signs or symptoms of the disease he or she was exposed to or came in contact with.

Category Z20, Contact with and (Suspected) Exposure to Communicable Diseases

The Z20 category codes for contact and exposure or suspected exposure to communicable disease may be used as the first-listed code to explain an encounter for testing. However, these codes may be used more commonly as secondary codes to identify a potential health risk. The types of communicable disease that the patient may have come in contact with include E. coli intestinal disease, tuberculosis, sexually transmitted disease, rabies, rubella, viral hepatitis, HIV, anthrax, varicella, and other and unspecified communicable diseases.

Category Z21, Asymptomatic Human Immunodeficiency Virus (HIV) Infection Status

The Z21 code indicates the patient has tested positive for the HIV virus but has not manifested symptoms of HIV or AIDS. The health record documentation may include "HIV positive." This code should not be confused with code B20, human immunodeficiency virus [HIV] disease or AIDS, which means the patient has the consequences of human immunodeficiency virus in the blood that causes the patient to have certain neoplasms or infections as a result of their immune compromised condition. A "code first" note appears under code Z21 to code HIV disease complicating pregnancy, childbirth, and the pueperium, if applicable, with O98.7-.

Category Z22, Carrier of Infectious Disease

The Z22 category codes describe colonization status or the presence on or in the body of a particular organism without it causing an illness in the patient. Codes within this category recognize carrier status for typhoid, diphtheria, specific bacterial diseases, sexually transmitted disease, viral hepatitis, and other viral and infectious diseases. Some of the commonly used codes in this category are Z22.330, carrier of group B streptococcus, Z22.321, Carrier or suspected carrier of Methicillin susceptible Staphylococcus aureus (MSSA), Z22.322, Carrier or suspected carrier Methicillin resistant Staphylococcus aureus (MRSA), and Z22.52, Carrier of viral hepatitis C. Many hospitals test patients routinely for MRSA colonization by performing a nasal swab test upon admission that can identify positive or negative MRSA colonization in the patient.

The category Z22 codes indicate that the patient is either a carrier or suspected carrier of an infectious disease but currently does not exhibit the symptoms of the disease. Status codes in the Z code classification are informational because the conditions they describe may affect the course of treatment. Remember, "status" is different from "history" in ICD-10-CM. The history codes indicate the patient no longer has the disease.

Categories Z23, Encounter for Immunization and Z28, Immunization Not Carried Out and Underimmunization Status

These codes are located in the Alphabetic Index under the main terms "Immunization," "Prophylactic," and "Vaccination."

> **EXAMPLE:** Immunization encounter: Z23, Need for prophylactic vaccination

Category Z23, Encounter for immunization is a three-character code that is used for any encounter when the purpose of the visit is to receive prophylactic inoculation against a disease.

A procedure code must also be used to show the inoculation occurred. Vaccinations and inoculation codes may be used as secondary codes during well-baby or well-child care visits if the service was given as part of routine preventive healthcare. The type of vaccine administered is not identified by diagnosis code Z23. Under category code Z23 is a "code first" note to code any routine child examination.

Category Z28, Immunization Not Carried Out and Underimmunization Status

Codes Z28.01 through Z28.9 describe specific reasons why an immunization or vaccination was not given. The reasons an immunization may not be given are medical contraindications, for example the patient has an acute or chronic illness or an allergy, or the patient is immune compromised, which are all reasons not to receive vaccinations. Other reasons are patient's decisions not to become immunized for reasons of belief or group pressure or simply because the patient refuses the vaccination. Other reasons identified with the codes are the fact that the patient has already had the illness the vaccine is intended to prevent or the immunization was not carried out because of the caregiver, parent or guardian's refusal to have it done. Tracking why an immunization was not given can be as important as tracking those that are given, according to the American Academy of Pediatrics. These codes identify the multiple reasons why a patient did not receive a routine immunization. Another important health status that can be identified with these codes is the fact that the person or child is "underimmunized." Code Z28.3, **Underimmunization** status, identifies the patient who has not received the vaccinations that are appropriate for the person's age. The doctor may describe this status in the record as "delinquent immunization status" or "lapsed immunization scheduled status."

Persons Encountering Health Services in Circumstances Related to Reproduction (Z30–Z39)

The codes from this section are used to describe healthcare services related to contraceptive and procreative management. Examples of codes in this section are codes that describe the status of the newborn at the time of the birth including the place where the infant was born and the type of delivery the mother experienced with this newborn. Other codes in this section identify how many infants were born to a mother, such as a single live birth, twins, triplets, and other types of multiple births. Codes in this section are also used to describe the supervision of pregnancy care provided to the pregnant woman during an uncomplicated, normal pregnancy.

Category Z30, Encounter for Contraceptive Management

Category Z30 includes codes for contraceptive management, such as initial prescription of contraceptives, counseling and instruction for natural family planning and other general contraceptive counseling and advice. Codes from this category are indexed under "Contraception, contraceptive" in the Alphabetic Index.

> **EXAMPLE:** Visit to physician for prescription of initial prescription of birth control pills: Z30.011, Encounter for initial prescription of contraceptive pills

Code Z30.2, Encounter for sterilization, is often assigned as an additional diagnosis when a sterilization procedure is performed during the same admission as a delivery. It may also be assigned as a principal diagnosis when the admission is solely for sterilization.

> **EXAMPLE:** Spontaneous delivery of full-term live infant with tubal ligation performed the day after delivery: O80, Encounter for full-term uncomplicated delivery; Z37.0, Outcome of delivery, single live birth; Z30.2, Encounter for sterilization with a procedure code to describe the specific delivery and sterilization procedure

> **EXAMPLE:** Patient desires permanent sterilization: Z30.2 with a procedure code for the specific sterilization procedure performed

Subcategory codes Z30.4 are used to report encounters for surveillance of contraceptives, which include encounters for repeat prescription for contraceptive pills as well as surveillance of injectable contraceptive. These subcategory codes are frequently used for office visits when the encounter is for the insertion of an intrauterine device (IUD) (Z30.430), for removal of an IUD (Z30.432), and for removal and reinsertion of an IUD (Z30.433). An encounter for routine checking of an IUD would be reported with code Z30.431, Encounter for routine checking of intrauterine contraceptive device.

Category Z31, Encounter for Procreative Management

Procreative management describes healthcare services related to producing an offspring. Services related to genetic testing and infertility services can be described with these codes. Screening for genetic carrier status is becoming more commonplace to identify individuals for certain serious genetic disease. For example, a couple may be screened either preconception or early in pregnancy to determine carrier status. If both partners are carriers, different pregnancy management may be instituted. Carrier status screening has become the professional standard of care for cystic fibrosis, Canavan disease, hemoglobinopathies, and Tay-Sachs disease. Because most of the individuals are noncarriers, it is inappropriate to use disease codes to describe the screening encounter; instead, subcategory codes Z31.43- is used to identify an encounter for genetic testing of female for procreative management and/or Z31.44- is used to identify the testing of the male partner for genetic disease carrier status. Other codes within category Z31 identify encounters for genetic counseling and advice on procreation as well as such specific codes as Z31.83 for an encounter for assisted reproductive fertility procedure cycle. Healthcare encounters for reversal of a previous tubal ligation or vasectomy, artificial insemination, procreative investigation and testing, and genetic counseling are also coded within this category.

Category Z32, Encounter for Pregnancy Test and Childbirth and Childcare Instruction

Subcategory code Z32.0, Encounter for pregnancy test, contains codes to identify an encounter when the result of a pregnancy test is positive, negative, or unknown. Other codes in this category describe encounters for childbirth and childcare instructions.

Category Z33, Pregnant State

Code Z33.1, Pregnant state, incidental, is used to identify the fact that a patient is pregnant. This code is used when the provider documents that the pregnancy is incidental or unrelated to the encounter. In that event, code Z33.1 is used in place of an obstetric code from Chapter 15. It is the provider's responsibility to state that the patient's condition being treated is not affecting the pregnancy.

Code Z33.2, Encounter for Elective Termination of Pregnancy

Category Z33.2 is used to code the healthcare encounter when a patient has requested an elective abortion or termination of pregnancy. A procedure code would be used to identify the abortion procedure performed. This code would not be used if the encounter was for the purpose of completing a procedure to terminate the pregnancy because of an early fetal death with retention of the dead fetus or because of a late fetal death that requires a pregnancy termination; it is also not applicable to the treatment of a patient with a spontaneous abortion.

Category Z34, Encounter for Supervision of Normal Pregnancy

Codes in category Z34 are assigned for supervision of a pregnancy. Codes Z34.0, Encounter for supervision of normal first pregnancy, and Z34.8, Encounter for supervision of other normal pregnancy, are generally used in outpatient settings and for routine prenatal visits. The fifth character with these codes identifies whether the patient is in her first, second, or third trimester of pregnancy. When a complication of the pregnancy is present, the code for that condition is assigned rather than a code from category Z34. These codes are not used with any other pregnancy code in Chapter 15 of ICD-10-CM because the Z34 code indicates the patient is pregnant and healthy, whereas the Chapter 15 codes indicate an obstetrical problem or condition exists. Code category Z34 is indexed under "Pregnancy, normal, supervision (of) (for)" in the Alphabetic Index to Diseases.

Category Z36, Encounter for Antenatal Screening of Mother

Code Z36, Encounter for **antenatal screening** of mother, describes the testing of the female during pregnancy for a variety of conditions and abnormalities. These codes, which are intended to describe the female, not the fetus, are used to indicate the screening was planned. Some of these screening procedures have become common during the antepartum period. If the screening test results are returned with abnormal findings or determine that a condition is present, the abnormal finding or condition should be coded as an additional code with the Z36 screening category code. The Z36 code is not used if the testing of the female is to rule out or confirm a suspected diagnosis because the patient has some sign or symptom. That is a diagnostic examination and the sign or symptom code is used to explain the reason for the test. The Z36 code also indicates that the screening examination was planned. A procedure code is required to confirm that the screening was performed.

Category Z3A, Weeks of Gestation

Codes from category Z3A are used on the mother's record to indicate the weeks of gestation for the current pregnancy. The coder must first assign the diagnosis codes for the complications of pregnancy, childbirth, and the puerperium (O00–O9A). These codes are used at any time during the patient's pregnancy and not just at the time of the delivery.

Category Z37, Outcome of Delivery

A code from category Z327, **Outcome of delivery**, should be included on every maternal record when a delivery has occurred. These codes are not to be used on subsequent postpartum records or on the newborn record. They are always secondary codes on the maternal record at the time of delivery. The Z37 code indicates whether the delivery produced a single or multiple birth and whether the infants were live births or stillbirths. The unspecified code, Z37.9, should not be used because the maternal health record will identify the details of the delivery. Codes in category Z37 are indexed under "Outcome of delivery" in the Alphabetic Index.

EXAMPLE: Spontaneous delivery of full-term live infant: O80, Encounter for full-term uncomplicated; Z37.0, Outcome of delivery, single live birth

Category Z37 codes are only assigned to the mother's health record. These codes should not appear on the baby's health record. Do not confuse the Z37 maternal codes with the Z38 liveborn infant codes that are used to describe the newborn's birth status.

Category Z38, Liveborn Infants According to Place of Birth and Type of Delivery

A code from categories Z38.0 through Z38.8 is used to identify all types of births and is always the first code listed on the health record of the newborn. The Z38 code is used "once in a lifetime" when the infant is born. The Z38 category code is used as the principal code on the initial record of the newborn infant. If the newborn is transferred to another institution, the Z38 code is not used at the second institution or on the infant's subsequent admissions or outpatient visits to any healthcare provider. The Z38 codes describe single or multiple live births, and single or multiple stillborns. Codes for these categories are indexed under "Newborn" in the Alphabetic Index. Using the Alphabetic Index and the main term "Newborn, born in hospital or born outside of hospital" the next information to be reviewed is the birth status of the infant: single, twin, triplet, quadruplet, quintuplet, or other multiple liveborn infant born to the same mother. If the infant was a single birth, the next information needed is whether the baby was born in or outside the hospital. If the infant was born inside the hospital, was the birth a vaginal or cesarean delivery? In addition to the Z38 category code, any disease or birth injury should also be coded as additional diagnoses, if applicable, on the infant's record.

Encounters for Other Specific Health Care (Z40–Z53)

CMS includes the following important note for categories Z40–Z53 at the beginning of this block of codes: "Categories Z40–Z53 are intended for use to indicate a reason for care in patients who may have already been treated for some disease or injury not now present, or who are receiving aftercare or prophylactic care consolidate the treatment or to deal with residual states."

Category Z40, Encounter for Prophylactic Surgery

A patient who has a genetic susceptibility to a disease, particularly if it is a malignancy, may request prophylactic removal of an organ to prevent the disease from occurring. These codes can be used to identify encounters for prophylactic organ removal, including breast, ovary, or removal of another organ. A note is included to "use additional code" to identify the risk factor leading to this surgery.

Category Z43, Encounter for Attention to Artificial Openings

Category Z43 describes attention to the artificial opening, which may include the following services:

* Closure of artificial openings

* Passage of sounds or bougies through artificial openings

- Reforming of artificial openings

- Removal or replacement of catheter from artificial openings

- Toileting or cleansing of artificial openings

Category Z43 codes may be first-listed diagnoses or used as additional diagnosis codes. These codes identify encounters for catheter cleaning, fitting, and adjustment services, and other care that is distinct from actual treatment. These codes are not used when there is a complication of the external stoma.

EXAMPLE:	Emergency department visit for a patient who needs replacement of a clogged gastrostomy tube: Z43.1, Encounter for attention to gastrostomy
EXAMPLE:	A patient is admitted for a scheduled closure of a colostomy: Z43.3, Encounter for attention to colostomy
EXAMPLE:	Encounter for replacement of cystostomy tube: Z43.5, Encounter for attention to cystostomy

Category Z47, Orthopedic Aftercare

Category Z47 is subdivided to describe particular orthopedic **aftercare**. Subcategory code Z47.1 is used to describe an encounter for aftercare following joint replacement surgery. An additional code is used with Z47.1 to identify the joint (Z96.6-). Subcategory Z47.2, Encounter for removal of internal fixation device is used to code the reason for the visit when a fixation device, such as a screw, plate, or pin for example, is removed from the body. Subcategory code Z47.3 is subdivided to identify aftercare following explantation of joint prosthesis, specifically shoulder joint, hip joint, or knee joint. The intent of these codes is to identify the healthcare encounter for the patient who has had their artificial joint removed, usually because of an infection in the joint or another complication. Other codes in this category identify encounters for orthopedic aftercare following surgical amputation, scoliosis surgery, or other specified orthopedic care.

Category Z48, Encounter for Other Postprocedural Aftercare

Subcategory Z48.0 would be used for an encounter for change or removal of nonsurgical and surgical wound dressing. Typically, these encounters occur in a physician's office, in an ambulatory clinic or center, or during a home healthcare visit. Code Z48.00 is intended to describe the encounter for the change or removal of a nonsurgical wound dressing. The encounter for the change or removal of a surgical wound dressing or packing is code Z48.01. An encounter for the purpose of removing sutures or staples would be reported with code Z48.02.

Broad categories exist for aftercare following organ transplant (Z48.2-) and surgical aftercare following surgery on specified body systems (Z48.8-). The aftercare codes are usually reported outside the acute care hospital setting to identify the postsurgical treatment after the initial treatment and surgery is completed. This postsurgical care may be received in a long-term care hospital or facility or through home care services.

Category Z49, Encounter for Care Involving Renal Dialysis

Z49 codes are used to identify the main reason for the encounter, for example, preparatory care for renal dialysis. Specifically the fitting and adjustment of an extracorporeal dialysis catheter or peritoneal dialysis catheter are included in subcategory Z49.0-. An encounter for adequacy testing for hemodialysis or peritoneal dialysis is coded with a subcategory code from Z49.3-. The note "Code also associated end-stage renal disease (N18.6)" appears under the category heading for Z49.

Category Z51, Encounter for Other Aftercare

Category Z51 includes codes for admissions or encounters for antineoplastic radiotherapy, antineoplastic chemotherapy, and immunotherapy; encounters for palliative care; and other specified aftercare.

Codes Z51.0, Encounter for antineoplastic radiation therapy, and codes from subcategory Z51.1, Encounter for antineoplastic chemotherapy and immunotherapy, are to be first-listed, followed by the diagnosis code when a patient's encounter is solely to receive radiation therapy, chemotherapy, or immunotherapy for the treatment of a neoplasm. If the reason for the encounter is more than one type of antineoplastic therapy, code Z51.0 and a code from subcategory Z51.1 may be assigned together, in which case one of these codes would be reported as a secondary diagnosis.

> **EXAMPLE:** Admission for chemotherapy for patient with metastasis to bone; patient has history of breast carcinoma with mastectomy performed 8 years ago: Z51.1, Encounter for antineoplastic chemotherapy; C79.51, Secondary malignant neoplasm of bone; Z85.3, Personal history of malignant neoplasm of breast. A procedure code would be assigned for the chemotherapy administration.

Code Z51.5 describes an encounter for palliative care. Code Z51.5 is a code for a patient receiving palliative care for a terminal condition. The terminal condition, such as carcinoma, COPD, Alzheimer's disease, or AIDS, should be the principal diagnosis. A code should also be assigned for the condition requiring palliative care. The code may be used during an inpatient admission or in any other healthcare setting when it is determined that palliative care should be initiated and no further treatment for the terminal illness is desired. There is no time limit or minimum for the use of this code assignment.

Code Z51.81, Encounter for therapeutic drug level monitoring, is the correct code to use when a patient visit is for the purpose of undergoing a laboratory test to measure the drug level in the patient's blood or urine or to measure a specific function to assess the effectiveness of a drug. Z51.81 may be used alone if the monitoring is for a drug that the patient is on for only a brief period, not long term. However, there is a "code also" note under this code to code any long-term (current) drug therapy (Z79.-) to indicate what drug is being monitored.

Category Z52, Donors of Organs and Tissues

Codes from category Z52, Donors, are used for living individuals who are donating blood, tissue, or an organ to be transplanted into another individual. Z52 codes are not used when the potential donor is examined (code Z00.5). Also, these codes are not used for cadaveric donations, that is, when a patient's organ(s) are harvested at the time of death according to the patient's stated wishes. These codes are only for individuals donating for others with the exception of Z52.01- for autologous blood donors. They are not used to identify cadaveric donations. Subcategory codes identify the donor of blood, skin, bone, bone marrow, kidney, cornea, and liver.

There are also codes for egg or oocyte donors that identify the age of the donor and whether the eggs are intended to be used for anonymous donations or for a designated recipient. Codes Z52.810–Z52.819 identify the age of the egg or oocyte donor (either younger than age 35 years or age 35 years or older) and specify whether the intended recipient is anonymous or designated.

Category Z53, Persons Encountering Health Services for Specific Procedures and Treatment, Not Carried Out

Code Z53.01 and Z53.09 state that a procedure and treatment was not carried out because of a contraindication. A contraindication is any medical condition that renders some form of treatment improper or undesirable. For example, the patient may have an infection, cardiac condition, or abnormal diagnostic test that would make performing the surgical procedure unsafe until the contraindication is resolved.

The patient may also decide, sometimes at the last minute before surgery begins, that he or she does not want the surgery or procedure performed at this time and the procedure is cancelled. Codes in subcategory Z53.20–Z53.29 identify when a patient decides not to have a procedure by leaving prior to being seen by healthcare provider or decides against the procedure for some reason. Two other codes, Z53.8 and Z53.9, are available to identify the scenarios where a procedure or treatment are not carried out for another reason or for an unspecified reason.

Persons with Potential Health Hazards Related to Socioeconomic and Psychosocial Circumstances (Z55–Z65)

Codes from the categories in this section are likely to be used to describe patients who require counseling or other social and supportive services for factors that are not specific health conditions but represent situations that influence physical and emotional health statuses.

Category Z59, Problems Related to Housing and Economic Circumstances

Codes in category Z59 are used primarily as additional diagnosis codes to further explain the socioeconomic factors that may be influencing the patient's need for healthcare services. The codes in this category may be used to describe circumstances that lead to the disruption of the family unit and create the need for specific healthcare services. For example, code Z59.0 identifies the patient as being homeless, which will impact the care and management of the patient by the healthcare provider.

Category Z62, Problems Related to Upbringing

Codes within this category identify circumstances such as current and past negative life events in childhood as well as current and past problems of a child related to upbringing. These circumstances may lead to counseling or other services for the patient. The personal history of physical and sexual abuse in childhood can be described with subcategory codes Z62.81-. Other problems that can be identified with codes in this category are parental overprotection, child in welfare custody, parent-child conflict, and other parent-child-sibling problems.

Category Z63, Other Problems Related to Primary Support Group, Including Family Circumstances

Category Z63 is one of several categories in ICD-10-CM that may be used when a patient or family member receives counseling services after an illness or injury, or when support is required to cope with family and social problems. These codes are not used in conjunction with a diagnosis code when counseling is considered integral to the treatment for the condition. Subcategory codes identify family circumstances that occur when a family member is absent, for example due to military deployment, disappearance or death of a family member, or disruption of the family due to divorce or separation. Other situations that may lead to counseling or other care include a dependent relative needing care at home, alcoholism and drug addiction in the family, or other family estrangement or inadequate family support.

Do Not Resuscitate (Z66)

This code may be used when it is documented by the provider that a patient is on **do not resuscitate (DNR)** status at any time during the stay. The DNR code Z66 will most likely be used on inpatient records to identify the decision made by the patient or according to the patient's documented wishes not to pursue resuscitation if the patient suffers a cardiopulmonary arrest. Usually the patient has a serious or terminal condition with a poor prognosis and may or may not be receiving palliative care at the time the DNR status identified.

Body Mass Index (Z68)

The **body mass index (BMI)** is the determination of a patient's weight in proportion to height. BMI measures are calculated as kilograms per meters squared. BMI can be used to characterize underweight as well as overweight status. For overweight individuals, codes in this category are used in conjunction with a code from category E66, Overweight and obesity, to provide specific information about the patient's status.

The BMI adult codes are for use for individuals 21 years of age and older. The codes for pediatric BMI use the value ranges for children currently represented in the Centers for Disease Control and Prevention (CDC) growth charts. The age group represented in the published CDC growth charts is 2 to 20 years old. The pediatric codes report percentiles as used on the growth charts.

For coding of the body mass index measurement, code assignments may be based on documentation from clinicians in addition to the patient's physician. Typically a dietitian will document the BMI number in a nutritional evaluation progress note. However, the dietitian's documentation can only supplement, not replace, the physician's documentation. The physician must document the medical diagnosis of overweight, obesity, or other nutritional problems to be coded. The BMI is reported as an additional diagnosis to the condition being evaluated. As with all additional diagnoses, the BMI should only be reported when it meets the definition of a reportable additional diagnosis.

The specific BMI values are contained in the following subcategory codes:

Z68.1	Body mass index [BMI] 19 or less, adult
Z68.2-	Body mass index [BMI] 20 to 29, adult
Z68.3-	Body mass index [BMI] 30 to 39, adult
Z68.4-	Body mass index [BMI] 40 or greater, adult
Z68.5-	Body mass index [BMI] pediatric

Persons Encountering Health Services in Other Circumstances (Z69–Z76)

The block of codes from Z69 to Z76 describe a variety of situations when a patient seeks counseling and other services related to health and lifestyle issues.

Category Z69, Encounter for Mental Health Services for Victims and Perpetrator of Abuse

These codes describe encounters for counseling for victims and perpetrators of abuse. Specific services include encounters for mental health services victims and perpetrators of parental child abuse (Z69.010–Z69.011) and nonparental child abuse (Z69.020–Z69.021). Other codes identify mental health services for victims and perpetrators of spousal or partner abuse (Z69.11–Z6.12) and other abuse such as rape victim counseling (Z69.81).

Category Z71, Persons Encountering Health Services for Other Counseling and Medical Advice, Not Elsewhere Classified

More counseling type services can be identified with codes from category Z71. These can be medical office or community mental health services for patients seeking relief from a dependence or other distress. Codes Z71.41 and Z71.42 are used to describe alcohol abuse counseling and surveillance services for the patient with alcoholism and the family members. Similar codes, Z71.51 and Z71.52, are used for drug abuse counseling and surveillance for the patient and the family members. A patient seeking human immunodeficiency virus (HIV) counseling would have code Z71.7 assigned for the encounter. Other codes in this category describe an encounter for a patient who has a feared condition which was not found (Z71.1), an encounter for a person who is seeking advice or treatment for another person (Z71.0), and an encounter when a person is seeking dietary counseling and surveillance (Z71.3). Code Z71.3 includes two "use additional code" notes to identify any associated underlying medical condition and body mass index, if known.

Category Z74, Problems Related to Care Provider Dependency

Category Z74 identifies the patient who is dependent on others for care on a daily basis. The codes here identify bed confinement status, which means, for example, that the patient is unable to ambulate or is bedridden (Z74.01), or that the patient has reduced mobility and is confined to a chair (Z74.09). Other codes in this category cover when the patient needs assistance with daily care, for example, with bathing, dressing, and meal preparation (Z74.1), and when the patient needs continuous supervision or is unable to be left alone (Z74.3).

Category Z75, Problems Related to Medical Facilities and Other Health Care

Category Z75 codes would be used to describe the situation for a patient who needs health services because other medical services are not available to this particular patient. For example, the patient may need to be hospitalized for a brief time because medical services are not available in the home (Z75.0) or the patient is awaiting admission to an adequate facility elsewhere (Z75.1). Other patients may need respite care in a long-term facility for a period of time while family members who usually provide care need a break or are unavailable for a time period (Z75.5).

Category Z76, Persons Encountering Health Services in Other Circumstances

The common theme to these codes is the individuals that would be described by these codes are not sick. Instead, the person needs a healthcare service for a specific reason. For example, a patient may simply need to obtain a repeat prescription for a medication, eyeglasses, or a device (Z76.0) Other situations may arise when a baby or child needs supervision and care in an alternative location when there are problems in the home or no one available to care for the child (Z76.1–Z76.2). A code, Z76.81, is used for an expectant parent(s)' prebirth or pre-adoption visit to a pediatrician's office in order to discuss future care for their child. Finally, a patient may be awaiting organ transplant status and needs to be seen by a provider who may also be providing healthcare for their illness, but the issue of waiting for the transplant surgery is also a concern (Z76.82).

Persons with Potential Health Hazards Related to Family and Personal History and Certain Conditions Influencing Health Status (Z77–Z99)

Many codes in this section are used on a daily basis for healthcare encounters in both hospital and ambulatory settings to identify common health issues in patients: family history of diseases, personal history of diseases, long-term current drug therapy, allergy status, acquired absence of limbs and organs, transplant status, presence of vascular implants, and grafts to name only a few.

Category Z77, Other Contact with and (Suspected) Exposures Hazardous to Health

Codes within subcategories Z77.01 to Z77.9 can be used to describe patients who seek medical care due to exposure or contact with nonmedical substances that pose a threat to their health. Such substances include, for example, arsenic, lead, uranium, and asbestos. Other hazardous substances included here are aromatic amines, benzene, as well as air, water, and soil pollution. Other hazards in the physical environment that may be damaging to a patient can be identified with codes here for exposure to mold, algae toxins, noise, radon, and other naturally occurring radiation. A commonly used code from this category may be Z77.22 for contact with and (suspected) exposure to environmental tobacco smoke, otherwise known as passive smoking, which has been recognized as a health risk for many people. These patients may be without symptoms due to the exposure but have other injuries from the same event.

Category Z79, Long Term (Current) Drug Therapy

Category Z79, Long term (current) drug therapy, contains status codes that are intended to be used in addition to Z51.81, Encounter for therapeutic drug level monitoring. Category Z79 codes only state that a patient is on a prescribed drug for an extended period of time. There is no definition or timeframe for long term. If a patient receives a drug on a regular basis and has multiple refills available for a prescription, it is appropriate to document long-term drug use. The code indicates a patient's continuous use of a prescribed drug for long-term treatment of a condition or for prophylactic use.

Category Z79 codes are not used to describe patients who have addictions to drugs. This category also is not used to describe the administration of medications to prevent withdrawal symptoms in patients with drug dependence—for example, methadone maintenance programs. Instead, assign the appropriate code for the drug dependence for this type of visit.

These Z79 codes are used for long-term drug treatment as a prophylactic measure (to prevent the recurrence of deep vein thrombosis), to treat a chronic disease (such as insulin for diabetes), or for treatment of a disease that requires long-term drug therapy (such as arthritis). Codes from category Z79 are not assigned for medications administered for a brief period of time to treat an acute illness or injury or to bring a chronic condition under better control. For example, a type 2 diabetic patient may receive insulin for a period of time when hospitalized to control the blood sugar while the patient is recovering from surgery or another illness. The use of insulin during this hospital stay is not coded with Z79.4.

Code Z51.81, Encounter for therapeutic drug level monitoring, is the correct code to use when a patient visit is for the purpose of undergoing a laboratory test to measure the drug level in the patient's blood or urine or to measure a specific function to assess the effectiveness of a drug. Z51.81 may be used alone if the monitoring is for a drug that the patient is on for only a brief period, not long term. However, there is a "use additional code" note after code Z51.81 to remind the coder to use an additional code for any long-term (current) drug therapy (Z79.-) to indicate what drug is being monitored. Likewise, under the category Z79 heading is a note to "code also" any therapeutic drug level monitoring with Z51.81.

EXAMPLE: The patient is on anticoagulants and the physician orders a prothrombin time (PT) to be obtained in the outpatient department: Z51.81, Encounter for therapeutic drug level monitoring; Z79.01, Long-term (current) use of anticoagulants and antithrombotics/ antiplatelets

Categories Z80–Z84, Family History of Primary Malignant Neoplasm, Mental and Behavioral Disorders, Certain Disabilities and Chronic Diseases, Other Specified Disorders and Other Conditions

Family history codes in ICD-10-CM, categories Z80-Z84, are used when a patient's family member(s) has a particular disease that puts the patient at higher risk of contracting the same condition. Physicians generally mean the same thing when using the term "family history."

Category Z80 describes a family history of primary malignant neoplasm. This risk factor is an important medical fact about a patient and may be the reason for increased monitoring and diagnostic testing of the patient with a family history of cancer. Specific codes are provided for the primary site of the neoplasm, such as digestive organs (Z80.0), lung (Z80.1), or breast (Z80.3) as well as family history of leukemia and other lymphoid, hematopoietic, and related tissue. The main term to use in the Alphabetic Index is "History, family, malignant neoplasm."

Category Z81 describes a family history of mental and behavioral disorders. Codes within this category identify family history of alcohol abuse and dependence (Z81.1), history of other psychoactive substance abuse (Z81.3), and other mental and behavioral disorders (Z81.8).

Category Z82 describes certain disabilities and chronic diseases leading to disablement. For example, codes are available to identify family history of stroke (Z82.3), family history of sudden cardiac death (Z82.41), and numerous other disabling conditions such as ischemic heart disease, asthma, arthritis, osteoporosis, polycystic kidney disease, and other congenital malformations, deformations, and chromosomal abnormalities.

Category Z83 codes identify a family history of certain other specific conditions that may describe a patient's reason for a healthcare encounter. These may be isolated illnesses or chronic conditions that the family member was diagnosed with; the patient possibly could have inherited the illness or condition or be at risk for developing it. For example, Z83.71, Family history of digestive disorders, colonic polyps, may be the reason a patient has a screening colonoscopy performed at an earlier age or with more frequency than individuals with average risk. Certain individuals are at greater risk of developing colon polyps if they have a family member in whom colon polyps have been diagnosed.

These Z codes are indexed under "History (personal) of" in the Alphabetic Index. Note the subterm "family" is indented under "History (personal) of" and is the point of reference for familial conditions.

> **EXAMPLE:** Family history of breast carcinoma: Z80.3 (describes a condition coded to C50 when present and treated)
>
> **EXAMPLE:** Family history of osteoporosis: Z82.62
>
> **EXAMPLE:** Family history of diabetes: Z83.3

Categories Z85–Z87, Personal History of Primary Malignant Neoplasm, Certain Other Diseases and Other Diseases and Conditions

As a reminder, the word "history" as used with all Z codes may not be consistent with the intent of the word "history" when used by a physician to describe a patient's condition.

Personal history in ICD-10-CM means the patient's past medical condition no longer exists and the patient is not receiving any treatment for the condition. However, the information is important because the condition has the potential for recurrence and the patient may require continued monitoring. A physician may use the word "history" to describe a current condition the patient is being treated for, such as history of diabetes mellitus or history of hypertension. If the patient is receiving treatment for the condition, it would not be classified as a "history" code in ICD-10-CM.

Personal history codes are frequently used in conjunction with follow-up Z codes and family history Z codes, as well as screening Z codes, to explain the reason for the visit or diagnostic testing. These codes are important information as their presence may alter the type of treatment the patient receives.

Categories Z85 through Z87 include codes for personal and family histories of malignant neoplasms and other health problems.

The personal history of malignant neoplasm (Z85) category includes primary cancer sites only, including leukemia and lymphoid, hematopoietic, and related tissues. There are no personal history codes for secondary neoplasm sites or carcinoma in situ sites. The instructional notes listed under each subcategory refer to specific code ranges for primary malignancy categories (categories C00–C96). Secondary and CA in situ malignancies are excluded from this range of codes. A patient with leukemia in remission should be classified to the C91–C95 categories with the fifth character identifying "in remission" status instead of the Z codes in this range. The history of leukemia or lymphatic or hematopoietic neoplasms codes in the Z85 subcategories means the patient is completely cured of the disease. Directional notes appear under the category heading of Z85, Personal history of malignant neoplasm to

1. Code first any follow-up examination after treatment of malignant neoplasm (Z08)

2. Use additional codes to identify:

    A. Alcohol use and dependence (F10.-)

    B. Exposure to environmental tobacco smoke (Z77.22)

C. History of tobacco use (Z87.891)

D. Occupational exposure to environmental tobacco smoke (Z57.31)

E. Tobacco dependence (F17.-)

F. Tobacco use (Z72.00)

Categories Z86 and Z87 identify certain other conditions that the patient may have a personal history of that is important to consider for future healthcare needs. Both category headings include the note to "code first any follow-up examination after treatment (Z09)" as these conditions are frequently the reason for follow-up examinations to assure the condition has not recurred in the patient. There are several conditions in the categories that are frequently documented by the physician in the health record and are used to explain the reason for the health encounter. For example, personal history of such serious health conditions such as the following:

- In-situ neoplasm of breast (Z86.000) or cervix uteri (Z86.001)

- Colonic polyps (Z86.010)

- Methicillin resistant Staphylococcus aureus infection (Z86.14)

- Combat and operational stress reaction (Z86.51)

- History of diseases of the circulatory system (Z86.7-) including pulmonary embolism, other venous thrombosis, transient ischemic attack, or cerebral infarction

In the Z87 category, codes are available to identify a patient's past medical condition that may have an impact on their current care or need for future services. For example, varied personal history conditions are coded as follows:

- Peptic ulcer disease (Z87.11)

- Dysplasia of female genital tract (Z87.41-)

- Urinary tract infections (Z87.440)

- Complications of pregnancy, childbirth and puerperium including pre-term labor (Z87.51–Z87.59)

- Nicotine dependence (Z87.891)

A set of subcategory codes, Z87.7, Personal history of (corrected) congenital malformation, is included here to be used to classify the patient with a known history of a congenital condition that has been repaired or corrected. An Excludes1 note appears under this subcategory to remind the coder that these codes would not be used if the congenital malformation has only been partially repaired and the patient still required medical treatment for it. Then the congenital condition would be coded instead. The congenital conditions in all body systems are included here, for example, malformations of the genitourinary tract, nervous system, digestive system, and heart and circulatory system.

Finally, in subcategory Z87.8 there are codes available for specific conditions that are important to note for a patient's health status. For example, personal history of healed traumatic fracture (Z87.81), traumatic brain injury (Z87.820), and anaphylaxis (Z87.892) are coded here.

Category Z88, Allergy Status to Drugs, Medicaments and Biological Substances and Subcategory Z91.0, Allergy Status, Other Than to Drugs and Biological Substances

Most of the codes in category Z88 and Z91.0 are exceptions to the general rule that a history code means the condition is no longer present. A person who has had an allergic reaction to food or a substance is always considered allergic to that substance. These Z codes indicate that the person is not currently exhibiting an allergic reaction but, instead, has the potential for a reaction if exposed to the substance in the future. The Z88 codes identify allergy status to drugs and biological substances such as penicillin, sulfonamides, anesthetic agent or serum, and vaccines for example. The Z91.0 category identifies food allergy status with six character codes for allergies to peanuts, milk products, and eggs for example. The other codes in category Z91 describe allergies to nonfood and nonmedicinals such as bee sting allergy and allergies to latex objects and radiographic dye or contrast materials. The main term "allergy" in the Alphabetic Index has subterms for drug, food, and other substances.

Category Z89, Acquired Absence of Limb

Codes within this category identify the status of the patient who has had an amputation of a limb that may be postprocedural or posttraumatic loss of the limb. The codes are specific to the limb and the laterality, for example, acquired absence of right finger(s) (Z89.021), acquired absence of left hand (Z89.112), or acquired absence of right great toe (Z89.411). The acquired absence of the leg below the knee is identified with codes for right leg, left leg, and unspecified leg (Z89.511–Z89.519). Likewise the acquired absence of the leg above the knee is identified with codes Z89.611–Z89.619. If a patient had an explantation or removal of a joint prosthesis with or without the presence of an antibiotic-impregnated cement spacer, the specific loss of a joint can be identified for the shoulder (Z89.231–Z89.239), the knee (Z89.521–Z89.529), and the hip (Z89.621–Z89.629.)

Category Z90, Acquired Absence of Organs, Not Elsewhere Classified

The status of an acquired absence may be postprocedural or posttraumatic loss of a body part; these situations should be classified to this category. Any congenital absence of an organ would be classified elsewhere in ICD-10-CM. Frequently these codes are used to describe patients who have had a malignant condition and had surgery to remove a diseased organ. For example, acquired absence of breast and nipple (Z90.10–Z90.13), kidney (Z90.5), and prostate (Z90.79). For acquired absence of the pancreas, a use additional note appears to remind the coder to use an additional code to identify any associated insulin use (Z79.4) or postpancreatectomy diabetes mellitus (E13.-). Some of the codes within this category are important for tracking Pap smear necessity. Women who have had a total hysterectomy with removal of the cervix (Z90.710) no longer require cervical Pap smears but do require vaginal smears to test for vaginal malignancies. Women with a cervical stump (Z90.711) following a hysterectomy still require cervical Pap smears. Code Z90.712 would identify the woman who has a surgically absent cervix but in whom the uterus remains. These conditions can be found in the Index under the main term Absence, followed by the organ name.

Category Z91, Personal Risk Factors, Not Elsewhere Classified

Other codes in category Z91 identify the fact that the patient has a personal history that presents hazards to health. Examples of commonly used codes in this category are **noncompliance** with medical treatment and regimen. Individual codes are available to describe a patient's noncompliance with dietary regimen (Z91.11). Other codes describe a patient's other noncompliance with medication regimen (Z91.14), a patient's noncompliance with renal dialysis (Z91.15), and a patient's noncompliance with other medical treatment and regimen (Z91.16). Any of these noncompliance activities can be a detriment to a patient's health status. Another risk to the patient can occur when the patient is noncompliant with his or her scheduled medications. Codes exist for the patient who takes less of their prescribed medication, which is identified as underdosing in ICD-10-CM. A patient may intentionally take less of their medication for financial reasons (Z91.120) or intentionally for another reason (Z91.128). In other situations the patient may take less of the medication unintentionally because of the patient's age-related debility such as forgetfulness or dementia (Z91.130) or unintentionally for other reasons (Z91.138). The codes for these conditions are located in the Alphabetic Index under the main term Noncompliance.

A patient with a history of fall(s) or identified as at risk for falling can be classified with code Z91.81. This code is used to identify patients at risk for falling or who have a history of falls with or without subsequent injuries. Falls are an important public health problem affecting about one-third of adults age 65 years and older annually. About 20 to 30 percent of those who fall will suffer moderate to severe injuries, including hip and other fractures and head trauma. Adults who are age 75 years or older and fall are more likely to be admitted to a long-term care facility for 1 year or longer. In this same population, more than 60 percent of deaths are from falls. Code Z91.81 can be used to identify patients who require closer monitoring to prevent falls, to justify specific diagnostic or therapeutic services to identify causes of falling, or to order preventive evaluation or services.

Category Z92, Personal History of Medical Treatment

Within this category are codes to identify the patient's personal history of antineoplastic chemotherapy (Z92.21), personal history of monoclonal drug therapy (Z92.22), personal history of estrogen therapy (Z92.23), personal history of inhaled steroid therapy (Z92.240), personal history of systemic steroid therapy (Z92.241), personal history of immunosuppressive therapy (Z92.25), and personal history of other drug therapy (Z92.299). Other codes for history of the particular condition for which the patient received chemotherapy or drug therapy could be used with these codes. Other facts about the patient can be described with other codes in this category, for example, the fact that the patient has received therapeutic radiation (Z92.3) or received tPA in a different facility in the past 24 hours (Z92.82), and the fact that the patient has a history of failed moderate or conscious sedation (Z92.83). All of these factors can have an impact on the patient's current and future healthcare needs.

Category Z93, Artificial Opening Status

Category Z93 is subdivided to identify the presence of an artificial opening, such as a tracheostomy (Z93.0), ileostomy (Z93.2), colostomy (Z93.3), cystostomy (Z93.5-), and so forth. These codes are indexed under "Status (post), artificial opening" in the Alphabetic Index.

EXAMPLE: Status post urinary tract: Z93.6, for nephrostomy or ureterostomy status

The exclusion note at the beginning of category Z93 instructs coders to use a code from subcategory Z43.- when the encounter or admission is for attention to or management of that artificial opening or when there are complications of the external stoma (J95.0-, K94.-, or N99.5-).

Category Z94, Transplanted Organ or Tissue Status

Category Z94 is used for homologous or heterologous (animal or human) organ, bone marrow, cornea, and stem cell transplants among other organs. If there are complications of the transplanted organ or tissue, the Alphabetic Index will direct the coder to the codes for the specific complications. This category of codes does not imply there is a problem with the transplanted organ or tissue.

These codes are indexed under "Transplant(ed) (status)" in the Alphabetic Index.

EXAMPLE: Status post kidney transplant (human donor): Z94.0, Kidney replaced by transplant

Another code, Z76.82, Awaiting organ transplant status, is included in another category of ICD-10-CM. Some patients who are on a waiting list for a heart transplant may be hospitalized due to the severity of their illness. Z76.82 is a status code to distinguish patients who are hospitalized while awaiting a new heart from patients who are hospitalized for direct treatment of their heart disease. This code could also be used to indicate that the patient is on any organ transplant waiting list.

Category Z95, Presence of Cardiac and Vascular Implants and Grafts

Category Z95 includes codes for a variety of postprocedural states, such as cardiac pacemaker in situ (Z95.0); automatic implantable cardiac defibrillator (Z95.810); aortocoronary bypass graft (Z95.1); presence of prosthetic heart valve (Z95.2); coronary angioplasty implant (stent) (Z95.5); heart assist device (Z95.811); and presence of fully implantable artificial heart (Z95.812). The Excludes1 note under this category reminds the coder that complications of cardiac and vascular devices, implants, and grafts are found in category T82.-. These postprocedural states are located in the Alphabetic Index under the main term "Status (post)."

Categories Z96, Presence of Other Functional Implants and Z97, Presence of Other Devices

These two categories identify other postprocedural states for the patient that specify what body part has been replaced with an implant or device. Examples of frequently used codes in these categories are presence of the following:

- Intraocular lens or pseudophakos, Z96.1
- Insulin pump (external)(internal), Z96.41
- Orthopedic joint implant identified by joint and laterality, Z96.6-
- Artificial limb (complete)(partial) identified by limb and laterality, Z97.1-
- Contraceptive (intrauterine) device, Z97.5

The presence of an implant or device is identified by a code found in the Alphabetic Index under the main term "Presence (of)."

Category Z98, Other Postprocedural States

Codes in this category identify a postsurgical or postprocedural status of the patient that can be important for future health care needs. Examples of frequently used codes in this category are

- Intestinal bypass and anastomosis status, Z98.0

- Cataract extraction status, Z98.4-

A note appears under this code to use additional code to identify the presence of an intraocular lens implant (Z96.1).

- Sterilization status for both tubal ligation and vasectomy status, Z98.5-

- Bariatric surgery status, Z98.84

- Transplanted organ removal status, Z98.85

An Excludes1 note appears with this code that an encounter for the removal of the transplanted organ should be coded to complication of transplanted organ (T86.-).

These postprocedural descriptions of a patient can be found in the Alphabetic Index under the main term "Status (post)."

Category Z99, Dependence of Enabling Machines and Devices, Not Elsewhere Classified

The last category in ICD-10-CM identifies the patient's dependence or required use of a machine or device to sustain life or function. The presence and dependence on cardiac devices are classified to category Z95. For example, many patients in both inpatient and outpatient settings would be identified for their special needs through the use of these codes:

- Dependence on respirator (ventilator)(mechanical ventilation), Z99.11

- Dependence on renal dialysis, Z99.2

- Dependence on supplemental oxygen, Z99.81

The main term for use in the Alphabetic Index for these scenarios is "Dependence on."

ICD-10-CM Review Exercises: Chapter 24

Assign the correct ICD-10-CM diagnosis codes to the following exercises.

1. This single newborn was born vaginally in the hospital. The baby is being treated for Rh incompatibility in a baby with documented type A+ blood and the mother's blood type documented as A-. What is the correct diagnosis code(s)?

   _____

2. Medical examination of four-year-old child prior to admission to preschool

   _____

3. Patient seen for fitting of right artificial leg after patient had below-knee amputation due to medical condition

   _____

4. Counseling visit for patient with alcohol dependence

   _____

(Continued on next page)

ICD-10-CM Review Exercises: Chapter 24 (Continued)

5. Personal history of lung carcinoma with past history of tobacco dependence

6. Presence of cardiac pacemaker and status post aortocoronary bypass surgery

7. The patient is having a screening colonoscopy and has a family history of colon carcinoma.

8. The encounter is for a patient who is receiving antineoplastic chemotherapy to treat primary carcinoma of the body of the pancreas

9. The encounter is for an elective termination of pregnancy.

10. The patient is a newborn triplet born in the hospital by cesarean delivery. The baby is premature born during the 35th week of the mother's pregnancy and has a low birth weight of 1,769 grams.

11. The patient was seen in the physician's office to determine if the patient has a sexually transmitted disease after being exposed to gonorrhea that was present in their partner.

12. The patient requests permanent sterilization because the patient does not want any more children because of the patient's past history with complications during pregnancies.

13. The patient was seen on an outpatient basis to donate bone marrow for a relative who needs a bone marrow transplant.

14. The patient was seen in the gynecologist's office for a routine gynecological examination with a cervical Papanicolaou smear.

15. The patient was seen in his oncologist's office for follow-up examination following chemotherapy treatment for a primary carcinoma of the breast that is no longer present.

16. The male patient, age 25, was brought to the emergency room after an explosion occurred at the industrial plant at work with other workers who were injured by the accident. This patient was not as close to the explosion as the other patients and had no signs or symptoms of an injury but was brought to the hospital to be examined as a precaution. After examination, the patient was found not to have any injury from the accident.

ICD-10-CM Review Exercises: Chapter 24 (Continued)

17. The patient was treated 10 days after following an accident when he was injured while cleaning windows at home when a glass windowpane broke. The patient had lacerations that were repaired. At this time the patient's arm was reexamined and a small piece of glass was found imbedded in soft tissue that was not previously found. The patient's primary care physician made a small incision and removed the sliver of glass. Code only the diagnosis for the retained glass fragment.

    _____

18. The two-year-old female patient was brought to the pediatrician's office by her mother and grandmother because the grandmother was concerned that the child had not received all of her immunizations because the patient's mother feared the vaccines would cause the child to develop a reaction. The physician counseled the mother about the risks and benefits of immunization and reassured her of the safety of them for children. The mother agreed to think about it and bring the patient back to the doctor's office the following week for possible vaccine administrations. The doctor describes the patient in her record as being delinquent with her immunization status.

    _____

19. The patient is a 45-year-old female who made an appointment with a psychologist to discuss the problems she is having in her marriage.

    _____

20. The patient is a 30-year-old female who is being seen by her obstetrician for normal prenatal care during the third trimester of her pregnancy. The patient has not had any complications of pregnancy and is expected to deliver in the next 3 weeks.

    _____

Chapter 25

Coding and Reimbursement

Learning Objectives

At the conclusion of this chapter, you should be able to:

1. Describe how the Medicare Severity Diagnosis-Related Groups (MS-DRGs) identify the levels of severity differences in a patient's condition

2. Briefly describe the hospital inpatient prospective payment system, including how base payment rates are determined and the formula for computing the hospital payment

3. Describe the purpose and activities of quality improvement organizations, comprehensive error testing programs, and recovery audit contractors

4. Explain medical necessity and its relationship to ICD-10-CM diagnosis codes

5. Explain the purpose of advance beneficiary notice

Key Terms

- Advance beneficiary notice (ABN)
- Comprehensive Error Rate Testing (CERT)
- Diagnosis-related group (DRG)
- Direct graduate medical education (DGME)
- Discharge disposition
- Disproportionate share hospital (DSH)
- Hospital inpatient prospective payment system
- Hospital's base rate
- Hospital's payment rate
- Indirect medical education (IME)
- Medical necessity
- Medicare Administrative Contractor (MAC)
- Medicare dependent hospital (MDH)
- Medicare Severity DRGs (MS-DRGs)
- Outlier

- Post-acute care setting
- Quality Improvement Organization (QIO)
- Recovery Audit Contractor (RAC)
- Relative weight
- Sole community hospital (SCH)

This text has included a thorough review of the characteristics and conventions of ICD-10-CM. While coding systems were originally established for statistical comparison and research purposes, in many cases the codes are used for reimbursement and other purposes. This chapter includes a brief discussion of some of the reimbursement purposes for coding; the hospital inpatient prospective payment system, Medicare payment review programs, and medical necessity.

Hospital Inpatient Prospective Payment System

The **hospital inpatient prospective payment system** (IPPS) is a method of payment undertaken by CMS to control the cost of inpatient acute care hospital services to Medicare recipients. Title VI of the Social Security Amendments of 1983 established the prospective payment system (PPS) to provide payment to hospitals for each Medicare case at a set reimbursement rate, rather than on a fee-for-service or per-day basis. The payment rates to hospitals, then, are established before services are rendered and are based on **diagnosis-related groups (DRGs)**.

For fiscal year 2008, Medicare adopted a severity-adjusted diagnosis-related group system called **Medicare Severity Diagnosis-Related Groups (MS-DRGs)**. This was the most drastic revision to the DRG system in 24 years. The goal of the new MS-DRG system was to significantly improve Medicare's ability to recognize severity of illness in its inpatient hospital payments. The new system is projected to increase payments to hospitals for services provided to the sicker patient and decrease payments for treating less severely ill patients. There are up to three levels of severity in the MS-DRG that reflect the differences in the patient's condition based on the additional diagnoses codes:

- MS-DRG with major complication or comorbidity (MCC). This level reflects the sickest patient with the highest level of severity and requires a significant amount of resources to treat both the principal diagnosis and the additional conditions the patient has.

- MS-DRG with complication or comorbidity (CC). This is a mid-level degree of severity based on these secondary diagnoses and requires additional resources for treating the principal and additional diagnoses.

- MS-DRG with no complication or comorbidity (non-CC). This means the patient did not have an additional condition that required significant additional resources other than what was needed to treat the condition the patient had.

MS-DRGs represent an inpatient classification system designed to categorize patients who are medically related with respect to diagnoses and treatment and who are statistically similar in their lengths of stay. Each DRG has a preset reimbursement amount that the hospital receives whenever the MS-DRG is assigned. Acute care hospitals receive Medicare IPPS payments on a per discharge basis for Medicare beneficiaries—one payment per one inpatient hospital stay. All outpatient diagnostic services and admission-related therapeutic services provided by the same hospital on the day of the patient's admission or within three days preceding the date of inpatient admission must be included on the inpatient hospital claim to Medicare and is paid as part of the MS-DRG payment. No separate payment is made for these outpatient services.

The Medicare patient's principal diagnosis and up to 24 additional diagnoses that include diagnoses that are recognized as major or other complication or comorbidity will determine the medical MS-DRG. If the patient had surgery or a significant procedure this will impact the MS-DRG assignment as well. Up to 25 procedure codes may be reported on the inpatient claim to Medicare and these will likely cause a surgical MS-DRG to be assigned. Each fiscal year, the Centers for Medicare and Medicaid Services (CMS) evaluates the composition of the MS-DRGs to determine if the DRG still includes clinically similar conditions that require similar amounts of resources to care for the patients. When the clinical and financial information about a particular MS-DRG proves that the group contains significantly different amounts of resources, CMS has the option to assign diagnosis and procedure codes to a different MS-DRG or create a new MS-DRG for a particular set of diagnoses or procedures.

The base payment rates for each DRG are determined from two basic sources. First, each MS-DRG is assigned a relative weight. The **relative weight** represents the average resources required to care for cases in that particular DRG relative to the national average of resources used to treat all Medicare cases. The average Medicare case is assigned a relative weight of 1.0000. Thus, cases in a MS-DRG with a weight of 2.0000, on average, require twice as many resources as the average Medicare case; on the other hand, cases in a MS-DRG with a weight of 0.5000, on average, require half as many resources as the average Medicare case. Each year, the relative weights of the MS-DRGs are updated to reflect changes in treatment patterns, technology, and any other factors that may change the relative use of hospital resources.

The second source that determines MS-DRG payment rate is the individual **hospital's payment rate** per case. This payment rate is based on a regional or national adjusted standardized amount that considers the type of hospital; designation of the hospital as large urban, other urban, or rural; and a wage index for the geographic area in which the hospital is located. This is called the base payment rate or standardized rate and is a dollar amount that includes a labor-related and non-labor-related portion. The labor-related portion is adjusted by the wage index for a geographic area to reflect the differences in the cost of employing individuals to work in the hospitals. The non-labor rate accounts for capital expenses and operating expenses that determine the cost of providing hospital services other than paying employees. The two factors together are called the hospital's wage-adjusted standard payment rate or the **hospital's base rate**. By submitting a claim for the inpatient services with the financial charges and the diagnoses and procedure codes to the Medicare contractor responsible for processing claims, the payment process begins. Based on the coded data on the claim, the Medicare contractor assigns each case to a specific MS-DRG.

Thus, the actual amount the hospital is reimbursed for each Medicare inpatient is determined by multiplying the hospital's individual base rate by the relative weight of the DRG, less any applicable deductible amount.

The formula for computing the hospital payment for each MS-DRG is as follows:

DRG Relative Weight × Hospital Base Rate = Hospital Payment

For any given patient in a MS-DRG, the hospital knows, in advance, the amount of reimbursement it will receive from Medicare. It is the responsibility of the hospital to ensure that its resource use is reasonably in line with the expected payment. In addition to the basic payment rate, Medicare provides for an additional payment for other factors related to a particular hospital's business. If the hospital treats a high percentage of low-income patients, it receives a percentage add-on payment applied to the MS-DRG-adjusted base payment rate. Another scenario that qualifies a hospital to receive this additional payment is when a hospital is located in an urban setting with 100 or more beds and receives more than 30 percent of the hospital's net revenue from state and other local government sources for indigent care. This add-on payment, known as the **disproportionate share hospital (DSH)** adjustment, provides for a percentage increase in Medicare payments to hospitals that qualify under either of two statutory formulas designed to identify hospitals that serve a disproportionate share of low-income patients.

Teaching hospitals with residents in approved residency programs receive what are called **direct graduate medical education (DGME)** payments that represent the direct costs of operating a residency program, including paying the residents' salaries and supervising physicians. In addition, an approved teaching hospital receives a percentage add-on payment for each Medicare discharge paid under IPPS. This is known as the **indirect medical education (IME)** adjustment. This percentage varies, depending on the ratio of residents to the inpatient beds.

Sole community hospitals (SCHs) can receive an additional operating payment. SCHs are hospitals that are (1) located at least 35 miles from another similar acute care IPPS hospital; (2) located in a rural setting located between 25 and 35 miles for another similar hospital and must meet one other criteria related to the admission patterns of the community residents; (3) located in a rural setting that experiences severe weather conditions that makes travel to similar hospitals inaccessible for at least 30 days in two out of three years; or (4) located in a rural setting that because of distances, roads, or weather conditions requires a travel time of at least 45 minutes between like hospitals. As the name of these hospitals implies, these hospitals are the sole source of healthcare in their area.

Medicare dependent hospitals (MDHs) receive additional operating payments. An MDH is a rural hospital with 100 or fewer beds, is not a SCH, and at least 60 percent of their discharges are Medicare patients. These hospitals are a major source of care for Medicare beneficiaries in their area. Together with SCHs, MDHs are afforded this special payment in order to maintain access to services for Medicare beneficiaries.

To assure the Medicare beneficiaries have access to high quality but expensive healthcare, additional payments are made for what is called an **outlier** or extremely costly care. The costs incurred by a hospital for a Medicare beneficiary are evaluated to determine whether the hospital is eligible for an additional payment as an outlier case. A fixed loss amount is set each year. Hospitals are paid 80 percent of their costs above the fixed loss threshold and 90 percent of costs above the outlier threshold for burn patients. This additional payment is designed to protect the hospital from large financial losses due to unusually expensive cases. Any outlier payment due is added to the DRG-adjusted base payment rate, plus any DSH, IME, and medical service add-on adjustments.

MS-DRG assignment is based on information that includes the following:

- Diagnoses (principal and secondary)
- Surgical procedures (principal and secondary)
- Discharge disposition or status
- Presence of major or other complications and comorbidities (MCC or CC) as secondary diagnoses

The **discharge disposition** of a patient, or where the patient goes after discharge from the hospital, has an impact on the hospital's payment for the inpatient admission. MS-DRG payments are reduced if the patient is transferred to another acute care hospital that receives IPPS payments or, for certain MS-DRGs, is transferred to another healthcare setting where Medicare payments are made for the patient's continued care. These **post-acute care settings** are healthcare settings where patient receive healthcare services after discharge from an acute care hospital include long-term care hospitals, rehabilitation or psychiatric hospitals, units in acute care hospitals, skilled nursing facilities, home health agencies, cancer hospitals, or children's hospitals. Hospitals receive a reduced payment for an IPPS patient who is transferred to another acute care hospital or to one of the post-acute care settings.

CMS evaluates the Medicare IPPS annually. CMS's Notice of Proposed Rulemaking is published in the *Federal Register* in late April or early May each year. This notice, on which the public may comment, announces the final decisions on all ICD-10-CM code changes in past years and includes proposed ICD-10-CM/PCS code changes after October 1, 2014 as well as proposed revisions to the DRG system. CMS's Final Rule announcing final revisions to the IPPS, including the DRG system, is published in the *Federal Register* in July or August, and the changes become effective October 1 each year.

Medicare Coding Reviews

CMS reviews acute IPPS and long term care hospital (LTCH) records for payment purposes. CMS contracts with Medicare Fiscal Intermediaries (FIs) and Medicare Administrative Contractors (MACs) to conduct medical and coding reviews to prevent improper payment of inpatient hospital claims. This review is done to ensure that billed items or services are covered and are reasonable and necessary as specified in section 1862(a)(1)(A) of the Social Security Act.

Quality Improvement Organizations

CMS contracts with one organization in each state to serve as that state's **Quality Improvement Organization (QIO)**. QIOs are not-for-profit private organizations staffed by physicians, nurses, and other healthcare professionals trained to review healthcare services and help Medicare beneficiaries review quality healthcare through quality improvement activities with healthcare providers in their state. CMS contracts with a QIO for a three-year period of time with an agreement called a scope of work as to what services the QIO will provide to Medicare beneficiaries or on their behalf.

Medicare contracts with QIOs to promote better patient care, better population health, and lower healthcare costs through improvement in the delivery of healthcare services. QIOs focus their work on the following:

1. Reviewing beneficiary complaints as well as serving as an advocate for beneficiaries and their families through quality improvement activities

2. Using evidence-based performance improvement tools to promote healthcare services

3. Working with nursing homes to reduce the occurrence of pressure ulcers

4. Working with hospitals to reduce central line catheter bloodstream infections

5. Promoting the use of electronic health records for care management

6. Increasing preventive services like flu and pneumococcal immunizations as well as colorectal and breast cancer screenings

7. Helping reduce readmissions to hospitals for Medicare beneficiaries by promoting community-based services to provide follow-up care for the hospitals

In addition, QIOs review all claims where hospitals submit an adjusted claim for a higher-weighted MS-DRG. This review ensures proper payment to the hospital and prevents improper payments through MS-DRG upcoding when the hospital submits a second bill when the hospital determines a different diagnosis or procedure code must be submitted. Finally, the QIO performs expedited coverage reviews requested by beneficiaries. This is usually a request from the patient to extend their hospital stay when their physician and hospital has determined the patient should be discharged from the hospital. The QIO attempts to resolve these discharge disputes between the patient and the physician and hospital (CMS 2012d).

Fiscal Intermediaries and Medicare Administrative Contractors

In 2012, CMS awarded Medicare claims processing contracts through a competitive bidding process to replace the claims contractors (fiscal intermediaries and carriers) with new contracted business called **Medicare Administrative Contractors (MACs)**. CMS contracted with a total of 19 MACs through three bidding cycles. As of October 2012, there were 15 MACs processing Part A and Part B Medicare claims for a particular jurisdiction. In the interim, four fiscal intermediaries and four carriers continued to process Part A and Part B Medicare claims. FIs and MACs are established insurance companies that process private insurance company claims in addition to Medicare claims.

FIs and MACs perform medical review of acute IPPS hospitals and LTCH claims to ensure that they are for covered, correctly coded, and reasonable and necessary services. These reviews are performed on either a prepayment or postpayment basis. The FI or MAC will conduct claim adjustments as needed. The FI or MAC conducts provider feedback, through their medical review departments, based on their review findings. They also conduct provider education through their provider outreach and education departments on issues related to submitting inpatient claims correctly as part of their goal to reduce the payment error rate.

Comprehensive Error Rate Testing Program

The **Comprehensive Error Rate Testing (CERT)** contractor reviews claims for the purpose of producing a national Medicare fee-for-service payment error rate. This is a rate for acute IPPS hospital and LTCH claims payment. The CERT contractor performs reviews on a postpayment basis. In order to determine the error rate by which Medicare FIs and MACs are paying acute IPPS hospital and LTCH claims appropriately, the review is conducted in accordance with coverage, coding, and medical necessity guidelines. The CERT contractor's clinical staff reviews the claim with the submitted medical record to determine if the claim submitted was coded correctly, met medical necessity requirements, and was paid appropriately. A statistically valid random sample of Medicare claims are reviewed on a postpayment basis.

Each hospital is notified when a claim has been selected for review in slightly different ways, depending on the review entity. The CERT contractor notifies providers that a claim is selected for CERT review via letter. The hospital provides copies of the selected reviews by mail or as directed to the CERT contractor. The provider must submit a copy of the record by the date requested. The FI or MAC reviews the claim and makes any necessary payment adjustments based on the review. The provider has the right to appeal the decision made by the CERT contractor through an established procedure. The CERT program provides Medicare with two measurements: how well the provider codes and submits the claim and how well the FI or MAC educates the provider community on how to submit claims correctly.

Recovery Audit Program Contractors

Despite the efforts of QIOs and other initiatives that CMS has undertaken, there are concerns that the Medicare Trust Fund may not be adequately protected against improper payments. Congress passed the Medicare Prescription Drug, Improvement, and Modernization Act of 2003 (MMA), which was designed to enhance and support Medicare's current efforts. Congress directed the Department of Health and Human Services (HHS) to conduct a three-year demonstration project using **Recovery Audit Contractors (RACs)** to detect and correct improper payments in the traditional Medicare fee-for-service program. Section 302 of the Tax Relief and Health Care Act of 2006 made the PAC program permanent and required the program be expanded to all 50 states no later than 2010.

The demonstration project began in 2005 and ended in 2008 with three contractors focusing on Medicare beneficiaries' healthcare claims in three states with large numbers of Medicare beneficiaries: New York, Florida, and California. The demonstration project allowed Medicare to evaluate the efficiency and effectiveness of the program in order to make improvements in the RAC program. Congress made the program permanent and CMS expanded the program to all states in 2010. The types of services included in RAC reviews are hospital inpatient admission, outpatient hospital visits, physician visits, skilled nursing facility admissions, home health services, and durable medical equipment provided. The RACs performed reviews of medical records with the corresponding Medicare claims to

- Detect improper Medicare payments, including both underpayments and overpayments

- Correct improper Medicare payments

Improper payments have been found for items and services that do not meet Medicare's coverage and medical necessity policies. Other payments were made in error based on the record being incorrectly coded. Finally, payments for services were found to be made in error based on the supporting documentation submitted that did not support the ordered service. An overpayment results in money collected from the provider paid by Medicare. An underpayment is made to the provider when the review determines the provider was owed additional money.

Each Recovery Audit Contractor is responsible for identifying overpayment and underpayments in approximately one-quarter of the country. The Recovery Audit Contractor in each jurisdiction is as follows:

Region A: Diversified Collection Services (DCS)
Region B: CGI
Region C: Connolly, Inc.
Region D: Health Data Insights, Inc.

RAC contractors review claims on a postpayment basis for potential overpayments and underpayments by the FI/MAC. The reviews are based on CMS regulations for billing, medical necessity, coverage determinations, and coding guidelines. The RAC contractor does not develop their own billing and coding policies. The claims are selected based on focused areas of review for both inpatient and outpatient records. Inpatient records are selected based on specific MS-DRGs targeted for review based on the RAC contractor's past experience with coding and sequencing errors. The inpatient record reviews are referred to as complex reviews. Outpatient records are selected based on experience primarily with billing errors using CPT/HCPCS codes. Each hospital is notified when a claim has been selected for review with an

"Additional Documentation Request" sent to the RAC coordinator at the hospital. The hospital must submit the record for each case identified for a review within a specified period of time. If the record is not submitted on a timely basis, the claim will be delayed and the payment made previously will be collected. The RAC contractor also performs what is called automated reviews strictly on the submitted outpatient claims based on experience with the use of CPT/HCPCS codes and the number of units charged for a particular procedure code using proprietary software. The RAC can only review claims submitted in the past three years.

If a particular record has been reviewed by another entity, such as the QIO or CERT contractor, the RAC contractor will not review the same case. When the RAC concludes that a billing or coding error has been made with an improper payment made, it will notify the FI/MAC to adjust the claim and recoup the payment from the providers. The error may be either an overpayment or an underpayment to the provider. The provider is notified of the finding and has the opportunity to appeal following an established appeal process that involves submitting documentation to support the provider's disagreement with the RAC decision. The appeals process used for the RAC is the same for all providers who want to appeal a Medicare's claim decision. There are five levels of appeals:

1. Appeal submitted to the claims processing contractor

2. Appeal submitted to a qualified independent contractor

3. Appeal submitted to an administrative law judge for a hearing

4. Appeal submitted to the Appeals Council Review

5. Final appeal may be submitted for a judicial review through the Federal District Court review process (CMS 2012e)

The examination of ICD-10-CM coding has been a major area of focus for the RACs because the diagnosis and procedure codes create the MS-DRGs, which are the basis of payment for acute-care hospitals. When ICD-10-CM coding is implemented, the examination of these codes will be the focus of RAC reviews for reimbursement purposes. ICD-10-CM/PCS and CPT coding in other healthcare organizations, such as rehabilitation hospitals and units and physician offices, determine reimbursement to the providers and therefore are a focus of attention during these providers' reviews. Certified coders are employed by RACs to perform coding reviews.

The types of errors found by the RAC that resulted in both overpayments and underpayments to the providers include the following:

- Codes for the incorrect number of ventilator hours that determined the MS-DRG

- Incorrectly coding cerebrovascular disease that determined the MS-DRG

- Selecting the incorrect principal diagnosis with an unrelated operating room procedure

- Incorrectly coding respiratory system diagnoses with ventilator procedures

- Incorrect discharge disposition that determines the transfer payment policy

The types of errors found by the RACs that resulted in overpayments to the providers include the following:

- Medically unnecessary admissions or unnecessary items or services

- Unbundling of CPT/HCPCS codes

- Incorrect number of units billed for outpatient services
- Incorrect codes for cardiac procedures that determined the MS-DRG
- Incorrect coding and billing for outpatient intravenous infusion and chemotherapy
- Incorrect coding for excisional debridements that determined the MS-DRG

The types of errors that resulted in underpayments to the providers include the following:

- Incorrectly coding small and large bowel procedures that determined the MS-DRG
- Incorrectly coding acute respiratory failure that determined the MS-DRG
- Incorrectly coding heart failure that determined the MS-DRG
- Incorrectly coding skin grafts and wound debridement (CMS 2012e)

Coding for Medical Necessity

Three factors help define the **medical necessity** of a diagnostic test, procedure, or treatment:

1. The likelihood that a proposed healthcare service will have a reasonable beneficial effect on the patient's physical condition and quality of life at a specific point in his or her illness or lifetime.

2. Healthcare services and supplies that are proven or acknowledged to be effective in the diagnosis, treatment, cure, or relief of a health condition, illness, injury, disease, or its symptoms and are consistent with the community's accepted standard of care. Under medical necessity, only those services, procedures, and patient care warranted by the patient's condition are provided.

3. The concept that procedures are only reimbursed as a covered benefit when they are performed for a specific diagnosis or specified frequency.

Accurate ICD-10-CM diagnosis coding is essential to establish the medical necessity of a particular service as required by Medicare's reasonable and necessary medical coverage policies. Other third-party payers also want to know the reason for the service before payment is determined. Medicare Administrative Contractors (MACs) that process Part A and Part B Medicare claims may develop local coverage decisions (LCDs), formerly known as local medical review policies (LMRPs). These policies ensure that claims submitted for certain services—typically outpatient services—have been deemed reasonable and necessary for the patient's condition. National coverage determinations (NCDs) also exist for other diagnostic and therapeutic services including many laboratory tests, for which Medicare payment is contingent on a particular condition being established as the reason the test was ordered. The coder must be certain that documentation contains all of the reasons why the physician ordered a diagnostic or therapeutic service. Then the coder must assign all of the appropriate ICD-10-CM diagnosis codes for the claim to be reviewed accurately for medical necessity and paid appropriately. The requirements for determining medical necessity have moved the coding personnel outside the traditional HIM department into hospitals' emergency departments, admitting or registration or access departments, central scheduling centers, and a variety of clinical departments performing many outpatient services, such as radiology and laboratory. The need to know if a patient's condition meets the medical necessity requirements of a particular service is essential prior to issuing an **advance beneficiary notice (ABN)**. An ABN is a statement signed by the patient when he or she is notified by the provider, prior to a service or procedure being performed, that Medicare may not reimburse the provider for the service, whereupon the patient indicates that he or she will be responsible for any charges. Medical necessity processing has brought the coding function closer to the point of care and, in some institutions, improved the documentation related to the reasons for outpatient therapy and testing services.

Review Exercises: Chapter 25

1. What was the goal of the MS-DRG system that replaced the DRG system?

2. What is the basic formula for calculating each MS-DRG hospital payment?

3. What are possible "add-on" payments that a hospital could receive in addition to the basic Medicare MS-DRG payment?

4. What additional factor is involved in the assignment of MS-DRGs besides principal and secondary diagnoses including the presence of major or other complications or comorbidities and discharge disposition or status?

5. What purpose are the reviews conducted by Quality Improvement Organizations designed to serve?

6. What is the name of the program that functions to detect and correct improper payments in the traditional Medicare fee-for-service programs?

7. How does Medicare or other third-party payers determine whether the patient has medical necessity for the tests, procedures, or treatment billed on a claim form?

8. How does a hospital qualify for a disproportionate share adjustment from Medicare?

9. What are the factors that Medicare uses to designate a hospital as a sole community hospital?

10. What are post-acute care settings?

Appendix A

Glossary of Coding Terms

Access location: Specifies the external site through which the internal organ is reached: skin or mucous membrane and external orifices

Additional significant procedure: The second, third, or other procedure performed that is surgical in nature or carries a procedural or an anesthetic risk or requires specialized training

Advance beneficiary notice (ABN): A statement signed by the patient when he or she is notified by the provider, prior to a service or procedure being done, that Medicare may not reimburse the provider for the service, wherein the patient indicates that he will be responsible for any charges

Aftercare: Aftercare visit Z codes are used to classify patient care encounters when the initial treatment of a disease has been performed and the patient requires continued care during the healing or recovery period, or for the long term consequences of a disease. The aftercare codes should not be used when the patient continues to receive for a current active illness when the diagnosis code is used instead

Alphabetic Index: Divided into two parts—the Index to Diseases and Injury and the Index to External Causes of Injury. Within the Index of Diseases and Injury there is a Neoplasm Table and a Table of Drugs and Chemicals. The Alphabetic Index in ICD-10-CM is formatted with main terms set in boldface are listed in alphabetical order. Main terms are entries printed in boldface type and flush with the left margin of each column in the Alphabetic Index

Bilateral procedure: A surgical or other procedure that was performed on two sides of the body, that is, on mirror images of the body such as two kidneys, two radial bones, and so on. Bilateral procedures impact ICD-10-PCS procedure coding. If a bilateral body part value exists for a particular body part, a single procedure code is assigned using the bilateral body part value. If no bilateral body part value exists, each procedure is coded separately using the appropriate body part value for right and left

Body part: Specific anatomical site where the procedure was performed

Body part key: List of anatomical terms with the corresponding PCS description that is used for the body part values in the ICD-10-PCS codes

Body system: The second character of a code defines the body system which is the general physiological system or anatomical region involved

Brackets: A punctuation mark [ ] found only in the Tabular List of ICD-10-CM to enclose synonyms, alternative wording, or explanatory phrases. Brackets are used in the Alphabetic Index to identify manifestation codes. *See also* **Slanted brackets; square brackets**

Canceled surgery: A surgical or other procedure that was started but not completed due to unforeseen circumstances; canceled procedures impact ICD-10-PCS procedure coding. A procedure may be canceled because of the patient's deteriorating medical condition during surgery, due to the patient's choice, due to malfunctioning equipment or the unavailability of staff

Category: A three-digit ICD-10-CM code that represents a single disease entity or a group of similar or closely-related conditions

Centers for Medicare and Medicaid Services (CMS):   The division of the Department of Health and Human Services that is responsible for developing healthcare policy in the United States and for administering the Medicare program and the federal portion of the Medicaid program and maintaining the procedure portion of the International Classification of Diseases, 10th revision, Procedure Classification System (ICD-10-PCS.)

Characters: The seven digits or letters of a code

Classification: A clinical vocabulary, terminology, or nomenclature that lists words or phrases with their meanings, provides for the proper use of clinical words as names or symbols, and facilitates mapping standardized terms to broader classifications for administrative, regulatory, oversight, and fiscal requirements

Classification system: A system for grouping similar diseases and procedures and organizing related information for easy retrieval. A system for assigning numeric or alphanumeric code numbers to represent specific diseases or procedures

"Code Also" note: Note appearing in ICD-10-CM, meaning that two codes may be required to fully describe a condition

Code first: An instruction notation found in the ICD-10-CM for categories in which primary tabulation (or first listing of the code) is not intended. The code, title and instructions are set in italic type to serve as notice not to assign that code as the principal or first listed code. The note requires listing the code for the underlying disease (etiology) first and the code for the manifestation second. The note will suggest underlying diseases but it is not all-inclusive

Coding: The transformation of verbal descriptions into numbers. The process of assigning numeric or alphanumeric representations to clinical documentation

Coding Clinic: A publication issued quarterly by the American Hospital Association and approved by the Centers for Medicare and Medicaid Services to give coding advice and direction for ICD-10-CM

Colon: A punctuation mark (:) that is used in the Tabular List of ICD-10-CM after an incomplete term that needs one or more additional terms or modifiers in order to be assigned to a given category or code

Combination codes: One code that describes both the etiology and manifestation of the disease, such as streptococcal pharyngitis, ICD-10-CM code J02.0. The underlying disease is the streptococcal infection and the manifestation is the pharyngitis

Comorbidity: Defined within the scope of the Medicare Acute Care Inpatient Prospective Payment System, an additional diagnosis that describes a pre-existing condition that, because of its presence with a specific principal diagnosis, will cause an increase in the patient's length of stay

Completeness: In the ICD-10-PCS system, there should be a unique code for all substantially different procedures

Complication: Defined within the scope of the Medicare Acute Care Inpatient Prospective Payment System, an additional diagnosis that describes a condition arising after the beginning of hospital observation and treatment and then modifies the course of the patient's illness or the medical care required

Complications/comorbidities: Illnesses or injuries that coexist with the condition for which the patient is primarily seeking healthcare. In the new Medicare-severity diagnosis-related groups (MS-DRGs), certain conditions that reflect more serious, resource intensive conditions are described as major complications/comorbidities (MCCs)

Connecting words: Subterms in the Alphabetic Index that appear after a main term to indicate a relationship between the main term and an associated condition or etiology

Cooperating Parties for the ICD-10-CM: A group of organizations (the American Health Information Management Association, the American Hospital Association, the Centers for Medicare and Medicaid Services, and the National Center for Health Statistics) that collaborates in the development and maintenance of the *International Classification of Diseases, Tenth Revision, Clinical Modification* (ICD-10-CM)

Current Procedural Terminology, Fourth Edition (CPT): A comprehensive, descriptive list of terms and numeric codes used for reporting diagnostic and therapeutic procedures and other medical services performed by physicians; published and updated annually by the American Medical Association

Department of Health and Human Services (HHS or DHHS): The cabinet-level federal agency that oversees all the health- and human-services-related activities of the federal government and administers federal regulations

Device: A graft, prostheses, implant, simple, mechanical, or electronic appliance that remains in the patient's body at the conclusion of the procedure

Device Aggregation Table: Table in ICD-10-PCS that crosswalks particular device character value definitions for specific root operations in a specific body part to the more general device character value to be used when the root operation covers a wide range of body parts and the device character represents an entire family of devices

Device Key: Key in ICD-10-PCS that includes brand names and generic names of devices to help the coder determine the PCS device description by referencing the name of the device used during a procedure

Diagnosis: A word or phrase used by a physician to identify a disease from which an individual patient suffers or a condition for which the patient needs, seeks, or receives medical care. All diagnoses affecting the current hospital stay must be reported as part of UHDDS

Diagnosis-related groups (DRGs): A unit of case-mix classification adopted by the federal government and some other payers as a prospective payment mechanism for hospital inpatients in which diseases are placed into groups because related diseases and treatments tend to consume similar amounts of healthcare resources and incur similar amounts of cost; in the

Medicare and Medicaid programs, one of more than 500 diagnostic classifications in which cases demonstrate similar resource consumption and length-of-stay patterns. Under the prospective payment system (PPS), hospitals are paid a set fee for treating patients in a single DRG category, regardless of the actual cost of care for the individual

Diagnostic and Statistical Manual of Mental Disorders, Fourth Revision, Text Revision (DSM-IV-TR): A nomenclature developed by the American Psychiatric Association to standardize the diagnostic process for patients with psychiatric disorders, which includes codes that correspond to ICD-9-CM codes; most recent version is fourth edition (text revision), or DSM-IV-TR, published in 2000 and revised in 2004 with updated clinical terms but very few coding changes

Disposition of patient: The destination of the patient upon leaving the hospital

Disproportionate share hospital (DSH): Healthcare organizations that meet governmental criteria for percentages of indigent patients or hospitals that serve a disproportionate share of low-income patients

Electronic appliances: Materials that assist, monitor, or take the place of or prevent a physiological function

Etiology and Manifestation: A coding convention that requires two codes for situations when one disease produces another condition. The first disease is considered the etiology and the second condition that it produces is called the manifestation

Excision: Cutting out or off, without replacement, a portion of a body part

Excludes1: Note that indicates that the conditions listed after it cannot ever be used at the same time as the code above the Excludes1 note

Excludes2: Note that means that two codes are applied when both conditions are present

Expandability: The structure of the codes allows for changes to be made easily by adding values as needed or using existing values to identify new procedures

Expected payer: The single major source expected by the patient to pay for this bill (for example, Blue Cross/Blue Shield, Medicare, Medicaid, workers' compensation)

External approach: An approach used when procedures are performed directly on the skin or mucous membrane

Family history: A family history is the identification of a medical condition that is currently or formerly present in a patient's family member that puts the patient at higher risk of contracting the same condition. The possibility of the patient contracting the same condition may alter the type of treatment the patient receives

Federal Register: The daily publication of the US Government Printing Office that reports all changes in regulations and federally-mandated standards, including HCPCS and ICD-10-CM codes

Follow-up code: A follow up code identifies the reason for healthcare services when the treatment of the patient's condition is completed, and the patient is undergoing surveillance or a "checkup" to determine if his or her disease-free status continues. A follow-up code means the condition has been fully treated and no longer exists

Grafts and prostheses: Biological or synthetic material that takes the place of all or a portion of a body part

Health Insurance Portability and Accountability Act of 1996 (HIPAA): The federal legislation enacted to provide continuity of health coverage, control fraud and abuse in healthcare, reduce healthcare costs, and guarantee the security and privacy of health information; limits exclusion for preexisting medical conditions, prohibits discrimination against employees and dependents based on health status, guarantees availability of health insurance to small employers, and guarantees renewability of insurance to all employees regardless of size; also known as Public Law 104-191 and the Kassebaum-Kennedy Law

Histology: The study of cell structures under a microscope

Hospital identification: The unique number assigned to each institution

ICD-10-CM Coordination and Maintenance (C&M) Committee: Committee composed of representatives from the National Center for Health Statistics (NCHS) and the Centers for Medicare and Medicaid Services (CMS) that is responsible for maintaining the United States' clinical modification version of the International Classification of Diseases, Ninth Revision (ICD-9-CM) code sets; holds open meetings that serve as a public forum for discussing (but not making decisions about) proposed revisions to ICD-10-CM

ICD-10-CM Official Guidelines for Coding and Reporting: A set of rules that have been developed to accompany and complement the official conventions and instructions provided within the ICD-9-CM system. Adherence to these guidelines when assigning ICD-10-CM diagnosis and procedure codes is required under the Health Insurance Portability and Accountability Act (HIPAA.) The guidelines are approved by the four organizations that make up the Cooperating Parties for ICD-10-CM. These guidelines have been developed to assist both the healthcare provider and the coder in identifying those diagnoses and procedures that are to be reported

Implant: Therapeutic material that is not absorbed, eliminated, or incorporated into a body part

Includes note: Includes or inclusion notes are used throughout the ICD-10-CM, the Tabular List, to further define or provide an example of a three character code. Includes notes are not exhaustive; that is, not every synonym or similar condition may be listed. Includes notes appear at the beginning of a chapter, section or directly below a category or subcategory code

Index: Provides an alphabetic listing of procedure titles in ICD-10-PCS

International Classification of Diseases, Ninth Revision, Clinical Modification (ICD-9-CM): A coding and classification system used in the United States to report diagnoses in all healthcare settings and inpatient procedures and services as well as morbidity and mortality information

International Classification of Diseases, Tenth Revision (ICD-10): The most recent revision of the disease classification system developed and used by the World Health Organization to track morbidity and mortality information worldwide (implemented by the United States on October 1, 2014)

International Classification of Diseases, Tenth Revision, Clinical Modification (ICD-10-CM): The replacement for ICD-9-CM, volumes 1 and 2, developed to contain more codes and allow greater specificity. ICD-10-CM will be used for diagnosis coding in all types of health care facilities and ambulatory settings

International Classification of Diseases, Tenth Revision, Procedure Coding System (ICD-10-PCS): A separate procedure coding system that replaces ICD-9-CM, volume 3, intended to improve coding accuracy and efficiency, reduce training effort, and improve communication with physicians. ICD-10-PCS will be used for inpatient hospital procedure coding

Instrumentation: Specialized equipment used to perform a procedure on an internal body part

Laterality: Right or left side

Main terms: Entries printed in boldface type and flush with the left margin of each column within Volume 2, the Alphabetic Index to Diseases and Injuries. Main terms represent (1) diseases, (2) conditions, (3) nouns, and (4) adjectives. This is the first place in ICD-10-CM that the coder uses to locate the ICD-9-CM code for the patient's disease, condition or procedure to be classified. Within ICD-10-PCS, the Index to Procedures, main terms identify the type of procedure performed

Medical necessity: Several factors are included in the determination of medical necessity: (1) The likelihood that a proposed healthcare service will have a reasonable beneficial effect on the patient's physical condition and quality of life at a specific point in his or her illness or lifetime. (2) Healthcare services and supplies that are proven or acknowledged to be effective in the diagnosis, treatment, cure, or relief of a health condition, illness, injury, disease, or its symptoms, and to be consistent with the community's accepted standard of care. Under medical necessity, only those services, procedures, and patient care warranted by the patient's condition are provided. (3) The concept that procedures are only reimbursed as a covered benefit when they are performed for a specific diagnosis or at a specified frequency

Medicare Prescription Drug, Improvement, and Modernization Act (MMA) of 2003: The federal legislation that includes language concerning the timeliness of data collection and contains information about the updating of ICD-9-CM twice a year, if needed, on April 1, as well as the traditional October 1st date for ICD-9-CM code changes

Medicare-Severity Diagnosis-Related Groups (MS-DRGs): For fiscal year 2008, Medicare adopted a severity-adjusted diagnosis-related group system called "Medicare-severity DRGs or MS-DRGs. This was the most drastic revision to the DRG system in 24 years. Medicare's goal with the new MS-DRG system was to significantly improve Medicare's ability to recognize severity of illness in its inpatient hospital payments. The new system is projected to increase payments to hospitals for services provided to the sicker patient and decrease payments for treating less severely ill patients

Method of approach: The surgical technique used to reach the operative site

Multiaxial: The ability of a nomenclature to express the meaning of a concept across several axes

National Center for Health Statistics (NCHS): The federal agency responsible for collecting and disseminating information on health services utilization and the health status of the population in the United States; developed the clinical modification to the International Classification of Diseases, Ninth Revision (ICD-9) and is responsible for updating the diagnosis portion of the ICD-10-CM

National Uniform Billing Committee (NUBC): The national group responsible for identifying data elements and designing the CMS-1500 or the Uniform Bill-04 (UB-04)

NEC: An abbreviation of "not elsewhere classified," this abbreviation in the Alphabetic Index represents "other specified." When a specific code is not available for a condition, the Alphabetic Index directs the coder to the "other specified" code in the Tabular List

Nonessential modifiers: A series of terms in parentheses that sometimes directly follow main terms and subterms in the Alphabetic Index to Diseases of ICD-10-CM. The presence or absence of these parenthetical terms in the diagnosis has no effect on the selection of the codes listed for that main term or subterm

NOS: An abbreviation of "not otherwise specified," NOS is the equivalent of unspecified. It is used only in Volume 1, Tabular List, of ICD-10-CM for both diseases and procedures. Codes describing "not otherwise specified" conditions or procedures are assigned only when the diagnostic or procedural statement, as well as the health record, does not provide enough information to assign a more specific code

Official Addendum to ICD-10-CM: The official document that notes the changes made to ICD-9-CM at least on an annual basis, traditionally on October 1st of every year. The National Center for Health Statistics publishes the addendum for the diagnosis classification. The Center for Medicare and Medicaid Services publishes the addendum for the procedure classification

Other diagnoses: Defined in UHDDS as all conditions that coexist at the time of admission, that develop subsequently, or that affect the treatment received or the length of stay

Overlapping lesion: A primary malignant neoplasm that overlaps two or more sites

Parentheses: A punctuation mark ( ) that encloses supplementary words or explanatory information that may or may not be present in the statement of a diagnosis or procedure. The words within the parentheses do not affect the code number assigned to the case. Terms in parentheses are considered nonessential modifiers

Personal history: A personal history is a description of the patient's past medical condition that no long exists and for which the patient is not receiving any treatment. However, the fact that the patient had the condition is important because the condition has the potential for recurrence and the patient may require continued monitoring

Personal identification: The unique number assigned to each patient that distinguishes the patient and his or her health record from all others

Physician identification: The unique number assigned to each physician within the hospital

Place of occurrence code: A code used to identify the place where an injury occurred. This code describes the physical location or place where the event occurred, not the patient's activity at the time of the event

Present on admission (POA): A data element required on the Uniform Bill-04 to be linked with all ICD-9-CM diagnosis codes according to present on-admission reporting guidelines. The purpose of the POA indicator is to differentiate between conditions that were present in the patient at the time of admission and the conditions that develop during the inpatient stay

Principal diagnosis: Defined in UHDDS as the condition established after study to be chiefly responsible for occasioning the admission of the patient to the hospital for care. The definition is used with ICD-9-CM coding to determine the first-reported diagnosis code

Principal procedure: The procedure performed for definitive treatment rather than for diagnostic or exploratory purposes or for treatment of a complication. Definition is used when applying ICD-9-CM procedure codes. When more than one procedure meets the criteria for principal procedures, the one most closely related to the principal diagnosis should be selected

Procedure (surgical or therapeutic): Any single, separate, systematic process upon or within the body that can be complete in itself; is normally performed by a physician, dentist, or other licensed practitioner; can be performed either with or without instruments; and is performed to restore disunited or deficient parts, remove diseased or injured tissues, extract foreign matter, assist in obstetrical delivery, or aid in diagnosis

Quality Improvement Organization (QIO):   Organizations that contract with Medicare to work with consumers, physicians, hospitals, and other caregivers to refine care delivery systems to make sure patients, particularly among underserved populations, receive the right care at the right time. The program also safeguards the integrity of the Medicare trust fund by ensuring payment is made only for medically-necessary services and investigates beneficiary complaints about quality of care. Under the direction of the Centers for Medicare and Medicaid Services (CMS), the program consists of a national network of QIOs responsible for each US state, territory, and the District of Columbia

Qualifier: The seventh character of ICD-10-PCS that specifies an additional attribute of the procedure, if applicable

Recovery Audit Contractors (RACs):   Organizations that contract with Medicare to perform reviews of medical records with the corresponding Medicare claim to (1) detect Medicare improper payments, including both underpayments and overpayments; and (2) correct Medicare improper payments. The demonstration project ended in 2008 and allowed Medicare to evaluate the efficiency and effectiveness of the program in order to make improvements in the RAC program before taking it into additional states as Medicare transitions the RAC program gradually through 2009. The examination of the ICD-9-CM coding is a major area of focus for the RACs as the diagnosis and procedure codes create the Medicare-severity diagnosis-related group (MS-DRG) that is the basis of payment for acute care hospitals. ICD-9-CM and CPT coding in other health care organizations, such as rehabilitation hospitals and units, physician offices, and so forth, determine reimbursement to the providers and, therefore, are a focus of attention during these providers' reviews

Rehabilitation: A structured program that results in controlling the alcohol or drug use and in replacing alcohol or drug dependence with activities that are nonchemical in nature

Release: Freeing a body part from an abnormal physical constraint by cutting or by use of force. Coded to the body part being freed in ICD-10-PCS

Repair: Restoring, to the extent possible, a body part to its normal anatomical structure and function. It also functions as the "not elsewhere classified (NEC)" root operation and is to be used when the procedure performed does not meet the definition of one of the other root operations in ICD-10-PCS

Reposition: Moving all or a portion of a body part to its normal location or other suitable location in ICD-10-PCS

Resection: Cutting out or off, without replacement, all of a body part. Includes all of a body part or any subdivision of a body part that has its own body part value in ICD-10-PCS

Root operation: The objective of the procedure being performed

Section: The first character of a code determines the broad procedure category, or section, where the code is located

"See" note: A cross-reference term in the Alphabetic Index to Diseases and Injuries that provides direction to the coder to look elsewhere in the code book before assigning a code. The *see* cross reference points to an alternative term. This is a mandatory instruction that must be followed to ensure accurate ICD-10-CM code assignment

"See also" note: A cross-reference term in the Alphabetic Index to Diseases and Injuries that provides direction to the coder to look elsewhere in the code book before assigning a code. The *see also* cross reference requires review of another term in the Index if all the needed information cannot be found under the first main term. This is a mandatory instruction that must be followed to ensure accurate ICD-10-CM code assignment

Significant procedure: A procedure that is surgical in nature or carries a procedural or an anesthetic risk or requires specialized training. Definition is used when applying ICD-9-CM procedure codes

Simple or mechanical appliances: Biological or synthetic material that assists or prevents a physiological function

Slanted brackets: A punctuation mark *[ ]* used in the Alphabetic Index to identify manifestation codes

Square brackets: A punctuation mark [ ] used in the Tabular List to enclose synonyms, abbreviations, alternative wording, or explanatory phrases

Standardized terminology: Each term in ICD-10-PCS has a specific meaning or definition

Status codes: Status codes indicate that a patient is either a carrier of a disease or has the sequelae or residual of a past disease or condition. The status code is informative because the status may affect the course of treatment and its outcome

Stereotactic radiosurgery: A form of radiation therapy that focuses high-powered x-rays on a small area of the body

Subterms: Entries printed below the main term within the Alphabetic Index to Diseases and Injuries of ICD-10-CM that affect the selection of an appropriate code for a given disease or procedure. The subterms form individual line entries arranged in alphabetic order and printed in regular type beginning with a lowercase letter. Subterms are indented one standard indentation to the right under the main term. Subterms describe essential differences in the site, cause, or clinical type. More specific subterms are indented farther to the right as needed, indented one standard indentation after the preceding subterm and listed in alphabetic order. Within Alphabetic Index to Procedures, subterms are listed under the main term and describe essential differences in site, diagnosis, or surgical technique

Tables: Each of the code Tables identifies the first three values of the code. Based on the first three values of the code identified in the Index, the corresponding Table is used to obtain the complete code by specifying the last four values. Each Table is composed of rows that specify the valid combinations of code values

Tabular List: Numerical listing of all of the codes in ICD-10-CM

Topography: A description of a region or a special part of the body

Transfer: Moving, without taking out, all or a portion of a body part to another location to take over the function of all or a portion of a body part. The root operation is used to represent those procedures where a body part is moved to another location without disruption of its vascular or nervous supply

Uniform Bill-04 (UB-04):   The single standardized Medicare form for standardized uniform billing, scheduled to be implemented in 2007 for hospital inpatients and outpatients; this form is used by the major third-party payers and most hospitals

Uniform Hospital Discharge Data Set (UHDDS): A minimum, common core set of data elements collected on individual acute-care short-term hospital discharges in Medicare and Medicaid programs. The standard was promulgated by the US Department of Health, Education, and Welfare in 1974. The intent of the standard was to improve the uniformity and comparability of hospital discharge data. The data set was revised in 1985 to improve data collection and since that time, the application of UHDDS definitions has been expanded to include all nonoutpatient settings. It applies now to acute-care, short-term-care, long-term-care and psychiatric hospitals; home health agencies; rehabilitation facilities; nursing homes; and other nonoutpatient settings

Use additional code: An instructional notation found in Tabular List, to indicate that an additional code may provide a more complete picture of the diagnosis or procedure if the health record provides supportive documentation. The instruction may appear at the beginning of a chapter and applies to all the codes in that chapter. It may appear at the beginning of a section, or it may appear in a subcategory and apply to the codes within that particular section or subcategory

Values: Individual letters and numbers occupying the seven digits or letters of the codes

World Health Organization (WHO): The United Nations specialized agency created to ensure the attainment by all peoples of the highest possible levels of health; responsible for a number of international classifications, including The International Statistical Classification of Diseases and Related Health Problems (ICD-10) and The International Classification of Functioning, Disability, and Health (ICF)

Appendix B

Microorganisms

Table of Microorganisms

Bacteria	Species	Common Diseases
Bacillus	B. anthracis	Cutaneous anthrax, eye infections, food-poisoning, intestinal anthrax, pulmonary anthrax
Bacteriodes	B. fragilis B. melaninogenicus	Abscess of brain, liver, bacteremia, endocarditis, gangrene, peritonitis
Bordetella	B. parapertussis B. bronchiseptica	Whooping cough
Brucella	B. melitensis B. abortus B. suis	Undulant fever, brucellosis
Chlamydia	C. trachomatis C. psittaci	Conjunctivitis, lymphogranuloma venereum, trachoma, cervicitis, salpingitis, urethritis
Clostridium	C. botulinum C. perfringens C. tetani C. septicum	Botulism, gas gangrene, lockjaw
Enterobacter		Urinary tract infection, pneumonia
Escherichia coli (E. coli)		Appendicitis, cystitis, infantile-diarrhea, peritonitis, pyelitis, pyelo-nephritis, postoperative wound infections
Haemophilus	H. aegyptius H. adrophilus H. ducreyi H. influenzae H. parainfluenzae	Chancres, conjunctivitis, endo-carditis, chronic sinusitis, influenza, meningitis, mastoiditis, pneumonia, upper respiratory disease
Klebsiella	K. ozaenae K. rhinoscleromatis K. pneumoniae	Disorder of smelling faculties, nodules of nose, pneumonia, severe enteritis, upper-respiratory disease
Mycobacterium	M. Leprae M. fortuitum	Cervical adenitis, leprosy, skin lesions, tuberculosis

Bacteria	Species	Common Diseases
Mycoplasma	M. hominis M. pneumoniae M. tuberculosis	Cervicitis, pneumonia, prostatitis, urethritis
Neisseria	N. meningitidis N. pneumoniae	Gonorrhea, meningococcal meningitis, pulmonary infections, tooth abscesses, urinary tract infection
Proteus	P. vulgaris P. mirabilis P. morganii P. rettgeri P. inconstans	Kidney disease, urinary tract infection
Pseudomonas	P. aeruginosa P. maltophilia P. cepacia	Chronic otitis media, upper-respiratory infections, urinary tract infection, wounds of burn sites, endocarditis
Rickettsiaceae	R. australis R. conorii R. prowazekii R. rickettsii R. typhi R. tsutsugamushi R. quintana	Spotted fever typhus, rickettsial pneumonitis
Salmonella	S. enteritis S. typhi S. arizonae S. cholerae—suis	Enteritis, endocarditis, liver infections, nephritis, meningitis, osteo-myelitis, typhoid fever, typhoid ulcers
Shigella	S. dysenteriae S. flexneri S. boydii S. sonnei	Dysentery
Staphylococcus	S. aureus S. epidermis S. saprophyticus	Diarrhea, food poisoning, conjunctivitis, meningitis, skin infections, pneumonia, septicemia
Streptococcus—alpha	Group D (enterococcus)	Urinary tract infection, wound-infection
Streptococcus—beta	Group A (S. pyogenes) Group B (S. agalactiae) Group C	Pharyngitis, tonsillitis wound and skin infections, septicemia Perinatal: pneumonia, meningitis, septicemia Pharyngitis, tonsillitis, sepsis, necrotizing fasciitis
Streptococcus pneumoniae		Pneumonia, septicemia, meningitis, otitis media
Streptococcus	S. viridans S. mitis S. bovis S. faecalis	Glomerulonephritis, puerperal fever, laryngitis, rheumatic fever, scarlet fever, sinusitis, tonsillitis
Treponema	T. pallidum T. pertenue T. carateum T. vincentii	Pinta (skin infection syphilis, trench mouth, yaw)

Classification of Bacteria

Gram-Negative Rods		
Aerobic Campylobacter Helicobacter Legionella Brucella Bordetella Francisella Pseudomonas	*Facultative Anaerobic* Enterobacteriaceae: 　Escherichia 　Salmonella 　Shigella 　Citrobacter 　Klebsiella 　Enterobacter 　Serratia 　Proteus 　Morganella 　Yersinia Vibrionaceae: 　Vibrio 　Aeromonas Pasteurellaceae: 　Haemophilus 　Gardnerella 　Pasteurella	*Anaerobic* Bacteroides Fusobacterium
Gram-Negative Cocci		
Aerobic Neisseria Branhamella (Moraxella)	*Facultative Anaerobic*	*Anaerobic* Veillonella
Gram-Positive Rods		
Aerobic Bacillus Corynebacterium Mycobacterium Nocardia	*Facultative* Lactobacillus Listeria Actinomyces	*Anaerobic* Clostridium
Gram-Positive Cocci		
Aerobic Peptostreptococcus	*Facultative Anaerobic* Staphylococcus Streptococcus	*Anaerobic* Peptococcus
Miscellaneous		
Arthropod Vector: No Arthropod Vector: Devoid of Cell Wall: Microaerophilic: Obligate Aerobic: Living Cells Required:	Rickettsia, Coxiella Chlamydia Mycoplasma, Ureaplasma Borrelia Leptospira Treponema	

Appendix C

Commonly Used Drugs

A coder's knowledge of drug names is essential. The administration of a medication may be a clue that a patient has a medical condition that is being treated and, therefore, qualifies as a condition to be coded. A patient may be admitted to the hospital or seen in the outpatient setting for one reason but, because of a preexisting comorbid condition, continues to receive treatment by drug therapy. Recognition of the drug and the condition it is treating is important for the coder to fully report the patient's treated diseases and conditions.

The following table lists commonly used drugs with the trade (brand) name and generic name given to each drug. A trade name usually is written starting with a capital letter; generic names are not capitalized. The functional classification or the purpose of each drug is listed as well as the conditions the drug is most likely used to manage or control.

Use Appendix C to become familiar with common drugs by using this independent study exercise.

Exercise

Make a reference list of drugs by functional classification. For each of these functional classes, use Appendix C to identify the drugs within each functional class by their trade names and generic names.

Functional Class

1. Angiotensin-converting enzyme (ACE) inhibitor
2. Analgesic
3. Antianginal
4. Antianxiety
5. Anticoagulant
6. Antidepressant
7. Antidysrhythmic
8. Antihypertensive
9. Antineoplastic
10. Antiplatelet
11. Antipsychotic
12. Beta-blocker
13. Bronchodilator
14. Calcium channel blockers
15. Diuretic
16. Sedative
17. Thrombolytic

Here is an example of this exercise. The coder identifies all the ACE inhibitor drugs by their (1) trade name and (2) generic name. Generic names sometimes follow a pattern. For example, generic names for ACE inhibitor drugs end with "pril." By knowing this pattern, it is easier to identify other drugs that are also ACE inhibitors.

1. ACE inhibitors

Trade Name	Generic Name
Accupril	quinapril
Altace	ramipril
Capoten	captopril
Lotensin	benazepril
Mavik	trandolapril
Monopril	fosinopril
Vasotec	enalapril
Zestril	lisinopril

Try this exercise independently with the other drug classes on the numbered list.

The list of drugs provided in Appendix C is by no means all the drugs that a coder should know. Every coder should have a drug reference book available for review, as there are thousands of drugs used for patient care and many new ones become available every year. Knowledge of drugs and their purposes is a skill every coder must develop.

Trade Drug Name	Generic Drug Name	Functional Classification	Used to Treat
Abilify	aripiprazole	Antipsychotic, neuroleptic	Schizophrenia
Accupril	quinapril	Antihypertensive angiotensin converting enzyme (ACE) inhibitor	Hypertension, congestive heart failure (CHF)
Actidose-Aqua, Charco-Aid, Liqui-Char	activated charcoal	Antidote	Poisoning
Adenocard, Adenoscan	adenosine	Antidysrhythmic	Supraventricular tachycardia, as a diagnostic aid to assess myocardial perfusion defects in coronary artery disease (CAD)
Adriamycin	doxorubicin	Antineoplastic	Wilms' tumor; bladder, breast, cervical, head, neck, liver, lung, ovarian, prostatic, stomach, testicular, thyroid cancer; Hodgkin's disease; acute lymphoblastic leukemia; myeloblastic leukemia; neuroblastomas; lymphomas; sarcomas
Agrylin	anagrelide	Antiplatelet	Essential thrombocytopenia, polycythemia vera, chronic myelogenous leukemia
Albuminar, Albutein, Buminate, Plasbumin	normal serum albumin	Blood derivative	Restores plasma volume in burns, hyperbilirubinemia, shock, hypoproteinemia, prevention of cerebral edema, cardiopulmonary bypass, acute respiratory distress syndrome (ARDS)
Aldactazide	combination of spironolactone and hydrochlorothiazide	Potassium-sparing diuretic and antihypertensive	Edema of CHF, hypertension, diuretic-induced hypokalemia, primary hyperaldosteronism, edema of nephrotic syndrome, cirrhosis of liver with ascites
Aldactone	spironolactone	Potassium-sparing diuretic	Edema of CHF, hypertension, diuretic-induced hypokalemia, primary hyperaldosteronism, edema of nephrotic syndrome, cirrhosis of liver with ascites
Aldomet	methyldopa, methyldopate	Antihypertensive	Hypertension, hypertensive crisis

Trade Drug Name	Generic Drug Name	Functional Classification	Used to Treat
Aldoril	Combination of methyldopa and hydrochlorothiazide	Antihypertensive	Hypertension, hypertensive crisis
Alkeran	mephalan	Antineoplastic	Multiple myeloma, malignant melanoma, advanced ovarian cancer
Allopurinol – Alloprim, Apo-Allopurinol	allopurinol	Antigout drug	Chronic gout, hyperuricemia associated with malignancies, recurrent calcium oxalate calculi, Chagas' disease, cutaneous/ visceral leishmaniasis
Altace	ramipril	Antihypertensive ACE inhibitor	Hypertension, CHF, reduction of risk of myocardial infarction (MI), stroke, death from cardiovascular disorders
Alupent	metaproterenol	Bronchodilator	Bronchial asthma, bronchopasms
Amikacin	amikin	Antibiotic/anti-infective	Severe systemic infections of central nervous system (CNS), respiratory, gastrointestinal (GI), genitourinary (GU), bone, skin, soft tissues caused by serious gram-negative bacterial organisms
Aminophylline	aminophylline	Bronchodilator, spasmolytic, pulmonary vasodilator, smooth muscle relaxant	Bronchial asthma, bronchospasm, Cheyes-Stokes respirations
Amoxil (Trimox, Wymox)	amoxicillin	Antibiotic, anti-infective	Skin, respiratory, GI, GU infections, otitis media, gonorrhea, gram-positive bacteria, gram-negative bacteria organisms
Ampicin, Marcillin, Omnipen, Polycillin, Prinacillin	ampicillin	Broad-spectrum antibiotic, anti-infective	Gram-positive and gram-negative organisms
Ancef	cefazolin	Antibiotic, anti-infective, cephalosporins	Gram-negative and gram-positive organisms, upper and lower respiratory tract infections, urinary tract infections (UTIs), skin infections, bone, joint, biliary, genital infections, endocarditis, surgical prophylaxis, septicemia

Trade Drug Name	Generic Drug Name	Functional Classification	Used to Treat
Angiomax	bivalirudin	Anticoagulant	Unstable angina in patients undergoing percutaneous transluminal coronary angioplasty (PTCA)
Apresoline, Hylazin	hydralazine	Antihypertensive, peripheral vasodilator	Essential hypertension
Ascriptin	Combination of aspirin, magnesium hydroxide, aluminum hydroxide, calcium carbonate	Nonnarcotic analgesic, anti-inflammatory, antipyretic	Rheumatoid arthritis, osteoarthritis, and other arthritic conditions
Atacand	candesartan	Antihypertensive, angiotensin receptor blocker (ARB)	Hypertension
Atarax, Vistaril	hydroxyzine	Anti-anxiety, antihistamine, sedative-hypnotic, antiemetic, anxiolytic	Anxiety preoperatively, postoperatively to prevent nausea, vomiting, to potentiate opioid analgesic, sedation, pruritus
Ativan	lorazepam	Sedative, hypnotic, anti-anxiety, anxiolytic	Anxiety, irritability in psychiatric or organic disorders, preoperatively, insomnia, adjunct to endoscopic procedures
Atro-Pen	atropine	Antidysrhythmic, anticholinergic parasympatholytic	Bradycardia, reversal of anticholinesterase agents, insecticide poisoning, blocking cardiac vagal reflexes, decreasing secretions before surgery, antispasmodic with GU, biliary surgery, bronchodilator
Augmentin	amoxicillin/clavulanate potassium	Broad-spectrum antibiotic, anti-infective	Sinus infections, pneumonia, UTI, skin infections, otitis media
Avapro	irbesartan	Antihypertensive, ARB	Hypertension, nephropathy in type II diabetes
AZT, Apo-Zidovudine, Azidothymidine, Novo-AZT, Retrovir	Zidovudine	Antiviral	Symptomatic/asymptomatic HIV infections (AIDS), confirmed Pneumocystis carinii pneumonia, prevention of maternal-fetal HIV transmission
Baclofen	baclofen	Skeletal muscle relaxant	Spinal cord injury, multiple sclerosis

Trade Drug Name	Generic Drug Name	Functional Classification	Used to Treat
Bactrim, Septra, Septra-DS	trimethoprim-sulfamethoxazole	Anti-infective, antibacterial	UTIs, acute and chronic prostatitis, otitis media, chronic bronchitis in adults, traveler's diarrhea, chancroid, Pneumocystis carinii pneumonitis
Benadryl	diphenhydramine	Antihistamine	Perennial and seasonal allergies due to inhalant allergens and foods; rhinitis, nighttime sedation, infant colic, nonproductive cough, motion sickness, and parkinsonism
Benicar	olmesartan medoxomil	Antihypertensive, ARB	Hypertension
Bentyl, Bentylol	dicyclomine	GI, anticholinergic	Peptic ulcer disease, infant colic, urinary incontinence
Betadine, Povidone Iodine, Bacitracin	betadine	Antiseptic	Disinfection of topical wounds, preoperative skin preparation
Bicillin	penicillin G benzathine	Broad-spectrum anti-infective	Respiratory infections, scarlet fever, erysipelas, otitis media, pneumonia, skin and soft-tissue infections, gonorrhea, gram-negative and gram-positive organisms
Blenoxane	bleomycin	Antineoplastic	Cancer of head, neck, penis, cervix, vulva, Hodgkin's disease, lymphosarcoma, reticulum cell sarcoma, testicular carcinoma, malignant pleural effusion
Brethine	terbutaline	Bronchodilator	Bronchial asthmas and reversible bronchospasm in bronchitis and emphysema, hyperkalemia
Bretylol	bretylium	Antidysrhythmic	Life-threatening ventricular tachycardia, cardioversion, ventricular fibrillation
Bronkosol	isoetarine	Bronchodilator	Bronchial asthma and reversible bronchospasm in bronchitis and emphysema
Bumex	bumetanide	Loop diuretic, antihypertensive	Edema in CHF, liver disease, renal disease, nephrotic syndrome, pulmonary edema, ascites, hypertension, anasarca
Buprenex	buprenorphine	Opioid analgesic	Moderate to severe pain

Trade Drug Name	Generic Drug Name	Functional Classification	Used to Treat
BuSpar	buspirone	Anti-anxiety, sedative	Anxiety disorders
Busulfex	busulfan	Antineoplastic	Chronic myelocytic leukemia
Campath	alemtuzumab	Antineoplastic	B-cell chronic lymphocytic leukemia
Capoten	captopril	Antihypertensive, ACE inhibitor	CHF, hypertension, diabetic nephropathy, MI
Cardene, Cardene SR	nicardipine	Antihypertensive, calcium channel blocker, antianginal	Stable angina pectoris
Cardizem, Cardizem CD, Cardizem SR	diltiazem	Calcium channel blocker	Angina pectoris due to coronary insufficiency, hypertension, vasospasm, atrial fibrillation, atrial flutter, paroxysmal supraventricular tachycardia
Catapres, Catapres-TTS	clonidine	Antihypertensive	Mild to moderate hypertension used alone or in combination, severe pain in cancer patients
Celestone	betamethasone	Corticosteroid	Immunosuppression, severe inflammation, prevention of neonatal respiratory distress syndrome by administering to mother
Chloromycetin	chloramphenicol	Antibiotic, anti-infective	Infections caused by H. influenzae, salmonella, Rickettsia, Neisseria, mycoplasma
Cipro	ciprofloxacin	Broad-spectrum anti-infective, antibacterial	Urinary tract infection (UTI), lower respiratory infection, bone and joint infection, chronic bacterial prostatitis, acute sinusitis, postexposure inhalation anthrax
Cleocin	clindamycin	Antibiotic, anti-infective	Infections caused by staphylococcus, streptococci, Rickettsia, Pneumocystis carinii, and other serious bacteria
Clinoril	sulindac	Nonsteroidal anti-inflammatory, antirheumatic	Mild to moderate pain, osteoarthritis, Rheumatoid, gouty arthritis, ankylosing spondylitis
Cogentin	benztropine	Antiparkinson agent, cholinergic blocker	Parkinson symptoms, acute dystonic reactions
Colace	docusate sodium	Laxative, stool softener	Soften stools

Trade Drug Name	Generic Drug Name	Functional Classification	Used to Treat
Compazine	prochlorperazine	Antiemetic, antipsychotic	Nausea, vomiting, psychotic disorders
Cordarone, Pacerone	amiodarone	Antidysrhythmic	Severe ventricular tachycardia, supraventricular tachycardia, atrial fibrillation, ventricular fibrillation, cardiac arrest
Corgard	nadolol	Antihypertensive, anti-anginal, beta-blocker	Stable angina pectoris, hypertension, prophylaxis of migraine headaches
Cortef, Hydrocortone	hydrocortisone	Corticosteroid	Severe inflammation, septic shock, adrenal insufficiency, ulcerative colitis, collagen disorders
Coumadin	warfarin sodium	Anticoagulant	Pulmonary emboli, deep vein thrombosis, MI, atrial dysrhythmias, postcardiac valve replacement
Cozaar	losartan	Antihypertensive, ARBs	Hypertension, nephropathy in type II diabetes
Cytoxan	cyclophosphamide	Antineoplastic	Hodgkin's disease, lymphomas, leukemia, cancer of female reproductive tract, breast, lung, prostate, multiple myeloma, neuroblastoma, retinoblastoma, Ewing's sarcoma
Dalmane	flurazepam	Sedative, hypnotic	Insomnia
Darvocet	Combination of propoxyphene-N and acetaminophen	Analgesic	Mild to moderate pain
Darvon	propoxyphene	Opiate analgesic	Mild to moderate pain
Decadron	dexamethasone	Corticosteroid	Inflammation, allergies, neoplasms, cerebral edema, septic shock, collagen disorders
Demerol	meperidine	Opioid analgesic	Moderate to severe pain, preoperatively and postoperatively
Desyrel	trazodone	Antidepressant	Depression
Diabinese	chlorpropamide	Antidiabetic	Stable type II (adult-onset) diabetes mellitus
Diamox	acetazolamide	Diuretic, carbonic anhydrase inhibitor, antiglaucoma, antiepileptic	Glaucoma, epilepsy, edema in CHF, drug-induced edema, acute mountain sickness

Trade Drug Name	Generic Drug Name	Functional Classification	Used to Treat
Diflucan	Fluconazole	Antifungal	Candidiasis—oropharyngeal, mucocutaneous, urinary; cryptococcal meningitis
Digoxin/ Digitoxin/ Digitalis	Digoxin/digitoxin/ digitalis (Note: Some drug manufacturers use the trade and generic name interchangeably for this drug.)	Cardiac glycoside, inotropic, antidysrhythmia	CHF, atrial fibrillation, atrial tachycardia, cardiogenic shock, paroxysmal atrial tachycardia, rapid digitalization in these disorders
Dilantin	phenytoin	Anticonvulsants, antidysrhythmic	Generalized tonic-clonic seizures, status epilepticus, nonepileptic seizures associated with Reye's syndrome or after head trauma, migraines, trigeminal neuralgias, Bell's palsy, ventricular dysrhythmias uncontrolled by antidysrhythmias
Dilaudid	hydromorphone	Opiate analgesic	Moderate to severe pain, nonproductive cough
Diovan	valsartan	Antihypertensive, ARB	Hypertension
Dolobid	diflunisal	Nonsteroidal anti-inflammatory/analgesic	Mild to moderate pain or fever including arthritis, 3 to 4 times more potent than aspirin
Dopamine	intropin	Adrenergic	Shock, increased perfusion, hypotension
Dulcolax	bisacodyl	Laxative	Constipation, bowel or rectal preparation for surgery or examination
Dyazide	Combination of hydrochlorothiazide and triamterene	Diuretic/antihypertensive	Edema and hypertension
Ecotrin	acetylsalicylic acid (aspirin)	Nonopioid analgesic, nonsteroidal anti-inflammatory, antipyretic, antiplatelet	Mild to moderate pain or fever including rheumatoid arthritis, osteoarthritis, thromboembolic disorders, transient ischemic attacks, rheumatic fever, post MI, prophylaxis of MI, ischemic stroke, angina
Elavil	amitriptyline	Antidepressant tricyclic	Major depression
Elitek	rabpuricase	Antineoplastic	Reduce uric acid levels in children who are receiving chemotherapy for leukemia, lymphoma, and solid tumor malignancies

517

Trade Drug Name	Generic Drug Name	Functional Classification	Used to Treat
Eloxitan	oxaliplatin	Antineoplastic	Metastatic carcinoma of colon or rectum
Elspar	asparaginase	Antineoplastic	Acute lymphocytic leukemia
Eminase	anistreplase	Thrombolytic enzyme	Acute MI for lysis of coronary artery thrombi
Epinephrine Pediatric, EpiPen, Bronkaid Mist, Primatene Mist, Adrenalin Ana-Guard	epinephrine	Bronchodilator, vasopressor	Acute asthmatic attack, hemostasis, bronchospasm, anaphylaxis, allergic reactions, cardiac arrest, adjunct in anesthesia, shock
Erythromycin Base Filmtab, Erythromycin Delayed-release, E-mycin, Eramycin	erythromycin	Antibiotic, anti-infective	Gonorrhea, mild to moderate respiratory tract, skin, soft-tissue infections, Legionnaire's disease, syphilis
Faslodex	fulvestrant	Antineoplastic	Advanced breast carcinoma in estrogen receptor-positive patients
Feosol, Slow Fe	ferrous sulfate	Hematinic, iron preparation	Iron-deficiency anemia, prophylaxis for iron deficiency in pregnancy
5-FU, Adrucil	fluorouracil	Antineoplastic, antimetabolic	Systemic: cancer of breast, colon, rectum, stomach, pancreas; Topical: multiple actinic keratoses, superficial basal cell carcinomas
Flexeril	cyclobenzaprine	Skeletal muscle relaxant	Adjunct for relief of muscle spasm and pain in musculoskeletal conditions
Fosamax	adendronate	Bone resorption inhibitor	Osteoporosis, Paget's disease
Garamycin	gentamicin	Anti-infective, aminoglycoside	Serious systemic infections of CNS, respiratory, GI, urinary tract, bone, skin, soft tissues caused by susceptible strains of Pseudomonas, E. coli, Proteus, Klebsiella, Serratia, Citrobacter and Staphylococcus, acute pelvic inflammatory disease
Gemzar	Gemcitabine	Antineoplastic	Adenocarcinoma of pancreas; non-small cell lung cancer
Glucophage	metformin	Oral antidiabetic	Stable type II (adult onset) diabetes mellitus

Trade Drug Name	Generic Drug Name	Functional Classification	Used to Treat
Halcion	triazolam	Sedative-hypnotic, anti-anxiety	Insomnia, sedative, hypnotic
Haldol	haloperidol	Antipsychotic, neuroleptic	Psychotic disorders, control of tics, vocal utterances in Tourette's syndrome, short-term treatment of hyperactive children showing excessive motor activity, control of severe nausea and vomiting in chemotherapy, organic mental syndromes with psychotic features, emergency sedation of severely agitated or delirious patients
HCTZ	hydrochlorothiazide	Thiazide diuretic, anti-hypertensive	Edema, hypertension, diuresis, CHF, idiopathic lower extremity edema therapy
Heparin	heparin	Anticoagulant, antithrombotic	Deep vein thrombosis (DVT), pulmonary emboli (PE), MI, open heart surgery, disseminated intravascular clotting syndrome, atrial fibrillation with embolization, prevention of DVT/PE, to maintain patency of indwelling venipuncture devices, anticoagulant in transfusion and dialysis procedures
Hepsera	adefovir dipivoxil	Antiviral	Chronic hepatitis B
Humira	adalimumab	Antirheumatic agent, immunodulator	Rheumatoid arthritis
Hydrodiuril, HCTZ	hydrochlorothiazide	Thiazide diuretic, antihypertensive	Edema, hypertension, diuresis, CHF, edema in corticosteroid, estrogen, nonsteroidal anti-inflammatory drugs (NSAIDs), idiopathic lower extremity edema therapy
Hygroton	chlorthalidone	Diuretic antihypertensive	Edema, hypertension, diuresis, edema in CHF, nephrotic syndrome
Imdur	isosorbide mononitrate	Antianginal, vasodilator	Chronic stable angina pectoris, prophylaxis of angina pectoris, CHF

Trade Drug Name	Generic Drug Name	Functional Classification	Used to Treat
Imuran	azathioprine	Immunosuppressive	Renal transplants to prevent graft rejection, refractory rheumatoid arthritis, refractory idiopathic thrombocytopenic purpura (ITP), glomerulonephritis, nephrotic syndrome, bone marrow transplant
Inderal, Inderal LA	propranolol	Antihypertensive, anti-anginal, anti-dysrhythmic, beta-blocker	Chronic stable angina pectoris, hypertension, supraventricular dysrhythmias, migraine, MI, pheochromocytoma, essential tremor, cyanotic spells related to hypertrophic subaortic stenosis, tetralogy of Fallot, dysrhythmias associated with thyrotoxicosis, alcohol withdrawal
Inspra	eplerenone	Antihypertensive	Hypertension
Insulin: Humulin, NPH, Novolin, Lente, Ultralente, Humalin	insulin: various forms	Antidiabetic, pancreatic hormone	Type I and II diabetes, many varieties of injectable insulin including beef, pork, and human are available for treatment of diabetes
Interleukin-2, IL-2, Proleukin	aldesleukin	Antineoplastic	Metastatic renal cell carcinoma in adults, phase II for HIV in combination with zidovudine, melanoma
Isoptin	verapamil	Calcium channel blocker, anti-hypertensive, antianginal	Chronic stable angina pectoris, vasospastic angina, dysrhythmias, hypertension, supraventricular tachycardia, atrial flutter or fibrillation
Isordil	isosorbide dinitrate	Antianginal, vasodilator	Chronic stable angina pectoris, prophylaxis of angina pain, CHF
Kaon	potassium gluconate	Electrolyte, mineral replacement	Prevention and treatment of hypokalemia
Kay Ciel, KCL, K-Dur, K-Lor, K-sol, K-tab, Slow-K	potassium chloride	Electrolyte, mineral replacement	Prevention and treatment of hypokalemia
Keflex, Keftab	cephalexin	Antibiotic, anti-infective, cephalosporin	Gram-negative infections, gram-positive infections, upper and lower respiratory tract infections, urinary tract, skin, and bone infections, otitis media

Trade Drug Name	Generic Drug Name	Functional Classification	Used to Treat
Kefzol	cefazolin	Antibiotic	Gram-negative and gram-positive organisms, upper and lower respiratory tract, urinary tract, skin infections, otitis media, tonsillitis, UTIs, bone, joint, biliary, genital infections, endocarditis, surgical prophylaxis, septicemia
Lanoxin	digoxin	Cardiac glycoside, inotropic, antidysrhythmia	CHF, atrial fibrillation, atrial tachycardia, cardiogenic shock, paroxysmal atrial tachycardia, rapid digitalization in these disorders
Lasix	furosemide	Loop diuretic	Pulmonary edema, edema in CHF, liver disease, nephrotic syndrome, ascites, hypertension
Leukeran	chlorambucil	Antineoplastic	Chronic lymphocytic leukemia, Hodgkin's disease, other lymphomas, macroglobulinemia, nephrotic syndrome, breast carcinoma, choreocarcinoma, ovarian carcinoma
Lexapro	escitalopram	Antidepressant	Major depressive disorder
Librium	chlordiazepoxide	Antianxiety	Anxiety, acute alcohol withdrawal, preoperatively for relaxation
Lipitor	atorvastatin	Antilipidemic	Primary hypercholesterolemia, dysbetalipoproteinemia, elevated triglyceride levels
Lithium carbonate	lithium	Antimanic, antipsychotic	Bipolar disorders (manic phase) prevention of bipolar manic-depressive psychosis
Lopressor	metoprolol	Antihypertensive beta blocker, antianginal	Hypertension, acute MI to reduce cardiovascular mortality, angina pectoris, heart failure
Lopurin	allopurinol	Antigout drug	Chronic gout, hyperuricemia associated with malignancies, recurrent calcium oxalate calculi, Chagas' disease, cutaneous/visceral leishmaniasis

Trade Drug Name	Generic Drug Name	Functional Classification	Used to Treat
Lotensin	benazepril	Antihypertensive ACE inhibitor	Hypertension
Lovastatin	mevacor	Antilipemic, cholesterol lowering agent	Adjunct in primary hypercholesterolemia, atherosclerosis, primary and secondary prevention of coronary events
Lovenox	enoxaparin	Anticoagulant, antithrombotic	Prevention of deep vein thrombosis, pulmonary emboli in hip and knee replacement
Mandol	cefamandole	Anti-infective, cephalosporin	Gram-negative and gram-positive infections, upper and lower respiratory tract, urinary tract, skin infections, peritonitis, septicemia, surgical prophylaxis
Mannitol, Osmitrol	mannitol	Diuretic, osmotic	Edema, decrease intraocular pressure, improve renal function in acute renal failure, chemical poisoning
Mavik	trandolapril	Antihypertensive ACE inhibitor	Hypertension, heart failure, post-MI, left ventricular dysfunction post-MI
Mellaril	thioridazine	Antipsychotic, neuroleptic	Psychotic disorders, schizophrenia, behavioral problems in children, anxiety, major depressive disorders, organic brain syndrome, dementia in elderly
Metamucil	psyllium	Laxative	Chronic constipation, ulcerative colitis, irritable bowel syndrome
Methotrexate	Folex, Rheumatrex	Antineoplastic	Acute lymphocytic leukemia, in combination for breast, lung, head, neck carcinoma, lymphosarcoma, gestational choriocarcinoma, hydratidiform mole, psoriasis, rheumatoid arthritis, mycosis fungoides
Micardis	telmisartan	Antihypertensive, ARB	Hypertension
Minipress	prazosin	Antihypertensive	Hypertension, refractory CHF, Raynaud's vasospasm
Monopril	fosinopril	Antihypertensive ACE inhibitor	Hypertension, CHF

Trade Drug Name	Generic Drug Name	Functional Classification	Used to Treat
Motrin	ibuprofen	Nonsteroidal anti-inflammatory, nonopioid analgesic and antipyretic	Rheumatoid arthritis, osteoarthritis, primary dysmenorrhea, gout, dental pain, musculoskeletal disorders, fever
Mustargen (Nitrogen mustard)	mechlorethamine	Antineoplastic	Hodgkin's disease, leukemia, lymphoma, lymphosarcoma, ovarian, breast, lung carcinoma, neoplastic effusions
Mycostatin	nystatin	Topical antifungals	Tinea cruris, tinea pedia, diaper rash, minor skin irritations
Mylanta	famotidine	Antacid, histamine receptor antagonist	Active duodenal ulcer, maintenance therapy for duodenal ulcer, Zollinger-Ellison syndrome, multiple endocrine adenomas, gastric ulcers, gastroesophageal reflux disease, heartburn
Myleran	busulfan	Antineoplastic	Chronic myelocytic leukemia
Mylicon	simethicone	Antiflatulent	Excess gas in the digestive system, flatulence
Natrecor	nesiritide	Vasodilator	Acutely decompensated CHF
Neoral, Sandimmune	cyclosporine	Immunosuppressant	Organ transplants to prevent rejection, rheumatoid arthritis, psoriasis
Neulasta	pegfilgrastim	Hematopoietic agent	Decrease infection in patients receiving antineoplastics who are myelosuppressive, to increase white blood cells in patients with drug-induced neutropenia
Nitroglycerin	nitroglycerin	Coronary vasodilator, antianginal	Stable angina pectoris, prophylaxis of angina, CHF associated with acute MI, controlled hypotension in surgical procedures
Nitropress, Sodium nitroprusside	Nitroprusside	Antihypertensive, vasodilator	Hypertensive crisis, to decrease bleeding by creating hypotension during surgery, acute CHF

Trade Drug Name	Generic Drug Name	Functional Classification	Used to Treat
Norpace	disopyramide	Antidysrhythmic	Premature ventricular contractions (PVCs), ventricular tachycardia, supraventricular tachycardia, atrial flutter and fibrillation
Norvasc	amlodipine	Antianginal, antihypertensive, calcium channel blocker	Stable angina pectoris, hypertension, vasospastic angina
Neupogen	filgrastim	Biologic modifier	To decrease infections in patients receiving chemotherapy who are myelosuppressive, to increase white blood cells in patients with drug-induced neutropenia, bone marrow transplantation
Oncovin	vincristine	Antineoplastic	Breast, lung cancer, lymphomas, neuroblastoma, Hodgkin's disease, acute lymphoblastic and other leukemias, rhabdomyosarcoma, Wilms' tumor, osteogenic and other sarcomas
Orinase	tolbutamide	Antidiabetic	Diabetes mellitus of stable type without acute complications
Paraplatin, Paraplatin-AQ	Carboplatin	Antineoplastic	Ovarian carcinoma
Paxil	paroxetine	Antidepressant	Major depressive disorder, obsessive-compulsive disorder, panic disorder, generalized anxiety disorder
Pegasys	peginterferon alfa-2A	Immunomodulator	Chronic hepatitis C
Pentamidine	nebupent, Pentam 300	antiprotozoal	Pneumocystis carinii infections
Periactin	cyproheptadine	Antihistamine, histamine receptor antagonist	Allergic reactions, urticaria, rhinitis, pruritus, cold
Persantine	dipyridamole	Coronary vasodilator, antiplatelet agent, beta-blocker	Prevention of transient ischemic attack, inhibition of platelet adhesion to prevent myocardial re-infarction, thromboembolism, with warfarin in prosthetic heart valves, prevention of coronary bypass graft occlusion with aspirin, angina pectoris

Trade Drug Name	Generic Drug Name	Functional Classification	Used to Treat
Phenergan	promethazine	Antihistamine, histamine receptor antagonist	Allergic rhinitis, control of nausea and vomiting, sedation, motion sickness, preoperative and postoperative sedation
Phenobarbital sodium	phenobarbital	Anticonvulsant	All forms of epilepsy, status epilepticus, febrile seizures in children, sedation, insomnia
Platinol, Platinol-AQ	cisplatin	Antineoplastic	Advanced bladder cancer, adjunctive in metastatic testicular cancer, adjunctive in metastatic ovarian cancer, head, neck cancer, esophagus, prostate, lung and cervical cancer, lymphoma
Plendil	felodipine	Antihypertensive, calcium channel blocker, antianginal	Hypertension, angina pectoris
Prednisone	prednisone	Corticosteroid	Severe inflammation, immunosuppression, neoplasms, multiple sclerosis, collagen disorders, dermatologic disorders
Prilosec	omeprazole	Antiulcer, proton pump inhibitor	Gastroesophageal reflux disease, severe erosive esophagitis, pathologic hypersecretory conditions, treatment of active duodenal ulcers with or without anti-infectives for Heliobacter pylori bacteria
Primacor	milrinone	Inotropic/vasodilator agent	Advanced CHF
Procanbid	procainamide	Antidysrhythmic	Life-threatening ventricular dysrhythmias
Procardia	nifedipine	Antianginal, antihypertensive, calcium channel blocker	Stable angina pectoris, vasospastic angina, hypertension
Prolixin	fluphenazine hydrochloride	Antipsychotic	Psychotic disorders, schizophrenia
Pronestyl	procainamide	Antidysrhythmic	Life-threatening ventricular dysrhythmias
Proventil, Ventolin	albuterol	Bronchodilator, adrenergic beta-agonist	Prevention of exercise-induced asthma, acute bronchospasm, bronchitis, emphysema, bronchiectasis or other reversible airway obstruction

Trade Drug Name	Generic Drug Name	Functional Classification	Used to Treat
Prozac	fluoxetine	Antidepressant	Major depressive disorder, obsessive-compulsive disorder, bulimia nervosa
Quinaglute, Quinalan, Quinora, Cin-Quin	quinidine	Antidysrhythmic	PVCs, atrial fibrillation, paroxysmal tachycardia, ventricular tachycardia, atrial flutter
Rapamune	sirolimus	Immunosuppressant	Organ transplants to prevent rejection, use with cyclosporine and corticosteroids
Relpax	eletriptan	Antimigraine agent	Acute treatment of migraine headache
Remodulin	treprostinil	Antiplatelet agent	Pulmonary arterial hypertension
ReoPro	abciximab	Platelet inhibitor	Used with heparin and aspirin to prevent acute cardiac ischemia following PTCA in patients at high risk for reclosure of affected arteries
Restoril	temazepam	Sedative-hypnotic	Insomnia
Rogaine (Minoxidil)	Minoxidil (Note: Some drug manufacturers use trade and generic name interchangeably for this drug.)	Alopecia agent, antihypertensive	Topically to treat alopecia. Originally developed as an antihypertensive but rarely used for that currently, reserved for severe, refractory hypertension unresponsive to other therapy
Riopan	magakdrate	Antacid	Heartburn, acid indigestion, peptic ulcer disease, duodenal, gastric ulcers, reflux esophagitis, hyperacidity
Septra, Septra DS	trimethoprim-sulfamethoxazole	Anti-infective, antibacterial	UTIs, otitis media, acute and chronic prostatitis, shigellosis, Pneumocystis carinii pneumonitis, chronic bronchitis, chancroid, traveler's diarrhea
Solu—Cortef	hydrocortisone sodium succinate	Corticosteroid	Severe inflammation, septic shock, adrenal insufficiency, ulcerative colitis, collagen disorders
Stadol	butorphanol	Opioid analgesic	Moderate to severe pain
Strattera	atomoxetine	Psychotherapeutic	Attention deficit hyperactivity disorder

Trade Drug Name	Generic Drug Name	Functional Classification	Used to Treat
Streptase	streptokinase	Thrombolytic enzyme	DVT, PE, arterial thrombosis, arterial embolism, arteriovenous cannula occlusion, lysis of coronary artery thrombi after MI, acute evolving transmural MI
Surfak	docusate calcium	Laxative, stool softener	Soften stools
Synthroid	levothyroxine	Thyroid hormone	Hypothyroidism, myxedema coma, thyroid hormone replacement, congenital hypothyroidism, thyrotoxicosis, congenital hypothyroidism, some types of thyroid cancer
Tagamet	cimetidine	Histamine receptor antagonist	Short-term treatment of duodenal and gastric ulcers and maintenance, management of gastroesophageal reflux disease (GERD) and Zollinger-Ellison syndrome
Tenormin	atenolol	Antihypertensive, anti-anginal	Hypertension, prophylaxis of angina pectoris, suspected or known MI
Teveten HCT	eprosartan mesylate/ hydrochlorothiazide	Antihypertensive, ARB	Hypertension
Theo-Dur, Theo-Sav, Theospan, Theostat, Theovent, Theo-X, T-Phyl, Uni-dur, Uniphyl	theophylline	Spasmolytic	Bronchial asthma, bronchospasm of COPD, chronic bronchitis
Thorazine	chlorpromazine	Antipsychotic, neuroleptic, anti-emetic	Psychotic disorders, mania, schizophrenia, anxiety, intractable hiccups in adults, nausea, vomiting, preoperatively for relaxation, acute intermittent porphyria, behavioral problems in children, nonpsychotic demented patients, Tourette's syndrome
Thyrolar	liotrix	Thyroid hormone	Hypothyroidism, thyroid hormone replacement
t-PA, tissue plasminogen activator	alteplase	Thrombolytic enzyme	Lysis of obstructing thrombi associated with acute MI, ischemic conditions requiring thrombolysis

Trade Drug Name	Generic Drug Name	Functional Classification	Used to Treat
TNKase	tenecteplase	Thrombolytic enzyme	Acute MI
Tobrax, TOBI	tobramycin	Anti-infective	Severe systemic bacterial infections of CNS, respiratory, GI, urinary tract, bone, skin, soft tissues, cystic fibrosis
Tolectin	tolmetin sodium	Anti-inflammatory	Used for relief of signs and symptoms of rheumatoid arthritis, osteoarthritis, and juvenile rheumatoid arthritis
Tonocard	tocainide	Antidysrhythmic	Life-threatening ventricular dysrhythmias (multifocal/ unifocal, PVCs), ventricular tachycardia
Traxene	chlorazepate	Antianxiety, anticonvulsant, sedative/hypnotic	Anxiety, acute alcohol withdrawal, adjunct in seizure disorder
Tylenol, APAP, Datril,	acetaminophen	Nonopioid analgesic/ antipyretic	Pain and/or fever
Unasyn	ampicillin sulbactam	Broad-spectrum anti-infective	Skin infections, intra-abdominal infections, pneumonia, meningitis, septicemia
Urokinase, Abbokinase	urokinases	Thrombolytic enzyme	Venous thrombosis, pulmonary embolism, arterial thrombosis, arterial embolism, arteriovenous cannula occlusion, lysis of coronary artery thrombi after MI
Valium	diazepam	Antianxiety, anticonvulsant, skeletal muscle relaxant	Anxiety, acute alcohol withdrawal, adjunct in seizure disorders, preoperatively as a relaxant, skeletal muscle relaxation, rectally for acute repetitive seizures
Vancocin	vancomycin	Anti-infective	Resistant staphylococcal infections, other staphylococcal infections, pseudomembraneous colitis
Vascor	bepridil	Antianginal	Stable angina pectoris
Vasotec	enalapril/enalaprilat	Antihypertensive, ACE inhibitor	Hypertension, CHF, ventricular dysfunction

Trade Drug Name	Generic Drug Name	Functional Classification	Used to Treat
Veetids	penicillin V potassium	Broad spectrum anti-infective	Respiratory infections, scarlet fever, erysipelas, otitis media, pneumonia, skin and soft-tissue infections, gonorrhea, gram-negative and gram-positive organisms
Velban	vinblastine sulfate	Antineoplastic	Used for palliative treatment of a variety of malignant and neoplastic conditions
Vfend	voriconazole	Antifungal	Serious fungal infections
Vicodin		analgesic, antipyretic	Relief of moderate to severe pain
Wellbutrin SR, Zyban	bupropion	Antidepressant, smoking deterrent	Depression (Wellbutrin), Smoking cessation (Zyban)
Wycillin	penicillin G procaine	Broad-spectrum anti-infective	Respiratory infections, scarlet fever, erysipelas, otitis media, pneumonia, skin and soft-tissue infections, gonorrhea, gram-negative and gram-positive organisms
Xanax	alprazolam	Anti-anxiety	Anxiety, panic disorders, anxiety with depressive symptoms
Xigris	drotrecogin alfa	Thrombolytic agent	Severe sepsis associated with organ dysfunction
Xylocaine	lidocaine	Antidysrhythmic	Ventricular tachycardia, ventricular dysrhythmias during cardiac surgery, MI, digitalis toxicity, cardiac catheterization
Zantac	ranitidine	Histamine receptor antagonist	Duodenal ulcer, Zollinger-Ellison syndrome, gastric ulcers, hypersecretory conditions, GERD, stress ulcers, erosive esophagitis (maintenance), active duodenal ulcers with Heliobacter pylori bacteria
Zaroxolyn	metolazone	Diuretic, antihypertensive	Edema, hypertension, CHF, nephrotic syndrome
Zebeta	bisoprolol	Antihypertensive	Hypertension

Trade Drug Name	Generic Drug Name	Functional Classification	Used to Treat
Zelnorm	tegaserod	5-HT4 receptor partial agonist, GI agent	Irritable bowel syndrome with primary symptom of constipation
Zestril	lisinopril	Antihypertensive, ACE inhibitor	Hypertension, adjunctive therapy of systolic CHF, acute MI
Zetia	ezetimibe	Antilipemic	Hypercholesterolemia
Zevalin	ibritumomab tiuxetan	Antineoplastic	Non-Hodgkin's lymphoma
Zithromax	azithromycin	Anti-infective	Mild to moderate infections of the upper respiratory tract, lower respiratory tract, uncomplicated skin and skin structure infections, nongonococcal urethritis or cervicitis, acute otitis media, acute pharyngitis/tonsillitis, community acquired pneumonia
Zocor	simvastatin	Antilipemic	Primary hypercholesterolemia, isolated hypertriglyceridemia, type III hyperlipoproteinemia, CAD
Zoloft	sertraline	Antidepressant	Major depression, obsessive-compulsive disorder, post-traumatic stress disorder, panic disorder
Zovirax	acyclovir	Antiviral	Mucocutaneous herpes simplex virus, herpes genitalis, varicella infections, herpes zoster, herpes simplex encephalitis
Zyloprim	allopurinol	Antigout drug	Chronic gout, hyperuricemia associated with malignancies, recurrent calcium oxalate calculi, Chagas' disease, cutaneous/visceral leishmaniasis

Appendix D

Morphology Terminology

Adenocarcinoma: Carcinoma derived from glandular tissue or in which the tumor cells form recognizable glandular structures. Adenocarcinomas may be classified according to the predominant pattern of cell arrangement, as papillary, alveolar, and so on, or according to a particular product of the cells, as mucinous adenocarcinoma.

Adenoma: A benign epithelial tumor in which the cells form recognizable glandular structures or in which the cells are clearly derived from glandular epithelium.

Adenoma, chromophobe: A tumor of the anterior lobe of the pituitary gland whose cells do not stain readily with either acid or basic dyes and whose presence may be associated with hypopituitarism.

Angioblastoma: Certain blood-vessel tumors of the brain; those arising in the cerebellum (cerebellar angioblastoma) may be cystic and associated with von Hippel-Lindau's disease; also, a blood-vessel tumor arising from the meninges of the brain or spinal cord (angioblastic meningioma).

Angioma: A tumor whose cells tend to form blood vessels (hemangioma) or lymph vessels (lymphangioma); a tumor made up of blood vessels or lymph vessels.

Angiosarcoma: A hemangiosarcoma.

Astrocytoma: A tumor composed of astrocytes; such tumors have been classified into Grades I–IV in order of increasing malignancy.

Carcinoma: A malignant new growth made up of epithelial cells tending to infiltrate the surrounding tissues and give rise to metastases.

Carcinoma, basal cell: An epithelial tumor that seldom metastasizes but has the potential for local invasion and destruction.

Carcinoma, cholangiocellular: Primary carcinoma of the liver originating in bile duct cells. Also called *cholangioma* and *cholangiocarcinoma*.

Carcinoma, embryonal: A highly malignant, primitive form of carcinoma, probably of germinal cell or teratomatous derivation, that usually arises in a gonad and rarely in other sites; a seminoma.

Carcinoma, epidermoid: Carcinoma in which the cells tend to differentiate in the same way that the cells of the epidermis do; that is, they tend to form prickle cells and undergo cornification.

Carcinoma, Merkel cell: An aggressive, neuroendocrine skin cancer; a lethal form of skin cancer with a 33 percent, disease-specific mortality. It appears as a painless, flesh colored or bluish-red nodule on the skin—often on the face, head or neck (skin surfaces most frequently exposed to sun)—and most often develops in older people. Merkel cell carcinoma tends to grow fast and spread quickly to other parts of the body.

Carcinoma, squamous cell: Carcinoma developed from squamous epithelium and having cuboid cells.

Cholangiocarcinoma: Cholangiocellular carcinoma.

Cholangioma: Cholangiocellular carcinoma.

Chondroma: A tumor or tumor-like growth of cartilage cells that may remain within the substance of a cartilage or bone (true chondroma, or enchondroma) or may develop on the surface of a cartilage (ecchondroma, or ecchondrosis).

Chondrosarcoma: A malignant tumor derived from cartilage cells or their precursors. Also called *chondroma sarcomatosum.*

Choriocarcinoma: An epithelial malignancy of trophoblastic cells, formed by the abnormal proliferation of cuboidal and syncytial cells of the placental epithelium, without the production of chorionic villi. Almost all cases arise in the uterus, developing from hydatidiform mole (50 percent), following an abortion (25 percent), or during a normal pregnancy (22 percent). The remainder occur in ectopic pregnancies and in genital (ovarian and testicular) and extragenital teratomas. Also called *chorioblastoma, chorioepithelioma, chorionic carcinoma* or *epithelioma, deciduocellular sarcoma,* and *syncytioma malignum.*

Cystadenocarcinoma: Carcinoma and cystadenoma.

Cystadenoma: Adenoma associated with cystoma.

Cystadenoma, mucinous: A multilocular tumor produced by the epithelial cells of the ovary and having mucin-filled cavities; the great majority of these tumors are benign. Also called *mucinous cystadenoma.*

Cystadenoma, serous: A cystic tumor of the ovary that contains thin, clear, yellow serous fluid and varying amounts of solid tissue, with a malignant potential several times greater than that of mucinous cystadenoma.

Cystoma: A tumor containing cysts of neoplastic origin; a cystic tumor.

Disease, Hodgkin's: A form of malignant lymphoma characterized by painless, progressive enlargement of the lymph nodes, spleen, and general lymphoid tissue; other symptoms may include anorexia, lassitude, weight loss, fever, pruritus, night sweats, and anemia. The characteristic histologic feature is presence of Reed-Sternberg cells.

Disease, von Recklinghausen's: A familial condition characterized by developmental changes in the nervous system, muscles, bones, and skin, and marked superficially by the formation of multiple pedunculated soft tumors (neurofibromas) distributed over the entire body, associated with areas of pigmentation. Also called *neurofibromatosis, multiple neuroma,* and *neuromatosis.*

Embryoma: A general term applied to neoplasms thought to derive from embryonic cells or tissues, including dermoid cysts, teratomas, embryonal carcinomas and sarcomas, nephroblastomas, hepatoblastomas, and so on.

Endothelioblastoma: A tumor derived from primitive vasoformative tissue with formation of usually small and slitlike vascular spaces lined by prominent endothelial cells, including hemangioendothelioma, angiosarcoma, lymphangioendothelioma, and lymphangiosarcoma.

Endothelioma: A tumor originating from the endothelial lining of blood vessels (hemangioendothelioma), lymphatics (lymphangioendothelioma), or serous cavities (mesothelioma).

Ependymoma: A neoplasm composed of differentiated ependymal cells; most ependymomas grow slowly and are benign, but malignant varieties do occur.

Fibroblastoma: A tumor arising from a fibroblast; such tumors are now differentiated as fibromas or fibrosarcomas.

Fibroma: A tumor composed mainly of fibrous or fully developed connective tissue. Also called *fibroid*.

Fibrosarcoma: A sarcoma derived from fibroblasts that produce collagen.

Glioma: A tumor composed of tissue that represents neuroglia in any one of its stages of development; sometimes extended to include all the primary intrinsic neoplasms of the brain and spinal cord, including astrocytomas, ependymomas, neurocytomas, and so on.

Hemangioma: An extremely common benign tumor, occurring most often in infancy and childhood, made up of newly formed blood vessels, and resulting from malformation of angioblastic tissue of fetal life. Two main types exist—capillary and cavernous.

Hemangiosarcoma: A malignant tumor formed by the proliferation of endothelial and fibroblastic tissue.

Hepatoma: A tumor of the liver, especially hepatocellular carcinoma.

Hypernephroma: Renal cell carcinoma whose structure resembles the cortical tissue of the adrenal gland.

Keloid: A sharply elevated, irregularly shaped, progressively enlarging scar due to the formation of excessive amounts of collagen in the corium during connective tissue repair.

Leiomyoma: A benign tumor derived from smooth muscle, most commonly of the uterus. Also called *fibroid*.

Leiomyosarcoma: A sarcoma containing large spindle cells of smooth muscle, most commonly of the uterus or retroperitoneal region.

Leukemia: A progressive, malignant disease of the blood-forming organs, characterized by distorted proliferation and development of leukocytes and their precursors in the blood and bone marrow. Leukemia is classified clinically on the basis of (1) the duration and character of the disease—acute or chronic; (2) the type of cell involved—myeloid (myelogenous), lymphoid (lymphogenous), or monocytic; or (3) increase or no increase in the number of abnormal cells in the blood—leukemic or aleukemic (subleukemic).

Leukemia, acute nonlymphocytic (ANLL): Leukemia occurring most commonly after treatment with alkylating agents characterized by pancytopenia, megaloblastic bone marrow, nucleated red cells in treatment, with a short survival time.

Leukemia, adult T-cell: A form of leukemia with onset in adulthood, leukemic cells with T-cell properties, frequent dermal involvement, lymphadenopathy and hepatosplenomegaly, and a subacute or chronic course; it is associated with human T-cell leukemia-lymphoma virus.

Leukemia, aleukemic: Leukemia in which the total white blood cell count in the peripheral blood is either normal or below normal; it may be lymphocytic, monocytic, or myelogenous. Also called *subleukemic leukemia*.

Leukemia, basophilic: A disorder resembling acute or chronic leukemia in which the basophilic leukocytes predominate.

Leukemia, chronic granulocytic: A form of leukemia occurring mainly between the ages of 25 and 60 years, usually associated with a unique chromosomal abnormality, in which the major clinical manifestations of malaise, hepatosplenomegaly, anemia, and leukocytosis are related to abnormal, excessive, unrestrained overgrowth of granulocytes in the bone marrow.

Leukemia, eosinophilic: A form of leukemia in which the eosinophil is the predominant cell. Although resembling chronic myelocytic leukemia in many ways, this form may follow an acute course despite the absence of predominantly blast forms in the peripheral blood.

Leukemia, hairy-cell: Leukemia marked by splenomegaly and by an abundance of large, mononuclear abnormal cells with numerous irregular cytoplasmic projections that give them a flagellated or hairy appearance in the bone marrow, spleen, liver, and peripheral blood. Also called *leukemic reticuloendotheliosis*.

Leukemia, leukopenic: *See* **leukemia, aleukemic.**

Leukemia, lymphatic: Leukemia associated with hyperplasia and overactivity of the lymphoid tissue, in which the leukocytes are lymphocytes or lymphoblasts. Also called *lymphoblastic leukemia, lymphocytic leukemia, lymphogenous leukemia, lymphoid leukemia*.

Leukemia, mast cell: A type of leukemia characterized by overwhelming numbers of tissue mast cells present in the peripheral blood.

Leukemia, monocytic: Leukemia in which the predominating leukocytes are identified as monocytes.

Leukemia, myelogenous: Leukemia arising from myeloid tissue in which the granular, polymorphonuclear leukocytes and their precursors are predominant. Also called *myelocytic leukemia, myeloid granulocytic leukemia*.

Leukemia, plasma cell: Leukemia in which the plasma cell is the predominant cell in the peripheral blood.

Lipoma: A benign tumor usually composed of mature fat cells.

Liposarcoma: A malignant tumor derived from primitive or embryonal lipoblastic cells that exhibit varying degrees of lipoblastic or lipomatous differentiation.

Lymphangioma: A benign tumor representing a congenital malformation of the lymphatic system, made up of newly formed lymph-containing vascular spaces and channels. Also called *angiomalymphaticum*.

Lymphangiosarcoma: A malignant tumor of lymphatic vessels, usually arising in a limb that is the site of chronic lymphedema.

Lymphoblastoma: Lymphoblastic lymphoma.

Lymphoma: Any neoplastic disorder of the lymphoid tissue; the term *lymphoma* often is used alone to denote malignant lymphoma.

Lymphoma, Burkitt's: A form of undifferentiated malignant lymphoma, usually found in central Africa—but also reported from other areas—and manifested most often as a large osteolytic lesion in the jaw or as an abdominal mass. The Epstein-Barr virus, a herpes virus, has been isolated from Burkitt's lymphoma and has been implicated as a causative agent.

Lymphoma, diffuse: Malignant lymphoma in which the neoplastic cells diffusely infiltrate the entire lymph node, without any definite organized pattern. Also called *lymphatic sarcoma* and *lymphosarcoma*.

Lymphoma, granulomatous: Hodgkin's disease.

Lymphoma, histiocytic: Malignant lymphoma characterized by the presence of large-sized tumor cells, resembling histiocytes morphologically but considered to be of lymphoid origin, that are irregular in shape with relatively abundant, frequently acidophilic cytoplasm. Also called *reticulum cell sarcoma*.

Lymphoma, lymphoblastic: A malignant lymphoma composed of a diffuse, relatively uniform proliferation of cells with round or convoluted nuclei and scanty cytoplasm that are cytologically similar to the lymphoblasts seen in acute lymphocytic leukemia.

Lymphoma, malignant: A group of malignant neoplasms characterized by the proliferation of cells native to the lymphoid tissues (lymphocytes, histiocytes, and their precursors and derivatives). The group is divided into two major clinicopathologic categories—Hodgkin's disease and non-Hodgkin's lymphoma.

Lymphoma, nodular: Malignant lymphoma in which the lymphomatous cells are clustered into identifiable nodules within the lymph nodes that somewhat resemble the germinal centers of lymph node follicles. Nodular lymphomas usually occur in older persons, commonly involving many (or all) nodes as well as possibly extranodal sites. Also called *Brill-Symmers'* or *Symmers' disease, follicular lymphoma*, and *giant follicle lymphoma*.

Lymphomas, non-Hodgkin's: A heterogeneous group of malignant lymphomas, the only common feature being an absence of the giant Reed-Sternberg cells characteristic of Hodgkin's disease. They arise from the lymphoid components of the immune system and present a clinical picture broadly similar to that of Hodgkin's disease, except the disease is initially more widespread, with the most common manifestation being painless enlargement of one or more peripheral lymph nodes.

Lymphosarcoma: A diffuse lymphoma.

Medulloblastoma: A cerebellar tumor composed of undifferentiated neuroepithelial cells that is highly radiosensitive.

Melanoblastoma: Malignant melanoma.

Melanoma: A tumor arising from the melanocytic system of the skin and other organs. When used alone, the term refers to malignant melanoma.

Melanoma, malignant: A malignant neoplasm of melanocytes, arising de novo or from a preexisting benign nevus, that occurs most often in the skin but also may involve the oral cavity, esophagus, anal canal, vagina, leptomeninges, and the conjunctiva or eye. Also called *melanotic carcinoma, melanoblastoma*, and *melanocarcinoma*.

Meningioma: A hard, slow-growing, usually vascular tumor occurring mainly along the meningeal vessels and superior longitudinal sinus, invading the dura and skull, and leading to erosion and thinning of the skull.

Mycosis fungoides: A chronic or rapidly progressive form of cutaneous T-cell lymphoma (formerly thought to be of fungal origin) that in some cases evolves into generalized lymphoma with a tendency for nodal, hematogenous, and visceral involvement.

Myeloma: A tumor composed of cells of the type normally found in the bone marrow. *See* **myeloma, multiple**.

Myeloma, multiple: A disseminated malignant neoplasm of plasma cells characterized by multiple bone marrow tumor foci and secretion of an M component, associated with widespread osteolytic lesions appearing radiographically as punched-out defects and resulting in bone pain, pathologic fractures, hypercalcemia, and normochromic, normocytic anemia. Spread to extraosseous sites occurs frequently in advanced disease. Depression of immunoglobulin levels results in increased susceptibility to infection. Bence Jones proteinuria is present in many cases and occasionally results in systemic amyloidosis. Renal failure resulting from calcium nephropathy or extensive cast formation occurs in about 20 percent of cases.

Myoma: A tumor made up of muscular elements.

Myxoblastoma: *See* **myxoma**.

Myxoma: A tumor composed of primitive connective tissue cells and stroma resembling mesenchyme.

Myxosarcoma: A sarcoma containing myxomatous tissue.

Neuroblastoma: A sarcoma of nervous system origin, composed chiefly of neuroblasts and affecting mostly infants and children up to 10 years of age. Most of such tumors arise in the autonomic nervous system (sympathicoblastoma) or in the adrenal medulla.

Neurofibroma: A tumor of peripheral nerves caused by abnormal proliferation of Schwann cells.

Neuroma: A tumor or new growth largely made up of nerve cells and nerve fibers; a tumor growing from a nerve.

Nevus: Any congenital lesion of the skin; for example, a birthmark.

Osteoblastoma: A benign, painful, rather vascular tumor of bone characterized by the formation of osteoid tissue and primitive bone. Also called *giant osteoid osteoma*.

Osteochondroma: Osteoma blended with chondroma, a benign tumor consisting of projecting adult bone capped by cartilage.

Osteoclastoma: Giant cell tumor of bone.

Osteoma: A tumor composed of bone tissue; a hard tumor of bonelike structure developing on a bone (homoplastic osteoma) and sometimes on other structures (heteroplastic osteoma).

Osteoma, osteoid: A small, benign, but painful, circumscribed tumor of spongy bone occurring especially in the bones of the extremities and vertebrae, most often in young persons.

Osteosarcoma: Osteogenic sarcoma.

Papilloma: A benign epithelial neoplasm producing finger-like or verrucous projections from the epithelial surface.

Pheochromocytoma: A usually benign, well-encapsulated, lobular, vascular tumor of chromaffin tissue of the adrenal medulla or sympathetic paraganglia. The cardinal symptom, reflecting the increased secretion of epinephrine and norepinephrine, is hypertension, which may be persistent or intermittent. During severe attacks, there may be headache, sweating, palpitation, apprehension, tremor, pallor or flushing of the face, nausea and vomiting, pain in the chest and abdomen, and paresthesias of the extremities.

Rhabdomyoma: A benign tumor derived from striated muscle.

Rhabdomyosarcoma: A highly malignant tumor of striated muscle derived from primitive mesenchymal cells and exhibiting differentiation along rhabdomyoblastic lines, including, but not limited to, the presence of cells with recognizable cross-striations.

Sarcoma: A tumor made up of a substance like the embryonic connective tissue; tissue composed of closely packed cells embedded in a fibrillar or homogenous substance. Sarcomas are often highly malignant.

Sarcoma, Ewing's: *See* **tumor, Ewing's**.

Sarcoma, Kaposi's: A multicentric, malignant neoplastic vascular proliferation characterized by the development of bluish-red cutaneous nodules, usually on the lower extremities, most often on the toes or feet, and slowly increasing in size and number and spreading to more proximal sites.

Sarcoma, osteogenic: A malignant primary tumor of bone composed of a malignant connective tissue stroma with evidence of malignant osteoid, bone, and/or cartilage formation. Also called *osteolytic sarcoma* and *osteoid sarcoma*.

Seminoma: A radiosensitive, malignant neoplasm of the testis, thought to be derived from primordial germ cells of the sexually undifferentiated embryonic gonad, occurring as a gray to yellow-white nodule or mass.

Teratoma: A true neoplasm made up of a number of different types of tissue, none of which is native to the area where it occurs; most often found in the ovary or testis.

Teratoma, malignant: A solid, malignant ovarian tumor resembling a dermoid cyst but composed of immature embryonal or extraembryonal elements derived from all three germ layers. Also called *immature teratoma* and *solid teratoma*.

Teratoma, mature: A benign teratoma of the ovary, usually found in young women. Also called *benign cystic teratoma, cystic teratoma*, and *dermoid cyst*.

Tumor, Ewing's: A malignant tumor of the bone that always arises in medullary tissue, occurring more often in cylindrical bones, with pain, fever, and leukocytosis as prominent symptoms. Also called *Ewing's sarcoma*.

Tumor, giant cell, of bone: A bone tumor composed of cellular spindle cell stroma containing scattered multinucleated giant cells resembling osteoclasts; symptoms may include local pain and tenderness, functional disability, and, occasionally, pathologic fractures.

Tumor, Krukenberg's: A special type of carcinoma of the ovary, usually metastatic from cancer of the gastrointestinal tract, especially of the stomach.

Tumor, mixed: A tumor composed of more than one type of neoplastic tissue, especially a complex embryonal tumor of local origin, which reproduces the normal development of the tissues and organs of the affected part.

Tumor, Wilms': A rapidly developing malignant mixed tumor of the kidneys, made up of embryonal elements. It usually affects children before the fifth year but may occur in the fetus and, rarely, in later life.

References and Bibliography

45 CFR 162. Final Rule 2009. HIPAA Administrative Simplification: Modifications to Medical Data Code Set Standards to Adopt ICD-10-CM and ICD-10-PCS. 2009 (January 16). http://edocket.access .gpo.gov/2009/pdf/E9-743.pdf.

American Congress of Obstetricians and Gynecologists. 2012. http://www.acog.org.

American Health Information Management Association. 2000. Where in the world is ICD-10? *Journal of AHIMA* 71(8): 52–57.

American Health Information Management Association. 2009a. AHIMA home page for ICD-10. http://www.ahima.org/icd10/.

American Health Information Management Association. 2009b. Analysis of the Final Rule: HIPAA Administrative Simplification: Modification to Medical Data Code Set Standards to Adopt ICD-10-CM and ICD-10-PCS. http://www.ahima.org/downloads/pdfs/advocacy /AnaylsisofFinalRulefortheAdoptionoftheICD-10-CMandICD-10-PCSCodeSets.pdf.

American Health Information Management Association and the American Hospital Association. 2003. ICD-10-CM Field Testing Project: Report on Findings. http://www.ahima.org/downloads/pdfs /resources/FinalStudy_000.pdf.

American Hospital Association. 1985–2012. *Coding Clinic for ICD-9-CM*. Chicago: American Hospital Association.

American Medical Association. 2003. *Complete Medical Encyclopedia*. New York: Random House Reference.

American Psychiatric Association. 2004. *Diagnostic and Statistical Manual of Mental Disorders—Text Revision*, 4th ed. Washington, D.C.: American Psychiatric Press.

Aquavella, J.V. 2013. Pseudophakic Bullous Keratopathy. http://emedicine.medscape.com /article/1194994-overview.

Averill, R.F., R.L. Mullin, B.A. Steinbeck, N.I. Goldfield, T.M. Grant, R.R. Butler. 2013. *Development of the ICD-10 Procedure Coding System (ICD-10-PCS)*. http://www.cms.gov/Medicare/Coding /ICD10/Downloads/pcs_final_report2013.pdf.

Barta, A. et al. 2008. ICD-10-CM primer. *Journal of AHIMA* 79(5):64–66.

Barta, A. and A. Zeisset. 2011. *Root Operations: Key to Procedure Coding in ICD-10-PCS*. Chicago: AHIMA.

Barta, A. 2012. *ICD-10-CM and ICD-10-PCS Preview Exercises, 2nd ed.* Chicago: AHIMA.

Barta, A., K. DeVault, and M. Endicott. 2012. *ICD-10-PCS Coder Training Manual, 2012 Instructor's Edition.* Chicago: AHIMA.

Beers, M.H. and R. Berkow, eds. 2000. *The Merck Manual*, 17th ed. Rahway, N.J.: Merck & Co.

Braunwald, E., A. Fauci, D. Kasper, S. Hauser, D. Longo, and J. Jameson. 2001. *Harrison's Principles of Internal Medicine.* New York: McGraw-Hill.

Bowman, S. 2008a. Brushing up on ICD-10-PCS. *Journal of AHIMA* 78(9):108–112.

Bowman, S. 2008b. Why ICD-10 is worth the trouble. *Journal of AHIMA* 79(3):24–29.

Canobbia, M.M. 1990. *Cardiovascular Disorders.* Mosby's Clinical Nursing Series. Vol. 1. St. Louis: Mosby-Year Book.

Centers for Disease Control. 2012. International Classification of Diseases, Tenth Revision, Clinical Modification (ICD-10-CM). http://www.cdc.gov/nchs/icd/icd10cm.htm.

Centers for Medicare and Medicaid Services. 2008. ICD-10 Overview. *Coordination and Maintenance Committee Meeting* (Baltimore, MD, September 24–25). http://www.cdc.gov/nchs/icd/icd9cm _maintenance.htm.

Centers for Medicare and Medicaid Services. 2010a. ICD-10-PCS Reference Manual. http://www .cms.gov/Medicare/Coding/ICD10/index.html.

Centers for Medicare and Medicaid Services. 2010b (March 5). *MLN Matters* number MM6851: Additional ICD-9 Codes Analysis and Processing Direction (Institutional Claims Only). http://www .cms.gov/MLNMattersArticles/downloads/MM6851.pdf.

Centers for Medicare and Medicaid Services. 2010c. Implementation of Recovery Auditing at the Centers for Medicare and Medicaid Services: FY 2010 Report to Congress as Required by Section 6411 of Affordable Care Act. http://www.cms.gov/Research-Statistics-Data-and-Systems/Monitoring -Programs/recovery-audit-program/downloads/FY2010ReportCongress.pdf.

Centers for Medicare and Medicaid Services. 2012a. ICD-10-CM Official Guidelines for Coding and Reporting. http://www.cdc.gov/nchs/icd/icd10cm.htm.

Centers for Medicare and Medicaid Services. 2012b. ICD-10-PCS Official Coding Guidelines. http:// www.cms.gov/Medicare/Coding/ICD10/2012-ICD-10-PCS.html.

Centers for Medicare and Medicaid Services. 2012c. ICD-10-PCS Reference Manual and Slides. http://www.cms.gov/Medicare/Coding/ICD10/2012-ICD-10-PCS.html.

Centers for Medicare and Medicaid Services. 2012d. Quality Improvement Organizations. http://www .cms.gov/Medicare/Quality-Initiatives-Patient-Assessment-Instruments/QualityImprovementOrgs /index.html.

Centers for Medicare and Medicaid Services. 2012e. Recovery Audit Program. http://www.cms.gov /Recovery-Audit-Program/01_Overview.asp#TopOfPage.

Davis, N.M. 2008. *Medical Abbreviations: 30,000 Conveniences at the Expense of Communication and Safety*, 14th ed. Warminster, PA: Neil M. Davis Associates.

Department of Health and Human Services. 1994. *Living with Heart Disease: Is It Heart Failure?* Consumer Version, Clinical Practice Guideline, Number 11. Rockville, MD: Agency for Health Care Policy and Research.

Department of Health and Human Services. 2010. *International Classification of Diseases, 9th Revision, Clinical Modification.* Washington, D.C.: U.S. Government Printing Office.

Department of Health and Human Services. 2010b. What Is Osteoarthritis? http://www.niams.nih.gov /Health_Info/Osteoarthritis/osteoarthritis_ff.pdf.

Department of Health and Human Services. 2011. What Is Pernicious Anemia? http://www.nhlbi.nih .gov/health/health-topics/topics/prnanmia/.

Department of Health and Human Services. 2012a. Acute Care Hospital Inpatient Prospective Payment System: Payment System Fact Sheet Series. http://www.cms.gov/Outreach-and-Education /Medicare-Learning-Network-MLN/MLNProducts/downloads/AcutePaymtSysfctsht.pdf.

Department of Health and Human Services. 2012b. Medicare Claim Review Programs: MR, NCCI Edits, MUEs, CERT, and Recovery Audit Program. http://www.cms.gov/Outreach-and-Education /Medicare-Learning-Network-MLN/MLNProducts/downloads/MCRP_Booklet.pdf.

Demirjian, B.G. 2012. Emphysema. http://emedicine.medscape.com/article/298283-overview.

DeVault, K., A. Barta, and M. Endicott. 2012. *ICD-10-CM Coder Training Manual, 2012 Instructor's Edition,* Chicago: AHIMA.

Devan, P.P. 2011. Mastoiditis. http://emedicine.medscape.com/article/2056657-overview.

DeNicola, L.K. 2012. Bronchiolitis. http://emedicine.medscape.com/article/961963-overview.

Dorland, W.A.N., ed. 2007. *Dorland's Illustrated Medical Dictionary,* 31st. Philadelphia: W. B. Saunders.

Ertl, L. 1992. Clinical notes: Intestinal ostomies. *Journal of AHIMA* 63(6):18–22.

Food and Drug Administration. 2010. Fatalities Reported to FDA Following Blood Collection and Transfusion: Annual Summary for Fiscal Year 2009. http://www.fda.gov/BiologicsBloodVaccines /SafetyAvailability/ReportaProblem/TransfusionDonationFatalities/ucm204763.htm#overall.

Gatti, J.M. 2011. Pathophysiology. http://emedicine.medscape.com/article/1015227-overview#a0104.

Graham, L.L. 1999. *Understanding Clinical Disease Processes for ICD-9-CM Coding.* Chicago: AHIMA.

Grimes, D. et al. 1990. *Infectious Diseases.* Mosby's Clinical Nursing Series. Vol. 3. St. Louis: Mosby-Year Book.

Harman, .B. 2006. *Ethical Challenges in the Management of Health Information.* Sudbury, MA: Jones and Bartlett Publishers.

Hazelwood, A.C. and C.A. Venable. 2009. *ICD-10-CM and ICD-10-PCS Preview,* 2nd ed. Chicago: AHIMA.

ICD-9-CM Coordination and Maintenance Committee. 1999–2012. Excerpts (agendas, proposals, and background materials) from the "Diagnoses and Procedures" portion of meeting minutes. http://www .cdc.gov/nchs/icd/icd9cm_maintenance.htm.

Illinois Department of Public Health. 2003. *Birth Defects and Other Adverse Pregnancy Outcomes in Illinois, 1997–2001.* Epidemiologic Report Series 03:02. Springfield, IL: Illinois Department of Health, Division of Epidemiologic Studies.

Ingenix. 2012. ICD-10-CM: The Complete Official Draft Code Set (2011 Draft). Salt Lake City: Ingenix.

Ingenix. 2012. ICD-10-PCS: The Complete Official Draft Code Set (2011 Draft). Salt Lake City: Ingenix.

Innes, K.K. and R. Roberts. 2000. Ten down under: Implementing ICD-10 in Australia. *Journal of AHIMA* 71(1):52–56.

Johnson, P. et al. 1999. Cardiac Troponin T as a marker for myocardial ischemia in patients seen at the emergency department for acute chest pain. *American Heart Journal* 137(6):1137–44.

Kizer, K.W. and M.B. Stegun. 2012. Serious Reportable Adverse Events in Health Care. AHRQ. http://www.ahrq.gov/downloads/pub/advances/vol4/Kizer2.pdf.

Kuehn, L. and T. Jorwic. 2012. *ICD-10-PCS An Applied Approach.* Chicago: AHIMA.

Li, H.H., and M.A. Kaliner. 2006. Allergic Asthma: Symptoms and Treatment. http://www.worldallergy.org/professional/allergic_diseases_center/allergic_asthma/.

Li, J.C. 2012. Benign Paroxysmal Positional Vertigo. http://emedicine.medscape.com/article/884261-overview.

Mayo Clinic Staff. 2009. Mitral valve stenosis: definition. http://www.mayoclinic.com/health/mitral-valve-stenosis/DS00420.

Mayo Clinic Staff. 2010. Osteomyelitis. http://www.mayoclinic.com/health/osteomyelitis/DS00759.

MedlinePlus. 2013. Health Topics. http://www.nlm.nih.gov/medlineplus/healthtopics.html.

Melloni, J. 2001. *Melloni's Illustrated Medical Dictionary*, 4th ed. Pearl River, N.Y.: The Parthenon Publishing Group.

National Center for Health Statistics. 2012. About the International Classification of Diseases, Tenth Revision, Clinical Modification (ICD-10-CM). http://www.cdc.gov/nchs/icd/icd10cm.htm.

National Center for Health Statistics. Report of the US Committee on Vital and Health Statistics. Uniform hospital abstract: minimum basic data set. Vital Health Stat. 4 (14). 1975. Updated by the Department of Health and Human Services. Health information policy council: 1984 revision of the Uniform Hospital Discharge Data Set. Office of the Secretary. Federal Register; vol 50 no 147. 1985.

National Heart, Lung, and Blood Institute. 2012. What Is Bronchoscopy? http://www.nhlbi.nih.gov/health/health-topics/topics/bron/.

National Pressure Ulcer Advisory Panel. 2012. Educational and Clinical Resources. http://www.npuap.org/resources/educational-and-clinical-resources/.

Nicholas, T. 1992. Clinical notes: Cardiac catheterization. *Journal of AHIMA* 63(3):25–26.

Prophet, S. 2002a. ICD-10 on the horizon. *Journal of AHIMA* 73(7):36–41.

Prophet, S. 2002b. Testimony before members of the National Committee on Vital and Health Statistics (NCVHS). Standards and Security Subcommittee, May 29, 2002. http://www.ahima.org/dc/comments.ncvhs.052902.cfm.

PubMed Health. 2010. Mitral stenosis. http://www.ncbi.nlm.nih.gov/pubmedhealth/PMH0001227.

PubMed Health. 2011. Rheumatoid lung disease. http://www.ncbi.nlm.nih.gov/pubmedhealth/PMH0001172/.

Puckett, C.D. 1998. *The Educational Annotation of ICD-9-CM,* 5th ed. Reno: Channel Publishing.

RAND Corporation. 2004. The Costs and Benefits of Moving to the ICD-10 Code Sets. http://www.rand.org/pubs/technical_reports/2004/RAND_TR132.pdf.

Riaz, K. 2012. Hypertension. http://emedicine.medscape.com/article/241381-overview.

Rice, M. and D. MacDonald. 1999. Appropriate roles of cardiac Troponins in evaluating patients with chest pain. *Journal of the American Board of Family Practice* 12(3):214–18.

Rogers, V. and A. Zeisset. 2004. *Applying Inpatient Coding Skills under Prospective Payment.* Chicago: AHIMA.

Schraffenberger, L. 2012. *Basic ICD-10-CM/PCS and ICD-9-CM Coding.* Chicago: AHIMA.

Segan, J. 2006. *Concise Dictionary of Modern Medicine.* New York: McGraw-Hill.

Shiel Jr., W.C. 2012. What is the difference between a symptom and a sign? http://www.medicinenet .com/symptoms_and_signs/article.htm.

Shohet, J.A. 2011. Otosclerosis. http://emedicine.medscape.com/article/859760-overview.

Skidmore-Roth, L. 2004. *Mosby's Nursing Drug Reference*. St. Louis: Mosby.

Stacy, G.S. 2011. Primary Osteoarthritis Imaging. http://emedicine.medscape.com /article/392096-overview.

Stedman, T. 2000. *Stedman's Medical Dictionary*, 27th ed. Baltimore: Williams & Wilkins.

University of Michigan Kellogg Eye Center. 2013. Cystoid Macular Edema (CME). http://www .kellogg.umich.edu/patientcare/conditions/cystoid.macular.edema.html.

Vertrees, S.M. 2012. Chorea in Adults Clinical Presentation. http://emedicine.medscape.com /article/1149854-clinical.

Way, L.W. 1996. *Current Surgical Diagnosis & Treatment,* 10th ed. New York: McGraw-Hill Professional Publishing Group.

Recommended Websites for Current ICD-10-CM and ICD-10-PCS Updates

AHIMA webpage for ICD-10 references: http://www.ahima.org/icd10/.

The Centers for Medicare and Medicaid Services for ICD-10 references: http://www.cms.gov /Medicare/Coding/ICD10/2012-ICD-10-PCS.html.

The Centers for Disease Control, Classification of Diseases, Functioning, and Disability for ICD-10 references: http://www.cdc.gov/nchs/icd/icd10cm.htm.

Note: A recommended AHIMA reference list for ICD-10-CM documents: ICD-10 Leadership Model Resource List. http://www.ahima.org/downloads/pdfs/about/ICD-10-Resources.pdf.

Coding Self-Test

Assign the appropriate ICD-10-CM and ICD-10-PCS codes (include procedure codes, external cause codes, and Z codes, where applicable) to the following:

1. Complete elective abortion, first trimester, 8 weeks, due to maternal rubella, with suspected damage to fetus affecting management of pregnancy; abortion by laminaria

   _____

2. Postpartum abscess of breast; patient discharged 5 days ago following spontaneous delivery of live triplets

   _____

3. Adenocarcinoma of descending colon with extension to mesenteric lymph nodes; permanent descending colon colostomy, open procedure with colostomy brought to the skin level

   _____

4. Paranoid schizophrenia

   _____

5. Obstructive hydrocephalus; cerebral ventricle to atrium shunt using synthetic substitute by open approach

   _____

6. Parkinsonism secondary to haloperidol neuroleptic drug therapy, initial encounter; drug was discontinued

   _____

7. Gangrene of lower leg due to uncontrolled type 1 diabetes

   _____

8. Newborn twin, male, delivered by cesarean delivery (in hospital) with syndrome of infant of diabetic mother

   _____

9. History of allergic reaction to penicillin

   _____

10. Chronic kidney disease, ESRD, dependence on renal dialysis; hemodialysis single session

_____

11. COPD with asthma

_____

12. Unstable angina

_____

13. Unexplained dizziness

_____

14. Hypertensive heart and kidney disease with chronic kidney disease, stage 3

_____

15. Iron deficiency anemia due to chronic blood loss

_____

16. Cystic pancreatitis

_____

17. Reye's syndrome

_____

18. Third-degree burn of chest and second-degree burn of right leg, initial encounter

_____

19. Organic brain syndrome due to cerebral arteriosclerosis

_____

20. Fracture of frontal bone with subarachnoid hemorrhage and concussion with no loss of consciousness due to motor vehicle accident collision with another car (patient driver of car), initial encounter

_____

21. Infiltrative tuberculosis of both lungs

_____

22. Ovarian retention cyst; laparoscopic partial oophorectomy, left side

_____

23. Lyme disease with associated arthritis

_____

24. Abnormal prothrombin time, cause to be determined

_____

25. Newborn born in community hospital transferred to university medical center. Code for the infant at the university medical center treated for hypoplastic left heart syndrome.

_____

26. Ingestion of 30 doxepin (Sinequan) tablets resulting in an overdose, determined to be a suicide attempt; tachycardia [Doxepin is a tricyclic antidepressant drug], initial episode of care

27. Fracture, right shoulder, humerus upper end (head), as the result of a fall from a chair she was standing on to reach a high shelf, occurred at her single family residence, kitchen while cooking; closed reduction, humeral head, with immobilization, initial episode of care. Patient is retired.

28. Inflamed seborrheic keratosis of right face; cryotherapy of lesion on right temple

29. Moderate mental retardation as the sequela of acute bacterial meningitis 10 years ago

30. Chlamydial vaginitis

31. Infiltrating duct breast carcinoma, right upper outer quadrant, with metastases to bone (female patient)

32. Diabetic hypoglycemic coma in a patient with uncontrolled type 1 diabetes

33. Secondary thrombocytopenia due to hypersplenism; total splenectomy, open

34. Pneumonia due to *Staphylococcus aureus;* fiberoptic bronchoscopy, tracheobronchial tree

35. Peptic ulcer of the lesser curvature of the stomach, acute, with hemorrhage; esophagogastroduodenoscopy (EGD) with closed biopsy of stomach

36. Rapidly progressive glomerulonephritis; percutaneous renal biopsy, right kidney

37. Coronary artery disease with previous autologous vein bypass grafts in the left anterior descending, left circumflex, and right posterior descending arteries. Procedure performed are coronary artery bypass grafts with double (left and right) internal mammary bypass to the left anterior descending and the left circumflex and a single aortocoronary bypass to the right posterior descending artery using saphenous vein graft with cardiopulmonary bypass

38. Patient with a history of bladder carcinoma seen for a follow-up examination related to his past partial cystectomy treatment; no recurrence found; cystoscopy with biopsy of bladder

39. Degenerative joint disease, bilateral knees; total knee replacement using metal prosthesis cemented, left knee

40. Malignant lymphoma, undifferentiated Burkitt type, Intrathoracic; percutaneous bone marrow biopsy, iliac

---

41. Postprocedural stricture of urethra with urinary retention; cystoscopic release of urethral stricture (female patient)

---

42. Chronic hidradenitis suppurativa, subcutaneous tissue, right axilla; wide excision of hidradenitis of right axilla; partial-thickness skin graft. Patient's own skin excised and grafted from patient's back to right axilla.

---

43. Heroin poisoning, accidental overdose; acute lung edema; multiple drug dependence including heroin and barbiturates, initial encounter

---

44. Positive tuberculosis skin test

---

45. Gunshot wound of chest with massive intrathoracic injury to right lung with laceration; shot by another person with a handgun who was charged with attempted homicide; injury occurred on a local residential street; patient died during an exploratory thoracotomy to examine right lung

---

46. Patient admitted for her first round of antineoplastic chemotherapy after a total abdominal hysterectomy and salpingo-oophorectomy for right ovarian carcinoma with known metastases to intra-pelvic lymph nodes; administration of antineoplastic chemotherapy by central vein infusion

---

47. Congenital hypertrophic pyloric stenosis corrected by open pyloromyotomy to dilate the pylorus of stomach in a four-week-old infant

---

48. Internal derangement of lateral meniscus, old tear, posterior horn, right knee; arthroscopy, right knee

---

49. Traumatic arthritis of left wrist secondary to old fracture-dislocation of lower end of radius, left

---

50. Pregnancy, preterm labor with preterm delivery at 35 weeks, single liveborn infant; postpartum fever of unknown origin; patient with known continuous marijuana drug dependence; spontaneous vaginal delivery

---

Index